SUDDEN DEATH

DEVELOPMENTS IN CARDIOVASCULAR MEDICINE

VOLUME 4

series ISBN 90-247-2336-1

SUDDEN
DEATH

edited by

H.E. KULBERTUS   *and*   **H.J.J.WELLENS**

University of Liège   *University of Limburg*
School of Medicine   *Department of Cardiology*
Division of Cardiology   *Annadal Hospital*
Liège   *Maastricht*

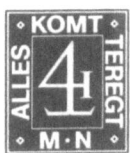

1980

MARTINUS NIJHOFF PUBLISHERS
THE HAGUE/BOSTON/LONDON

Distributors:

for the United States and Canada

Kluwer Boston, Inc.
160 Old Derby Street
Hingham, MA 02043
USA

for all other countries

Kluwer Academic Publishers Group
Distribution Center
P.O. Box 322
3300 AH Dordrecht
The Netherlands

Library of Congress Cataloging in Publication Data   ㏄ℙ

Main entry under title:

Sudden death.

   (Developments in cardiovascular medicine; 4)
   Includes index.
   1. Cardiac arrest – Congresses. 2. Sudden death – Congresses. I. Kulbertus, Henri.
II. Wellens, H.J.J. III. Series. [DNLM: 1. Death, Sudden. 2. Heart diseases – Morta-
lity. WI DE997PE v. 4 / WG205 S943]
RC685.C173S82   616.1'29   79-27584

ISBN-13:978-94-009-8836-1   e-ISBN-13:978-94-009-8834-7
DOI: 10.1007/978-94-009-8834-7

FOREWORD

Over the last ten years, it has become increasingly obvious that sudden death represents the major challenge confronting cardiology in the last part of the XXth Century.

Careful epidemiologic studies have established the magnitude of this overall important problem of public health. The frequent association of sudden death with coronary artery disease has been demonstrated. Some of the electrophysiologic mechanisms underlying lethal arrhythmias have been unveiled. In addition, clinical markers permitting identification of high risk individuals have emerged. Finally, different studies have raised some hope as to the ability of therapeutic interventions to protect these patients against a premature and possibly evitable demise.

Over the years, a sizable amount of new and relevant information, both basic and clinical, has become available. We felt therefore that a conference on sudden death might be timely. It was decided to organize a small gathering during which experts from different disciplines in cardiology could sit together in a quiet retreat to share their knowledge and discuss issues pertaining to research and therapy that might be of benefit to patients. The conference was held in Liège, on May 7, 8 and 9, 1979. This three day meeting in which representatives from seven different countries participated was extremely stimulating. The discussions were very lively and sometimes reflected the divergence of opinion which may persist on some topics.

In spite of its frequency, sudden death is clearly a difficult subject to investigate. It is apparent that the search for a perfectly reliable animal model which would permit the study of the mechanisms of sudden death and the assessment of protective interventions still meets with huge difficulties. Likewise, pathologists are often disappointed by their inability to detect over-acute histological changes induced by myocardial ischemia.

On the whole, the conference probably raised as many, and possibly more, questions than it solved. Some of them arose from a lack of universal agreement on very simple matters. It is amazing for example that a consensus is still lacking regarding the definition of sudden death. Even more, it appeared that the definition of ventricular fibrillation might need a reassessment. Most of the European participants who recognize ventricular fibrillation and torsades de pointe as two separate entities were reluctant to accept that what they are used to call ventricular fibrillation can be a self-terminating event. It seemed acceptable to all participants that the patients with the most damaged hearts were also those who were the most likely to die suddenly. Therefore, any clinical method which depicts severe and diffuse coronary lesions and/or poor left ventricular function may be expected to identify high risk individuals. It became apparent that if warning arrhythmias are correlated with a high risk of dying, their independent contribution to prognosis still remains unclear. In addition, and this is an intriguing clinical problem, it is difficult to decide upon the optimal duration of ambulatory monitoring to depict these arrhythmias after myocardial infarction. Longer monitoring periods do allow to recognize their presence in an increasing proportion of patients to such an extent that prolonged monitoring may disclose malignant arrhythmias in almost every post-infarction subject thus, losing much of its predictive significance.

Production of repetitive ventricular responses following induced ventricular ectopic beats might very well identify hearts with electrical instability and provide a tool for assessment of drug therapy. However, several participants expressed the view that the technique should be submitted to further appraisal before being accepted as a routine practice in clinical cardiology.

Prevention of sudden death after myocardial infarction may prove to be a most difficult enterprise. Lethal arrhythmias may indeed result from different mechanisms. Ventricular fibrillation may be the consequence of an inhomogeneity of excitability and conduction related to the scar of the previous necrosis. It may also be related to recurrent ischemic episodes or reperfusion phenomena. The search for a miracle drug, which might solve all these problems satisfactorily is therefore probably unrealistic.

The conference critically reviewed some large scale secondary prevention trials. The implementation of randomized designs raises a large number of questions which were clearly outlined. At present, much remains to be done before we can delineate the optimal individual drug regimen to be applied in high risk patients.

Coronary artery disease is not the only possible cause of sudden cardiac death. Other aetiologies are of importance either because of the number of patients involved (conduction disorders, cardiomyopathies, pre-excitation), or because their underlying mechanisms have an intrinsic interest which encroaches upon basic cardiac physiopathology (the long QT syndrome).

The purpose of this book is to bring forward a broad overview and current assessment of a critically important question which involves the life of hundreds of thousands of individuals each year. It is our hope that it will be of help to all those who share an interest in the epidemiology, causes, mechanisms and prevention of sudden cardiac death.

July 1979

H.E. KULBERTUS   H.J.J. WELLENS

ACKNOWLEDGMENTS

It is our pleasant duty to thank all those who, in one way or the other, have contributed to the success of the meeting.

First of all, we express our grateful appreciation to the speakers who kindly accepted to participate in the Symposium and who produced their manuscripts on time. The Symposium was made possible by the generous financial support of ICI Belgium. We wish to express our deepest gratitude to Dr. Lassance and Mr. Lambo for their understanding of our wishes and their endeavours to meet them.

The preparation of the conference and later on of the book involved a great deal of secretarial work; Mrs. B. Vervier achieved it with kind dedication and remarkable efficiency. She surely deserves our most sincere thanks. We would finally like to pay a tribute to Mr. Commandeur and Martinus Nijhoff Publishers for their invaluable efforts in the production of this book.

H.E. KULBERTUS   H.J.J. WELLENS

CONTENTS

Section 4. Prevention of sudden death

Section 5. Sudden death in noncoronary heart disease

LIST OF CONTRIBUTORS

Appel, R. Division of Cardiology, University of Miami School of Medicine, PO Box 016960, Miami, Florida, 33101, U.S.A.

Attuel, P. Service de Cardiologie, Hôpital Lariboisière, 2, rue Ambroise Paré, 75475 Paris, Cedex 10, France.

Bär, F. W. Department of Cardiology, University of Limburg, Annadal Hospital, Maastricht, The Netherlands.

Bogaert, M.G. Heymans Institute of Pharmacology, University of Gent, Gent 9000, Belgium.

Castellanos, A. Division of Cardiology, University of Miami School of Medicine, PO Box 016960, Miami, Florida 33101, U.S.A.

Conde, C.A. Division of Cardiology, University of Miami School of Medicine, PO Box 016960, Miami, Florida 33101, U.S.A.

Coumel, Ph.* Service de Cardiologie, Hôpital Lariboisière, 2, rue Ambroise Paré, 75475 Paris, Cedex 10, France.

Davies, M.J. Department of Histopathology, St. George's Hospital Medical School, Cranmer Terrace, London SW 17, ORE, United Kingdom.

Davis, H. University of Rochester Medical Center, PO Box 653, 601 Elmwood Avenue, Rochester, N.Y. 14642, U.S.A.

De Camilla, J. University of Rochester Medical Center, Box 653, 601 Elmwood Avenue, Rochester, N.Y. 14642, U.S.A.

de Leval-Rutten, F. Institut Provincial E. Malvoz, 4, Quai du Barbou, 4020 Liège, Belgium.

Detre, K. University of Pittsburgh, Department of Epidemiology, Graduate School of Public Health, Pittsburgh, Pennsylvania 15261, U.S.A.

Dubois, M. Institut Provincial E. Malvoz, 4, Quai du Barbou, 4020 Liège, Belgium.

Durrer, D. Department of Cardiology and Clinical Physiology, Wilhelmina Gasthuis, Amsterdam, The Netherlands.

El-Sherif, N.* State University of New York, Downstate Medical Center, Veterans Administration Medical Center, Brooklijn, N.Y. 11209, U.S.A.

Epstein, S. E.* Cardiology Branch, Building 10, Room 7 B-15, National Heart, Lung and Blood Institute, National Institutes of Health, Bethesda, Maryland 20014, U.S.A.

Farre, J. Fundacion Jimenez Diaz, Servicio de Cardiologia, Ciudad Universitaria, Madrid, Spain.

Gallagher, J.J.* Department of Medicine, Duke University Medical Center, Durham, North Carolina 27710, U.S.A.

Gilmour, R.F. Jr, Krannert Institute of Cardiology, Department of Medicine, Indiana University School of Medicine, The Veterans Administration Hospital, Indianapolis, Indiana 46202, U.S.A.

Gomes, J.A.C. State University of New York, Downstate Medical Center, Veterans Administration Medical Center, Brooklyn, N.Y. 11209, U.S.A.

Greene, L.H.* Division of Cardiology, Harborrien Medical Center, 325 Ninth Avenue, Seattle, Washington 98104, U.S.A.

---

* These contributors were active participants in the symposium held in Liège, on May 7, 8 and 9, 1979.

Greenspan, A.M. Electrophysiology Laboratory, 666 White Building, Hospital of the University of Pennsylvania, 3400 Spruce Street, Philadelphia, Pennsylvania 19104, U.S.A.

Harker, L.A. Division of Hematology, Harborview Medical Center, Seattle, Washington 98108, U.S.A.

Harrison, L. Department of Medicine, Duke University Medical Center, Durham, North Carolina 27710, U.S.A.

Heilman, M.S. Department of Medicine, Sinaï Hospital of Baltimore, The Johns Hopkins University School of Medicine, Baltimore, Maryland 21105, U.S.A.

Hjalmarson, Å.* Department of Medicine I, Sahlgren's Hospital, University of Göteborg, S-41345 Göteborg, Sweden.

Horowitz, L.M. Electrophysiology Laboratory, 666 White Building, Hospital of the University of Pennsylvania, 3400 Spruce Street, Philadelphia, Pennsylvania 19104, U.S.A.

Ideker, R.E. Department of Pathology and Medicine, PO Box 3712, Duke University Medical Center, Durham, North Carolina 27710, U.S.A.

James, Th. N.* Department of Medicine, University of Alabama Medical Center, Birmingham, Alabama 35294, U.S.A.

Janse, M.J.* Department of Cardiology and Clinical Physiology, Wilhelmina Gasthuis, Amsterdam, The Netherlands.

Josephson, M.E.* Electrophysiology Laboratory, 666 White Building, Hospital of the University of Pennsylvania, 3400 Spruce Street, Philadelphia Pennsylvania 19104, U.S.A.

Julian, D.G.* University of Newcastle upon Tyne, Regional Cardiothoracic Centre, Freeman Hospital, Newcastle upon Tyne, United Kingdom.

Kang, P.S. State University of New York, Downstate Medical Center, Veterans Administration Medical Center, Brooklyn N.Y. 11209, U.S.A.

Karagueuzian, H.S. Department of Pharmacology, College of Physicians and Surgeons, Columbia University, New York 10032, U.S.A.

Kasell, J. Department of Medicine, Duke University Medical Center, Durham, North Carolina 27710, U.S.A.

Kelen, G.J. State University of New York, Downstate Medical Center, Veterans Administration Medical Center, Brooklyn, N.Y. 11209, U.S.A.

Khan, R.G. State University of New York, Downstate Medical Center, Veterans Administration Medical Center, Brooklyn, N.Y. 11209, U.S.A.

Kléber, A.G. Department of Cardiology and Clinical Physiology, Wilhelmina Gasthuis, Amsterdam, The Netherlands.

Klein, G.J. Department of Medicine, Duke University Medical Center, Durham, North Carolina 27710, U.S.A.

Kulbertus, H.E.* Institut Provincial E. Malvoz and the Division of Cardiology, Institute of Medicine, University of Liège, 66 Bvd de la Constitution, 4020 Liège, Belgium.

Kuller, L.H.* University of Pittsburgh, Graduate School of Public Health, Department of Epidemiology, Pittsburgh, Pennsylvania 15261, U.S.A.

Langer, A. Department of Medicine, Sinaï Hospital of Baltimore, Baltimore, Maryland 21205, U.S.A.

Leclercq, J.F. Service de Cardiologie, Hôpital Lariboisière, 2, rue Ambroise Paré, 75475 Paris, Cedex 10, France.

Lie, K.I.* Department of Cardiology and Clinical Physiology, Wilhelmina Gasthuis, Amsterdam, The Netherlands.

Manger Cats, V. Department of Cardiology and Clinical Physiology, Wilhelmina Gasthuis, Amsterdam, The Netherlands.

Mallon, St. M. Division of Cardiology, University of Miami School of Medicine, PO Box 016960, Miami, Florida 33101, U.S.A.

Maron, B.J. Cardiology Branch, Building 10, Room 7B-15, National Heart, Lung and Blood Institute, National Institutes of Health, Bethesda, Maryland 20014, U.S.A.

Martins, J.B. University of Iowa Hospitals, Iowa City, Iowa 52242, U.S.A.

Milosevic, D. Service de Cardiologie, Hôpital Lariboisière, 2, rue Ambroise Paré, 75475, Paris, Cedex 10, France.

Mirowski, M.* Department of Medicine, Sinaï Hospital of Baltimore, The Johns Hopkins University School of Medicine, Baltimore, Maryland 21205, U.S.A.

Morsink, H. Department of Cardiology and Clinical Physiology, Wilhelmina Gasthuis, Amsterdam, The Netherlands.

Moss, A. J.* University of Rochester Medical Center, PO Box 653, 601 Elmwood Avenue, Rochester, N.Y. 14642, U.S.A.

Mower, M.M. Department of Medicine, Sinaï hospital of Baltimore, Baltimore, Maryland 21215, U.S.A.

Myerburg, R.J.* Division of Cardiology, University of Miami School of Medicine, PO Box 016960, Miami, Florida 33101, U.S.A.

Perper, J.A. University of Pittsburgh, Graduate School of Public Health, Department of Epidemiology, Pittsburgh, Pennsylvania 15261, U.S.A.

Petit, J.M. Institut Provincial E. Malvoz, 4, Quai du Barbou, 4020 Liège, Belgium.

Pisa, Z.* WHO, Geneva, Switzerland.

Pitt, B.* Department of Medicine, Division of Cardiology, University of Michigan School of Medicine, Ann Arbor, Michigan 48109, U.S.A.

Popple, A.W. Department of Histopathology, St. George's Hospital Medical School, Cranmer Terrace, London S.W. 17 ORE, United Kingdom.

Reid, Ph. R. Division of Cardiology and Clinical Pharmacology, The Johns Hopkins Hospital, 601 North Broadway, Baltimore, Maryland 21205, U.S.A.

Ritchie, J.L.* Department of Medicine, University of Washington School of Medicine, Division of Cardiology, Veterans Administration Medical Center, 4435 Beacon Avenue S., Seattle, Washington 98108, U.S.A.

Ross, D. Department of Cardiology, University of Limburg, Annadal Hospital, Maastricht, The Netherlands.

Rosengarten, M. Service de Cardiologie, Hôpital Lariboisière, 2, rue Ambroise Paré, 75475, Paris, Cedex 10, France.

Ruffy, R. Washington University Medical Center, St. Louis, Missouri 63178, U.S.A.

Schaeffer, A.H. Division of Cardiology and Clinical Pharmacology, The Johns Hopkins Hospital, 601 North Broadway, Baltimore, Maryland 21205, U.S.A.

Schwartz, P.J.* Istituto di Ricerche Cardiovascolari, "Giorgio Sisini," dell' Universita di Milano, Via F. Sforza 35, 20122 Milano, Italy.

Sheps, D.S. Division of Cardiology, University of Miami School of Medicine, PO Box 016960, Miami 33101, U.S.A.

Smith, W.M. Department of Medicine, Duke University Medical Center, Durham, North Carolina 27710, U.S.A.

Spielman, S.R. Electrophysiology Laboratory, 666 White Building, Hospital of the University of Pennsylvania, 3400 Spruce Street, Philadelphia, Pennsylvania 19104, U.S.A.

Sung, F.J. Division of Cardiology, University of Miami School of Medicine, PO Box 016960, Miami, Florida 33101, U.S.A.

Talbot, E. University of Pittsburgh, Graduate School of Public Health, Department of Epidemiology, Pittsburgh, Pennsylvania 15261, U.S.A.

Thomas, A.C.* Department of Histopathology, St. George's Hospital Medical School, Cranmer Terrace, London SW 17, ORE, England.

Vanagt, E.J. Department of Cardiology, University of Limburg, Annadal Hospital, Maastricht, The Netherlands.

van Capelle, F.J.L. Department of Cardiology and Clinical Physiology, Wilhelmina Gasthuis, Amsterdam, The Netherlands.

Van Durme J.P.* Department of Cardiology, University Hospital, 9000 Gent, Belgium.

Verrier, R.L.* Cardiovascular Research Laboratory, Department of Medicine, Harvard School of Public Health, 665, Huntington Avenue, Boston, Massachusetts 02115, U.S.A.

Wallace, A.G. Department of Medicine, Duke University Medical Center, Durham, North Carolina 27710, U.S.A.

Wellens, H.J.J.* Department of Cardiology, University of Limburg, Annadal Hospital, Maastricht, The Netherlands.

Wilms-Schopman, F. Department of Cardiology and Clinical Physiology, Wilhelmina Gasthuis, Amsterdam, The Netherlands.

Winkle, R. A.*Cardiology Division, Stanford University Medical Center, Stanford, California 94305, U.S.A.

Wit, A.L.* Department of Pharmacology, College of Physicians and Surgeons of Columbia University, 630 West 168th Street, New York, N.Y. 10032, U.S.A.

Zeiler, R.H. State University of New York, Downstate Medical Center, Veterans Administration Medical Center, Brooklyn, N.Y. 11209, U.S.A.

Zipes, D.P.* Krannert Institute of Cardiology, Department of Medicine, Indiana University School of Medicine, The Veterans Administration Hospital, Indianapolis, Indiana 46202, U.S.A.

SECTION 1
EPIDEMIOLOGY AND PATHOLOGY OF SUDDEN DEATH

1.1. SUDDEN DEATH: A WORLDWIDE PROBLEM

Z. PISA

Sudden death is, according to our present knowledge, most frequent in industrial countries of North America and Europe. The majority of victims have significant coronary heart disease(1, 2, 3, 4);however, acute myocardial infarction, or acute thrombosis, are found at autopsy in only a small percentage of the cases (3).

It is well established that the significant part of ischemic heart disease (IHD) mortality occurs suddenly (5). It might be useful, therefore, to start our discussion with some data on the changing pattern in mortality for coronary heart disease in countries during the last decade.

With Epstein (6), we made an analysis of the trends in ischemic heart disease mortality (410–414, ICD 8th rev.) in 27 countries for which there are reliable mortality statistics available. Besides the United States (Figure 1), there is a significant decline in mortality in Canada, Australia, New Zealand, Japan, Belgium, Finland, Italy and Norway. There are, however, countries, like Yugoslavia (Figure 2), other countries of northern and eastern

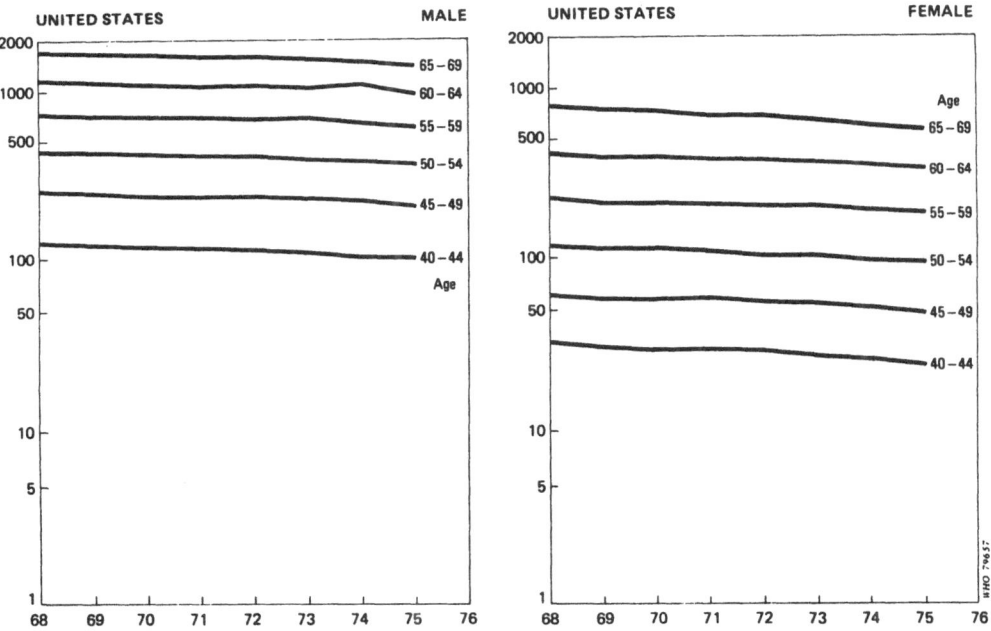

Figure 1. USA Mortality trends for IHD (ICD 410–414); age-specific rates per 100,000 population in 1969–1975.

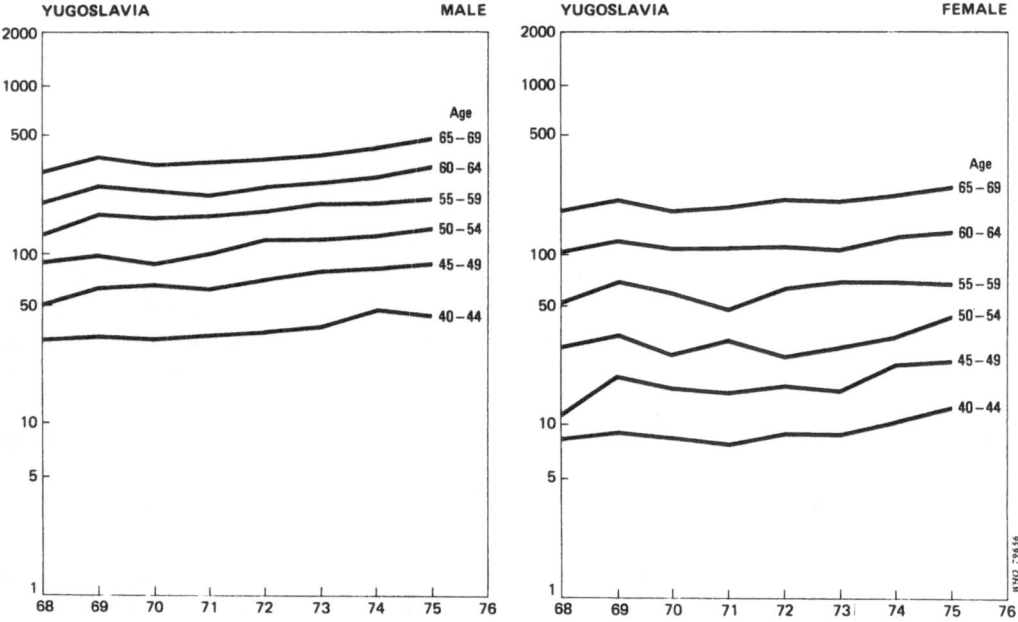

Figure 2. Yugoslavia. Mortality trends for IHD (ICD 410–414); age-specific rates per 100,000 population in 1968–1975.

Europe and even the Republic of Ireland, where the mortality is still on the increase. The remaining countries of southern and western Europe do not show any clearcut pattern.

The most distressing fact is that, at the present time, we do not have enough hard evidence available to be able to explain the reasons for these changing trends in coronary heart disease mortality. As a matter of fact, we are not even sure if the change in mortality reflects a similar change in morbidity. A conference organized last October by the National Heart, Lung, and Blood Institute in Bethesda, which discussed the reasons for the decreasing trends in cardiovascular diseases mortality in the United States, recommended – among other items – that systems monitoring the incidence of coronary heart disease should be established in different countries and population areas. Such monitoring systems should facilitate the interpretation of changes in mortality and morbidity and their relation to eventual changes in the levels of the established risk factors in the populations.

WHO is now collaborating closely with several leading institutes around the world in designing such a monitoring system. Advantage is being taken of our previous experience with the WHO project, Myocardial Infarction Community Registers (7). If applied on a large-scale population basis, these monitoring systems might be a significant breakthrough in collection of reliable information on the incidence of ischemic heart disease and, when extended, on other cardiovascular diseases, and eventually on non-communicable diseases in general.

If properly prepared, such an international project might contribute significantly to the knowledge about the epidemiology and natural history of sudden death.

The reviews of the extensive literature on sudden death agree unanimously that there is a great inconsistency in definitions of sudden death, and that therefore comparisons and uniform interpretation of results from different studies are, at the present time, extremely difficult (8, 9, 10). The definitions range between instantaneous death and death occurring up to 24 hours after the onset of symptoms.

The definitions for which WHO committees were partly or fully responsible during the last twenty years present a similar picture. In 1959 the Expert Committee on Hypertension and Coronary Heart Disease defined sudden death as "instantaneous death that is occurring within a few minutes of the onset of clinical manifestations" (11). In the 8th, as well as 9th, revision of the International Classification of Diseases, sudden death (cause unknown) is included in an ill-defined category (12, 13). The 9th revision, however, also introduces cardiac arrest (ICD 427.5) which figures under cardiac dysrhythmias (ICD 427). In 1969/70, the Scientific Council on Atherosclerosis and Ischemic Heart Disease of the International Society of Cardiology, and the Councils on Atherosclerosis and Epidemiology of the American Heart Association and WHO, proposed the definition: Sudden unexpected (natural) death is defined as death occurring instantaneously or within an estimated 24 hours of the onset of acute symptoms or signs (14). In the WHO sponsored pathological study the definition used was "non-violent death occurring unexpectedly within six hours in an apparently healthy subject, or in a sick person whose condition was either steady or improving" (15).

In 1979, the Task Force of the International Society and Federation of Cardiology and WHO on Nomenclature and Criteria for Diagnosis of IHD (16), defines "the primary cardiac arrest as a sudden event, presumably due to electric instability of the heart where evidence which allows other diagnosis is lacking. If no resuscitation is applied, or if resuscitation is unsuccessful, primary cardiac arrest is referred to as sudden death". The report, in a footnote, states: "The definition of sudden death was purposely omitted by the Committee because sudden death is a consequence of cardiac arrest, which is the real manifestation of ischemic heart disease. The definition used should be operational." This implies that in any future it would be preferable to record the time of death from the onset of symptoms for each case.

This approach was used in the project on the Myocardial Infarction Community Registers (7). The aim was to register each person suspected of having a myocardial infarction in a defined population. That also meant analysing each case of sudden death occurring there.

The project has been carried out in 21 population areas; 19 in Europe, one in Israel and one in Australia. For operational reasons data were collected from the population between the ages 20–64 years, which comprised $3\frac{1}{2}$ million inhabitants. The total population covered comprised 7 million inhabitants. All the centres utilized the standardized protocol, and data were pooled and centrally analysed in the WHO office in Geneva. During the year 1971 more than 10,000 cases of acute myocardial infarction (AMI) were registered.

The project avoided the definition of sudden death, but recorded the time elapsed between the onset of symptoms and eventual death. The following diagnostic categories were used in fatal cases:

– *Definite* (myocardial infarction): positive post-mortem findings required.

– *Possible*: a past history of chronic coronary heart disease, or autopsy evidence of chronic ischemic heart disease.

– *Not an infarct*: another diagnosis has been made.

– *Insufficient information*: remaining fatal cases which were notified were included.

In the present analysis, the information on definite and possible cases was combined and five centres were excluded where the percentage of cases with insufficient information on the time of death exceeded 20%.

The annual age-standardized attack rate of acute myocardial infarction per thousand population for males and females of the age group 20–64, together with first hour death rates, are presented in Table 1. The highest attack rate, for men as well as women, was in Helsinki, 7.3 for males and 1.6 for females. The lowest was in Bucharest, 1.5 and 0.3. The first hour death rate was highest for men in Helsinki, 1.59, and lowest in Göteborg, 0.19. For women, the highest was in London, 0.35, and the lowest in Göteborg, 0.02.

Table 1. Annual age-standardized rates per 1000 population 20–64 years in MI Community Registers areas (7).

CENTRE	SEX	ATTACK RATE	FIRST HOUR DEATH RATE
GOTHENBURG	M	2.6	0.19
	F	0.6	0.02
PRAGUE	M	3.5	0.73
	F	0.6	0.09
BUCHAREST	M	1.5	0.26
	F	0.3	0.02
BUDAPEST	M	2.9	0.70
	F	0.8	0.20
DUBLIN	M	4.7	0.51
	F	1.3	0.12
HEIDELBERG	M	2.6	0.41
	F	0.4	0.07
HELSINKI	M	7.3	1.59
	F	1.6	0.21
LONDON	M	4.3	0.76
	F	1.2	0.35
NIJMEGEN	M	4.8	0.86
	F	1.0	0.19
TAMPERE	M	6.2	1.22
	F	·1.1	0.11
WARSAW	M	3.1	0.36
	F	0.9	0.06
LUBLIN	M	2.6	0.20
	F	0.5	0.04
KAUNAS	M	2.6	0.54
	F	0.4	0.05
BODEN	M	4.1	0.88
	F	1.4	0.23
PERTH	M	4.6	0.62
	F	1.4	0.14
TEL AVIV	M	3.8	0.38
	F	1.3	0.16

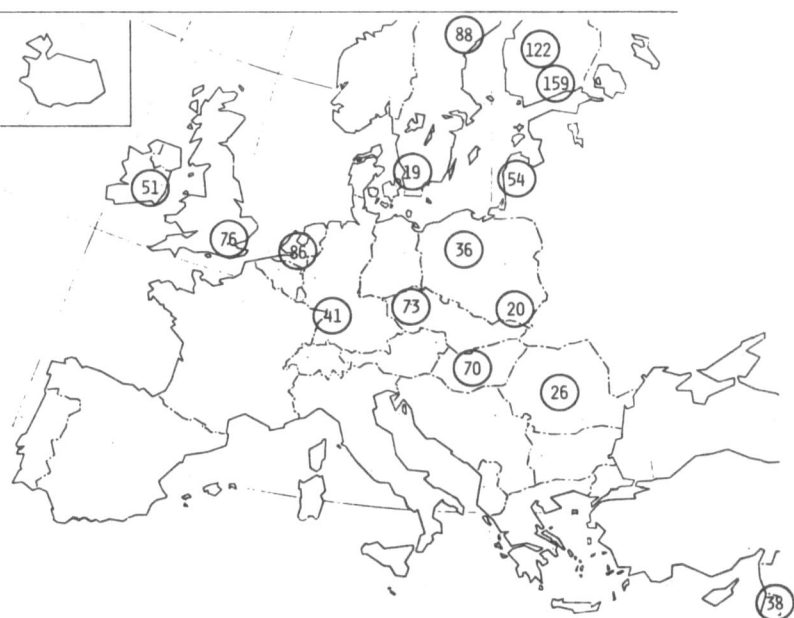

Figure 3. First hour annual death rates per 100,000 population in Myocardial Infarction Community Registers areas (7). Males, age-standardized rates 20–64 years.

Figure 3 presents the first hour death rates per 100,000 population in males in European centres. The highest first hour death rates are in the north of Europe (with the exception of Göteborg). For males these first hour death rates would be placed among the five first leading causes of death in any of these countries. Only death rates for coronary heart disease, cerebrovascular diseases and malignant neoplasms would, in general, be preceding the death rates for sudden death alone.

The correlations between the attack rates of AMI with the first hour death rates are highly significant for men (Figure 4) as well as for women (Figure 5). It shows that the proportion of sudden death to the events is constant in areas with low as well as high myocardial infarction (MI) attack rates. The first hour death rate also increases with age. Figure 6 shows the proportion of patients dying in relation to the time elapsed from onset of symptoms, and compares males in the age groups 45–54 and 55–64. The mortality during the 24 hours is generally higher in the older age group. The percentage of those who die during the first hour is also larger in the age group between 55–64. The difference is highly significant (p < 0.001). The percentage of first hour deaths for the older age group was only reached during the fourth hour after onset of symptoms in the younger age group. Similar findings, i.e. lower death rates in a time unit, were also seen in younger women.

The WHO Myocardial Infarction Community Registers study provided us with further information which shows how difficult it is to deal with the problem of sudden death with our present stress on curative approaches in health services.

From the 1114 subjects who died during the first half-hour, only 47 were seen before death

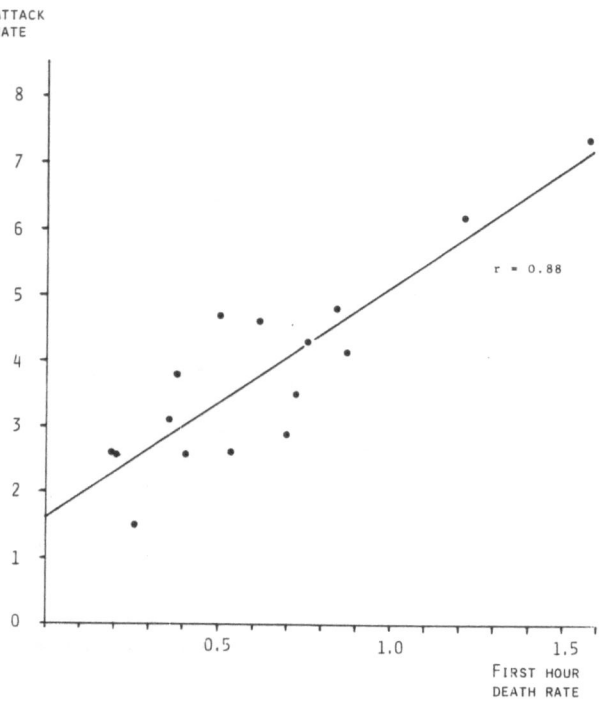

Figure 4. Correlation between the annual MI attack rates and first hour death rates per 1000 population in MI Community Registers listed in Table 1; males, age-standardized rates 20–64 years.

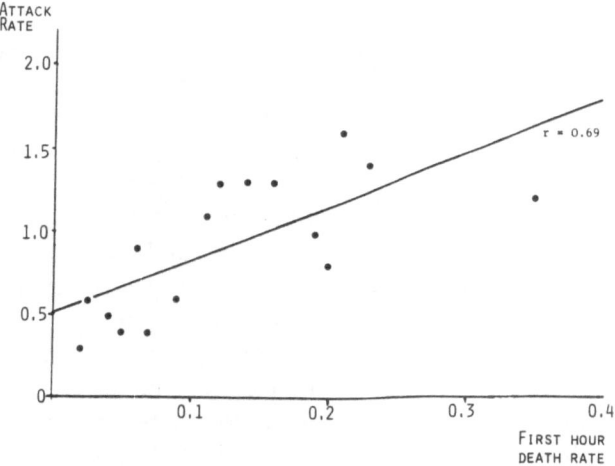

Figure 5. Correlation between the annual MI attack rates and first hour death rates per 1000 population in MI Community Registers listed in Table 1; females, age-standardized rates 20–64 years.

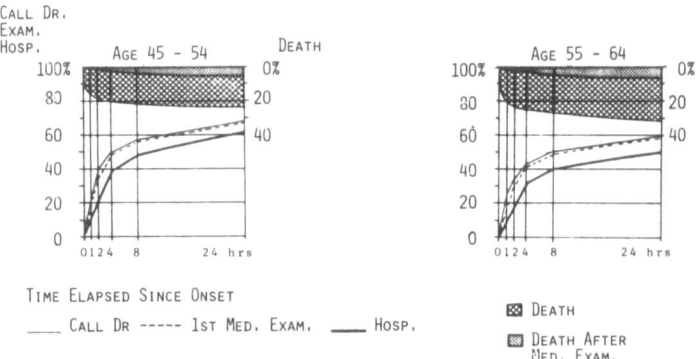

Figure 6. Proportion of patients in relation to events since onset of attack for males in age groups 45–54 years and 55–64 years; all centres combined (7).

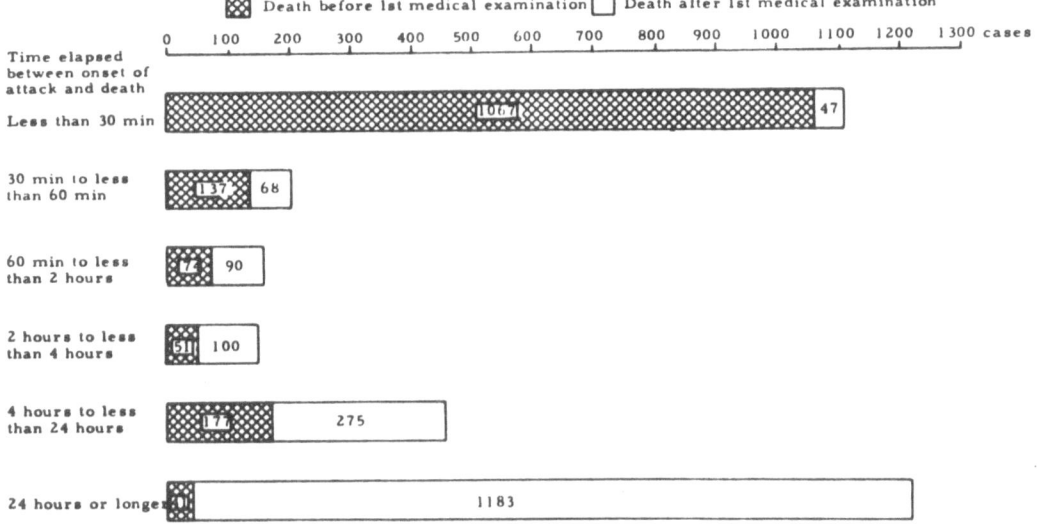

Figure 7. Number of deaths according to medical examination and time elapsed since onset of attack in MI Community Registers (7); all centres combined; patients diagnosed as "AMI none" excluded.

by a medical person (Figure 7). Even in the second half-hour, from the 205 cases, only 68, that means only one-third, were seen by a medical person before dying. Of the 24-hour deaths, 73 % occurred before the first medical examination was possible. Figure 7 also summarizes the problems in dealing with sudden death. It also shows the percentage of patients who, in a given time unit, called for medical help, were examined and hospitalized. The most important factor in the delays to provide medical help is the patient's delay in calling the doctor. However, the situation is often such that a patient does not even have the opportunity to do so.

It will be extremely difficult to influence the mortality of coronary heart disease, and specifically that of sudden death, by some curative and organizational measures which would be introduced only after the event. Remarkable results are being reported from Seattle (17) where the full participation of the community is ensured. The 180,000 inhabitants of Seattle are already trained in cardiac resuscitation (18) and encouraging results have, therefore, also been achieved in saving persons from dying suddenly. Nevertheless, irrespective of how impressive these results are, and how successful is the approach to the community, the only solution to the problem of sudden death is more research into its etiology and pathogenesis so that preventive measures could be introduced in time to avoid the occurrence of the event.

REFERENCES

1. Scott RF, Briggs TS: Pathologic findings in pre-hospital deaths due to coronary atherosclerosis. Amer J Card 29:782–787, 1972.
2. Friedman M, Manwaring JH, Rosenman RH: Instantaneous and sudden deaths. JAMA 225:1319–1328, 1973.
3. Reichenbach LD, Moss NS, Meyer E: Pathology of the heart in sudden cardiac death, Amer J Card 39:865–872, 1977.
4. Janushkevichius ZJ, Bloozhas JN, Stalioraityte EJ, Baubiniene AV, Milashauskiene MA, Grabauskas VJ, Mazheika AA, Ryzhakovaite MV, Kamarauskiene DB, Ragaishis JR: Sudden out-of-hospital coronary death and chronic lesions of coronary arteries and myocardium: Morphological data of kaunas male population study. Acta Med Scand suppl. 33:615–64, 1978.
5. Kuller L: Sudden death in arteriosclerotic heart disease. The case for preventive medicine, Amer J Card 24:617–628, 1969.
6. Epstein FH, Pisa Z: International comparisons in ischaemic heart disease mortality. Proceedings of the "Conference on the decline in coronary heart disease mortality", National Heart, Lung, and Blood Institute, NIH, Bethesda, Md, October 24–25, 1978 (in press).
7. Myocardial infarction community registers. Public health in Europe no 5, World Health Org. Regional Office for Europe, 1976.
8. Paul O, and Schatz M: On sudden death. Circulation 43:7 10, 1971.
9. Biörck G, and Wikland B: "Sudden death" what are we talking about? Circulation 45: 256–258, 1972.
10. Strasser T: Definizioni e limiti. Proceedings of the intern symp on coronary sudden death; Rome, January 29, 1977, Ciba-Geigy, Milano, 1977.
11. Hypertension and coronary heart disease: Classification and criteria for epidemiological studies; WHO Tech Rep Series 168, 1959.
12. Manual of the international statistical classification of diseases, injuries and causes of death, 8th rev, WHO, Geneva, 1967.
13. Manual of the international statistical classification of diseases, injuries and causes of death, 9th rev, WHO, Geneva, 1977.
14. Cardiovascular diseases unit, World Health Organization and Scientific Council on Arteriosclerosis and Ischaemic Heart Disease of Int Soc of Cardiol: Opinions and practices concerning the use of the term "Sudden Death", 1972, Unpublished.
15. Kagan AR, Sternby NH, Uemura K, Vanecek R, Vihert AM: Atherosclerosis of the aorta and coronary arteries in five towns, Bull Wld Hlth Org 53:489–499, 1976.
16. Nomenclature and criteria for diagnosis of ischaemic heart disease. Report of the Joint International Society and Federation of Cardiology/World Health Organization Task Force on Standardization of Clinical Nomenclature. Circulation 59:607–609, 1979.
17. Weaver WD, Lorch GS, Alvarez HA, Cobb LA: Angiographic findings and prognostic indicators in patients resuscitated from sudden cardiac death. Circulation 54:895–900, 1976.
18. Cobb LA: A community's experience with the pre-hospital emergency care; a working paper for the WHO Working Group on the development of coronary care in the community, Brussels, February 12–15, 1979.

1.2. SUDDEN DEATH DUE TO ARTERIOSCLEROTIC HEART DISEASE: A STUDY OF WOMEN

E. TALBOTT, L.H. KULLER, K. DETRE and J.A. PERPER

1. INTRODUCTION

Numerous studies have described the distribution of sudden and unexpected deaths due to arteriosclerotic heart disease in the community (1). Other studies have determined the extent of coronary artery disease, acute pathology in the coronary arteries and myocardial pathology related to sudden death (1–3). More recent analytical studies have either ascertained the risk factors related to sudden death among "normal individuals" or for survivors of a heart attack, myocardial infarction or angina pectoris (4–5). The most recent studies have focused on clinical trials of either primary prevention of sudden death or modification of the natural history of angina pectoris and myocardial infarction patients (6–10).

No specific definition of sudden death has ever been universally accepted (11). Investigators usually define their cases by length of survival, degree of prior disability, whether the death is witnessed or not and by a prior history of heart disease.

Table 1. Descriptive epidemiology. A) Narrative.

1. Sudden death defined by length of survival, whether witnessed or not, history of heart disease and prior disability: About one third sudden deaths unwitnessed
2. About 20–25% of heart attacks result in sudden death
3. Sudden deaths about 5 times more frequent in men than women: Incidence increase with age
4. Incidence of sudden death; similar among Blacks and Whites
5. About half of sudden deaths in community have prior history of clinical heart disease
6. Most sudden and unexpected deaths occur at home while victim is involved in *usual activities*
7. High frequency of prodromal symptoms; in days to weeks prior to a sudden death especially unusual increase in fatigue out of proportion to activities
8. Many sudden death victims saw a physician within days to weeks prior to sudden death, usually for no specific symptomalogy
9. Specific precipitating factors identified in some sudden deaths, but generally no specific event identified
10. Declining death rates due to ASHD may suggest a decrease in *sudden deaths*

Some of the most common findings from the descriptive population studies are listed in Table 1. Probably the most striking finding has been the relative paucity of sudden death among women as compared to men (11–14). Sudden death due to arteriosclerotic heart disease is about five times higher in men than women. This was true for both blacks and whites in the Baltimore study (Table 2).

The incidence of heart attack and various diagnostic subgroups has been measured prospectively in the Framingham study (Table 3) (15). It is interesting to note that in the Fram-

Table 2. Incidence of sudden ASHD deaths by age, race and sex – Baltimore/10,000/year.*

	Age 45-54			Age 55-64		
		No heart disease			No heart disease	
Race, sex	All	Total	Within 15 min	All	Total	Within 15 min.
WM	22.0	14.0	3.0	45	17	4.0
WF	5.0	2.0	0.6	10	5.0	1.0
BM	20.0	14.0	2.0	36	21	2.0
BF	4.0	1.0	0.5	12	5.0	1.0
RATIO						
WM/WF	4.4	7.0	5.0	4.5	3.4	4.0
WM/BM	1.1	1.0	1.5	1.3	0.8	2.0
BM/BF	5.0	14	4.0	3.0	4.2	2.0
BF/WF	1.2	2.0	1.2	0.8	1.0	1.0

* Classified according to the following sets of criteria: 1) all ASHD sudden deaths; 2) those with no history of heart disease; and 3) no history of heart disease, and death witnessed as occurring within 15 minutes.

Table 3. Incidence of selected cardiovascular diseases: Framingham Study (white men and women)/100,000 year.

CLINICAL DISEASE	WHITE MEN				WHITE WOMEN			
	35-44	45-54	55-64	65-74	35-44	45-54	55-64	65-74
Coronary Heart Disease	40	94	209	202	06	27	98	127
Angina Pectoris: Uncomplicated	08	27	75	56	04	15	58	65
Myocardial Infarction	19	43	93	116	02	08	18	34
Sudden Death: From CHD	03	11	29	13	-	02	04	14
Sudden & Unexplained Death	03	10	27	13	-	02	04	14
Congestive Heart Failure	04	19	39	61	04	06	27	39
Intermitt Claudication	03	16	51	57	02	04	19	31

ingham study there was not a single sudden and unexpected death in a woman under the age of 45 (15). A review of other current studies substantiates the rarity of sudden and unexpected deaths in women under the age of 45.

The clinical manifestations of arteriosclerotic heart disease are different in men and women. Women have a much lower incidence of all heart disease (Table 3) (15). A higher percentage of all heart attacks in women were characterized by angina pectoris rather than either myocardial infarction or sudden death. The reasons for this disparity in clinical presentation have not been fully explained. Many believe that at least some of the cases of angina in women may be a misclassification of symptoms, or that women may have more angina with minimal coronary atherosclerosis. The prognosis of angina pectoris is much better in women than men (16, 17). In young women especially, the prognosis of angina pectoris was very good and does not differ substantially from the normal population of women free of angina pectoris (16).

It is possible that the differences in clinical manifestations of heart attack between men and women may be related to the "acute" pathology of the clinical entities (thrombosis, hemorrhage in the plaque, ruptured plaque, etc.). All clinical types of atherosclerotic heart disease, myocardial infarction, angina pectoris, and sudden deaths are characterized by fairly extensive coronary atherosclerosis. Unfortunately few studies have correlated the extent of coronary artery disease and the clinical types of disease especially in women. Individuals have been noted to have angina pectoris with relatively normal coronary arteries (18, 19). The prognosis of such patients was excellent.

Epidemiological-pathological studies such as the International Atherosclerosis Project have shown that women have less coronary atherosclerosis than men (20). The difference in the extent of disease was greater for the coronary than for the thoracic or abdominal aorta. Sex differences in the extent of disease were greater for New Orleans whites than blacks (20). However this racial difference was not consistent in other countries.

The death rates attributed to ischemic heart disease or arteriosclerotic heart disease based on United States Vital Statistics have been much higher in the "all other women category" which is predominantly black as compared to white (Table 4) (23). However a careful evaluation of deaths certified in Baltimore in 1972 failed to demonstrate any substantial differences in the age specific death rates due to arteriosclerotic heart disease (22). The large differences noted in the Vital Statistics appeared to be due to the misclassification of deaths related to heart failure, hypertension and renal disease to ischemic heart

Table 4. Death rates for females for ischemic heart disease, for specified age groups, by color: United States, 1976.

COLOR AND YEAR	ALL AGES	25-34 YEARS	35-44 YEARS	45-54 YEARS	55-64 YEARS	65-74 YEARS	75-84 YEARS	85 YEARS AND OVER
FEMALE 1976[1]	259.2	1.9	14.6	68.8	245.9	754.4	2,469.4	6,324.1
FEMALE, WHITE 1976[1]	272.0	1.4	11.7	58.5	226.7	630.7	2,485.3	6,596.1
FEMALE, ALL OTHER 1976[1]	176.9	4.9	33.1	148.2	421.8	983.0	2,277.8	3,590.9

[1] Excludes deaths of non-residents of the United States.
Source: Division of Vital Statistics, National Center for Health Statistics.

disease. Little difference was noted in the incidence of sudden death or myocardial infarction among black and white women in Baltimore (Table 2). The International Atherosclerosis Project results did suggest a slightly greater prevalence of coronary atherosclerosis among black as compared to white women in New Orleans (20).

The death rates due to heart attack have been declining rapidly for both men and women (21). The decline has been consistent across all age groups and for both blacks and "all others" (Table 5). The specific reasons for the decline in mortality have not been determined. No reliable data on either the trends in incidence or case-fatality exist.

Table 5. Percent change between 1968 and 1976 in death rates for all causes and for ischemic heart disease, for specified age groups, by color and sex: United States.

AGE	TOTAL			WHITE			ALL OTHER		
	BOTH SEXES	MALE	FEMALE	BOTH SEXES	MALE	FEMALE	BOTH SEXES	MALE	FEMALE
ALL CAUSES									
ALL AGES	-8.1	-10.0	-5.6	-6.8	-9.2	-3.7	-16.7	-15.9	-17.6
25-34 years	-13.4	-10.6	-19.9	-9.7	-7.8	-15.1	-24.5	-19.9	-33.3
35-44 years	-20.5	-18.3	-24.2	-19.2	-18.1	-21.4	-28.6	-23.0	-36.0
45-54 years	-15.5	-15.6	-15.2	-15.2	-16.0	-13.7	-21.2	-17.7	-25.8
55-64 years	-13.4	-14.7	-10.7	-12.8	-14.8	-8.4	-18.3	-13.9	-23.1
65-74 years	-16.0	-14.1	-18.0	-15.7	-13.9	-17.5	-19.6	-16.5	-22.7
75-84 years	-11.6	-6.9	-14.0	-11.9	-6.8	-14.5	-7.3	-5.9	-8.0
85 years and over	-20.9	-17.2	-22.3	-20.0	-16.1	-21.5	-28.4	-25.7	-29.2
ISCHEMIC HEART DISEASE									
ALL AGES	-11.1	-14.3	-6.6	-10.0	-13.5	-5.1	-17.7	-18.1	-17.1
25-34 years	-31.3	-26.0	-42.4	-25.0	-23.2	-36.4	-44.1	-33.1	-53.3
35-44 years	-28.9	-27.3	-35.7	-26.6	-26.6	-28.2	-40.4	-33.1	-51.7
45-54 years	-21.3	-21.1	-22.0	-20.8	-21.1	-19.6	-26.7	-22.3	-33.5
55-64 years	-21.0	-20.4	-22.1	-20.4	-20.4	-20.1	-25.9	-20.4	-32.4
65-74 years	-23.1	-20.2	-26.8	-22.9	-19.9	-26.8	-25.2	-22.5	-27.8
75-84 years	-16.1	-12.8	-17.3	-16.2	-12.6	-17.6	-12.1	-11.2	-12.7
85 years and over	-20.8	-18.5	-21.6	-19.8	-17.1	-20.6	-30.2	-29.9	-29.5

Source: Division of Vital Statistics, National Center for Health Statistics.

Unfortunately there is no reliable information about trends of sudden death. However since sudden death accounted for such a high percentage of total arteriosclerotic heart disease deaths, it would be surprising if the incidence of sudden death was also not declining.

Analytical studies that determine the relationship between risk factors and heart attack can be divided into two specific types: 1) risk factors for the initial heart attack and 2) determinants of the natural history following a heart attack.

The incidence of sudden and unexpected death is very low in women as previously noted. Few longitudinal studies have specifically attempted to measure the risk factors for sudden death among women because of this relatively low incidence (15). In general, the major risk factors such as smoking, blood pressure, serum cholesterol have been associated with all clinical manifestations of ischemic heart disease in men (4). We can probably presume that the same relationship is present in women (23), although again no data to substantiate this finding is available.

In the Framingham study among women aged 45 or over and free of clinical heart disease in 1965 there were 63 heart attacks through 1975 (23). The risk of heart attack was directly related to the levels of low density lipoprotein cholesterol, blood pressure and history of diabetes (24) and inversely related to the levels of HDL cholesterol (Table 6). Neither relative weight nor triglyceride levels were prospectively related to the risk of heart attack among women. Cigarette smoking was not a major cardiovascular risk factor in this older age group for either men or women. Among women with a history of diabetes, the risk of heart attack at each level of high density lipoprotein cholesterol was the same as for men. Other studies have also shown an increased incidence, case-fatality and mortality among women with diabetes or hyperglycemia. The number of sudden deaths was too small for a specific analysis (25, 26).

Table 6. Standardized logistic regression coefficients for incidence of coronary heart disease: The Framingham Study.

Characteristics*	Standardized Logistic Regression Coefficients†			
	Univariate		Multivariate	
	Men	Women	Men	Women
High-density lipoprotein cholesterol	-0.488‡	-0.741‡	-0.610‡	-0.650‡
Low-density lipoprotein cholesterol	0.288§	0.303§	0.332‖	0.260§
Triglyceride	0.048	0.276‖	-0.092	-0.106
Systolic blood pressure	0.323‖	0.400‖	0.327‖	0.216
ECG-left ventricular hypertrophy	0.279‡	0.207‖	0.245‖	0.159§
Relative weight	0.029	0.283§	-0.016	0.031
Diabetes	-0.024	0.474	-0.114	0.390‡

* Measured at Examination 11.
† Estimated by method of Walker-Duncan (20).
‡ $P < 0.001$.
§ $P < 0.05$.
‖ $P < 0.01$.

Source: Tavia Gordon; William P. Castelli M.D.; Marthana C. Hjortland, PH.D.; William B. Kannel, M.D., F.A.C.P.; and Thomas R. Dawber, M.D., F.A.C.P.; Diabetes, Blood Lipids, and the Role of Obesity in Coronary Heart Disease Risk for Women: The Framingham Study, Ann Intern Med vol 87, (4), October 1977.

Men have a higher risk of heart attack including sudden death than women at every level of major known risk factors except for the possible interaction between diabetes and HDL previously described (17). It appeared therefore, that the differences in response to the levels of the risk factors rather than the prevalence of the risk factor level in the population actually account for the differences in the incidence of heart attack between men and women.

A study in Helsinki, Finland (27) attempted to compare risk factors among sudden and not sudden ASHD deaths, myocardial infarction, and angina pectoris. The data regarding the risk factors was unfortunately collected after the event and from hospital charts. Thirty-nine sudden deaths among women were included in the analysis. A history of hypertension and heavy cigarette smoking was more prevalent among the sudden deaths than for the other clinical manifestations of heart attack among women.

A similar type of study in Göteborg (28), Sweden compared women with ischemic heart disease and a population sample. Only ten women died suddenly outside of the hospital with myocardial infarction and four other women were classified as having heart disease deaths outside of the hospital. Diabetes, cigarette smoking and high triglyceride levels were more prevalent among women who had a myocardial infarction than in the population sample. Very little information was reported about the sudden deaths of women who died outside of the hospital.

There are no studies of the distribution of the extent of coronary artery disease among "healthy men and women". The relationship between extent of coronary artery disease and the risk of sudden death for either men or women can not be determined. As noted, pathology studies report that women have less coronary artery disease than men. Deaths due to arteriosclerotic heart disease for both men and women have more extensive coronary artery disease than deaths due to other causes (29). There was also no difference in the extent of coronary artery disease between men and women in New Orleans who died due to coronary artery disease (20). We might presume that the lower risk of sudden death among women was therefore a function of the prevalence of severe coronary atherosclerosis.

The early studies of the pathology of sudden and unexpected deaths have been previously reviewed. The studies done in the 1950's and 1960's primarily concentrated on deaths referred to medical examiner's or coroner's offices and were generally concerned about the distribution of the specific cause of death, activity at onset, and "acute pathology".

A detailed study of sudden death in Rochester, Minnesota over a 25 year period was recently reported (30). Sudden deaths occurred within one hour of onset and unexpected deaths were sudden deaths without a prior history of heart attack. Eighty-three percent of 349 sudden deaths were autopsied including 73 women who died suddenly and unexpectedly without a prior history of heart disease. The sudden and unexpected deaths usually had extensive coronary artery disease. No differences in the extent of coronary artery disease between men and women who died suddenly was reported. Only five of the sudden deaths in women were under the age of 50.

There have been no studies to date that have identified a specific precipitating event or major "environmental determinant" of sudden death among women. Also, no studies have followed "normal women" with frequent ECG monitoring in order to determine the relationship between cardiac arrhythmias and sudden death. The relatively low incidence of sudden death among women would probably preclude this type of study.

The natural history of heart attacks among women has been evaluated in several studies (16, 17, 31). The studies have generally not determined the specific risk of sudden death following a myocardial infarction.

During the first 14 years of the Framingham Study eighteen women died due to coronary heart disease (16). Eleven of these eighteen deaths had a prior history of heart disease. In addition seven (39 %) of the eighteen deaths occurred outside of a hospital and were classified as sudden deaths. The history of myocardial infarction was similar for men and women but as previously noted women with angina pectoris especially at a young age had a much better prognosis than men.

The Health Insurance Plan of Greater New York study (17) has determined the natural history of angina pectoris and myocardial infarction. There were 129 women with a myocardial infarction and 118 with angina pectoris. Among patients with a first myocardial infarction, the percentage dead at one month was similar for men (16.7%) and women (18.3%). The probability of survival whether measured from the time of the heart attack or for those who survived one month was similar for men and women. The prognosis of men with angina or myocardial infarction was apparently the same but women with angina pectoris had a better prognosis than those with a myocardial infarction. The highest mortality for both men and women occurred within the first few months after the myocardial infarction or episode of angina pectoris. The survivorship improved substantially with length of time after the myocardial infarction. Approximately 82% of the deaths among women and 86% of the male deaths in the follow-up cohort were due to heart attacks. Only 69 % of the angina deaths in women were due to arteriosclerotic heart disease. Previous studies have suggested that for women about 60% of the cardiac deaths were sudden.

Risk factors related to the long term prognosis following a myocardial infarction were evaluated at the time of a "baseline examination", approximately 6 months after the myocardial infarction or initial diagnosis of angina pectoris. The risk of death following a myocardial infarction or angina pectoris among women was increased by elevated blood pressure, serum cholesterol over 270 mg %, history of diabetes and presence of an abnormal ECG.

A community study of acute heart attacks in Edinburgh, noted that 28 % (31) of all first heart attacks in men and 23 % in women were sudden deaths. The percentage of first heart attacks that were sudden deaths increased substantially with age from 10.7% at 20–49 yrs to 36.5 % at 60–69 yrs. The percentage of all heart disease deaths within the first four weeks was about 60 % for both men and women. Among women, 38.9 % of deaths within the first four weeks occurred within the first hour and 80 % of the sudden deaths occurred within one hour.

The results were consistent with the Framingham study, the prognosis, both short term and long term following a myocardial infarction was similar for men and women. The women who had angina pectoris however seemed to enjoy a better prognosis.

Unfortunately there have been few detailed follow-up studies of women who have had coronary arteriography. Based on the clinical observation, there is probably a fairly large number of women with modest coronary artery disease and angina pectoris. This group of women probably accounts for both the better prognosis of women with angina pectoris and the lower sex-ratio of angina as compared to myocardial infarction or sudden death.

Similarly other determinants of natural history such as cardiac arrhythmias or left ventricular function have not been analyzed in a large cohort of women. As the prognosis after a myocardial infarction is similar among men and women, future longitudinal follow-up studies and clinical trials should probably include both men and women.

The study of sudden death among women, particularly the initial event, sudden and unexpected deaths, may yield important clues to both the understanding of the etiology of atherosclerosis and the "precipitation of sudden death". This applies specifically to some of the psychosocial variables which may be involved. As noted, sudden and unexpected death among women under the age of 45 is rare. Prospective studies unfortunately will not yield enough information from so few deaths for detailed analysis. Either cross-sectional community or so-called historical prospective studies of large cohorts of women appear to be the only feasible study design.

The cross-sectional studies of sudden death in women can determine:

1) What were the social demographic characteristics of sudden death?
2) Where do women die suddenly and during what types of activities?
3) Are there any specific precipitating factors for sudden death?
4) What is the relationship of sudden death to hormonal determinants, such as age at menopause, number of children, history of artificial menopause, use of hormones?
5) Are there any unusual habits that discriminate women who die suddenly as compared to controls, such as smoking, drinking alcoholic beverages, etc.?

2. METHODS

During the past 15 years we have completed several studies of sudden death due to natural causes in a defined community. The first study investigated all sudden, non-traumatic deaths in Baltimore residents (age 20–64) who died between 1964–1965 (32, 33). The basic aims of the study were to measure the causes of deaths, differences in the frequency and causes of sudden death by race, sex and socioeconomic status and the relationship between sudden and unexpected deaths due to arteriosclerotic heart disease and total arteriosclerotic heart disease mortality. No detailed pathological examination was included as part of the study.

The second study (22) was a pathologic and retrospective historical study of sudden death and myocardial infarction (age 25–64) in Baltimore between June 1970 and June 1972. This study consisted of a detailed epidemiologic and pathologic study of the factors that lead to the onset of a sudden death and myocardial infarction. The major emphasis was on the period of time just prior to a sudden death or myocardial infarction.

The third study was limited to women between the ages of 25–64 who died suddenly with no prior history of heart disease between September 1973 and April 1975 in Allegheny County, Pennsylvania (34). Sixty-four deaths were included during the 18 month period. The basic aims of the study were to identify the risk factors related to sudden death among women especially the previously noted increased prevalence of a psychiatric history among white women who died suddenly in Baltimore.

The fourth study will be completed shortly. A detailed epidemiological pathological study of sudden death among women in Allegheny County (age 25–64) between 1977 and 1979 (17 months). The aims of the study were to further substantiate the reported psychiatric history among women who died suddenly and to quantify the pathology of sudden death among women with and without a prior psychiatric history.

3. RESULTS

The percentage of all sudden non-traumatic deaths due to arteriosclerotic heart disease was 61 % in our initial studies. A higher percentage of sudden deaths in men was due to arterio-sclerotic heart disease than in white women. A much lower percentage of sudden deaths were due to arteriosclerotic heart disease among blacks (Table 7). Spain has done a detailed study of causes of sudden deaths analyzed at the Westchester County Coroner's Office, 91 % of the sudden deaths among men and only 48 % for women were due to arteriosclerotic heart disease.

Table 7. Percentage of all sudden deaths due to ASHD age 40–64 Baltimore: 1967 study – by length of survival and whether witnessed.

	WM	WF	BM	BF	T
UNWITNESSED	74	53	42	52	59
WITNESSED					
<2 Hr	84	93	45	58	72
2-24 Hr	69	56	34	21	51
TOTAL SUDDEN DEATH	76	66	41	45	61

In the 1970 Baltimore study, 118 arteriosclerotic heart disease sudden deaths and 116 sudden deaths due to other causes had a detailed post-mortem examination; 73 % of white men and 58 % among white women were due to arteriosclerotic heart disease.

Over half (58 %) of 40 arteriosclerotic heart disease sudden deaths among white women without a prior history of heart disease as compared to 36 % of 15 sudden white male deaths were unwitnessed. In approximately two years in Baltimore (1970–1972) only 9 sudden deaths among women without a history of heart disease (age 25–64) were witnessed and died within 15 minutes. In the 1973–1975 Allegheny County study, 53 % of the 64 sudden cardiac deaths among the women were unwitnessed.

There were 80 ASHD sudden deaths among white women in the 1970–1972 Baltimore study, 35 (44 %) had a definite prior history of heart disease and 51 (64 %) a history of heart disease, hypertension or diabetes (Table 8). The distributions of prior cardiovascular diseases was similar for white men and women.

Table 8. Distribution of ASHD sudden deaths by history of disease: by race and sex.

RACE/ SEX	TOTAL	HEART DISEASE NO.	%	HYPERTENSION* NO.	%	DIABETES* NO.	%	HYPERTENSION & DIABETES* NO.	%	HEART DISEASE NO.	HYPERTENSION OR DIABETES %
WM	305	161	53	33	11*	9	03*	3	01*	206	68
WF	80	35	44	13	16	1	01	2	03	51	64
BM	105	38	36	19	18	2	02	3	03	62	60
BF	30	17	57	4	13	2	01	1	03	24	80
OTHER	2			1	50					1	50
TOTAL	522	251	49	70	13	14	03	9	02	344	66

* Those without heart disease.
Sixty-five percent of not sudden death had a history of clinical heart disease.

Sudden and unexpected death due to arteriosclerotic heart disease is rare among both black and white women. Sudden deaths among white women in an urban community were more likely to be unwitnessed. A lower percentage of sudden deaths in women are probably due to arteriosclerotic heart disease than in men, suggesting that detailed post-mortem studies are probably necessary to substantiate the causes of death especially for unwitnessed deaths in which the length of survival or circumstances of the deaths can not be determined.

A higher percentage of all arteriosclerotic heart disease deaths were more sudden in men than women (Table 9). Most sudden deaths among women occur at their home, (73 % of

Table 9. Percentage of ASHD deaths that were sudden by age, race, sex: Baltimore 1972–74.

RACE/SEX	25-44	45-54	55-64	TOTAL
WM	68	70	61	63
WF	88	63	43	49
BM	73	78	68	72
BF	71	40	46	47
TOTAL	72	68	57	61

sudden deaths with and 85 % without a prior history of heart disease). Only a very small percentage occurred at work, during recreation or in the street or community facilities. Over half the sudden deaths occurred while the women were apparently relaxing at home (Table 10). However, about one third of ASHD sudden deaths without a prior history of disease occurred during sleep. The relatively high percentage of ASHD sudden deaths that were unwitnessed limits the interpretation of the activity at onset. Other studies however have generally substantiated these results.

Table 10. Distribution of ASHD sudden deaths and living myocardial infarction patients by activity at onset – white women Baltimore 1970–72.

HISTORY OF HEART DISEASE		N %	SLEEPING %	EATING %	RELAXING AT HOME %	DRIVING %	RIDING IN CAR %	WORKING %	OTHER %
YES	SUDDEN DEATH	30	17	-	57	-	-	03	13
	M.I.	35	29	03	47	-	-	15	08
NO	SUDDEN DEATH	40	30	03	35	-	-	21	11
	M.I.	74	17	03	54	01	-	16	09

The frequency of prodromal symptoms prior to a sudden ASHD death and the frequency of visits to a physician within weeks prior to death were similar for men and women. About half of the women who died suddenly had reported a history of an unusual increase in fatigue in the two weeks prior to their sudden death and 15 % had seen a physician within seven days prior to death. The reasons for the marked increase in fatigue have not been determined. In previous studies we have suggested that it might be a symptom of angina pectoris, left ventricular failure or depression.

Risk factors such as elevated blood pressure and cholesterol cannot be measured in a retrospective community sudden death study. In the 1973–1975 Allegheny County study information about smoking, drinking of alcoholic beverages, disease, marital status, and pregnancy history was obtained from the next of kin or other friend or relative and for a neighbourhood control for each sudden death. A similar type of information was also collected in the 1970–1972 Baltimore study. The ASHD sudden deaths in the two Allegheny County studies had no prior history of heart disease.

In the 1970–1972 Baltimore study 9 (23 %) or 39 women who died suddenly due to ASHD had a prior history of a "psychiatric disorder" as compared to none of the controls (Table 11). There was no difference in the prevalence of diabetes or hypertension between the sudden deaths and controls. In the Allegheny County study of 1973–1975, the high prevalence of prior psychiatric history was again noted; 12 (19 %) gave a history of either being hospitalized for psychiatric disorders or being treated by a physician and at the time of the death being on a major psychotherapeutic drug. The preliminary results of our third study in Allegheny County are very interesting. To date 13 (19 %) of 70 ASHD sudden deaths and only 1 (2 %) of 59 controls have a prior history of psychiatric disorder based on the same definition as in the previous study in Allegheny County (Table 11).

The specific psychiatric diagnosis for the 12 deaths in the 1973-1975 studies includes depression (6), schizophrenia (2) and a history of nervous breakdowns (4). All but one of the 12 deaths had been on a major psychotherapeutic drug.

Several previous studies have suggested that there may be an increased frequency of sud-

Table 11. Prior history of psychiatric disease among women who died suddenly due to ASHD and living controls (no prior history of heart disease).

STUDY		N	PSYCHIATRIC HISTORY	
			NO.	%
BALTIMORE STUDY				
1970-72	CASES	39	9	23
	CONTROLS	39	0	-
ALLEGHENY COUNTY				
1973-75	CASES	64	12	19
	CONTROLS	64	0	-
ALLEGHENY COUNTY *				
1977-78	CASES	70	13	19
	CONTROLS	59	1	2

* Study not completed.

den death among patients with psychiatric diseases, stress or users of various psychotherapeutic drugs (36–40).

A recent report from the Framingham study classified women by "type A or B behavior" (41). Type A women had a higher prevalence of coronary heart disease. A further follow-up study has shown that type A women have an increased risk of heart attacks (42). The number of sudden and unexpected deaths among women was too low for any specific type of analysis. Women who were classified in the Framingham study as "emotionally labile" also had a higher prevalence of heart attack.

In the Baltimore study of sudden deaths there was no increased prevalence of a psychiatric history among either the women who had a myocardial infarction and survived or for those who had died but not suddenly due to arteriosclerotic heart disease.

Cigarette smoking has been associated with an increased risk of both myocardial infarction and sudden death especially among men (15). The relationship between cigarette smoking and heart attacks among women has been controversial especially for the older age group. In both the Baltimore and Pittsburgh studies of sudden death among women there was about a two fold excess risk associated with cigarette smoking (Table 12). In the Pittsburgh study of 1973–1975 the risk among one pack a day or greater cigarette smokers was about 3.5 fold.

In the initial Allegheny County study, heavy drinkers of alcoholic beverages have had a much higher prevalence of sudden death (26.5 %) than in the controls (6.3 %), relative risk 2.5. Consumers of large quantities of alcohol die suddenly from a variety of diseases including a poorly defined syndrome called alcohol fatty liver sudden death. Therefore unless detailed and careful post-mortem examinations are done the alcohol history may be spurious and due to a misclassification of the cause of death.

Table 12. History of current cigarette smoking among white women who died suddenly due to ASHD and living controls (no previous history of heart disease).

STUDY	N	CURRENT CIGARETTE SMOKERS	
		NO.	%
BALTIMORE STUDY			
1970-72 SUDDEN DEATHS	39	26	66
CONTROLS	39	13	33
ALLEGHENY COUNTY			
1973-75 SUDDEN DEATHS	64	48	75
CONTROLS	64	28	44

3.1. Marital Status – Pregnancy History and Use of Oral Contraceptives

In both the Baltimore and Allegheny County studies, a higher percentage of women who died suddenly were unmarried as compared to the controls. The Baltimore study especially included a complete ascertainment of all sudden deaths so the differences by marital status could not be attributed to selective referral of sudden deaths to either a coroner's or medical examiner's office.

In the original Allegheny County study, eleven (19.6 %) of the ever married women in the sudden death group and only 2(3.5%) of the ever married control women had had no children. Preliminary data from the more recent Allegheny County study of 1977–1979 substantiates this initial finding (Table 13).

Ten of the eleven nullipara women were compared with their controls. The mean age at marriage of the cases was 26.8 years as compared to 21.2 for the controls. The cases therefore

Table 13. Preliminary data. Sudden death in women: number of children born to ever-married (between 17 and 44 years of age) cases and controls. Allegheny County 1977–1978.

NO. CHILDREN	N=61		N=56	
NO. CHILDREN	CASES		CONTROLS	
	NO.	%	NO.	%
0	11	18%	3	5.4
1	9	14.7	6	10.7
2	23	37.7	22	39.3
3	8	13.1	12	21.4
4	3	4.9	8	14.3
5	5	8.2	0	0
6+	2	3.2	5	8.9
TOTAL	61	100%	56	100%
	Aver. No. Children: 2.09		Aver. No. Children: 2.64	

had been married for an average of only 15 years during their childbearing period as compared to 22 years for the controls. Why did the nullipara women who died suddenly get married at a later age? The most plausible hypothesis is related to selection for marriage including certain behavioral and social characteristics. The late age of marriage and higher prevalence of nulliparity may be related to the psychiatric history, suggesting unusual behavioral characteristics of women who died suddenly due to arteriosclerotic heart disease.

Thirteen women died suddenly and unexpectedly under the age of 45 in the preliminary analysis of the 1977–1979 Allegheny County study. Twelve of the thirteen were included in a detailed pathology study. Six of the thirteen deaths were due to arteriosclerotic heart disease. All of the women who died suddenly due to arteriosclerotic heart disease were cigarette smokers. Four of the six women had either been taking oral contraceptives or birth control pills. Every death had either been on birth control pills or had a hysterectomy (Table 14). None of the seven non-ASHD deaths had been on birth control pills nor any of the controls. Of the women who died suddenly due to ASHD, 2 had two coronary arteries with greater than 50% stenosis and 1 had three and 2 had four vessel disease, right coronary, left main, left anterior descending, and left circumflex.

Table 14. Characteristics of young women who died suddenly due to ASHD. Ages 25–44. (Autopsy deaths only. One out of 6 ASHD sudden deaths died in Emergency room of hospital and was not autopsied.)

	N	ESTROGEN INTAKE	HYSTERECTOMY	CIGARETTE SMOKING
ASHD SUDDEN	5	3 Birthcontrol pills 1 Estrogen replacement	2	5(4)Greater 1 Pack/day
OTHER SUDDEN	7	0	0	6(5)Greater 1 Pack/day
LIVING CONTROL	5	0	0	1 (½ pack per day)

The relationship between the use of oral contraceptives and both cardiovascular deaths and myocardial infarction has been reported in several studies (43–47). The combined increased risk of both cigarette smoking and use of oral contraceptives has also been suggested (46, 47). The previous studies have either not separated sudden from non-sudden deaths or lacked adequate autopsy verification of the cause of death. One half of all sudden and unexpected deaths in women under the age of 45 were not due to arteriosclerotic heart disease in this study.

Spain has reported a preliminary study of women who died following a myocardial infarction and had been on oral contraceptives (47). The deaths generally had ulcerated atherosclerotic plaques or adherent thrombus and a few healing fibrous plaques. The lesions were reported to be similar to the ulcerated atheroma produced experimentally in chickens by estrogens. In the present Allegheny County Study all of the women who died suddenly and who were on oral contraceptives or estrogen replacement had extensive coronary atherosclerosis. The results did not mean that estrogen increased the extent of atherosclerosis;

rather, women with extensive atherosclerosis, perhaps due to other risk factors, such as hyperlipoproteinemia, may be at increased risk of sudden death if taking oral contraceptives or estrogen replacement and smoking cigarettes.

The analysis of the Framingham study suggests that the risk of heart attack increased after the menopause. The effect appears to be independent of age. Several studies including the Framingham study noted an increase in cholesterol, blood pressure and weight following the menopause (49, 50). Plasma cholesterol levels rose substantially among women after the age of 40–45, as compared to men. Whether this increase in risk factors is a function of hormonal change or environmental factors including diet remains to be determined. The relatively rapid increase in risk of heart attack shortly after the menopause is probably not due to changes in these risk factors since the incubation period would be too short. Later changes in risk of heart attack among women with increasing age however may be due to changes in risk factors.

The relationship between estrogen therapy, oral contraceptives, artificial menopause, hormonal patterns and risk of heart disease has been reviewed by several investigators (43). There is still some controversy about these relationships. Women who have had an artificial menopause appear to have an increased risk of heart attack and have severe atherosclerosis. Women taking oral contraceptives were at an increased risk of both myocardial infarction and cardiovascular death. The association is strongest for cigarette smokers. There is no evidence that post-menopausal estrogen replacement therapy is related to either an increase or decrease in heart attacks among women (51). For men, however, there is fairly strong evidence that estrogen therapy following a myocardial infarction increased the risk of subsequent cardiovascular death (43).

The initial studies of sudden death in Allegheny County estimated the relative risk of sudden death for women based on a combination of risk factors. The major risk factors for sudden death were cigarette smoking, heavy to moderate alcohol consumption, psychiatric history, and having no children. Women who had three or more of these risk factors (28 of 46) had an 11.7 fold relative risk as compared to the controls (4 of 64).

4. PATHOLOGY

Most of the previous pathology studies of sudden death have been limited to deaths autopsied by medical examiners or the coroner's office. The prevalence of atherosclerosis has also been measured in several community pathology studies previously described. The most important points from the previous pathology studies were: 1) a high percentage of sudden deaths in women are not due to arteriosclerotic heart disease, 2) women who die suddenly have a similar extent of coronary artery stenosis as men, 3) women who die from other causes have less atherosclerosis than age matched men, 4) the frequency of acute pathology such as thrombosis may be similar for men and women.

Detailed pathology studies were included in the 1970–1972 Baltimore study and the current Allegheny County study. The results of the Allegheny County study are still preliminary. Twenty-four sudden deaths due to arteriosclerotic heart disease (2 with a previous history of heart disease, and 15 sudden deaths due to other causes among white women) were included in the Baltimore study.

The methods for studying the coronary arteries and myocardium have been previously described. Women who died suddenly due to arteriosclerotic heart disease in the 1970–1972 study had a lower prevalence of severe atherosclerosis ($\geq 75\%$) coronary artery stenosis than men. The prevalence of acute pathology, hemorrhage in plaque, acute thrombosis or ruptured plaque was similar among white men and women. Only five post-mortem studies were included for black women.

There were approximately 100 sudden deaths among white women in the current Allegheny County study (March 1977 to October 1978). All had no prior clinical history of heart disease. Sixty-four of the 100 sudden deaths had been included in the detailed post-mortem study including 46 of 80 due to arteriosclerotic heart disease (Table 15). The study represents almost a complete ascertainment of all sudden non-traumatic deaths among white women aged 25–64 without a prior history of heart disease during a 17 month period.

Table 15. March 1, 1977 – October 31, 1978. Sudden death in women aged 25–64 in Allegheny County, N = 89. (Eleven additional cases to be completed [ASHD]).

Sudden death causes	Autopsied	Not autopsied	Total
ASHD			
Non-psychiatric	38	19	57
Psychiatric	8	5	13
Non-ASHD			
Non-psychiatric	15	1	16
Psychiatric	3	0	3
Total	64	25	89

Eight of the thirteen ASHD sudden death cases with a psychiatric history were autopsied (60 %). The principal difference between autopsied ASHD psychiatric cases and non-autopsied ASHD psychiatric cases is age at demise. The mean age of the former being 53.5 years and of the latter 60.8 years. The admitting diagnosis was most commonly a diagnosis of depression or a "nervous breakdown" (particularly earlier cases).

The distribution of risk factors, specifically hypertension and cigarette smoking among sudden deaths with a psychiatric history are no greater than in previous non-psychiatric ASHD sudden death populations.

The degree of coronary narrowing is very much different in the ASHD sudden death psychiatric population than in the remaining ASHD cases. As shown previously in Table 16, three of the cases have no major vessel with 50 % involvement or greater and another has but one vessel with 50 % stenosis. Three of these four women died while in their sleep. The remaining woman died within 15 minutes of onset of symptoms (witnessed cases).

There exists the possibility of an acute precipitating event (or life stressor) contributing to the fatal event in each of the cases (Table 17). Case number five was in the throes of an acute agitated depression as a result of her mother's death three months prior to her own demise. Case six was fired four months before her death from a job as a dock loader at an airline. She had been involved in a lengthy court discrimination suit. Yet another woman (number

Table 16. Distribution of extent of coronary artery stenosis by age and psychiatric history: ASHD sudden deaths (1977–78).

NUMBER OF ARTERIES ≥ 50% STENOSIS

PSYCHIATRIC HISTORY	AGE	N	0	1	2	3	4
NO	25-44	5	-	-	2	1	2
NO	45-54	16	-	-	4	8	4
YES	45-54	4	2	1	-	1	0
NO	55-64	17	1	1	4	6	5
YES	55-64	4	1	-	-	1	2
TOTAL	ALL	46	4	2	10	17	13

[1] Psychiatric history – Data on coronary arteries not available for analysis at time of study report.

7) lost her hotel management job when the building she worked in burnt to the ground. This occurred three months prior to her death. Case number eight had been hospitalized the year before, for a "nervous breakdown" and according to the husband, lived in dread of having to return for more treatment.

The reports of "stressful life events" are of course often a result of hindsight, i.e. elicited after the fact, from relatives who would like to seize upon a reason for their loved one's demise. Numerous studies have reported on increased mortality of the surviving partners following the death of their spouses. The mechanism for such deaths remains obscure.

Eight deaths with a prior history of psychiatric disease have been included in the detailed pathology study. The distribution of the extent of coronary artery stenosis was remarkably different between the sudden ASHD deaths with and without a prior history of psychiatric disease. Four of the eight psychiatric history related deaths had either no coronary artery stenosis or only one coronary artery with greater than 50% coronary artery stenosis as compared to 2 of 37 without a prior history of psychiatric disease (Table 18). Detailed postmortem examination including extensive toxicology failed to identify another cause of death. Therefore the women who died suddenly and had a psychiatric history did not apparently have severe coronary artery disease.

The specific causes of death for these women with minimal coronary artery disease and a psychiatric history is a puzzle. It is also difficult to generalize about the non-autopsied deaths because they tended to be witnessed and occurred in relatively few minutes. The study of these deaths is particularly difficult because of their rarity. Only 13 sudden "cardiac deaths" with a psychiatric history were identified among a population of close to 2,000,000 in 17

Table 17. Sudden death due to ASHD psychiatric cases by diagnosis, autopsy and medication histories and other risk factors, N = 13.

AUTOPSIED ASHD PSYCHIATRIC CASES		DIAGNOSIS	VALIDATION/ DATE OF ADMISSION	CURRENT PSYCHOTROPHIC MEDICATION HISTORY	CURRENT SMOKING OR HBP
3-4 Vessel Narrowing ≥ 50%			Hospitalized		
CASE	AGE				
1	47	alcoholism	1973	None	1+ pk/day
2	55	nervous breakdown (ECT)	1948	None	2+ pks/day
3	59	nervous breakdown	1955	None	1-2 pks/day
4	53	nervous breakdown	June 78	Haldol	NO
0-1 Vessel Narrowing ≥ 50%					
5	57	agitated depression	5/31/78	Thorazine	NO
6	51	anxiety reaction	1963 & 1968	None	2+ pks/day
7	52	depression	1973	Triavil	NO
8	52	nervous breakdown	Dec. 1976- April 1977	None	HBP/Diabetic
NOT AUTOPSIED ASHD PSYCHIATRIC CASES					
9	63	nervous breakdown	1967	None	HBP
10	62	agitated depression	1967	Triavil	NO
11	52	depression (ECT)	1963 & 1977	None	2+ pks/day
12	63	paranoid phychosis	1971 & 1974	None	1-2 pks/day
13	64	depression	1978	None	HBP

months. They may however represent an important clue to the relationship between psychosocial factors, cardiac arrhythmias, and sudden death.

The women who died suddenly without a history of psychiatric disease had more extensive coronary artery stenosis than those sudden deaths due to other causes. However out of 16 who died from other causes, 6 had 3–4 arteries with greater than 50% narrowing. Therefore the extent of coronary artery disease does not completely discriminate between sudden death due to ASHD and other causes. The specific cases of the sudden death due to other causes is shown in Table 19.

5. DISCUSSION

Sudden and unexpected death due to arteriosclerotic heart disease has been studied extensively during the past 20 years. The descriptive studies have substantiated the relationship

Table 18. Comparison of extent of coronary artery stenosis among women who died suddenly due to ASHD and from other natural causes (excluding psychiatric history).

NO. OF ARTERIES WITH > 50% STENOSIS*

AGE		N	0	1	2	3	4
24-44	ASHD	5	0	1	1	1	2
	OTHER	7	4	0	2	1	0
45-54	ASHD	16	0	0	4	8	4
	OTHER	3	0	1	1	-	1
55-64	ASHD	17	1	1	4	6	5
	OTHER	5	2	0	0	2	1
TOTAL	ASHD	37	1	1	10	15	10
	OTHER	16	6	1	3	3	3

* Left main, anterior descending, circumflex and right coronary artery.

Table 19. Non-ASHD sudden deaths by cause of death, N = 19.

C.O.D.	NUMBER
AORTIC ANEURYSM	2
BRONCHOPNEUMONIA	3
EMPHYSEMA	2
MYOCARDITIS	1
BERRY ANNEURYSM	2
SUBARACHNOID HEMORRHAGE	3
FATTY LIVER	2
HEPATIC FAILURE	1
HEMOPERITONEUM	1
GLOMERULONEPHRITIS	1
G.I. HEMORRHAGE	1
TOTAL	19

with age, and a much higher incidence in men. A few studies report that the incidence of sudden death is similar among blacks and whites.

The pathology studies have consistently noted an extensive degree of coronary atherosclerosis, acute pathology, such as thrombosis and hemorrhage in a plaque, and both myocardial pathology and cardiomegaly. The few prospective longitudinal studies suggest that the risk factors for sudden deaths and for myocardial infarction are similar especially for men. Studies of the natural history of heart attack, both short and long term, have identified some of the risk factors for sudden death including the extent of coronary artery disease, left ventricular function and cardiac arrhythmias.

Clinical trials have attempted to evaluate the methods of reducing sudden deaths by modification of risk factors, coronary bypass surgery, antiarrhythmic drugs, and platelet inhibitors. These studies have all given us a broad brush approach to the problem of sudden death. The specific reasons why a sudden death occurs at a certain point in time and the initial pathophysiology and the so-called unidentified risk factors within the broad category of risk are still unresolved. Sex, men as compared to women, is still the most powerful risk factor. However it has been been rather difficult to study because of the rarity of sudden death among women.

The present studies show that sudden and unexpected death among women less than 45 is primarily related to heavy cigarette smoking, use of estrogen preparations, either as oral contraceptives or as replacement therapy. The women who died suddenly had extensive coronary artery disease. We might hypothesize that women who had coronary artery disease primarily on the basis of elevated risk factors such as hyperlipoproteinemia or hypertension are the population at risk for sudden death precipitated by cigarette smoking and taking of hormonal preparations. Such women are fortunately few in the population and therefore the risk of sudden death among young women given the high prevalence of cigarette smoking and hormonal use especially of oral contraceptives is low. It is also possible however that cigarette smoking or contraceptive pills enhance atherosclerosis independent of the other risk factors. Unfortunately, it is probably extremely difficult or impossible to test this hypothesis in humans.

Over half of the sudden deaths among women less than 45 were not due to arteriosclerotic heart disease. It was interesting to note that the cigarette smoking history was similar in both the ASHD and other sudden deaths but the contraceptive and estrogen preparation history was very different. Studies of sudden death among young women probably require detailed postmortem examination as well as careful follow back interviews.

In women who die suddenly over the age of 45, we have previously noted a high prevalence of nulliparity and longer period of time from marriage to birth of first child. The higher prevalence of nulliparity may be a measure of hormonal factors related to atherosclerosis. However it also could be a measure of selection for both marriage and having children. Women who marry at a late age and remain nulliparius may have certain social, psychological and risk factor characteristics that increase their likelihood of sudden death such as cigarette smoking, diabetes, obesity and hypertension.

All three studies of sudden death have noted a high prevalence of prior psychiatric history. The current Allegheny County study has now shown that some women with a psychiatric history who die suddenly apparently from "heart disease" have minimal coronary artery stenosis. However, results are based on only eight sudden deaths with a psychiatric history that were included in the autopsied series. The cause of death and its relationship to specific pathophysiology and to the psychiatric history is therefore still undetermined.

Women who have psychiatric disorders may be an interesting population to study with regard to the relationship between the brain and cardiac function especially cardiac arrhythmia. The risk of sudden death will probably be too low among these women to make it feasible to do longitudinal studies to determine the risk of sudden death.

Finally, the accuracy of the causes of sudden death for women may be suspect without a detailed post-mortem examination. The accuracy of the cardiovascular disease death rates for women is probably not as good as for men. A previous study has also suggested that this may be especially true for black women. It is probably important that post-mortem studies be done in cases of sudden and unexpected death among women if an accurate cause of death is to be determined. Even with a detailed post-mortem examination there were still sudden deaths in which the cause of death could not be determined.

REFERENCES

1. Kuller L: Sudden and unexpected non-traumatic deaths in adults: A review of epidemiological and clinical studies. J Chron Dis 19:1165–1192, 1966.
2. Spain DM, Bradess VA, Mohr C: Coronary atherosclerosis as a cause of unexpected and unexplained death: An autopsy study from 1949–1959. JAMA 174:384–388, 1960.
3. Spain DM, Bradess VA: Sudden death from coronary atherosclerosis: Age, race, sex, physical activity, and alcohol. Arch Intern Med 100:228–231, 1957.
4. Kannel WB, Doyle JT, McNamara PM, Quickenton P, Gordon T: Precursors of sudden coronary death: Factors related to the incidence of sudden death. Circulation 51:606–613, 1975.
5. Kuller LH: Heart disease and rehabilitation: State of the art 1978. Presented at the Natural History of Coronary Heart Disease at Mount Sinai Medical Center, New York, 1978.
6. The Multiple Risk Factor Intervention Trial Group: Statistical design considerations in the NHLI multiple risk factor intervention trial (MRFIT). J Chron Dis 30:261–275, 1977.
7. Detre K, Murphy ML, Hultgren H: Effect of coronary bypass surgery on longevity in high and low risk patients. Report from the V.A. Cooperative Coronary Surgery Study. Lancet 2:1243–1245, 1977.
8. The Anturane Reinfarction Trial Research Group: Sulfinpyrazone in the prevention of cardiac death after myocardial infarction. The Anturane Reinfarction Trial. N Engl J Med 298:289–294, 1978.
9. Elwood PC, Cochrane AL, Burr ML, Sweetnam PM, Williams G, Welsby E, Hughes SJ, Renton R: A randomized controlled trial of acetyl salicylic acid in the secondary prevention of mortality from myocardial infarction. Br Med J 1:436–440, 1974.
10. The Coronary Drug Project Research Group: The coronary drug project. Design, methods and baseline results (AHA Monograph no 38). Circulation 47 (suppl 1), 1973.
11. Kuller LH, Perper JA, Cooper MC: Sudden and unexpected death due to arteriosclerotic heart diseases. In: Modern trends in cardiology, Oliver MF (ed), London, Butterworths, 1974, p 292–332.
12. Hagstrom RM, Federspiel CF, Ho YC: Incidence of myocardial infarction and sudden death from coronary heart disease in Nashville, Tennessee. Circulation 44:884–890, 1971.
13. Margolis JR, Gillum RF, Feinleib M, Brasch RC, Fabsitz RR: Community surveillance for coronary heart disease: The Framingham cardiovascular disease survey. Methods and preliminary results. Am J Epidemiol 100:425–436, 1974.
14. Dawber TR: Risk factors for atherosclerotic disease. Michigan, Upjohn, 1975.
15. Kannel WB, Gordon T: The Framingham Study: An epidemiological investigation of cardiovascular disease. Section 26, Washington, DC, US Government Printing Office, 1970.
16. Gordon T, Kannel WB: Premature mortality from coronary heart disease. The Framingham Study. JAMA 215:1617–1625, 1971.
17. Weinblatt E, Shapiro S, Frank CW: Prognosis of women with newly diagnosed coronary heart disease – A comparison with course of disease among men. Am J. Public Health 63:577–592, 1973.
18. Potts KH, Stein PD, Houk PC: Transmural myocardial infarction with arteriographically normal appearing coronary arteries. Chest 62:549–552, 1972.
19. Glancy DL, Marcus ML, Epstein SE: Myocardial infarction in young women with normal coronary arteriograms. Circulation 44:495–502, 1971.
20. McGill HC (ed): The geographic pathology of atherosclerosis. Baltimore, The Williams & Wilkins Company, 1968.
21. National Center for Health Statistics: Chartbook for the conference on the decline in coronary heart disease mortality: Ischemic heart disease. US Department of Health, Education and Welfare, Public Health Service

National Center for Health Statistics, Division of Vital Statistics, Hyattsville, Maryland, 1978.

22. Kuller L, Perper J, Cooper M: Demographic characteristics and trends in arteriosclerotic heart disease mortality: Sudden death and myocardial infarction. In: Sudden Coronary Death Outside Hospital. Prineas RJ, Blackburn H (eds), Dallas, The American Heart Association, 1975, p III-1–III-15.

23. Gordon T, Castelli WP, Hjortland MC, Kannel WB, Dawber TR: Diabetes, blood lipids, and the role of obesity in coronary heart disease risk for women. The Framingham Study. Ann Intern Med 87:393–397, 1977.

24. Garcia MJ, McNamara PM, Gordon T, Kannell WB: Morbidity and mortality in diabetics in the Framingham population. Sixteen year follow-up study. Diabetes 23:105–111, 1974.

25. Tansey MJB, Opie LH, Kennelly BM: High mortality in obese women diabetics with acute myocardial infarction. Br Med J 1:1624–1626, 1977.

26. Ostrander LD: Hyperglycemia and vascular disease in Tecumseh, Michigan. In: Early diabetes, Camerini-Davalos RA, Cole HS (eds), New York, Academic Press, 1970, p 365–373.

27. Romo M: Factors related to sudden death in acute ischaemic heart disease. A community study in Helsinki. Department of the Finnish Heart Association and the Department of Medicine, University Central Hospital, Helsinki, Finland, 1972. (Also published as supplement 547 to Acta Medica Scandinavica).

28. Bengtsson C: Ischaemic heart disease in women. Acta Med Scand suppl 549:5–128, 1973.

29. Perper JA, Kuller LH, Cooper M: Arteriosclerosis of coronary arteries in sudden, unexpected deaths. In: Sudden Coronary Death Outside Hospital, Prineas RJ, Blackburn H (eds), Dallas, The American Heart Association, 1975, p III-27–33.

30. Titus JL, Oxman HA, Connolly DC, Nobrega FT: Sudden unexpected death as the initial manifestation of coronary heart disease: Clinical and pathological observations. Singapore Med J 14:291–293, 1973.

31. Armstrong A, Duncan B, Oliver MF, Julian DG, Donald KW, Fulton M, Lutz W, Morrison SL: Natural history of acute coronary heart attacks: A community study. Br Heart J 34:67–80, 1972.

32. Kuller LH, Lilienfeld A, Fisher R: Epidemiological study of sudden and unexpected deaths due to arterio-sclerotic heart disease. Circulation 34: 1056–1068, 1966.

33. Kuller L, Lilienfeld A, Fisher R: An epidemiological study of sudden and unexpected deaths in adults. Medicine 46:341–359, 1967.

34. Talbott E, Kuller LH, Detre K, Perper J: Biologic and phychosocial risk factors of sudden death from coronary disease in white women. Am J Cardiol 39:858–864, 1977.

35. Dynes JB: Cause of death in schizophrenia. Behav Neuropsychiatry 1:12–14, 1969.

36. Wolpert A, Yaryura-Tobias JA, Kertzner L: Silent myocardial infarction in a chronic psychotic population. Dis Nerv Syst 32:280–283, 1971.

37. Engel GL: Sudden and rapid death during psychological stress. Folklore or folk wisdom? Ann Intern Med 74:771–782, 1971.

38. Lehman HE, Ban TA (eds): Toxicity and adverse reaction studies with neuroleptics and antidepressants. Quebec Psychopharmacological Research Association, 1965.

39. Leestma JE, Koenig L: Sudden death and phenothiazines: A current controversy. Arch Gen Psychiat 18:137–148, 1968.

40. Haynes SG, Feinleib M, Levine S, Scotch N, Kannel WB: The relationship of psychosocial factors to coronary heart disease in the Framingham Study. II. Prevalence of coronary heart disease. Am J Epidemiol 107:384–402, 1978.

41. Haynes SG, Feinleib M, Kannel WB: Prospective study of psychosocial factors and coronary heart disease in Framingham. Abstracts of papers presented at the eleventh meeting of the Society for Epidemiologic Research. Am J Epidemiol 108:229, 1978.

42. McGill HC Jr, Stern MP: Sex and atherosclerosis. Atherosclerosis Rev 4:157–242, 1979.

43. Inman WHW, Vessey MP: Investigation of deaths from pulmonary, coronary, and cerebral thrombosis and embolism in women of child-bearing age. Br Med J 2:193–199, 1968.

44. Mann JI, Vessey MP, Thorogood M, Doll R: Myocardial infarction in young women with special reference to oral contraceptive practice. Br Med J 2-241–245, 1975.

45. Mann JI, Doll R, Thorogood M, Vessey MP, Waters WE: Risk factors for myocardial infarction in young women. Br J Prev Soc Med 30:94–100, 1976.

46. Shapiro S, Rosenberg L, Slone D, Kaufman DW, Stolley PD, Miettinen OS: Oral-contraceptive use in relation to myocardial infarction. Lancet 1:743–746, 1979.

47. Spain DM, Glagov S, Gross EM: Pathogenesis of oral contraceptive associated myocardial infarction. Abstracts of the 50th Scientific Sessions, American Heart Association, III-125, 479, 1977.

48. Kannel WB, Hjortland MC, McNamara PM, Gordon T: Menopause and risk of cardiovascular disease. The

Framingham Study. Ann Intern Med 85:447–452, 1976.

49. Hjortland MC, McNamara PM, Kannel WB: Some atherogenic concomitants of menopause: The Framingham Study. Am J Epidemiol 103:304–311, 1976.

50. Weiss N: Relationship of menopause to serum cholesterol and arterial blood pressure: The United States' health examination survey of adults. Am J Epidemiol 96:237–241, 1972.

51. Pfeffer RI, Whipple GH, Kurosaki TT, Chapman JM: Coronary risk and estrogen use in postmenopausal women. Am J Epidemiol 107:479–487, 1978.

1.3. A PATHOLOGIST'S VIEW OF SUDDEN CARDIAC DEATH

A.C. THOMAS, M.J. DAVIES and A.W. POPPLE

The initial pathological examination of the heart of a case of sudden cardiac death usually results in the case being placed in one of three categories. In descending order of frequency these are:

1) Ischaemic heart disease – (coronary atherosclerosis).
2) Gross macroscopic abnormality such as hypertrophic cardiomyopathy, aortic valve stenosis or other cardiac condition carrying a clearly defined clinical or epidemiological risk of sudden death.
3) Hearts apparently normal on macroscopic examination.

1. ISCHAEMIC HEART DISEASE

In the United Kingdom cases of sudden ischaemic death come to autopsy by the thousand every year. Surprisingly little accurate morphological data emerge due to the sheer volume of work imposed on the pathologists carrying out the autopsies for H.M. Coroner. The legal forensic system is designed to exclude unnatural death not to derive scientific data about natural disease.

From the literature it is possible to derive the information that a proportion of patients dying suddenly from ischaemic heart disease have a recent occlusive thrombus in a major coronary artery. The reported incidence of this finding varies widely (Table 1). A comparative study from five centres in the United States (1) found an incidence between 17 and 46 % in 868 autopsies. This range closely mimics the scatter in the overall world literature of 4–64 % (Table 1). This wide range may reflect different selection of case material, different temporal definition of sudden death, varying standards of methodology used to examine the coronary arteries or even an actual geographic variation in the incidence of occlusive thrombi.

A major variant in case selection is the time between onset of pain and death. Instantaneous death is usually taken as occurring within one hour; in contrast deaths up to 24 hours are still classified by many as sudden. A few studies have suggested that the incidence of thrombi is very low in instantaneous as compared with later "sudden" deaths (2) while others find little difference. Other variants vitiating strict comparability between series are the proportion of males to females, smokers against non-smokers and the levels of hypertension all of which may alter the incidence of occlusive thrombi.

The methods of examining the coronary arteries vary widely and are rarely strictly

Table 1. Frequency of recent occlusive coronary thrombosis in sudden death due to ischaemic heart disease.

Author		Place	Definition of Sudden	Number of Cases	Thrombosis %
Friedman et al.	(2)	San Francisco	< 1 min	27	4
Kuller et al.	(3)	Baltimore	<24 hrs	486	15
Lie and Titus	(1)	Minnesota	< 6 hrs	120	17
Spain and Bradess	(4)	U.S.A.	< 1 hr	189	18
Titus et al.	(5)	Minnesota	< 1 hr	286	19
Perper et al.	(6)	Pennsylvania	<24 hrs	171	22
Haerem	(7)	Oslo	<10 min	47	30
Myers and Dewar	(8)	Newcastle	< 1 min	10	30
Mitchell and Schwartz	(9)	Oxford	< 6 hrs	–	31.6
Davies and Popple	(10)	London	< 6 hrs	120	33
Baba and Bashe	(11)	Ohio	<24 hrs	121	38
Myers and Dewar	(8)	Newcastle	<24 hrs	66	42
Rissanen et al.	(12)	Finland	<24 hrs	141	44
Scott and Briggs	(13)	New York	< 1 hr	183	46
Liberthson et al.	(14)	Miami	<15 min	220	58
Friedman et al.	(2)	San Francisco	<24 hrs	37	59
Crawford et al.	(15)	London	< 1 hr	75	64

comparable. Two fundamental points should be met by acceptable studies. Every 4 mm segment of the whole epicardial coronary tree must be examined and the degree of stenosis in each segment accurately measured by morphometry of post-mortem angiograms, by visual grids on microscopic sections or by a quantitating microscope. Such measurements correlate well with the degree of stenosis measured by coronary arteriography in life (16). Naked eye assessment of cross sections of uninjected coronary arteries in the post-mortem room is less than ideal. The otherwise detailed autopsy protocol recommended by the American Heart Association and sponsored by the Scientific Council on Atherosclerosis and Ischaemic Heart Disease of the International Society of Cardiology however, still uses a visual grading of stenosis (17).

Ostensibly there should be no difficulty in pathologists agreeing on the definition of an occlusive recent thrombus. In practice the close association between complex atheromatous lesions and thrombi can lead to the latter being missed unless close serial histological sections are examined. In one study (14), for example, distinctions are made between acute occlusion due to thrombus, a ruptured plaque and intramural haemorrhage; in contrast others (2) would probably regard all these as being the result of different planes of section through an occlusive thrombus.

A proportion of those cases with recent occlusive coronary thrombi will have demonstrable regional myocardial infarction at autopsy. Those who do not either have survived for an insufficient time period for necrosis to be demonstrable by morphological means or have sufficient collateral flow to prevent significant myocardial necrosis. Where there is recent total coronary occlusion, death can be reasonably related to this vascular event and exactly analogous to experimental ligation of a major coronary artery in the dog which will also lead to a high proportion of deaths from ventricular fibrillation within one hour.

In the majority of patients with occlusive coronary thrombi fatal arrhythmias are most likely to arise within the area of ischaemic ventricular muscle itself. In a minority of cases quite different and alternative pathophysiological mechanisms have been invoked. Thrombosis of the right coronary artery, which in the majority of hearts supplies the posterior descending coronary artery, and hence the atrioventricular (AV) nodal artery, is clinically associated with AV block beginning some 24 hours after the onset of chest pain and lasting three to four days before normal conduction returns. While often regarded as indicating temporary nodal ischaemia the time course and experimental work in dogs show this to be more likely mediated by diffusion of potassium ions from adjacent dead muscle (18). James (19) has suggested that right coronary artery thrombosis may be more likely to result in sudden death from nodal malfunction. Our own study of sudden death (10) shows that there is a slight increase of the number of right coronary thrombi as compared to left anterior descending occlusions than in non-sudden acute myocardial infarction deaths. In the former 36 % of those with thrombi are in the right coronary artery, in the latter only 34 %. One series (8) reported right coronary thrombi in 48 % of sudden death cases actually reversing the preponderance of occlusions in the left anterior descending coronary usually found in acute myocardial infarction. In contrast other series do not find any right preponderance but the overall trend is to suggest that right coronary occlusion is indeed more common in sudden death (Table 2) than late hospital infarct deaths.

Table 2. Site of occlusive coronary thrombus in acute myocardial infarction and sudden ischaemic death.

		No.	Main Left	LAD	R	LC
Acute Myocardial Infarction (Hospital Deaths)						
Plotz	(20)	1495	71	834	379	211
Davies et al.	(21)	460	15	219	160	63
		1955	86	1053 (54 %)	539 (28 %)	274 (14 %)
Sudden Death						
Friedman et al.	(2)	21	1	11	7 (33 %)	2
Davies and Popple	(10)	39	0	18	16 (41 %)	9
Myers and Dewar	(8)	40	0	12	19 (48 %)	9
Crawford et al.	(15)	48	0	27	15 (31 %)	6
Bashe et al.	(22)	46	3	16	19 (41 %)	8
		194	4	84 (43 %)	76 (39 %)	34 (18 %)

Occlusion of the left anterior descending coronary artery proximal to the first septal branch may lead to extensive antero-septal infarction and bilateral bundle branch lesions leading to sudden death (23, 24) from conduction disturbance. Occlusion of the main left coronary artery is also associated with sudden death on the basis that infarction of the bulk of the left ventricle follows (25) but this is, in fact, rare. Perper and his colleagues (6) found no example in 171 cases of sudden cardiac death.

Despite the variation in the morphological data reported in the literature one clear fact emerges that a second and large group of sudden ischaemic deaths do *not* have any major recent pathological event in the coronary arteries as an explanation for death to occur on the particular day.

Some clinical support for there being at least two sub-groups in ischaemic sudden death comes from patients resuscitated in the street by flying squad teams. Here only a proportion subsequently develop the clinical picture of acute myocardial infarction (14, 26, 27).

For the pathologist the problems of this second group without occlusive thrombi are to define the extent and degree of stenosis present, to define the lowest quantitative limit of disease which can reasonably be taken to cause death and, if possible, to demonstrate some recent subtle change in myocardium or coronary vessels as the immediate precursor of death.

The technical problems of such morphological studies of the coronary artery tree and myocardium are again considerable. For a coronary artery study to be acceptable there must be quantitative assessment of the lumen size of every 0.4 cm cross segment of the whole epicardial coronary artery tree. The majority of methods used are at best semi-quantitative with visual assessment of the lumen as no stenosis, more than $\frac{3}{4}$ lumen remaining, more than $\frac{1}{2}$ lumen remaining and less than $\frac{1}{4}$ lumen remaining being the usually adopted grading (17).

We personally have elected to study accurately and in detail, using a quantitating microscope, a series of ischaemic sudden deaths as compared with age, sex matched controls. Our technique accurately and reproducibly measures the lumen area of the vessel as a percentage of the total area within the internal elastic lamina. Our experience is that this method correlates extremely well with data from coronary arteriograms in life particularly with degrees of stenosis over 70 %. Below 50 % stenosis the correlation is less good; areas of diffuse intimal disease may score up to 50 % stenosis by post-mortem quantitation and be regarded as normal by selective coronary arteriograms in life.

Values are measured for every 0.4 cm segment of the whole epicardial coronary tree. In all 80 patients comprising 50 males and 30 females dying of ischaemic heart disease were studied. As a control the next age and sex matched patient dying of malignancy or accident without any clinical evidence of vascular disease was used. The test and control groups, not surprisingly but encouragingly, are statistically distinguishable. Taking the worst *single* area of stenosis at any point in the coronary tree, 85% stenosis best separates the groups (Figure 1). Taking a mean value of the three worst areas of stenosis a figure of over 87% best separates the groups. Taking an individual area of over 75% stenosis as significant stenosis and expressing the results conventionally as single, double or triple vessel disease the test and control groups are rough inverted mirror images (Table 3). The background level of atherosclerosis in the population studied is clearly high. Areas of stenosis in the range of 50–70% are commonplace in the control group. These results agree in general with the numerous semi-quantitative studies published and confirm that in the majority of ischaemic deaths widespread stenosis is present but it would appear that 85 % stenosis is a significant critical level. In a minority of patients only one vessel has reached this critical level but even in such cases 50–70 % foci of stenosis are invariably found in other vessels.

The answers to the actual mechanism of death in this group of patients without occlusive recent thrombi can only come from 24 hour ECG monitoring and by epidemiology. The

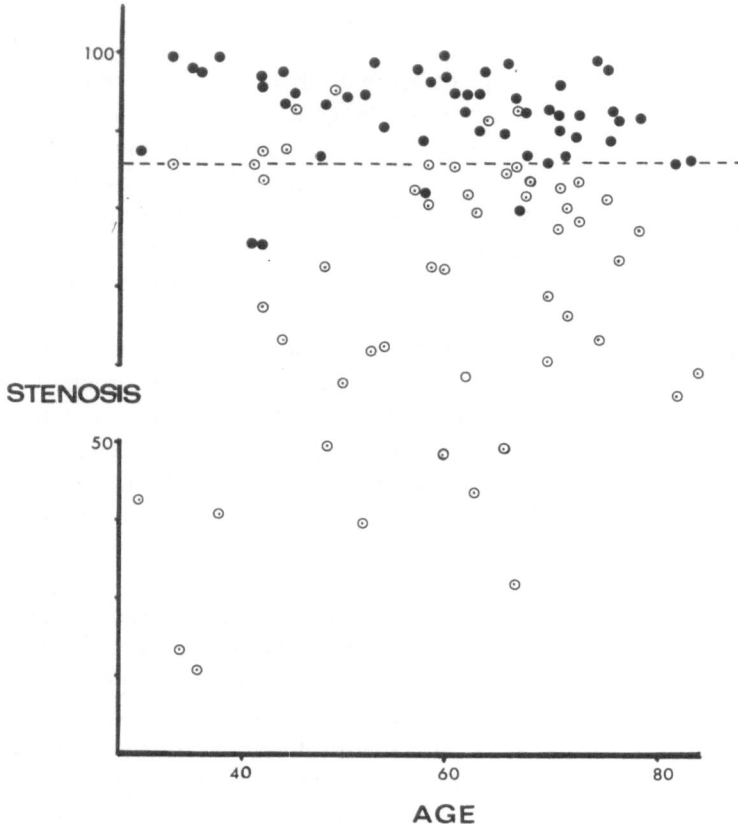

Figure 1. Data for the single worst area of coronary stenosis plotted for age in males. Closed circles represent patients dying of ischaemic heart disease, open circles are age matched controls dying of non-cardiac causes. A dotted line at 85 % stenosis best separates the two groups.

Table 3. Frequency of arteries with more than 75 % stenosis in any one 0.4 cm. segment. Age, sex matched material.

No. of Arteries	Test	n = 80	Controls
0	1*		42
1	11 (14 %)		17
2	18		15
3	50		6 (8 %)

* ? Wrongly certified death

fortuitous cases where arrhythmias occurring just prior to death in ambulatory patients are recorded seem most likely to provide the clues (28, 29, 30). The actual rhythm present within minutes of collapse in most cases of ischaemic sudden death is ventricular fibrillation (14).

The proportion of patients dying suddenly from ischaemic heart disease reported in the literature to have acute myocardial necrosis varies widely. The major determinant of this variation is the sensitivity of the method used to demonstrate necrosis. A classic transmural or subendocardial regional infarct visible at naked eye and best accurately delineated by macroscopic enzyme techniques on 1 cm transverse slices (1, 31, 32, 33, 34) is found in from 12 to 47% of ischaemic sudden deaths. As stressed by Reichenbach and Moss (35) such relatively large areas of necrosis involve interstitial tissues as well as myocardial cells and are true infarctions. In our experience (36) these lesions are closely related to occlusive thrombi although others (11) record a less consistent association.

There are numerous histological techniques designed to demonstrate early infarction where the lesion is either less than eight hours old and not visible macroscopically or there are lesser degrees of tissue destruction. The latter (35) involves only the myocardial cells while the interstitial tissues are spared but does lead to focal scarring and is best known as focal myocardial necrosis or myofibrillary degeneration.

The numerous histological or histochemical methods described to demonstrate dying muscle cells all claim to be more specific or sensitive than those preceding them. Essentially they fall into two groups, those showing alteration of myofibrillary arrangement by staining with acid or basic fuchsin stains where contraction bands within individual cells are shown (37, 38) or actual myocardial distortion in the "wavy" fibre seen on conventional stains (39). The problem of such methods is their extreme sensitivity and frequent positive results in control material where agonal changes occurring as a *result* of dying over some minutes are shown. Use of these methods has been claimed, however, to demonstrate that up to 85 % of patients dying suddenly have myocardial necrosis (1, 35, 40, 41).

Patients dying of ischaemic heart disease without recent thrombotic occlusion of a major coronary artery thus represent a myocardium which is at times focally or diffusely underperfused due to stenosis of the coronary arteries. The myocardium has an enhanced electrical instability, in some, for purely pathophysiological reasons, in others associated with varying degrees of myocardial cell necrosis. To ascribe a single factor to the cause of death for any individual patient within this spectrum is unwise.

The risk of sudden death in any patient with coronary atherosclerosis can be regarded as representing a balance between the degree of arterial obstruction and the level of electrical stability in the myocardium. Factors influencing the former are the actual degree of stenosis at any point and the number of such stenotic foci. Factors influencing the latter are poorly understood but electrical stability may be influenced by, for example, hard or soft water environment or by increased sympathetic tone. An indication that the actual degree of coronary stenosis is not the sole determinant of life or death comes from the overlap of the degree of coronary atherosclerosis in control subjects with those judged to die as a result of atheroma. Some 10 % of "control" males over 40 years of age have an equivalent degree of coronary disease to the 10th centile of the sudden ischaemic death males. This high proportion of subjects in the normal population seems too high to be explicable simply on competing causes of death. To paraphrase J.S. Tolkein there are "some that deserve death and are alive, some that deserve life and are dead" with regard to their coronary artery disease.

Amongst other attempts to define a more immediate morphological cause for death has been an analysis of the conduction system (1, 14); this well controlled study showed no obvious morphological basis for death.

Non-occlusive mural thrombi in coronary vessels have been found to be more common in sudden ischaemic deaths and suggested as a possible source of micro-emboli (42). Platelet thrombi in small vessels within the myocardium are also described as more common (43). These findings suggest that an increasing thrombotic tendency in patients with coronary atherosclerosis may precede death but more controlled data is needed.

A very small minority of ischaemic cardiac deaths are due to non-atherosclerotic arterial disease. Anomalous coronary artery anatomy is often entirely benign but on occasion causes death. The simplest anomaly of one orifice giving rise to both major arteries is not dangerous unless associated with other defects. If the main left coronary artery arises in the right sinus and passes behind the pulmonary trunk it may become obliterated leading to extensive collateral flow. Coronary arteries arising in the pulmonary trunk allow development of shunts from left to right and lead to myocardial ischaemia with sudden death (44).

Dissecting aneurysms confined to the coronary arteries occur both in Marfan's syndrome and spontaneously, particularly in pregnant women, leading to sudden death (45, 46, 47, 48). Coronary artery emboli, formerly most associated with bacterial endocarditis, are now a not uncommon cause of death as a complication arising from aortic prosthetic valves. Coronary ostial stenosis due to syphilitic aortitis (49) is a classic cause of sudden death but is now rare. Coronary arteritis may be a complication of generalised disease as in polyarteritis nodosa and nodal artery involvement is associated with sudden death (50, 51, 52). In young infants arteritis confined to the coronary arteries may cause sudden death from haemopericardium or myocardial necrosis (53).

2. NON-VASCULAR SUDDEN CARDIAC DEATH

A wide range of pathological conditions which can be recognised by simple macroscopic examination of the heart is associated with sudden death although the actual mechanism is not always clear. Left ventricular hypertrophy, particularly due to pressure overload as in severe aortic valve stenosis, may be complicated by, and even present as, sudden death. Cases seen in forensic practice are associated with total heart weights of over 550 gms, that is some 50 % increase in isolated left ventricular weight. This degree of left ventricular hypertrophy is associated with a high incidence of demonstrable myocardial necrosis due to a failure of subendocardial perfusion without significant pathology of the coronary arteries. In systemic hypertension similar degrees of left ventricular hypertrophy are often associated with a greater than average extent of coronary atherosclerosis.

Hypertrophic obstructive cardiomyopathy (HOCM) is a classic cause of sudden death both in symptomatic, clinically diagnosed cases and in asymptomatic previously fit individuals unaware of any cardiac disorder. Teare's original description of the disease originated from its frequency in forensic practice due to sudden death. The magnitude of risk

Table 4.

	Sudden death undiagnosed HOCM	Cardiac death non-sudden HOCM diagnosed/symptomatic	Death non-cardiac HOCM coincidental finding
Male	39	10	5
Female	7	6	6
	46	16	11
Heart weight	478 ± 136	526 ± 123	470 ± 95
s/p ratio	1.8 (1.4–2.6)	1.9 (1,6–2.3)	2.2 (1.7–2.3)

of sudden death for individuals known to have HOCM and clinically symptomatic is variable but perhaps the most reasonable estimate is that of a multicentre study where 26 in 190 patients died suddenly over five years (54). The actual mechanism still seems controversial and uncertain. Our own study (Table 4) of previously undiagnosed HOCM compared with known cases where death was due to other causes such as coincidental malignancy, post-operative, or from cardiac failure does not reveal any difference in septal/posterior wall ratio, in total or isolated ventricular weights or in the presence of a plaque of endocardial thickening on the septum opposite the anterior cusp of the mitral valve indicating left ventricular outflow obstruction. This experience is identical to that of Maron and his colleagues (55). In our experience there is a striking male preponderance in the group dying suddenly. A tendency for sudden death to run in some families with HOCM and not in others is also described (56). The failure of morphological data to separate those cases of undiagnosed HOCM dying suddenly from diagnosed cases who do not may be nothing more than selection since pathologists use the septal asymmetry as the key to diagnosis and may not recognise HOCM in its absence. The level of pathological autopsy diagnosis of HOCM in previously fit subjects dying suddenly remains erratic. Over 15 years we have received numerous examples of HOCM as "mysterious" sudden deaths unrecognised by the pathologist and the entity is still described as idiopathic cardiomegaly or attributed to unrecognised hypertension.

The relation between the floppy mitral valve and sudden death continues to cause controversy. A small proportion of patients with mitral valve prolapse due to floppy valves appear to have episodic ventricular ectopic beats and may die suddenly (57, 58, 59, and 60). Numerous theories have been advanced to explain the association but few have any possibility of confirmation by morphology in the dead heart. Pathological studies show the floppy valve to be remarkably frequent in autopsy surveys occurring in up to 5 % of individuals over 65 years of age (61). Echocardiographic surveys are not in gross disagreement with this figure, if it is assumed that the majority of patients with mitral prolapse have floppy mitral valves. In view of this frequency the actual risk of sudden death to any individual with mitral prolapse must be infinitesimally small.

Pathological studies in forensic practice do produce occasional cases of sudden death where the only abnormality is a floppy mitral valve, without ruptured chordae, with no significant coronary atherosclerosis and no abnormality of morphology in the left ventricle. Three cases seen personally in whom electrocardiograms were available all showed infero-lateral T wave inversion, in accord with previous work (62), suggesting that this appearance delineates those patients with floppy valves at risk from arrhythmia.

3. SUDDEN CARDIAC DEATH WITH A MACROSCOPICALLY NORMAL HEART WITHOUT CORONARY ARTERY DISEASE

Hearts falling in this third group often provide practical problems for the forensic pathologist under pressure to provide an instant cause of death. There is a distressing, if understandable, tendency to "find" some degree of atherosclerosis in the coronary arteries. The practice in Japan of applying the eponym "Pokkuri Disease" (63) is desirable and allows quantitation of the frequency of the problem. The term "spontaneous cardiac arrhythmia" would be applicable in the United Kingdom but is unpopular in many Coroners' courts.

The practical approach by the pathologist is first to exclude a diffuse myocardial disease such as myocarditis and then to consider primary disorders of rhythm or conduction.

All forms of myocarditis are complicated by a wide spectrum of atrial and ventricular arrhythmias and conduction defects. It is therefore not surprising that sudden death is a feature. The commonest form, usually known as non-specific acute myocarditis, is charac-terised by varying degrees of myofibre necrosis with a florid interstitial pleomorphic in-flammatory cell infiltrate. Since Coxsackie virus is known to produce this picture in ex-perimental animals as well as in man most cases are assumed to be viral although actual proof is often lacking. Studies of the conduction system show heavy involvement, especially of the bundle branches (64). A particularly florid myocarditis is characterised by serpigenous areas of necrosis around which giant cells of myogenic origin are found. This form of myo-carditis is rapidly fatal and cases are frequently encountered in forensic practice with a total history of only a few hours. The aetiological agent is unknown but evidence of organ specific autoimmune disease and an occasional association with thymic tumours are known (65). Sarcoidosis is easily recognised histologically and does occasionally cause sud-den death from involvement of the conduction system with minimal involvement of other organs (66, 96). Non-specific myocarditis virtually confined to the Purkinje fibres of the ventricle (67) or the AV node is described (68).

Where the heart appears normal macroscopically and myocardial disease has been excluded, histologically primary disease of rhythm and conduction should be considered. Sudden death is associated with a number of characteristic, often familial, electrocardio-graphic abnormalities; in some the conduction system is morphologically normal in others not.

A long QT interval is inherited as an autosomal dominant or recessive when associated with auditory nerve deafness (69, 70, 71, 72). The risk of sudden death is significant; a typical family study (73) showed six cases in 14 members from three generations in one family; of the six cases three have died suddenly. Detailed examination of the conduction system has not revealed a specific morphological abnormality other than reports of changes in small arteries (74). Electron dense granules within the mitochondria of myocardial cells are reported (73) which may suggest a basic biochemical defect in cell membranes.

The pre-excitation syndromes can now be regarded with certainty as due to accessory extra-conduction pathways. Providing meticulous techniques are used and the whole of both AV rings and the septum are sectioned excellent correlation between morphology and electrophysiological function is obtained (75, 76). In the AV rings the accessory conduction paths probably represent persistent remnants of embryonic ring tissue from the central portion of which the normal conduction system forms.

Familial and congenital defects of conduction fall into two groups. In the first the abnormality is simply a gap in the conduction system and there is no progression of the conduction abnormality as seen in electrocardiograms. Examples are congenital AV block either due to absence of the atrial portion of the AV node, or of the penetrating main bundle and congenital right bundle branch block due to absence of the first segment of the right bundle branch (77, 78). It is now recognised that an undue proportion of such defects occur in the infants of mothers with systemic lupus erythematosus (79). Sudden death is not a common complication of congenital AV block in which the prognosis is remarkably benign but syncopal attacks may begin in middle age (80).

Bundle branch or AV block may, however, also reflect a familial increasing loss of conduction fibres in which the electrocardiogram changes progressively, culminating in complete AV block with syncope and appreciable risk of sudden death (81, 82, 83). One family in whom three members died suddenly had bizarre vacuolated conduction fibres (84). In a family with 78 members, ten died suddenly and hypoplasia and atrophy of the main AV bundle were found (83).

Destruction of the conduction system by a wide range of acquired pathological processes may also progress to AV block and result in sudden death. Mesotheliomas of the AV node, microscopic cystic masses seldom over 0.5 cm. in diameter, are strategically placed to destroy the AV node. The "tumour" is most likely to be derived from mesothelial cell nests carried in from the posterior wall of the heart with the developing AV node in the foetus. Numerous case reports record sudden death as a common presenting feature of this tumour (85, 86, 87, 88).

The main bifurcating bundle of His runs on the crest of the muscular interventricular septum and is vulnerable to haemodynamic stresses in aneurysms of the membranous septum (89), to extension of calcium from aortic or mitral valves (90) and extension of aortic root inflammation as in bacterial endocarditis (91) or to the aortitis of ankylosing spondylitis (92, 93); in all such cases sudden death may be an occasional complication.

The entity of bilateral bundle branch fibrosis, whether of the Lenegre type or Lev type, will produce right bundle branch block and left axis deviation as part of the progression to ultimate AV block. In this earlier stage there is a small but appreciable risk of sudden death (94, 95).

To the pathologist, examination of the conduction system in cases of sudden death where the heart looks normal on macroscopic examination is seldom conclusive unless electrocardiograms are available as part of the investigation of earlier syncope or palpitations. Our experience over 15 years is shown in Tables 5 and 6. None of the patients were over 50 years

Table 5. 24 patients without macroscopic abnormality of the heart or vessels – previous ECG data obtained. All under 50 years of age.

ECG Abnormality	No.	Conduction System Morphology
Pre-excitation	6	Anomalous Pathways
Long QT Interval	1	Normal
Episodic Supraventricular Tachycardia	2	Normal
Multifocal Ventricular/Atrial Ectopics	2	Normal
Ventricular Ectopic Beats	7	Normal
A-V Block (Partial)	1	Mesothelioma A-V Node
Bundle Branch Block (Partial or Complete)	3	Fibrosis or Hypoplasia of Bundle Branches

Table 6. 34 patients dying suddenly – no EEG data available. No macroscopic cause apparent – myocardium normal. Ages 5–49.

Clinical Data	
Palpitations Alone	12
Palpitations and Syncopal or Fainting Attacks	4
Syncopal Attacks Alone	3
Family History of Sudden Death	3
No Complaints Known	11
Siblings with Long QT	1
	34
Conduction System Morphology	
Mesothelioma A-V Node	2
Anomalous Conduction Path (Mahaim Type)	10
Absent Right Branch	2
Hypoplasia Main Bundle/Branches	2
Fibrosis Bundle Branches	3
Normal	15
	34

of age at death; the youngest was five. In those patients with electrocardiograms perhaps the most difficult and interesting group are those with simple ventricular ectopic activity. The limits of morphology are however very plain from Tables 5 and 6. The three patients with partial bundle branch block may represent cases similar to those reported in families with sudden deaths (83).

Cases where no electrocardiographic data are available and only scanty clinical information was obtained have morphological findings in the conduction system equally difficult to interpret. The incidence of Mahaim type anomalous paths seems strikingly high but many of these cases were children where these paths are normally more common. In the absence of detailed electrophysiological study their relation to the death is only speculatory. In none of the 57 patients in either groups have changes been observed in small arteries.

REFERENCES

1. Lie JT, Titus JL: Pathology of the myocardium and the conduction system in sudden coronary death. Circulation 52 (suppl 3):41–52, 1975.
2. Friedman M, Manwaring JH, Rosenman RH, Donlon G, Ortego P, Grube SM: Instantaneous and sudden deaths – clinical and pathological differentiation in coronary artery disease: J Am Med Assoc 225:1319–1328, 1973.
3. Kuller LH, Perper JA: Myocardial infarction and sudden death in an urban community. Bull NY Acad Med 49:532–543, 1973.
4. Spain DM, Bradess VA: Sudden death from coronary heart disease. Survival time, frequency of thrombi and cigarette smoking. Dis Chest 58:107–110, 1970.
5. Titus JL, Oxman HA, Connolly DC, Nobrega FT: Sudden unexpected death as the initial manifestation of coronary heart disease. Clinical and pathological observations. Singapore Med J 14:291–293, 1973.
6. Perper JA, Kuller LH, Cooper M: Arteriosclerosis of coronary arteries in sudden unexpected deaths. Circulation 52 (suppl 3):27–33, 1975.
7. Haerem JW: Mural platelet microthrombi and major acute lesions of main epicardial arteries in sudden death. Atherosclerosis 19:529–541, 1974.
8. Myers A, Dewar HA: Circumstances attending 100 sudden deaths from coronary artery disease with coroner's necropsies. Br Heart J 37:1133–1143, 1975.
9. Mitchell JRA, Schwartz CJ: Arterial disease. Oxford, Blackwell, 1965.
10. Davies MJ, Popple A: In press. Histopathology, 1979.
11. Baba N, Bashe WJ, Keller MD, Geer JC, Anthony JR: Pathology of atherosclerotic heart disease in sudden death – organising thrombus and acute coronary vessel lesions. Circulation 52 (suppl 3):53–59, 1975.
12. Rissanen V, Romo M, Siltanen P: Pre-hospital sudden death from ischaemic heart disease – a post-mortem study. Br Heart J 40:1025–1033, 1978.
13. Scott RG, Briggs RS: Pathological findings in pre-hospital deaths due to coronary atherosclerosis. Am J Cardiol 29:782–787, 1972.
14. Liberthson RR, Nagel EL, Hirschman JC, Nussenfeld SR, Blackborne BD, Davies JH: Pathophysiologic observations in pre-hospital ventricular fibrillation and sudden cardiac death. Circulation 49:790–797, 1974.
15. Crawford T, Dexter D, Teare RD: Coronary artery pathology in sudden death from myocardial ischaemia. Lancet 1:181–185, 1961.
16. Hutchins GM, Bulkley BH, Ridolfi RL, Griffith LSC, Lohr FT, Piasio MA: Correlation of coronary arteriograms and left ventriculograms with post-mortem studies. Circulation 56:31–37, 1977.
17. Schwartz CJ, Lovell RH, Oliver MF, Paul O: Methodological considerations for the study of sudden cardiac death. An autopsy protocol. Circulation 52 (suppl 3): 78–95, 1975.
18. Jackrel J, Miller JA, Schechter FG, Minkowitz S, Stuckey JH: Atrioventricular conduction following ligation of the anterior septal artery in the dog. An electrocardiographic, histopathologic and histochemical study. Am J Cardiol 25:552–561, 1970.
19. James TN: Pathogenesis of arrhythmias in acute myocardial infarction. Am J Cardiol 24:791–799, 1969.
20. Plotz M: Coronary heart disease. London, Cassell, 1957.
21. Davies MJ, Woolf N, Robertson WB: Pathology of acute myocardial infarction with particular reference to occlusive coronary thrombi. Br Heart J 38:659–664, 1976.
22. Bashe WJ Jr, Baba N, Keller MD, Geer JC, Anthony JR: Pathology of atherosclerotic heart disease in sudden death II. The significance of myocardial infarction. Circulation 52 (suppl 3):63–77, 1975.
23. Sutton RS, Davies MJ: The conduction system in acute myocardial infarction associated with heart block. Circulation 38:987–992, 1968.
24. Becker AE, Lie KI, Anderson RH: Bundle branch block in the setting of acute anteroseptal myocardial infarction – clinicopathological correlation. Br Heart J 40,773–783, 1978.
25. Ferris JA: The pathology of fatal dysrhythmias – a Canadian Approach. Forensic Sci 8:23–28. 1976.
26. Baum RS, Alvarez H, Cobb LA: Survival after resuscitation from out of hospital ventricular fibrillation. Circulation 50:1231–1235, 1974.
27. Schaffer WA, Cobb LA: Recurrent ventricular fibrillation and modes of death in survivors of out-of-hospital ventricular fibrillation. New Engl J Med 293:259–262, 1975.
28. Bleifer SB, Bleifer DJ, Hansmann DR, Sheppard JJ, Karpman HL: Diagnosis of occult arrhythmias by Holter electrocardiography. Prog Cardiovasc Dis 16:569–599, 1974.
29. Gradman AH, Bell PA, Debusk RF: Sudden death during ambulatory monitoring; clinical and electro-

cardiographic correlations. Report of a case. Circulation 55:210–221, 1977.

30. Pool J, Kunst K, Vanwermeskerken JL: Two monitored cases of sudden death outside hospital. Br Heart J 40:627–629, 1978.

31. Jestaedt R, Sandritter W: Erfahrungen mit der TTC (triphenyltetrazolium-chlorid). Reaktion für die pathologisch-anatomische Diagnose des frischern Herzinfarktes. Zeitschrift für Kreislaufforschung 48:802–809, 1959.

32. Lie JT, Pairolero PC, Holley KE, Titus JL: Macroscopic enzyme mapping verification of large homogenous experimental myocardial infarcts of predictable size and location in dogs. J Thorac Cardiovasc Surg 69:599–605, 1975.

33. Anderson JA, Hansen BF: The value of the nitro BT method in fresh myocardial infarction. Frequency and location of fresh myocardial infarction in a consecutive series of autopsies. Am Heart J 85:611–619, 1973.

34. Anderson KR, Popple A, Parker DJ, Sayer R, Trickey RJ, Davies MJ: An experimental assessment of the macroscopic enzyme techniques for the autopsy demonstration of myocardial infarction. J Path 1979 (in press).

35. Reichenbach DD, Moss NS: Myocardial necrosis and sudden death in humans. Circulation 52 (suppl 3): 60–62, 1975.

36. Davies MJ, Fulton WFM, Robertson WB: The relation of coronary thrombosis to ischaemic myocardial necrosis. J Path 127:99–110, 1979.

37. Lie JT, Holley KE, Kamoa WR, Titus JL: New histochemical method for morphological diagnosis of early stages of myocardial ischaemia. Mayo Clinic Proc 46:319–327, 1971.

38. Nayar A, Olsen EGJ: The use of basic fuchsin stain in the recognition of early myocardial ischaemia. Cardiovasc Res 8:391–394, 1974.

39. Bouchardy B, Majno G: Histopathology of early myocardial infarcts: A new approach. Am J Path 74:301–317, 1974.

40. Reichenbach DD, Moss NS, Myer E: Pathology of the heart in sudden death. Am J Cardiol 39:865–872, 1977.

41. Lie JT: Histopathology of the conduction system in sudden death from coronary heart disease. Circulation 51:446–452, 1975.

42. Frink RJ, Trowbridge JO, Rooney PA: Non-obstructive coronary thrombosis in sudden cardiac death. Am J Cardiol 42:48–52, 1978.

43. Haerem JW: Platelet aggregates in intramyocardial vessels of patients dying suddenly and unexpectedly of coronary artery disease. Atherosclerosis 15:199–213, 1972.

44. Ogden JA: Congenital anomalies of the coronary arteries. Am J Cardiol 25:474–479, 1970.

45. Claudon DG, Claudon DB, Edwards JE: Primary dissecting aneurysm of coronary artery – a cause of myocardial ischaemia, Circulation 45:259–266, 1972.

46. Palomino SJ: Dissecting intramural hematoma of left coronary artery in the puerperium: A case report and survey of the literature. Am J Clin Path 51:119–125, 1969.

47. Shaver PJ, Carrig TF, Baker WP: Post partum coronary artery dissection. Br Heart J 40:83–86, 1978.

48. Guthrie W, Maclean H: Dissecting aneurysms of arteries other than the aorta. J Path 108:219–235, 1972.

49. Heggveit HA: Syphilitic aortitis – a clinicopathological autopsy of 100 cases. Circulation 29:346–355, 1964.

50. Holsinger DR, Osmundson PU, Edwards JE: The heart in polyarteritis nodosa. Circulation 25:610–618, 1962.

51. James TN, Birk RE: Pathology of cardiac conduction system in polyarteritis nodosa. Arch Intern Med 117: 561–567, 1966.

52. Thiene G, Valente M, Rossi L: Involvement of the cardiac conduction system in panarteritis nodosa. Am Heart J 95:716–724, 1978.

53. Kegal SM, Dorsey TJ, Towen M, Taylor WF: Cardiac death in mucocutaneous lymph node syndrome. Am J Cardiol 40:282–286, 1977.

54. Goodwin JF, Krikler DM: Sudden death in cardiomyopathy. Adv Cardiol 25:98–106, 1978.

55. Maron BJ, Roberts WC, Edwards JE, McAllister HA Jr, Foley DD, Epstein SE: Sudden death in patients with hypertrophic cardiomyopathy: characterisation of 26 patients without functional limitation. Am J Cardiol 41:803–810, 1978.

56. Maron BJ, Lipson LC, Roberts EC, Savage DD, Epstein SE: Malignant hypertrophic cardiomyopathy: identification of a sub-group of families with unusually frequent premature death. Am J Cardiol 41:1133–1140, 1978.

57. Barlow JB, Bosman CK, Pocock WA, Marchand P: Late systolic murmurs and non-ejection (mid-late) systolic clicks. Analysis of 90 patients. Br Heart J 30:203–218, 1968.

58. Marshall CE, Shappell SD: Sudden death and the ballooning posterior leaflet syndrome. Detailed anatomic and histochemical investigation. Archs Path 98:134–138, 1974.

59. Jeresaty RM: Sudden death in the mitral valve prolapse – click syndrome. Am J Cardiol 37:317–318, 1976.

60. Leichtman D, Nelson R, Gobel FL, Alexander CS, Cohn JN: Bradycardia with mitral valve prolapse, a potential mechanism of sudden death. Ann Intern Med 35:453–457, 1976.

61. Davies MJ, Moore BP, Braimbridge MV: The floppy mitral valve – a study of incidence pathology and complications in surgical necropsy and forensic material. Br Heart J 40:468–482, 1978.

62. Campbell RWF, Godman MG, Fiddler GI, Marquis RM, Julian DG: Ventricular arrhythmias in syndrome of balloon deformity of mitral valve. Definition of possible high risk group. Br Heart J. 38:1053–1057, 1976.

63. Gotoh K: A histopathological study on the conduction system of the so-called 'Pokkuri disease' (sudden unexpected cardiac death of unknown origin in Japan). Jap Circ J 40:753–768, 1976.

64. Morales AR, Adelman S, Fine G: Vancella myocarditis – a case of sudden death. Archs Path 91:29–31, 1971.

65. Davies MJ, Pomerance A, Teare RD: Idiopathic giant cell myocarditis – a distinctive clinicopathological entity. Br Heart J 37:192–196, 1975.

66. Morales AR, Levy S, Davies J, Fine G: Sarcoidosis of the heart. Pathology Annual. Edited by Sheldon C Sommers. Appleton-Century Crofts, 1974.

67. Sevy S, Kelly J, Ernst H: Fatal paroxysmal tachycardia associated with focal myocarditis of the Purkinje system in a 14 month child. J Pediat 27:796–800, 1968.

68. Robboy SJ: Atrioventricular node inflammation – mechanism of sudden death in protracted meningococemia. New Engl J Med 286:1091–1093, 1972.

69. Fraser GR, Froggatt P, James TN: Congenital deafness associated with ECG abnormalities, fainting attacks and sudden death. A recessive condition. Q Jl Med 33:361–384, 1964.

70. Johansson BW, Jorming B: Hereditary prolongation of the QT interval. Br Heart J 34:744–751, 1972.

71. Cascos AS, Sanchez-Harguindey L, Derabago P: Cardio-auditory syndromes. Br Heart J 31:26–33, 1969.

72. Phillips H, Ichinose H: Clinical and pathologic studies in the hereditary syndrome of a long QT interval, syncopal spells and sudden death. Chest 58:236–243, 1970.

73. Moothart RW, Pryor R, Hawley RL, Clifford NJ, Blount SG Jr: The heritable syndrome of prolonged QT interval, syncope, sudden death. Electron microscope observation. Chest 70:623–626, 1976.

74. James TN: Small arteries of the heart. Circulation 56: 2–14, 1977.

75. Becker AE, Anderson RH, Durrer D, Wellens HJ: The anatomic substrates of the Wolf-Parkinson-White syndrome. A clinicopathological correlation in seven patients. Circulation 57:870–879, 1978.

76. Durrer D, Wellens HJ: The Wolf-Parkinson-White syndrome anno 1973. Euro J Cardiol 1:347–367, 1974.

77. Anderson RH, Arnold CG, Wenick MD, Losekoot TG, Becker AE: Congenitally complete heart block. Circulation 56:90–101, 1977.

78. Esscher E, Hardell LI, Michaelsson M: Familial isolated complete right bundle branch block. Br Heart J 37: 745–748, 1975.

79. McCue CM, Mantakas ME, Tingelstad JB, Ruddy S: Congenital heart block in newborns of mothers with connective tissue disease. Circulation 56: 82–90, 1977.

80. Campbell M, Emmanuel R: Six cases of congenital block followed for 34–40 years. Br Heart J 29:577–587, 1967.

81. Simonsen EE, Madesen EG: Four cases of right sided bundle branch block and one case of atrioventricular block in three generations of a family. Br Heart J 32:501–504, 1970.

82. Gazes PC, Culler R, Taber E, Kelly RE: Congenital familial cardiac conduction defects. Circulation 32: 32–35, 1965.

83. Lynch HT, Mohiuddin S, Moran J, Kaplan A, Sketch M, Zencka A, Runco V: Hereditary progressive atrioventricular conduction defect. Am J Cardiol 36:297–301, 1975.

84. Gault JH, Cantwell J, Lev M, Braunwald E: Fatal familial cardiac arrhythmias. Histologic observations on the cardiac conduction system. Am J Cardiol 29:548–553, 1972.

85. Hopkinson JM, Newcombe CP: Heart block due to epithelial heterotopia. J Path 104:218–220, 1971.

86. James TN, Galakhov I: Fatal electric instability of the heart associated with benign congenital polycystic tumour of the atrioventricular node. Circulation 56:667–678, 1977.

87. Bharati S, Bicoff JP: Sudden death caused by benign tumour of the atrioventricular node. Arch Intern Med 136: 244–248, 1976.

88. Sophir IM, Spitz WU: Endodermal inclusions of the heart; so-called mesotheliomas of the atrioventricular node. Arch Path 92:180–186, 1971.

89. Thery C, Lekieffre J, Dupuis C: Atrioventricular block secondary to a congenital aneurysm of the membranous septum. Histological examination of conduction system. Br Heart J 37:1097–1101, 1975.

90. Rytand DA, Lipsitch LS: Clinical aspects of calcification of mitral annulus. Arch Intern Med 78: 544–564, 1946.

91. Demoulin JC, Boniver J, Casters P, Nicolas R, Kulbertus HE: Complete heart block in bacterial endocarditis. Acta Cardiol 30:59–66, 1975.
92. Cosh JA, Barritt DW, Jayson MI: Cardiac lesions of Reiters syndrome and ankylosing spondylitis. Br Heart J 35:553, 1973.
93. Harvey DB, Hollenberg M, Kunkel F, Scheinman MM: Ankylosing spondylitis with complete heart block. Arch Intern Med 136:1046–1050, 1976.
94. Denes P, Dhingra RC, Wu D, Wyndham CR, Amat-y-Leon F, Rosen KM: Sudden death in patients with chronic bifascicular block. Arch Intern Med 173: 1005–1010, 1977.
95. Mac Anulty JH, Rahimtoola SH, Murphy ES, Kaufman S, Ritzmann LW, Kanarek P, De Mots H: A prospective study of sudden death in high risk bundle branch block. New Engl J Med 299:209–215, 1978.
96. Lie JT, Hunt D, Valentine, PA: Sudden death from cardiac sarcoidosis with involvement of conduction system. Am J Med Sci 267:123–128, 1974.

1.4. NEURAL PATHOLOGY OF THE HEART IN SUDDEN DEATH

Th. N. JAMES

When sudden death occurs unexpectedly and cannot be explained by usual findings or circumstances, most now believe that the terminal event was a lethal disturbance of the electrical activity of the heart. By contrast to occasionally fatal instability, there is normally a remarkable stability of cardiac rhythm and conduction which is marvelously durable under a continuing barrage of changes in demand on the work of the heart. Many different factors contribute to this durable stability. Familiar ones include changes in the contractile property of myocardium and in the pattern of coronary flow. It is not generally appreciated how important autonomic neural control is to almost every facet of this stable performance, including not only cardiac contraction and coronary flow, but also every component of the heart's electrophysiological function. Nerves influence the rate at which the heart beats, the nature of its rhythm, the speed and route by which it conducts its electrical impulse, and the process by which both the atrial and ventricular myocardium becomes repolarized.

Distortions of the neural control of the heart may be either transient, prolonged or permanent. Depending on other circumstances existing at the time (e.g., acute myocardial ischemia or other anatomical or functional abnormalities of the conduction system), even brief periods of abnormal neural influence can be serious and sometimes fatal. Sudden acceleration or sudden slowing of heart rate, or temporary impairment of AV (atrioventricular) conduction can each or all be direct consequences of variations in neural control of the heart.

There are at least two reasons why those interested in cardiac structure have generally paid so little attention to the matter of neural control of cardiac electrical stability. First, abnormal neural function may be transient and unassociated with any presently detectable abnormalities in structure. Second, there has been relatively little interest in either normal or abnormal neuroanatomy of the heart as it may relate to cardiac rhythm or conduction. One notable exception to this usual lack of anatomical interest has been the pioneering work of Lino Rossi, who has for some time maintained that a variety of diseases do involve the nerves of the heart and that this is functionally important (1).

In this presentation I wish to review some personal experience with examination of the cardiac conduction system and its neural elements in a variety of examples of sudden unexpected death not explained by careful usual necropsy examinations. Almost by definition of the work (study of sudden unexpected death), one is confronted with little if any useful clinical information except observation of the terminal event. Occasionally, victims of such death have had one or more warning episodes of syncope, and even more rarely, some of them were investigated for possible cardiac causes. But in the majority, retrospective conjecture is all that is possible concerning what the form of cardiac electrical instability may have been. Such conjecture can at least provide working hypotheses, and for that purpose we are fortunate in having an abundance of experimental electrophysiological observations as well as clinical studies in patients who have various forms of documented arrhythmia or heart block. Many aspects of such research are being presented by other participants in this symposium.

1. NORMAL ANATOMY OF THE NEURAL STRUCTURES OF THE HEART

Both vagal and sympathetic nerves fill the heart, but their finer distribution is difficult to define even with histochemical methods such as cholinesterase stains or fluorescent properties. From physiological studies there are some general considerations of fundamental importance which must be held in mind with any anatomical discussions. For example, vagal influence on both mechanical and electrical properties of the atria is much more profound than is vagal influence on the ventricles. There have been some sophisticated demonstrations of various changes in ventricular properties caused by vagal influence, but these pale in comparison with what is easily and dramatically demonstrable for the atria. On the other hand, sympathetic neural influence on the ventricles is readily and unequivocally demonstrable, as it is for the atria. Sympathetic neural influence on the ventricles includes not only the stimulation of ventricular contractility but also modulation of the speed and pattern of ventricular repolarization (2, 3), whereas the vagi are more important in modulating atrial repolarization (4).

In addition to cholinergic and adrenergic nerves, there are many ganglia in the heart (5). Again based in part on findings from physiological studies, it is unlikely that any significant numbers of sympathetic ganglia are located in the heart. Virtually all cardiac ganglia are vagal. Cardiac sympathetic nerves are postganglionic and their parent ganglia are long distances (anatomically speaking) from the heart. There may be some autonomic reflex arcs with both afferent and efferent limbs entirely contained within the heart itself. If so, these are probably cholinergic or vagal in nature, but their existence presently remains debatable. There are, incidentally, almost no ganglia below the level of the atrioventricular sulci. Ganglia are particularly abundant in the region between coronary sinus and posterior margin of AV node, at the posterior margin of the sinus node and along its caval margin, less numerous at the anterior margin of the sinus node, are scattered in the upper portion of the interatrial septum, and are prominently seen near the origin of both coronary arteries. There are also many ganglia in the connective tissue lying between the aorta and pulmonary artery. Between the origins of the aorta and pulmonary artery there is an interesting cluster of chemoreceptor tissue which receives its blood supply from the main left coronary artery (6–8). These chemoreceptors are histologically similar to carotid body.

What may be plausibly summarized is that both vagal and sympathetic nerves innervate and control the atria, that sympathetic nerves certainly have profound influence on the ventricles, and that virtually all cardiac ganglia are vagal. Some chemoreceptors of the heart receive their blood supply from the left coronary artery.

2. SECONDARY INVOLVEMENT OF CARDIONEURAL STRUCTURES, INCLUDING APOPLEXY OF THE HEART

There is no form of vascular accident to the brain which does not have its explicit counterpart within the heart (9). This includes focal hemorrhage with ischemic degeneration from coronary occlusion or from coronary embolism. The sinus node and the AV node are control centers of cardiac electrical activity analogous to various control centers in the brain, and they are similarly vulnerable to the entire panorama of vascular accidents. Along with the myocardial cells responsible for automaticity and conduction, their neighboring nerves are afflicted by the same disease processes. The sudden heart block which is often observed in acute posterior myocardial infarction may be either transient or sustained. When it is a more prolonged and sometimes fatal complication, the focal hemorrhagic degeneration includes abundant neural elements in the vicinity of the AV node (9, 10).

Other diseases which may damage both the myocardial cells and their accompanying nerves in the sinus node and AV node, leading to various forms of cardiac electrical instability, include lupus erythematosus (Figure 1) (11), polyarteritis nodosa (12), amyloidosis (13), thrombotic thrombocytopenic purpura (14), congenital homocystinuria (15), and several heritable neuromuscular and musculoskeletal disorders (16, 17, 18). It may be anticipated

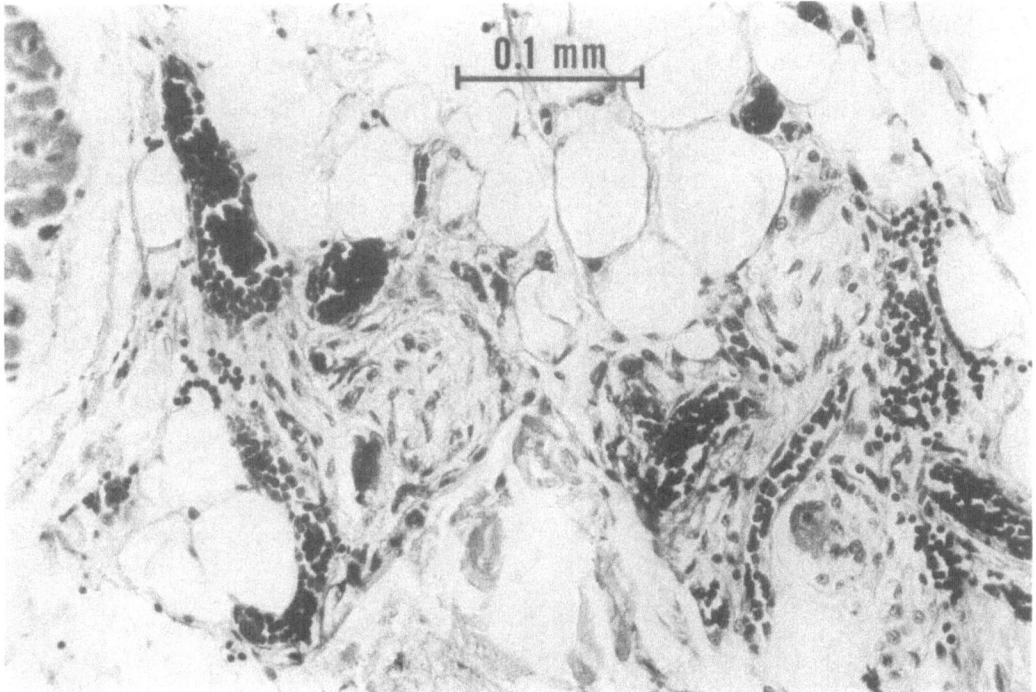

Figure 1. Congested nerves and ganglia in this photomicrograph are from near the AV node of a patient dying with arrhythmias due to disseminated lupus erythematosus. Magnification here and in subsequent photomicrographs is indicated with a reference bar. Goldner trichrome stain, here and in all subsequent photomicrographs.

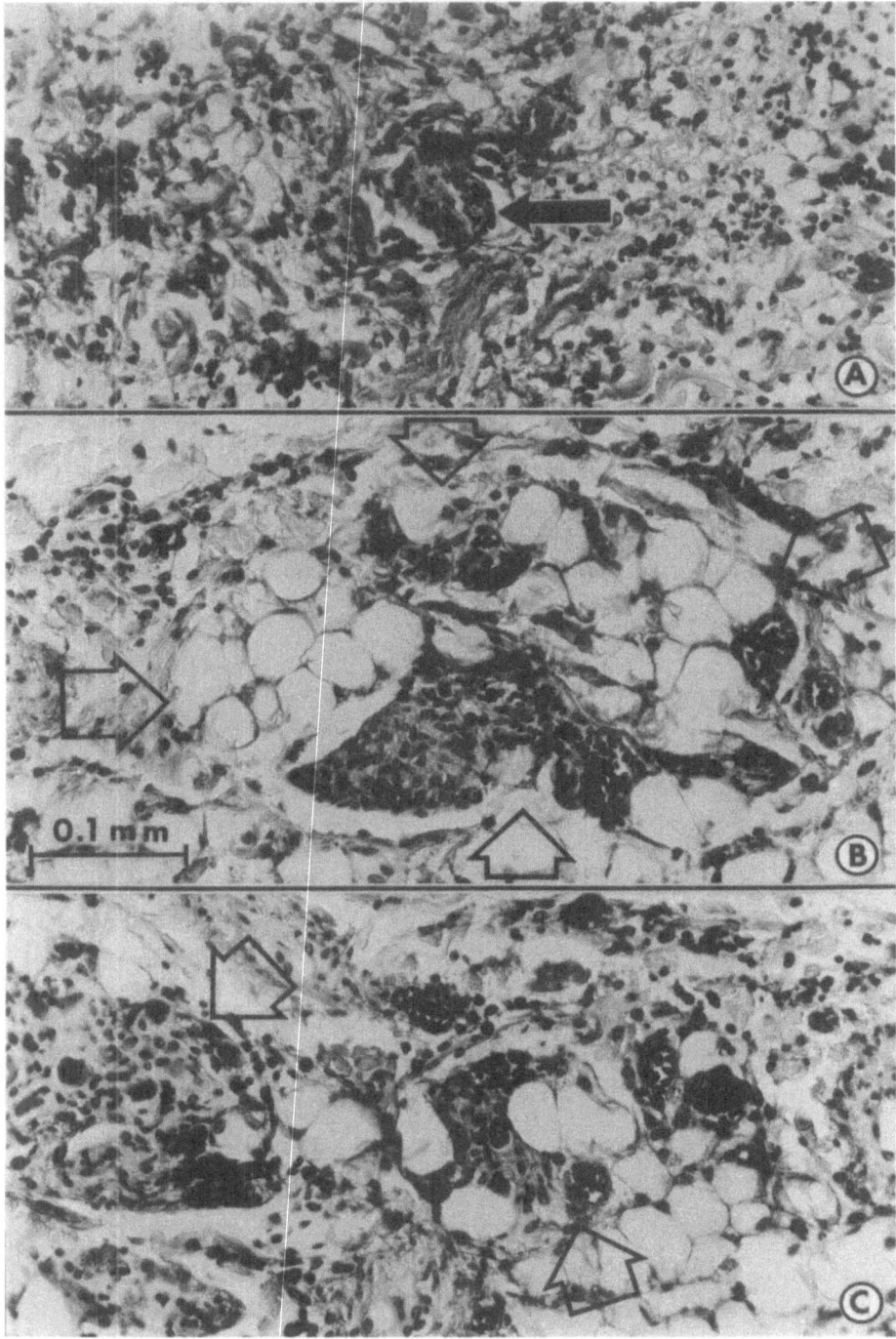

Figure 2. These three photomicrographs are from the heart of a child dying with arrhythmias and heart block due to diphtheritic myocarditis; details of the case have been reported previously (19). Neural abnormalities shown here include degenerative and vesicular neuritis (arrow in *A*, area with four arrows in *B*) and two ganglia with degenerating neurons (arrows in *C*).

that neural lesions within the heart may be especially numerous or severe in patients with the latter groups of diseases, and when sought, they are easily demonstrable. There are, furthermore, some diseases known to have a special affinity for nerves and ganglia, such as diphtheria (Figure 2). While the neural damage associated with diphtheria has been studied in many different parts of the body, the extent of diphtheritic damage to cardioneural structures has received less attention but is extensive (19, 20).

3. PRIMARY DISEASES OF NERVES AND GANGLIA WITHIN THE HEART

There is increasing evidence that nerves and ganglia of the heart may be the specific target of some diseases, and that this rather selective neuropathology can be an important contribution to the pathogenesis of some examples of cardiac electrical instability and of sudden unexpected death (21). Disease involving the nerves and ganglia of the heart is focal in nature with some neural elements appearing to be spared. It is this focal or erratic and asymmetrical involvement which may be especially important in causing electrophysiological abnormalities and instability. For example, the transplanted heart appears to function reasonably well under most circumstances (there are some important exceptions), but in transplantation the neural ablation is of necessity complete and leaves no asymmetry or inhomogeneity of neural influence.

Inhomogeneity of sympathetic neural influence on the ventricular myocardium can lead to serious abnormalities of repolarization (2, 3). In pharmacological experiments, certain simple aliphatic aldehydes have powerful sympathomimetic actions while other very closely related compounds specifically prolong ventricular repolarization (22, 23). Both in the pharmacological experiments (22, 23) and in human examples of asymmetrical sympathetic neural influence on the ventricular myocardium (21), there is marked QT prolongation, increased ventricular vulnerability, and the easy production of dangerous ventricular arrhythmias.

One naturally occurring clinical expression of this type of increased ventricular vulnerability was first recognized in congenitally deaf children (24, 25) but is now known to occur even more often in individuals with normal hearing (26–28). The grotesque prolongation of the QT interval in electrocardiograms of such patients is unmistakable. Similar QT abnormalities can be produced in dogs by rendering ventricular sympathetic neural control asymmetrical (2, 3). There have now been several clinical examples of "normalizing" the long QT interval and terminating recurring syncopal attacks by unilateral (usually left) stellate ganglionectomy (29–31). A logical interpretation would be that some extracardiac abnormality led to unbalanced sympathetic neural influence and prolonged the ventricular vulnerability. However, in a recent investigation of the hearts from eight individuals who had died suddenly and were known to have the prolonged QT syndrome (three were deaf and five heard normally, none being from the same family), there was impressive inflammatory degeneration of nerves and ganglia within each heart (21) (Figures 3–8).

Along with the QT prolongation indicative of abnormal ventricular repolarization, another frequent clinical finding in such patients is sinus bradycardia (25). This is particular-

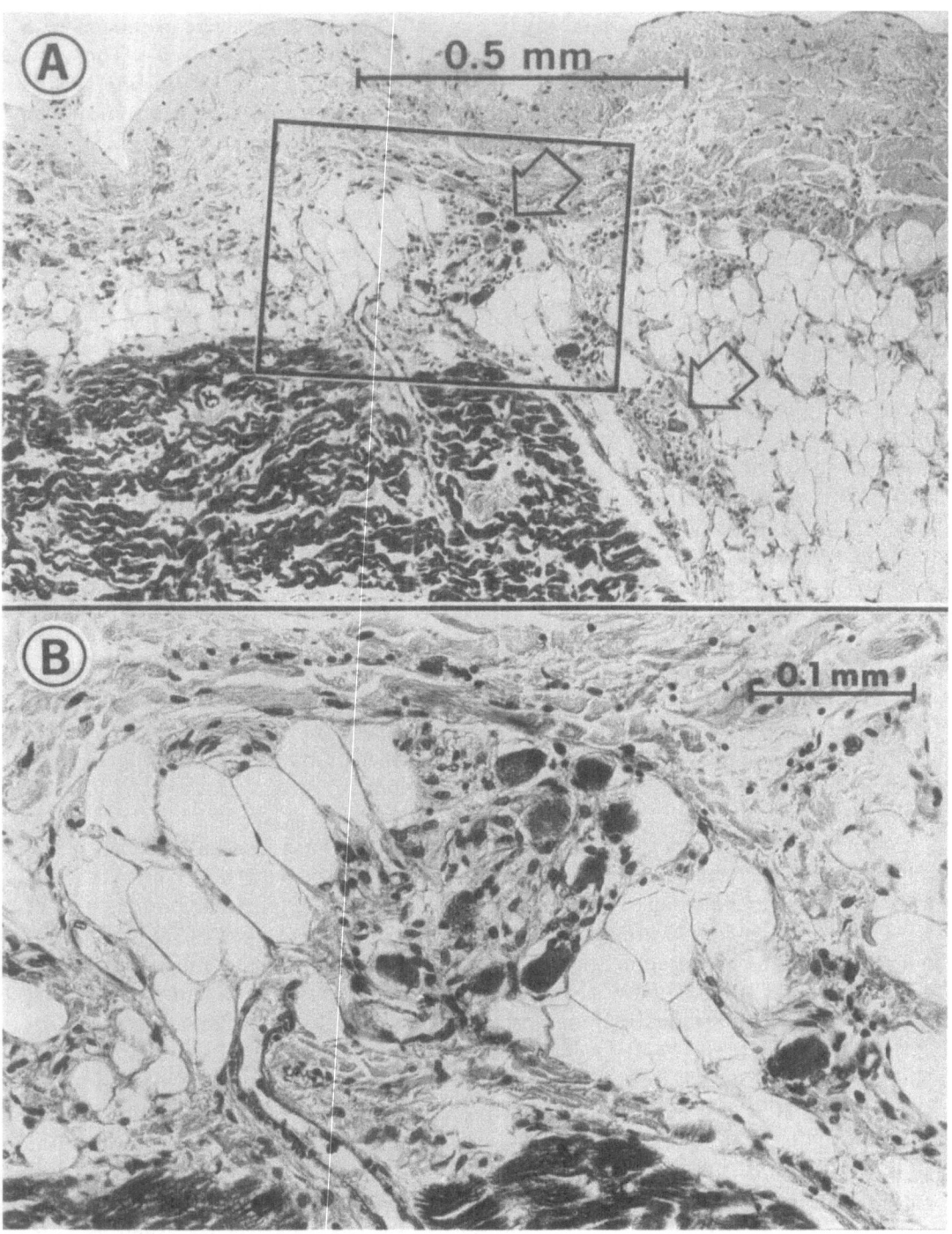

Figure 3. Inflammatory degeneration of a ganglion (two arrows in *A*) near the sinus node is shown here from the heart of one patient dying with the long QT syndrome (normal hearing). Boxed area in *A* is seen at higher magnification in *B*.

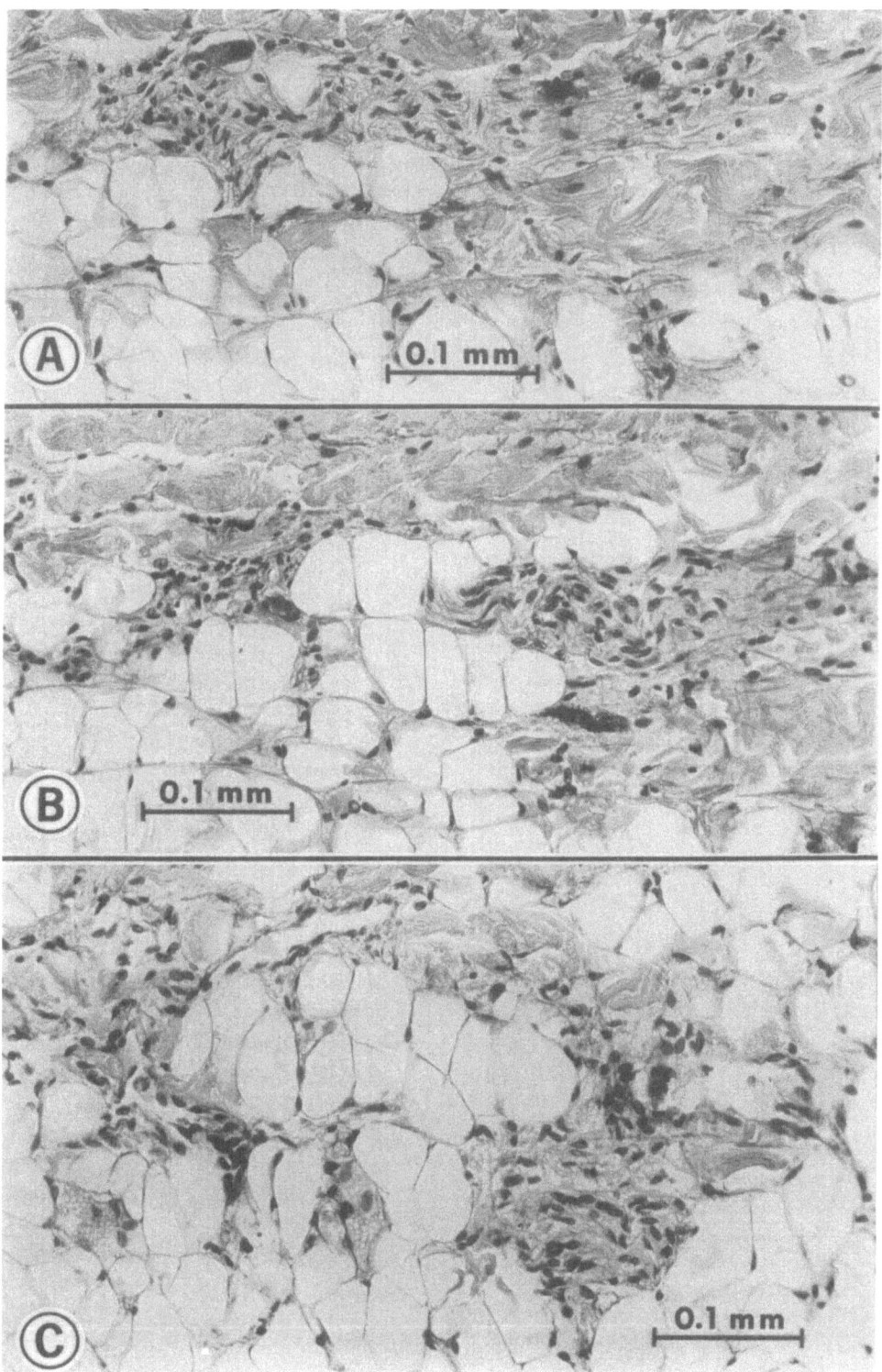

Figure 4. Vesicular degeneration of nerves and ganglia near the sinus node is shown here from the heart of a second patient dying with the long QT syndrome. Patient was not deaf.

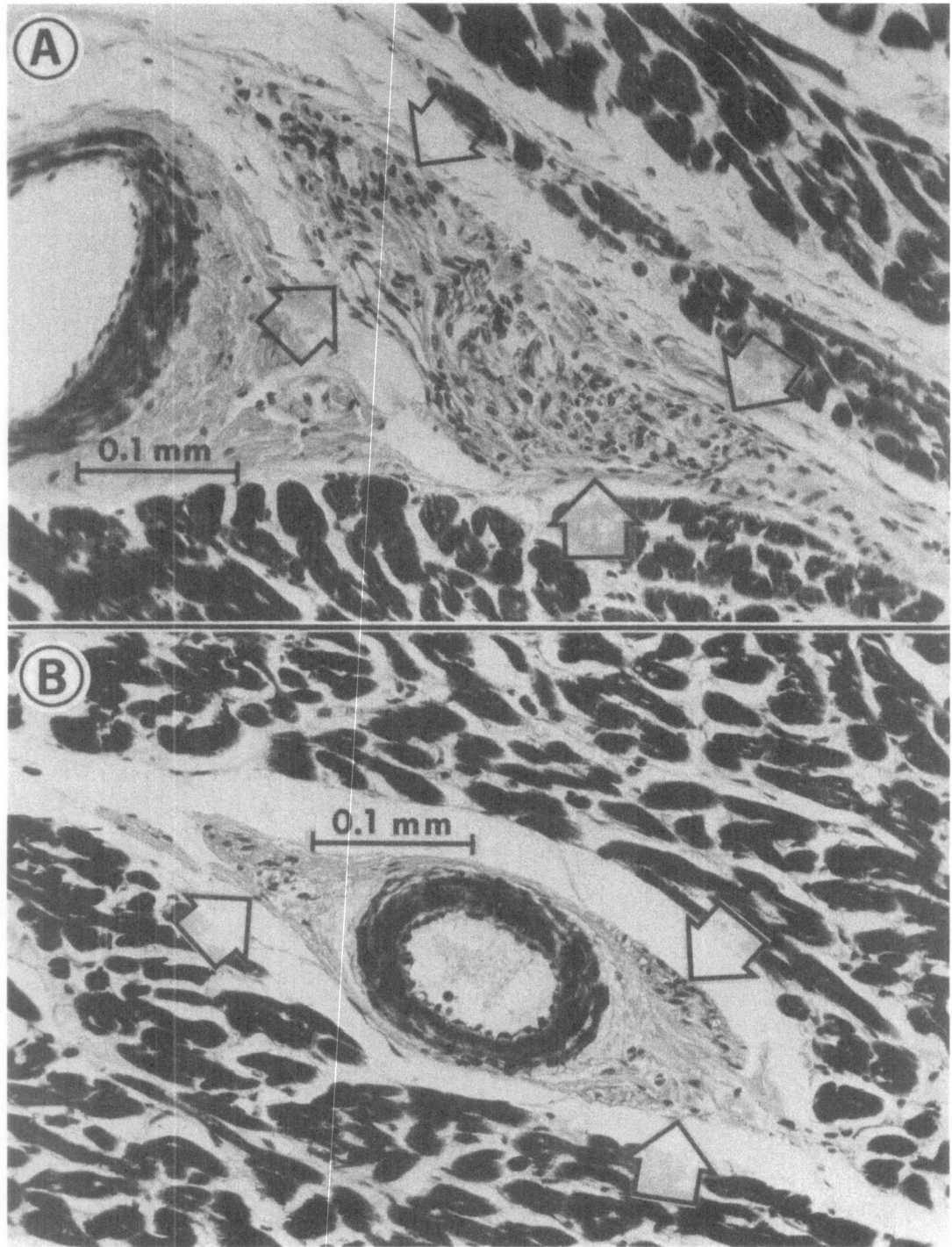

Figure 5. Degeneration and scirrhous fibrosis of small nerves (arrows) near coronary branches in the ventricular myocardium are shown here from a third normally hearing patient who died suddenly as part of the long QT syndrome.

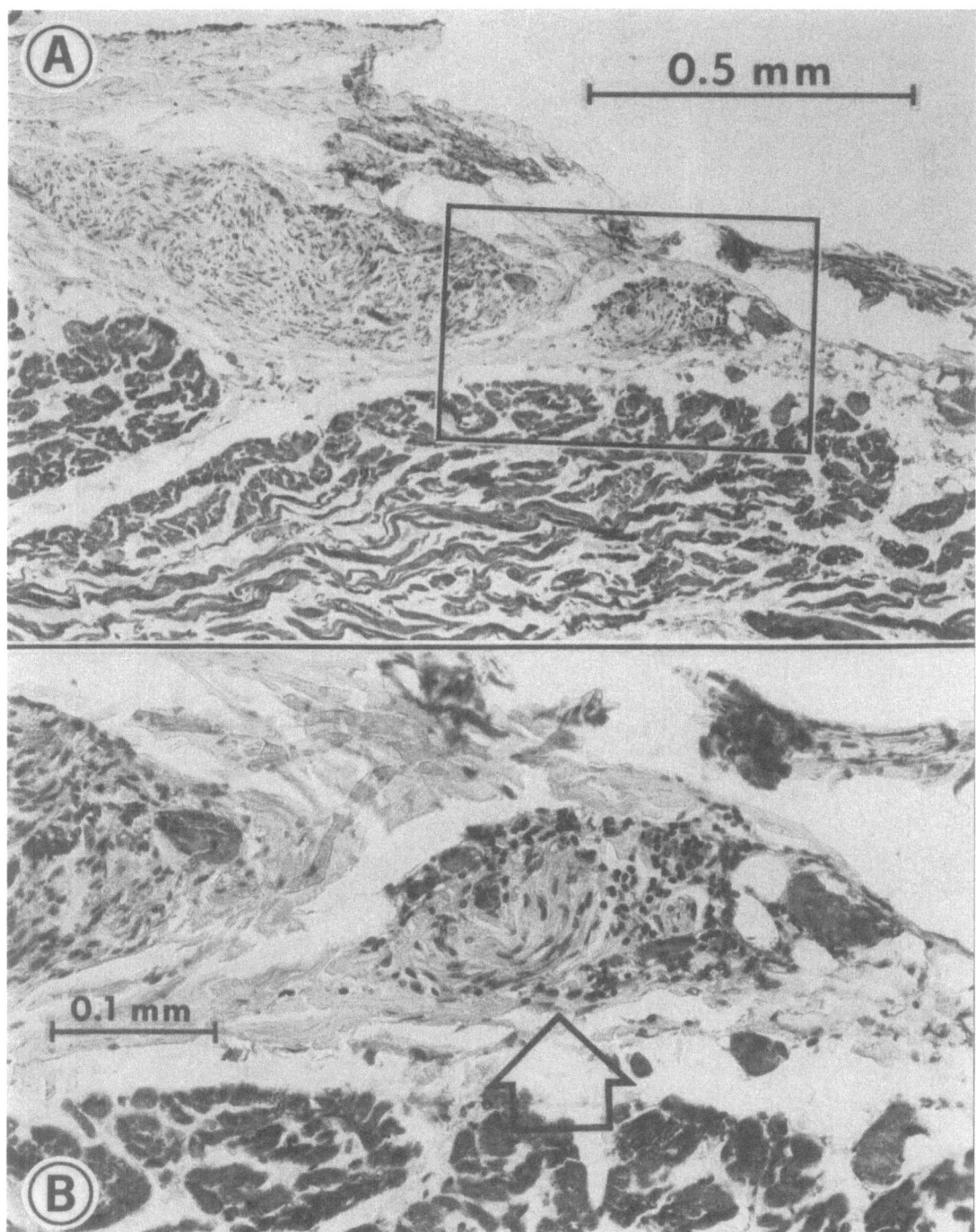

Figure 6. Ganglionitis and neural degeneration are illustrated in these photomicrographs from near the sinus node of a deaf child with the long QT syndrome and sudden death. A large nerve is seen in the upper left portion of *A*, and the boxed area includes a ganglion with inflammation, indicated with an arrow in the enlarged version in *B*.

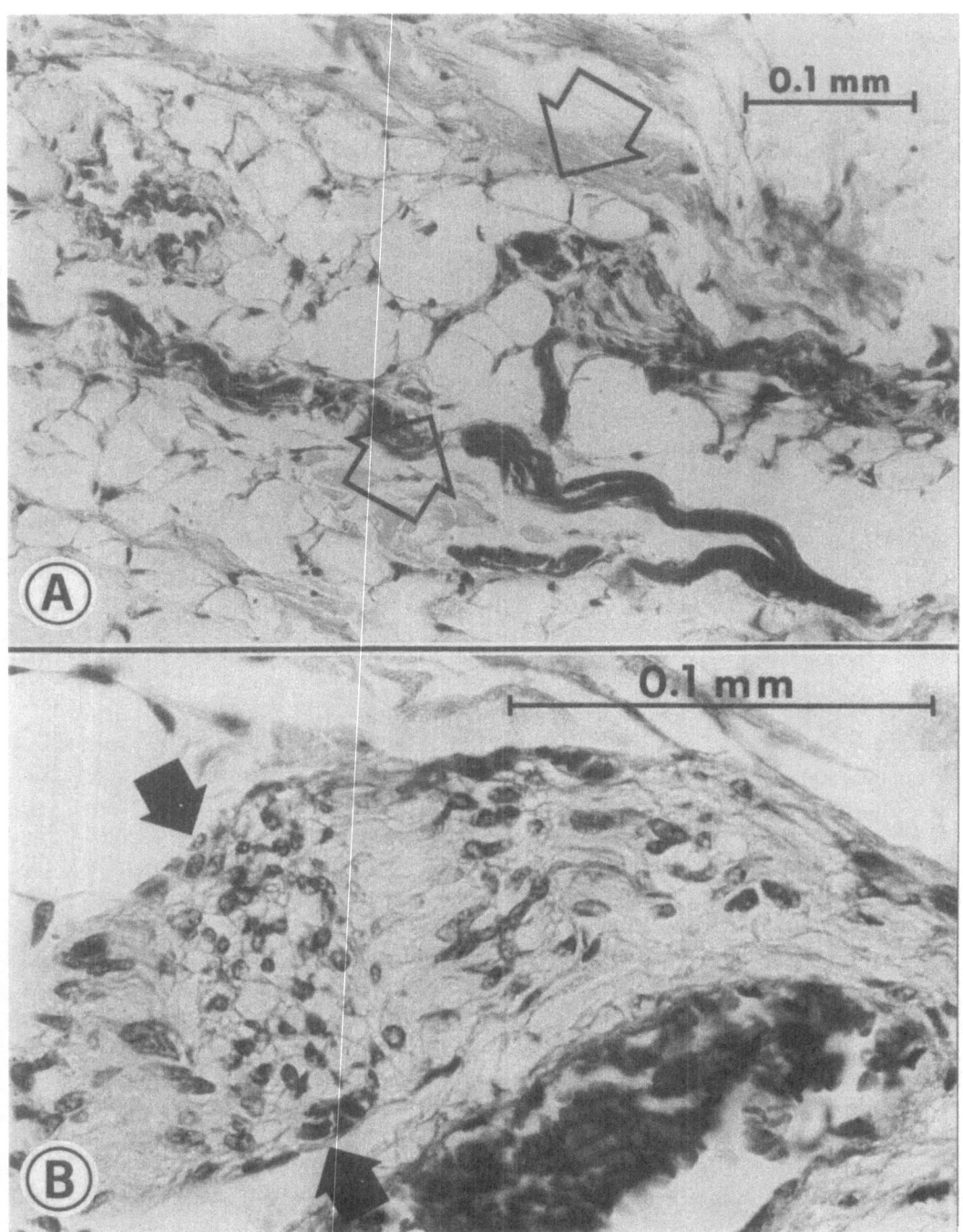

Figure 7. Vesicular neural degeneration and ganglionitis is shown here from the heart of a second deaf patient who had the long QT syndrome and died suddenly. A ganglion and nerve are indicated with arrows in *A*, with a few sinus node fibers seen beneath them. Vesicular degeneration of the nerve in *B*, marked with arrows, is from near the AV node.

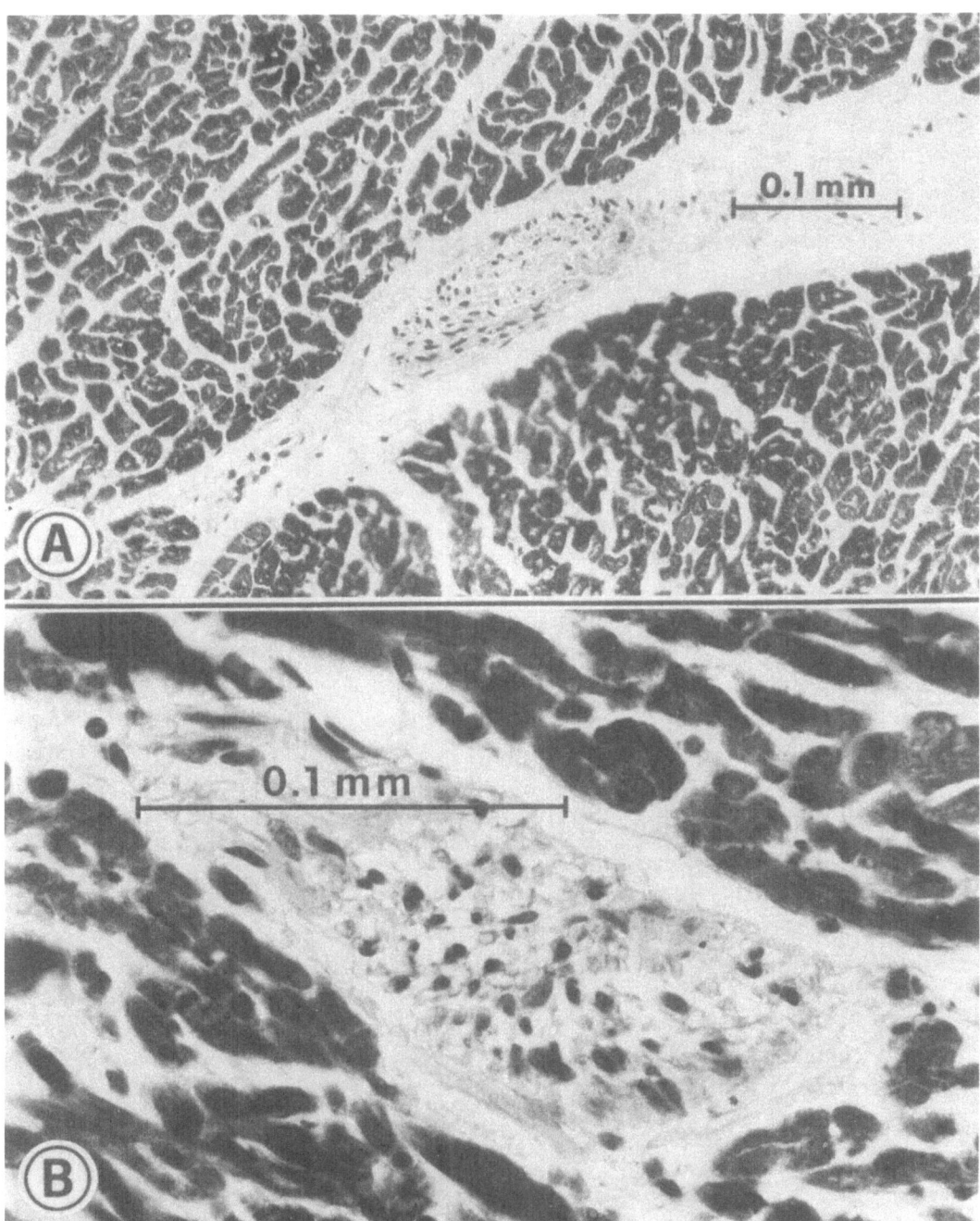

Figure 8. Fibrosis and degeneration of two small nerves within ventricular myocardium are shown here from a fourth normally hearing child who died suddenly with the long QT syndrome.

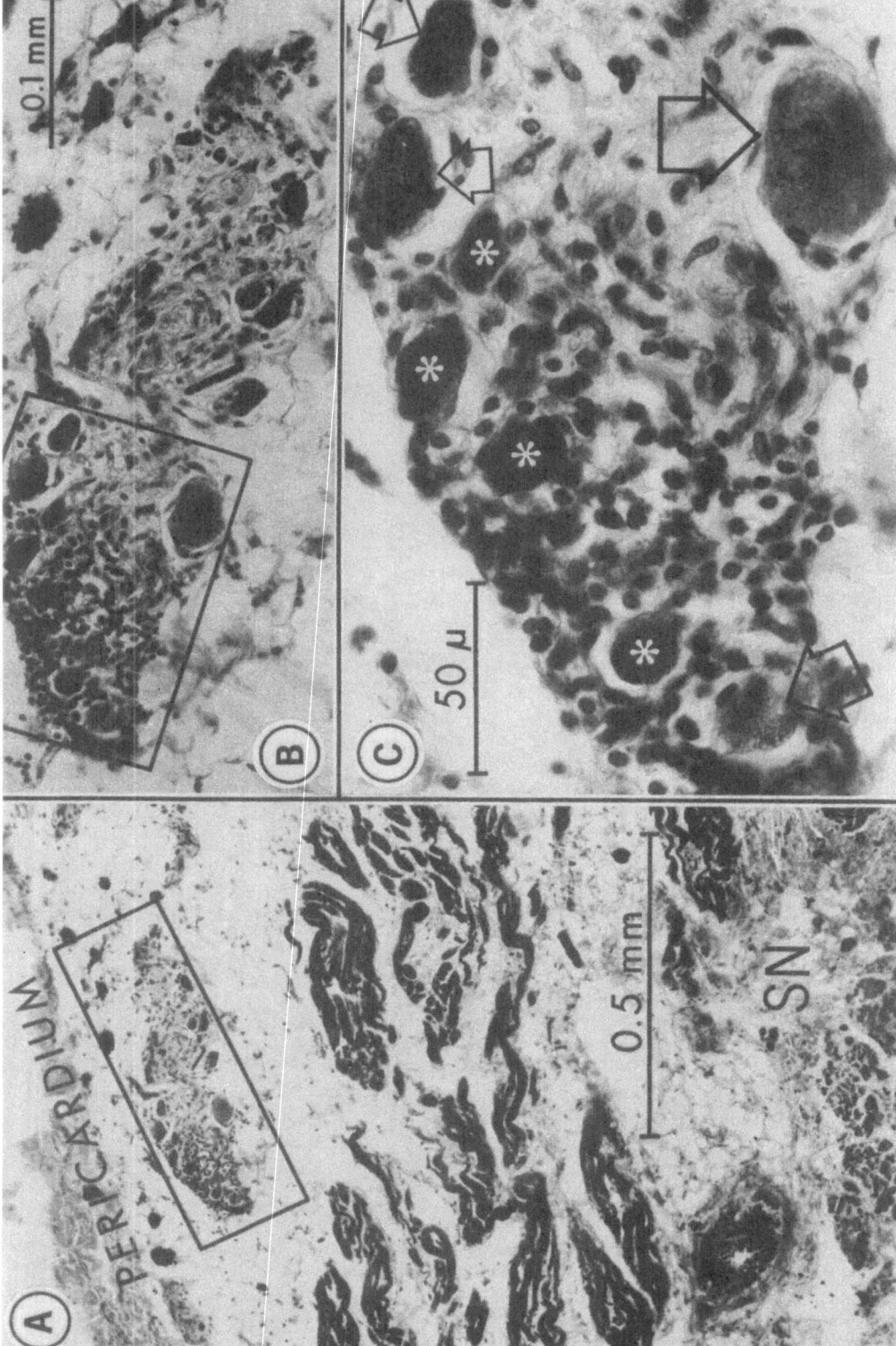

ly conspicuous in childeren with the disease. While the sinus node artery is abnormally thickened in the hearts of some patients dying with a long QT syndrome (21, 25, 28), loss of sympathetic neural influence may be an additional explanation for the sinus bradycardia. Experimentally, normal sinus rate is to some extent maintained by sympathetic neural control, but an optimal rate for AV junctional escape pacemakers is even more dependent on adrenergic neural control (32). In the absence of such sympathetic influence, the AV junctional pacemaker may escape erratically and with a long lag time. This could be still an additional hazard in the absence of normal sinus rate or rhythm, especially if there is associated prolongation of ventricular repolarization; the erratic escape rhythm may offer just the inappropriately timed "premature" beat necessary to fall within the vulnerable period of the ventricles.

In addition to cardioneural disease associated with abnormal ventricular repolarization (long QT interval) and sudden death, I have seen in other examples of sudden unexpected death an almost isolated form of ganglionitis in the heart and this was not known to be associated with any abnormality of ventricular repolarization (Figure 9). Here neither the etiology nor the electrophysiological influence of the ganglionitis is known.

What the etiology of any of the primary cardioneural diseases may be is presently uncertain. They may represent some form of heritable degeneration, an attractive possibility in view of the widely assumed hereditary nature of long QT syndromes. On the other hand, there is only circumstantial evidence that long QT syndromes are heritable in nature. It is an equally plausible hypothesis to suspect that the cardioneural disease, including its functional consequences such as QT prolongation, represents some chronic infection such as a herpes virus (33). There are abundant clinical examples now of certain viruses which slowly produce disease (the varicella-zoster virus), or may recur (herpes labialis) in some individuals over periods of many years. In such patients there may be some hereditary predisposition, or there may not be, the infection in families simply being directly transmitted rather than inherited.

4. FUNCTIONAL CONSEQUENCES OF CARDIAC NEUROPATHIES

Certain balances are essential in the normal neural control of the heart. Two extremes to consider are the simultaneous massive discharge of vagal and sympathetic systems which occurs in some reflexes (8), as contrasted to the absence of neural control following cardiac transplantation. In addition there is an appreciable normal imbalance during resting control conditions, but a different normal imbalance during stressful states. For example, vagal influence on atrial myocardium is normally dominant while sympathetic nerves dominate

---

Figure 9. Ganglionitis near the sinus node is illustrated here from the heart of a previously healthy young woman who died suddenly and unexpectedly. She was not deaf and did not have a long QT interval. The ganglion boxed in *A* is near the sinus node (SN) and is seen at higher magnification in *B*. Boxed area in *B* is magnified still more in *C*. Asterisks indicate shrunken degenerating neurons, while those marked with open arrows show various degrees of abnormal enlargement or possible swelling.

neural influence in the ventricles. Some autonomic neural influence is more concentrated in certain regions of the heart (sinus node, AV node) than in others (ordinary working myocardium). Given these various unbalancing influences, there is still an uncanny ability for the heart to "right itself" and for its electrical stability to be preserved by opposing actions of its vagal and sympathetic neural control.

When the heart accelerates from sympathetic drive, the vagus acts as a check rein to modulate the tachycardia. When the heart slows from vagal influence, various compensatory mechanisms can include sympathetic neural enhancement of ventricular contraction to preserve effective cardiac output and optimal coronary flow. Some of these balancing adjustments occur almost instantaneously, an advantage offered by many neurophysiological processes, while others begin slowly but may be more long lasting.

In the face of these advantageous balancing tendencies for normal neural control of the heart, there are by contrast many other factors which can cause undesirable forms of imbalance. Among such factors one can include processes which are not primarily neural in nature but which may either enhance or impair neural function. Hypercalcemia, for example, can augment vagal influence on cardiac rate and rhythm. The various effects of pheochromocytoma are sympathomimetic events familiar to all clinicians. Morphine and digitalis have some vagomimetic actions, atropine and quinidine and many antihistamines impair vagal effects, guanethidine and bretylium block adrenergic neuronal activity, and an increasing array of pharmacologic compounds block adrenergic β-receptors.

All of the examples just cited may be considered physiological or pharmacological (i.e. not anatomical) distortions, at least within the context of our present ability to detect such structural variations. There will surely come a time when the structure of membrane receptors and transmembrane ionic channels can more readily be directly visualized. But even today there are many cardiac neuropathies susceptible to study by presently available anatomical techniques. It is widely recognized that some diseases, such as diabetes and Chagas' myocarditis, have conspicuous affinity for damaging cardiac nerves, and these results can be seen. What is just beginning to be appreciated is the prevalence of a wide variety of both secondary and primary neuropathies of the heart, as outlined in the two preceding sections. Because of the focal nature of such cardioneuropathies, they inevitably unbalance neural control of the heart.

Asymmetry of vagal influence on the atria facilitates both the onset and perpetuation of atrial fibrillation (34). Anything which causes dispersion of refractory periods in the ventricular myocardium, such as bradycardia (35), can increase the likelihood of ventricular arrhythmias. While vagal influence can cause such bradycardia, asymmetry of sympathetic neural influence has an even more directly dangerous effect on ventricular myocardium by increasing its vulnerability, including a tendency to ventricular fibrillation as discussed relative to patients with the long QT syndromes (25).

Classes of neural responses in the heart can be generally grouped as either tonic or episodic. The fact that atropine increases the heart rate of normal subjects at rest illustrates that there is a constant degree of vagal "tone", although the level of this neural activity is further modified by cyclic events such as normal breathing. More powerful episodic neural influence occurs as part of many autonomic reflexes, originating both within the heart and elsewhere. Over all of these neural events and processes the brain acts as a modulator. Not only are tonic neural events integrated there, but most reflexes relay from there, and both conscious and subconscious mental processes superimpose their additional important effects.

Thinking and emotions profoundly influence nearly every element of neural control of the heart. Without delving into the mechanisms of being frightened to death or worried into sickness, there are indisputable cardioneural consequences of becoming angry, apprehensive, grief-stricken or excited. Prolonged electrocardiographic monitoring studies have repeatedly proven the temporal relationship of emotional events to electrical instability of the heart. Every experienced cardiologist has come to appreciate the clinical value of reassurance in treating patients with angina, myocardial infarction or pulmonary edema. While the association of disturbing thoughts or emotions with many forms of cardiac electrical instability is well established, the pathophysiological processes involved are less well defined. Further anatomical studies of the nerves of the heart may prove useful in clarifying this pathogenesis.

One can appreciate the value of such clinicopathological correlations from the three following facts. First, nerves and ganglia of the heart are often anatomically abnormal; second, such lesions are conspicuous in the vicinity of crucial control centers such as the sinus node and AV node, and third, cardiac neuropathies are demonstrable in many victims of sudden unexpected death. Combining such clinicopathological observations with experimental findings obtained from selective elimination or enhancement of either vagal or sympathetic neural influence within either sinus node (36–38) or the AV node and His bundle (39–41) will permit the construction of important clinical hypotheses. More careful postmortem study of the heart, including particularly the conduction system and the cardiac nerves and ganglia, is therefore to be encouraged, especially when the patient died suddenly or unexpectedly or when specific disturbances of cardiac rhythm or conduction had recently been documented. From careful correlation of such clinical, experimental and postmortem investigations, we can anticipate more rapid progress in our understanding of how nerves control the heart and how they may either stabilize or distort its electrical activity.

ACKNOWLEDGMENT

This work was supported in part by the National Heart, Lung and Blood Institute (Program Project Grant HL 11, 310 and SCOR on Ischemic Heart Disease no 1 P 17 17, 667) and by the Philip B. Hofmann Fund for Medical Research.

REFERENCES

1. Rossi L: Histopathology of cardiac arrhythmias (second edition). Casa Editrice Ambrosiana, Milano, 1978.
2. Abildskov JA: Adrenergic effects on the QT interval of the electrocardiogram. Am Heart J 92: 210–216, 1976.
3. Burgess MJ: Relation of ventricular repolarization to electrocardiographic T wave-form and arrhythmia vulnerability. Am J Physiol 5:H391-H402, 1979.

4. James TN, Urthaler F, Isobe JH: Neurogenic influence on the P-Tp segment. Am J Cardiol 32:799–807, 1973.
5. James TN: Cardiac innervation: Anatomic and pharmacologic relations. Bull NY Acad Med 43:1041–1086, 1967.
6. Becker AE: The glomera in the region of the heart and great vessels. Pathol Eur 1:410–424, 1966.
7. Eckstein RW, Shintani F, Rowen HE Jr, Shimomura K, Ohya N: Identification of left coronary blood supply of aortic bodies in anesthetized dogs. J Appl Physiol 30:488–492, 1971.
8. James TN, Isobe JH, Urthaler F: Analysis of components in a hypertensive cardiogenic chemoreflex. Circulation 52:179–192, 1975.
9. James TN: De Subitaneis Mortibus. XXVIII. Apoplexy of the heart. Circulation 57:385–391, 1978.
10. James TN: De Subitaneis Mortibus. XXIV. Ruptured interventricular septum and heart block. Circulation 55:934–946, 1977.
11. James TN, Rupe CE, Monto RW: Pathology of the cardiac conduction system in systemic lupus erythematosus. Ann Intern Med 63:402–410, 1965.
12. James TN, Birk RE: Pathology of the cardiac conduction system in polyarteritis nodosa and its variants. Arch Intern Med 177:561–567, 1966.
13. James TN: Pathology of the cardiac conduction system in amyloidosis. Ann Intern Med 65:28–36, 1966.
14. James TN, Monto RW: Pathology of the cardiac conduction system in thrombotic thrombocytopenic purpura. Ann Intern Med 65:37–43, 1966.
15. James TN, Carson NAJ, Froggatt P: De Subitaneis Mortibus. IV. Coronary vessels and conduction system in homocystinuria. Circulation 49:367–374, 1974.
16. James TN: Observations on the cardiovascular involvement (including the cardiac conduction system) in progressive muscular dystrophy. Am Heart J 63:48–56, 1962.
17. Rossi L, James TN: Neurovascular pathology of the heart in progressive muscular dystrophy. Panminerva Med 6:357–360, 1964.
18. James TN, Fisch C: Observations on the cardiovascular involvement in Friedreich's ataxia. Am Heart J 66:164–175, 1963.
19. James TN, Reynolds EW Jr: Pathology of the cardiac conduction system in a case of diphtheria associated with atrial arrhythmias and heart block. Circulation 28: 263–267, 1963.
20. Morales AR, Vichitbandha P, Chandruang P, Evans H, Bourgeois CH: Pathological features of cardiac conduction disturbances in diphtheritic myocarditis. Arch Pathol 91: 1–7, 1971.
21. James TN, Froggatt P, Atkinson WJ, Lurie PR, McNamara DG, Miller WW, Schloss GT, Carroll JF, North RL: De Subitaneis Mortibus. XXX. Observations on the pathophysiology of the long QT syndromes with special reference to the neuropathology of the heart. Circulation 57:1221–1231, 1978.
22. Moore JI, Swain HH: Sensitization to ventricular fibrillation. I. Sensitization by a substituted propiophenone, U-0882. J Pharmacol Exp Ther 128:243–252, 1960.
23. James TN, Bear ES: Cardiac effects of some simple aliphatic aldehydes. J. Pharmacol Exp Ther 163:300–308, 1968.
24. Jervell A, Lange-Nielsen F: Congenital deaf-mutism, functional heart disease with prolongation of the Q-T interval, and sudden death. Am Heart J 54:59–68, 1957.
25. Fraser GR, Froggatt P, James TN: Congenital deafness associated with electrocardiographic abnormalities, fainting attacks and sudden death. A recessive syndrome. Q J Med 33:361–385, 1964.
26. Romano C, Gemme G, Pongiglione R: Aritmie Cardiache Rare Dell'eta' Pediatrica. II. Accessi sincopali per fibrillazione ventricolare parossistica. (Presentazione del primo case della letteratura pediatrica italiana.) Clin Pediat 45:656–683, 1963.
27. Ward OC: A new familial cardiac syndrome in children. J Irish Med Assn 54:103–106, 1964.
28. James TN: Congenital deafness and cardiac arrhythmias. Am J Cardiol 19: 627–643, 1967.
29. Moss AJ, McDonald J: Unilateral cervicothoracic sympathetic ganglionectomy for the treatment of long QT interval syndrome. N Engl J Med 285:903–904, 1971.
30. Schwartz PJ, Malliani A: Electrical alternation of the T-wave: Clinical and experimental evidence of its relationship with the sympathetic nervous system and with the long Q-T syndrome. Am Heart J 89:45–50, 1975.
31. Coyer BH, Pryor R, Kirsch WM, Blount SG Jr: Left stellectomy in the long QT syndrome. Chest 74: 584–586, 1978.
32. Urthaler F, Millar K, Burgess MJ, Abildskov JA, James TN: Comparative dependence on adrenergic neural tone by automaticity in the sinus node and in the AV junction. J Pharmacol Exp Ther 187:269–279, 1973.
33. Warren KG, Brown SM, Wroblewska Z, Gilden D, Koprowski H, Subak-Sharpe J: Isolation of latent herpes simplex virus from the superior cervical and vagus ganglions of human beings. New Eng J Med 298:1068–1069, 1978.

34. Moe GK, Abildskov JA: Atrial fibrillation as a self-sustaining arrhythmia independent of focal discharge. Am Heart J 58:59–70, 1959.

35. Han J, Millet D, Chizzonitti B, Moe GK: Temporal dispersion of recovery of excitability in atrium and ventricle as a function of heart rate. Am Heart J 71:481–487, 1966.

36. James TN: Cholinergic mechanisms in the sinus node with particular reference to the actions of hemocholinium. Circ Res 19:347–357, 1966.

37. James TN, Bear ES, Lang KF, Green EW, Winkler HH: Adrenergic mechanisms in the sinus node. Arch Intern Med 125:512–547, 1970.

38. Urthaler F, James TN: Cholinergic and adrenergic control of the sinus node and AV junction. Chapter 9 in Neural Regulation of the Heart, Randall WC (ed), Oxford University Press, New York, 1977, p 247–288.

39. James TN, Bear ES, Frink RJ, Lang KF, Tomlinson JC: Selective stimulation, suppression or blockade of the AV node and His bundle. J Lab Clin Med 76:240–256, 1970.

40. Urthaler F, Katholi CR, Macy J Jr, James TN: Mathematical relationship between automaticity of the sinus node and the AV junction. Am Heart J 86:189–195, 1973.

41. Urthaler F, Katholi CR, Macy J Jr, James TN: Electrophysiological and mathematical characteristics of the escape rhythm during complete AV block. Cardiovasc Res 8:173–186, 1974.

SECTION 2
THE ELECTROPHYSIOLOGY OF LETHAL ARRHYTHMIAS

SECTION 2A
ANIMAL MYOCARDIAL INFARCTION MODELS

2.1. STUDIES ON VENTRICULAR ARRHYTHMIAS IN ANIMAL MODELS OF ISCHEMIC HEART DISEASE: WHAT CAN WE LEARN?

H.S. KARAGUEUZIAN and A.L. WIT

Sudden cardiac death often is a direct consequence of ventricular fibrillation. Individuals who have ventricular fibrillation may have a high incidence of ventricular premature depolarizations and tachycardia prior to its occurrence. The ventricular fibrillation may be related to this high incidence of other ventricular arrhythmias, at least in some instances (1). Since sudden death most often occurs in the setting of atherosclerotic heart disease the ventricular arrhythmias and the fibrillation are most likely caused by cardiac ischemia. Myocardial infarction may or may not be present. A significant number of individuals resuscitated from ventricular fibrillation have shown no evidence of infarction (2) but sudden death also occurs in individuals with fresh or old myocardial infarcts (3).

Since sudden death is often associated with and caused by ventricular arrhythmias, improved understanding of why and how arrhythmias occur in ischemic heart disease might eventually aid in therapy. These arrhythmias are a result of alterations in electrophysiology of cardiac fibers in the ischemic regions. Investigations into the nature of these alterations are important. However, it is difficult, and often impossible, to do many of the necessary studies in patients aimed at elucidating the mechanisms causing ischemic arrhythmias because of the unpredictable quality of the syndrome and the serious clinical situation which is associated with it. Because of these constraints, animal models must be used to learn more about the pathophysiology of these arrhythmias. The ideal animal model in which to study arrhythmias associated with sudden death should have the following characteristics; 1) it should develop atherosclerotic heart disease and chronic ischemic heart disease, 2) it should develop chronic ventricular arrhythmias, 3) it should spontaneously develop ventricular fibrillation with or without accompanying myocardial infarction, 4) it should have a heart which is large enough to permit electrical recordings to be easily made from various localized regions, 5) the anatomy of the coronary arteries and ventricular conducting system should be similar to the human heart.

Although attempts have been made to develop such a model, no readily usable model which has all these characteristics exists. However, this is not to say that nothing can be done in the laboratory to answer questions on how arrhythmias and arrhythmic death occur. There are a large number of animal models which can be used to investigate the effects of ischemia on cardiac electrophysiology. Each model has its own advantages and disadvantages. To derive the most useful information from each model the investigator must realize the limitations of the model he is studying, ask only questions that studies with the model can answer and be prudent in extrapolating experimental data to the clinical setting. When done in this manner studies on experimental animals can provide important information which can improve our understanding of clinical arrhythmias, caused by ischemia. Results from experimental studies on animals can also stimulate the clinical electrophysiologist and lead to discoveries of phenomena in the human heart which might not have been noticed had they not been seen in the experimental animal. But there is also a reciprocal relationship between the clinical and laboratory electrophysiologist. In some instances observations in the clinic provide questions that can only be answered by investigations on animal models. In this chapter we will discuss several examples of how experiments on animal models have shown some of the mechanisms which probably underlie arrhythmias caused by ischemia in humans.

1. CARDIAC ARRHYTHMIAS IN THE CANINE HEART AFTER CORONARY ARTERY OC-CLUSION

Sudden arrhythmic death often occurs soon after the onset of myocardial infarction (4). Myocardial infarction in humans may be caused by occlusion of a coronary artery resulting from rupture of an atherosclerotic plaque, coronary artery spasm or other mechanisms (5, 6). The result of such an occlusion is the deprivation of a region of the myocardium of its normal blood supply. In the canine, myocardial infarction can be produced experimentally by depriving a region of the myocardium of its normal blood supply. This has been done in anesthetized animals with the chest open by ligating either the left anterior descending or circumflex coronary artery (7), or in the unanesthetized animal by using balloon occluders (8) or ameroid constrictors (9). These techniques used to occlude the artery obviously do not resemble the natural process which causes coronary occlusion in humans. However, the end result is still cessation of blood flow to a region of the myocardium and these animal models are, therefore, useful for determining how ischemia affects the electrical activity of previously normal myocardium. However, it must be kept in mind that in humans a long period of chronic ischemia may precede the complete coronary occlusion. Such chronic ischemia may alter myocardial electrophysiology prior to the complete occlusion and influence the response of the cells to complete occlusion when it occurs. This possibility has not yet been explored in the experimental laboratory.

Despite the fact that experimental coronary artery occlusion in the dog does not exactly duplicate the process occurring in humans useful information has come from this experimental approach and this information has improved our understanding of the mechanisms which cause ischemic ventricular arrhythmias. Such information has been obtainable because electrical activity can be recorded from ischemic regions of the ventricle during coronary artery occlusion.

1.1. Continuous electrical activity and ventricular arrhythmias

One important observation which has resulted from occluding the coronary arteries of dogs is the relationship between "continuous electrical activity" in ischemic myocardium and the occurrence of ventricular arrhythmias. Studies in several laboratories have described the

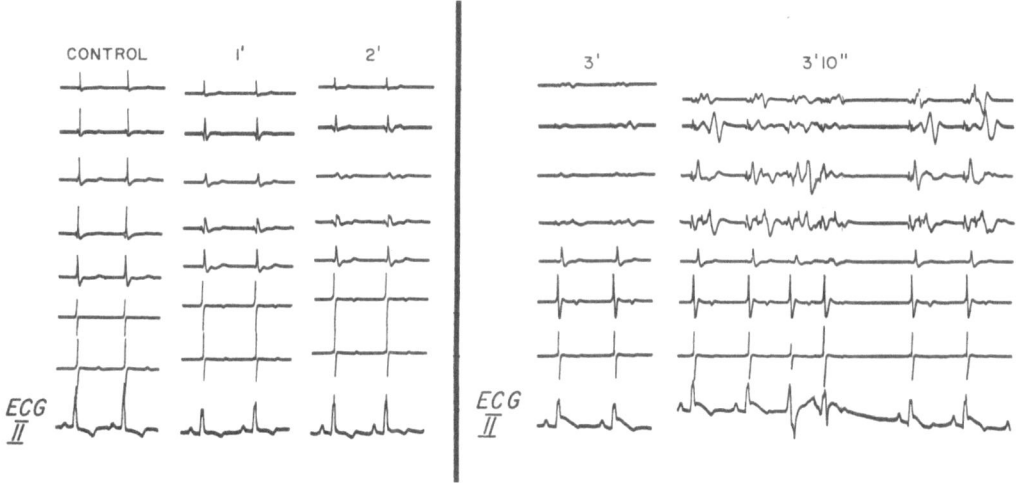

Figure 1. The immediate effects of coronary artery occlusion on bipolar electrograms recorded from the epicardium of the canine heart. In each panel bipolar electrogram recordings from 7 different regions are shown in the first seven traces. The bottom trace is a lead II ECG. The top 5 electrograms were recorded from the region which became ischemic after the left anterior descending coronary artery was occluded, the sixth and seventh electrograms were recorded from non-ischemic myocardium. At the left recordings taken prior to coronary artery occlusion are shown (control). At all sites electrograms appear as large amplitude spikes of short duration. To the right of the control records are records obtained 1 min, 2 min, 3 min and 3 min and 10 sec after complete occlusion of the LAD near its origin. There is a progressive decrease in amplitude and increase in duration of the electrograms recorded from the ischemic region and no change in the electrograms recorded from non-ischemic regions. ST segment changes on the ECG can be seen after 3 min. At 3 min, 10 sec amplification of the signals recorded from the ischemic region has been increased. Discrete spikes of electrical activity are no longer evident. In the top 4 traces the electrograms have become fragmented and continuous electrical activity is evident. This is associated with the occurrence of ventricular premature depolarizations. (Reproduced from 13.)

effects of coronary artery occlusion on the extracellular, bipolar electrogram, recorded from ventricular muscle as it becomes ischemic after coronary occlusion (10–14) (Figure 1). In general, as ischemia progresses the amplitude of the electrogram (which when recorded from normal ventricular myocardium is a "spike" of 1 to 10 mV in amplitude and about 5 msec in duration) decreases and the duration increases. Within minutes the electrogram is no longer a discrete "spike" but becomes fragmented into multiple spikes. Finally, the electrogram associated with a single ventricular impulse may be composed of multiple low amplitude deflections that occur for several hundred milliseconds and activity at the recording site may continue for a longer time period than the duration of the T wave of the ECG (Figure 1). When this happens ventricular arrhythmias occur. The ventricular arrhythmias which can be induced in the canine heart 3–7 days after coronary occlusion are also associated with similar continuous electrical activity in the ischemic region (15, 16). Although there is a definite relationship between the occurrence of continuous electrical activity and ventricular arrhythmias the exact electrophysiological mechanism for these arrhythmias is still not completely certain. The most favored hypothesis is that continuous electrical activity indicates the occurrence of reentry.

The studies described above most certainly influenced clinical investigators in their studies on ischemic arrhythmias in humans, and this is one of the important features of experimental animal studies. Although it has not been possible to record electrograms from ischemic human ventricular myocardium within the first few minutes after the onset of ischemia which causes ventricular arrhythmias it has been possible to record electrograms from chronic ischemic regions, in aged ventricular infarcts, and aneurysms (17, 18). Electrograms recorded from such regions have shown fragmentation, and continuous electrical activity similar to that which was shown in the canine experiments (18) has been evident during ventricular arrhythmias (Figure 2). Therefore, it appears that the electrophysiological mechanisms causing at least some ischemic related arrhythmias in humans are similar to those in the canine heart and these arrhythmias in humans may be caused by reentry. This is an example where animal investigation provided the stimulus that resulted in an important clinical observation.

1.2. Subendocardial cardiac fibers surviving in infarcts and ventricular arrhythmias

In the dog, after occlusion of the left anterior descending (LAD) coronary artery, a delayed phase of ventricular arrhythmias occurs 6–10 hours later and may persist for several days (10). Ventricular arrhythmias in humans also may not occur for many hours after the onset of the initial symptoms indicative of coronary occlusion (19). Extensive electrophysiological and anatomical studies on the canine heart have defined the origin and electrophysiological mechanism for these ventricular arrhythmias in the dog (20–24). Four types of observations

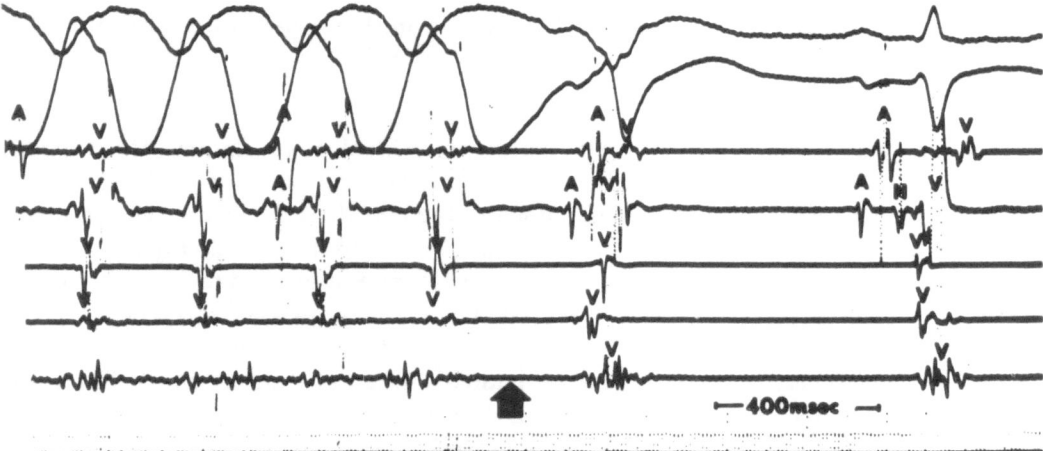

Figure 2. Continuous electrical activity recorded with an electrode catheter from the endocardial surface of a myocardial infarct in a human heart. The top two traces are ECG leads V_1 and V_2. Beneath these are electrograms recorded from the region of the coronary sinus, the His bundle, the right ventricle, the border of the left ventricular aneurysm and the endocardial surface of the aneurysm. The electrograms are shown during a period of ventricular tachycardia. Continuous electrical activity is evident on the endocardial surface of the aneurysm (bottom trace). The tachycardia terminates at the arrow. The electrogram recorded from the endocardial surface of the aneurysm is fragmented but continuous activity throughout diastole is no longer evident. (Reproduced from 18.)

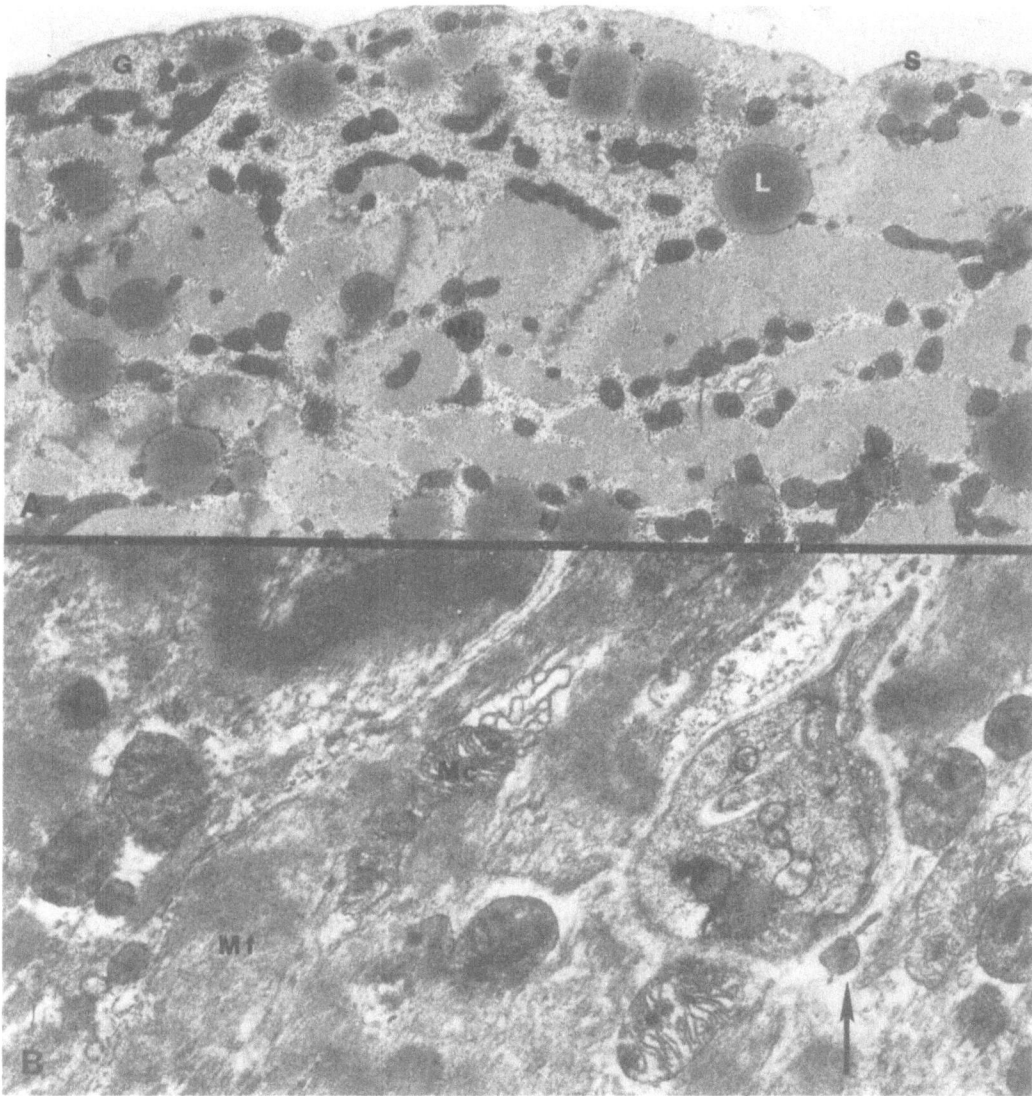

Figure 3. Electron micrographs of a surviving subendocardial Purkinje fiber (A) and a disrupted ventricular muscle cell (B) in the infarcted anterior papillary muscle of a dog 24 hours after coronary artery ligation. In A, the surviving Purkinje fiber is characterized by an intact sarcolemma (S), normal mitochondria (Mc) and the presence of glycogen (G). Note the accumulation of lipid droplets (L). In B, glycogen is absent, the myofibrils (Mf) appear indistinct, dark granules are present in the swollen mitochondria (Mc) and sarcolemmal discontinuities are present (arrow). (A, ×9600, B, ×13,000.) (Reproduced from 26.)

have indicated that the arrhythmias occur because of automaticity in subendocardial Purkinje fibers which survive on the endocardial surface of the infarcts. These experimental observations are as follows: 1) Histological and ultrastructural studies have shown intact Purkinje fibers on the endocardial surface of infarcts (20, 25). Large amounts of lipid droplets

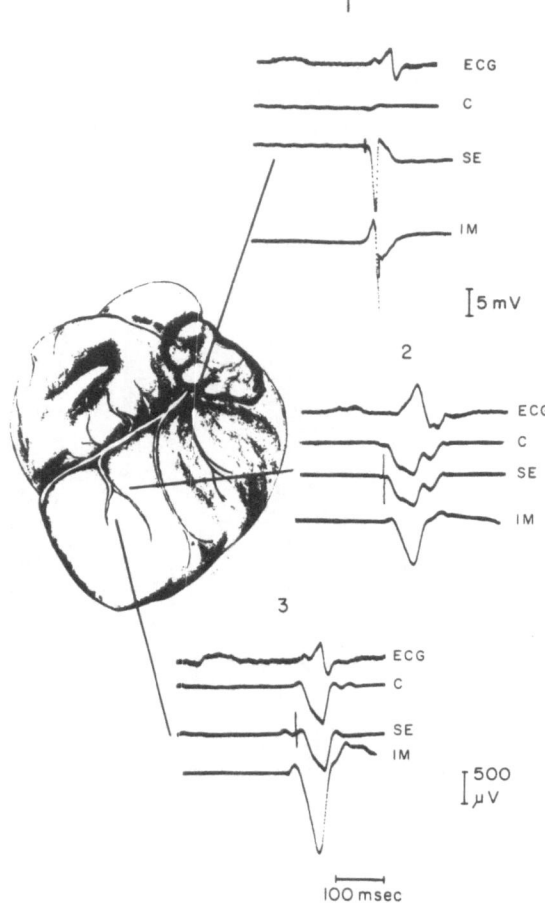

Figure 4. Bipolar recordings from infarcted and noninfarcted myocardium in the in situ canine heart 24 hours after coronary artery ligation. The extensive left ventricular infarct is depicted as the unshaded area adjacent to the anterior descending coronary artery, which has been ligated near its origin. Noninfarcted regions are shaded. In each section on the right, the top trace is a lead II electrocardiogram (ECG). The second trace (C) shows the potential recorded within the left ventricular cavity with bipolar electrodes; the third and fourth traces are subendocardial (SE) and intramural (IM) bipolar electrograms recorded from the designated areas. Calibrations at the right apply only to the electrograms and not the ECG. The 5 mV calibration is for Panel 1 only. The 500 uV calibration is for Panels 2 and 3. Panel 1 shows recordings from a noninfarcted region of the left ventricle. A low-amplitude wave was recorded from within the left ventricular cavity; this wave occurred simultaneously with the QRS complex of the surface ECG. An early, rapid deflection, 2 msec in duration, signifying Purkinje fiber activation is seen in the subendocardial electrogram and is followed by a deflection of greater amplitude and duration coincident with the QRS complex, denoting activation of ventricular muscle. A large amplitude deflection signifying ventricular muscle activity is seen in the intramural electrogram. Panel 2 shows recordings from sites within the infarct for a ventricular premature depolarization. Panel 3 shows recordings from sites within the infarct for a sinus beat. Amplification of electrograms in Panels 2 and 3 is 10 times that shown for the noninfarcted area in Panel 1. Again, a slow wave lasting the duration of the QRS complex of the ECG was recorded within the left ventricular cavity. Similar slow deflections are seen in the subendocardial and intramural recordings; there is no evidence of ventricular muscle activity. However, in the subendocardial recordings a rapid deflection (2 msec in duration) that signifies subendocardial Purkinje fiber activity is seen prior to the slow deflection. The late low amplitude positive deflections seen in the intramural electrograms may indicate some residual local activity in these regions. (Reproduced from 20.)

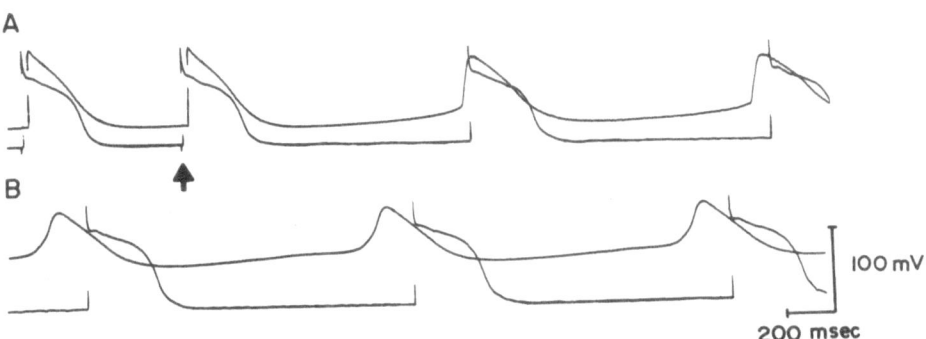

Figure 5. Transmembrane potentials recorded from subendocardial Purkinje fibers in an isolated preparation of infarcted canine myocardium. The top trace in each panel shows action potentials recorded from a fiber on the endocardial surface of the infarct, the bottom trace in each panel shows action potentials recorded from a fiber in an adjacent noninfarcted region. In Panel A, the first two impulses are elicited by electrical stimulation of the preparation. The stimulus is turned off at the arrow. Spontaneous diastolic depolarization develops in the Purkinje fiber in the infarct and results in automatic firing. In B, which shows recordings from the same 2 cells several minutes later, it is evident that impulses are arising in the automatic Purkinje fibers in the infarct (top trace) and are conducting into the non-infarcted region. (Reproduced from 21.)

seen in the cytoplasm of these fibers suggest that they are ischemic. Ventricular muscle cells beneath these Purkinje fibers show structural changes indicative of necrosis (Figure 3). 2) Electrograms have been recorded from Purkinje fibers on the endocardial surface of canine infarcts 24 hours to several days after coronary occlusion (20, 23, 24). At this time, electrograms can usually not be recorded from intramural ventricular muscle in the infarcted region (Figure 4). 3) Transmembrane potentials have been recorded from Purkinje fibers on the endocardial surface of isolated preparations of infarcted canine myocardium (20–22). Sontaneous diastolic depolarization is often evident in the recordings (Figure 5). 4) Earliest activation during ventricular arrhythmias 24 hours after LAD occlusion often occurs in Purkinje fibers on the subendocardial surface of the infarcts, indicating the arrhythmias arise in this region (23, 24).

The demonstration in an experimental animal model that arrhythmias may arise because of automaticity in surviving cells on the endocardial surface of infarcts stimulated studies in humans to determine whether a similar mechanism for ischemic arrhythmias exists in the human heart. Some evidence now suggests that it may. This evidence includes the following observations: 1) Histological and ultrastructural studies have shown intact Purkinje fibers surviving on the endocardial surface of some anteroseptal human infarcts. These fibers contain lipid droplets as was seen in the canine fibers (26) (Figure 6). However, unlike in the canine heart, variable amounts of subendocardial ventricular muscle cells also survive. Beneath this endocardial rim of intact myocardial fibers is necrotic myocardium. It must be stressed that all human infarcts do not have this structural characteristic. In all likelihood the structure of the infarct depends on the location of the coronary occlusion, the events preceding the occlusion, and the factors which cause the occlusion. 2) Transmembrane potentials have been recorded from cardiac fibers on the endocardial surface of preparations isolated from human infarcts and aneurysms (Figure 7). Although some of these potentials appear to be characteristic of Purkinje fibers, others may have been recorded from ventricular muscle cells (27). Some of the surviving fibers exhibit phase 4 depolarization and automatic impulse initiation (Figure 7). These preparations were isolated from infarcts that were older than those studied from the canine heart. The observation that spontaneous diastolic depolarization occurs in fibers surviving on the endocardial surface of

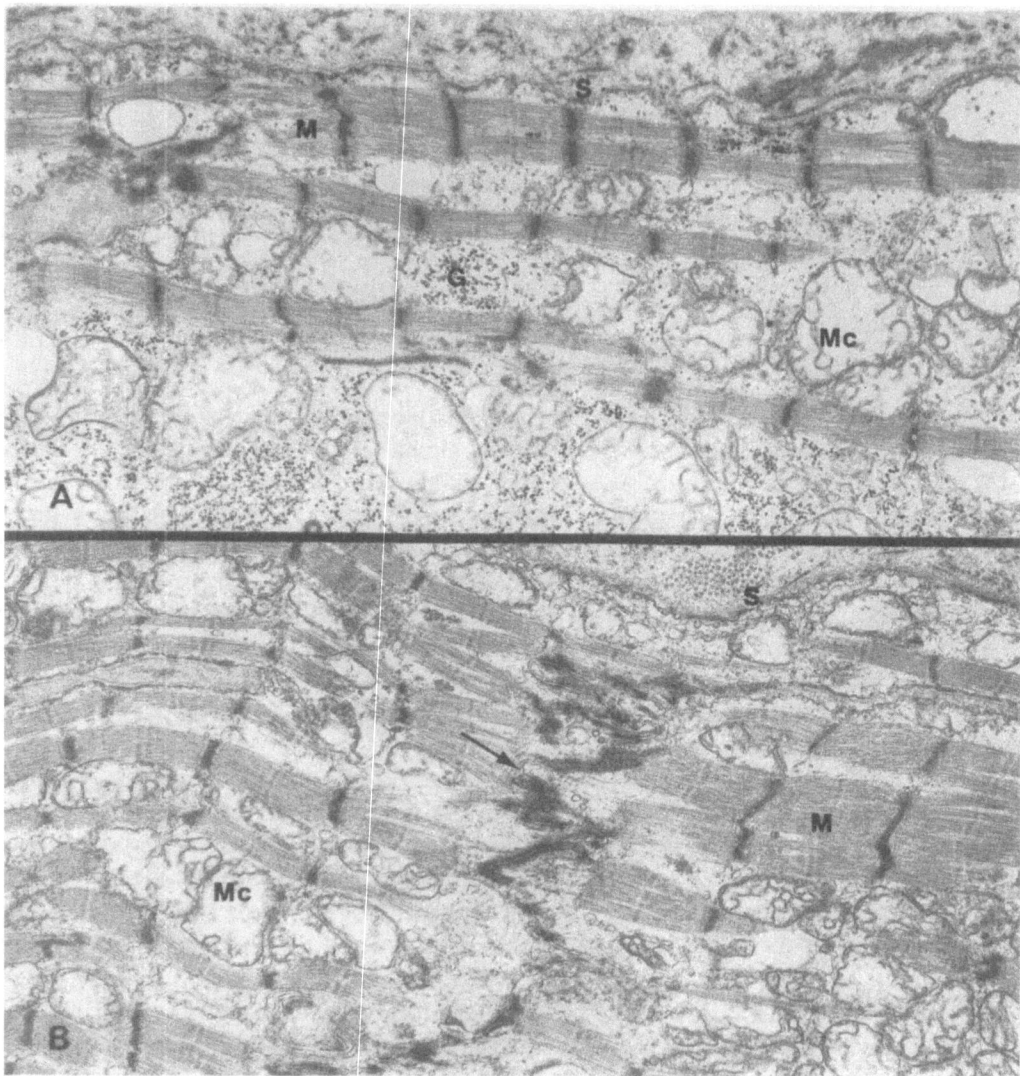

Figure 6. Electron micrographs of intact subendocardial cells in the anterior papillary muscle of a 12-month-old human infarct. A shows a surviving subendocardial Purkinje fiber overlying the area of fibrosis of the healed infarct. S is the intact sarcolemma; M shows distinct myofilaments; Mc are vacuolated mitochondria. Glycogen is still present. B shows a ventricular muscle cell trapped in the fibrous scar of the healed infarct. The sarcolemma (S) is also intact; myofibrils (M) are distinct; Mc are vacuolated mitochondria and the arrow indicates an intercalated disc. The appearance of this cell is identical to that of intramural ventricular muscle cells in on-infarcted regions (×9000). (Reproduced from 26.)

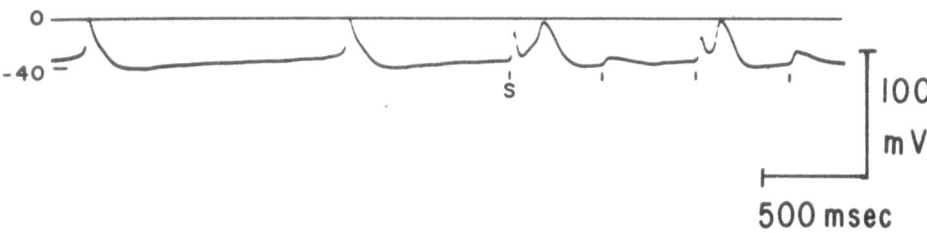

Figure 7. Transmembrane potentials recorded from the endocardial surface of a human infarct. At the left the fiber is spontaneously active and phase 4 depolarization is evident. At S stimulation at a basic cycle length of 450 msec is begun. The first and third stimuli excite the fiber. From these records it is not possible to determine whether this is a Purkinje fiber or a ventricular muscle fiber. (Reproduced from 27.)

aneurysms in human hearts is not proof that these fibers are the cause of ventricular arrhythmias. In fact, some of the patients from whom these aneurysms were obtained did not have ventricular arrhythmias (27). 3) Earliest activation during some ventricular arrhythmias caused by ischemia and infarction may occur on the endocardial surface of the infarcted region, in the cardiac fibers which survive there (28). This suggests that some arrhythmias arise on the endocardial surface of infarcts. 4) Electrophysiological studies in the catheterization laboratory indicate that many of the ventricular tachycardias which occur on the first day after the onset of symptoms of infarction are caused by automaticity. These arrhythmias can neither be initiated nor terminated by electrical stimulation of the ventricles. Overdrive suppression is evident after a period of stimulation at rates more rapid than the tachycardia (29). However, it has not been shown that these are the arrhythmias which arise in the fibers surviving on the subendocardial surface of the infarcts.

Therefore, the studies on humans do suggest that some clinical arrhythmias caused by ischemia arise in fibers on the endocardial surface of infarcts and that some arrhythmias are caused by automaticity. The mechanisms are similar to those first identified in the studies on the canine heart, indicating that despite the differences between experimentally and clinically occurring myocardial infarction, studies on animal models can provide meaningful information on the mechanisms of arrhythmias.

2. CARDIAC ARRHYTHMIAS IN THE CANINE HEART AFTER CORONARY OCCLUSION AND REPERFUSION

Ventricular arrhythmias and sudden death may not be caused only by permanent coronary occlusion but may also be related to temporary occlusion followed by reperfusion of the ischemic region through the previously occluded artery. Temporary coronary occlusion most likely occurs clinically because of coronary spasm (30). Experimental studies on the canine have indicated that the duration of the period of occlusion prior to reperfusion may have an important influence on the subsequent pathophysiology of the arrhythmias. Occlusions of 15–45 minutes do not cause myocardial infarction but following release of the occlusion ventricular fibrillation invariably occurs within minutes, either abruptly without warning or preceded by short bursts of tachycardia (19, 31). The mechanism for these arrhythmias is still unknown but when laboratory studies do provide the answers, the information may have important relevance to some types of arrhythmias which cause sudden death, particularly those which are not associated with myocardial infarction.

Occlusion of a coronary artery for longer periods of time followed by reperfusion has a different effect on the electrophysiology of the ventricles than occlusion for the short periods described above. Longer periods of occlusion do result in infarction but the anatomy and the electrophysiological properties of the infarct are different from infarcts caused by permanent occlusion. The arrhythmias associated with long periods of occlusion followed by reperfusion are described in detail in the next section.

2.1. Ventricular tachycardia after long periods of coronary occlusion followed by reperfusion

Paroxysmal ventricular tachycardia may occur in humans with ischemic heart disease and with myocardial infarcts or ventricular aneurysms. Electrocardiographically such tachycardias often begin with a premature ventricular depolarization. This may be the event which initiates the tachycardia. Tachycardia may last for a long period of time before terminating abruptly. Wellens et al. (32, 33), and later, other investigators (34–36) have done an extensive series of electrophysiological studies on patients who have a clinical history of such episodes of tachycardia. It has been demonstrated that ventricular tachycardia can be induced in these patients by premature stimuli applied to the ventricle through an electrode catheter (Figure 8). The stimulated premature depolarization which initiates tachycardia must occur at a critical time period in the cardiac cycle, stimuli occurring earlier or later do not initiate tachycardia. Once initiated, tachycardia can be terminated by single or multiple stimuli applied to the ventricle. It has been concluded that such tachycardias which can be initiated and terminated by stimulating the ventricle are caused by reentry because it was previously shown in studies on isolated preparations of cardiac tissue that reentry can be initiated and terminated in this way (37–39).

More detailed electrophysiological studies on ventricular arrhythmias initiated and terminated by premature depolarizations are important since such tachycardias might lead to ventricular fibrillation and sudden death, and such tachycardias may respond to antiarrhythmic drugs differently than other types of ventricular arrhythmias. Studies designed to determine the mechanism of this arrhythmia can be best accomplished in animal models since electrical recordings can be readily obtained from all regions of the ventricle and a variety of experimental interventions can be done which cannot be done in humans. With this in mind we have developed a canine model of this arrhythmia (40, 41).

In initial experiments we investigated whether prolonged periods of ventricular tachycardia could be induced by premature ventricular depolarizations in dogs with infarcts caused by permanent ligation of the left anterior descending coronary artery (LAD) 10–15 mm from its origin by the method described by Harris (7). Pentipolar plaque electrodes were sutured to the left atrial appendage (for recording an atrial electrogram) and to the anterior surface of the right ventricle near the right ventricular outflow tract (for stimulating the ventricles). The chest was then closed and during the closure 2 circular silver electrodes with a diameter of 2.5 mm were sutured subcutaneously, one on the dorsal and one on the

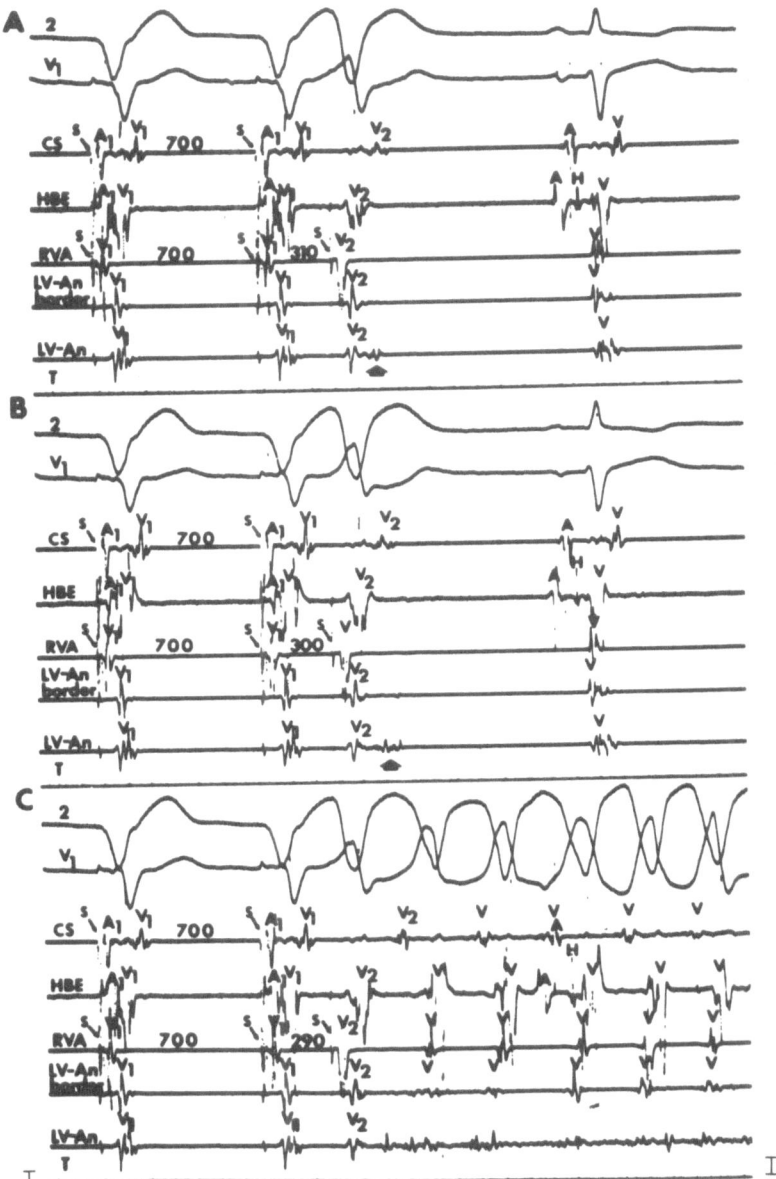

Figure 8. Initiation of ventricular tachycardia by premature ventricular stimulation in a patient with a ventricular aneurysm. In each panel is shown from top to bottom electrocardiographic leads 2 and V_1; electrogram from the coronary sinus (CS), His bundle recording site (HBE), right ventricular apex (RVA), the border of a left ventricular aneurysm (LV-An) and, the endocardial surface of the aneurysm (LV-AN) and time lines T at 10 msec intervals. The ventricles and atria were paced at a basic cycle length of 700 msec (A_1, V_1) and after every eighth paced complex premature ventricular stimuli were applied at progressively shorter coupling intervals to the basic drive (V_2). In A and B ventricular extrastimuli delivered at coupling intervals of 310 and 300 msec respectively did not induce tachycardia even though fractionation of the electrogram recorded from the aneurysm occurred. At a critical coupling interval of 290 msec (C) fractionation of the electrogram in the aneurysm spanned diastole and ventricular tachycardia ensued. (Reproduced from 47.)

ventral aspect of the thorax for recording the electrocardiogram. The dogs were then permitted to recover from the anesthesia. All the surviving dogs developed spontaneous ventricular arrhythmias 24–48 hours following surgery which subsided by the second or third
day. Beginning on day 2 (48 hours postoperatively) and on each of 7 subsequent days the
animals were studied in a conscious state while standing in a sling. The ventricles were
driven at cycle lengths of 400, 350 and 300 msec. After each 12 regularly driven impulses, a
single premature stimulus was applied to the ventricle. Premature impulses were also induced during sinus rhythm. The interval between the last driven impulse and the induced
premature impulse was shortened gradually until the ventricle no longer responded to the
premature stimulus. In the dogs with permanent coronary artery occlusion stimulated,
single premature ventricular depolarizations most often induced single or multiple (2–10)
non-driven ventricular depolarizations which followed the stimulated ventricular depolarizations with short coupling intervals (Figure 9). Such repetitive activity could be induced on each of 5 days after the time of coronary occlusion and could not be induced thereafter. Long periods of induced tachycardia rarely occurred. In only 2 of 10 animals was sustained ventricular tachycardia, which lasted more than several minutes, induced. The results, therefore, indicate that long periods of ventricular tachycardia cannot easily be induced by premature depolarizations in hearts with anteroseptal infarcts caused by permanent
occlusion of the LAD.

Since the anatomy of an infarct may determine, at least partly, the types of arrhythmias
which occur after infarction we did a second series of experiments in dogs with infarcts with
a different structure. The infarcts caused by permanent occlusion of the LAD described
above involved the anterior septum, and anterior free wall. They involved at least the inner
two-thirds of the ventricular wall in most animals and in 2 dogs were transmural. On the
endocardial surface 2–4 layers of intact subendocardial Purkinje fibers were found (20–25).
The infarcted myocardium was homogeneous and all muscle cells within the borders of the
infarct were necrotic or replaced by fibroblasts (depending on the age of the infarct when
it was examined) (41). To alter the structure of this infarct we occluded the LAD 10–15 mm
from its origin for two hours and then released the occlusion, allowing reperfusion of the
ischemic region. The two hour period of occlusion was sufficiently long to cause death of
some myocardial cells (42). However, since in the dog all myocardial cells in an ischemic
region do not die immediately and simultaneously after a coronary artery occlusion, but
rather, cell death continues for at least several hours (43, 44), reperfusion was able to
salvage or prevent death of some ischemic myocardium (45, 46). This resulted in a hetero-
geneous infarct (Figure 10). These infarcts extended over the same area of the left ventricle
as the infarcts produced by permanent occlusion but unlike infarcts caused by permanent
coronary artery occlusion, regions of non-infarcted myocardium were found throughout
the infarct. These regions of non-infarcted myocardium either appeared completely sur-
rounded by infarcted myocardium or were continuous with non-infarcted myocardium
bordering the infarct (Figure 10). On the endocardial surface of reperfused infarcts two to
four layers of subendocardial Purkinje fibers and an additional 5-15 layers of ventricular
muscle cells were intact and presumably viable.

Dogs with reperfused infarcts were instrumented in exactly the same way as the dogs

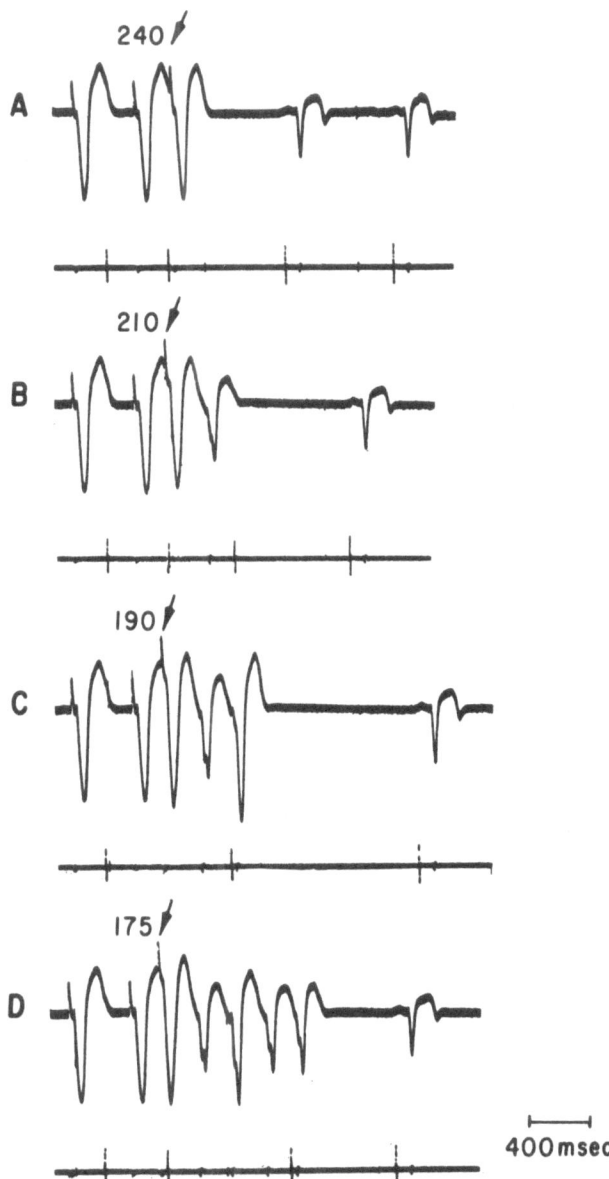

Figure 9. Effects of ventricular stimulation on ventricular rhythm of a dog, 3 days after permanent coronary artery occlusion. In each panel the upper trace is the ECG and the lower trace is an atrial electrogram. The ventricles are being driven at a cycle length of 400 msec; in A, a stimulated ventricular premature impulse (arrow) at a coupling interval of 240 msec is followed by a pause and then by sinus rhythm. In B, the coupling interval of the premature impulse is 210 msec. This is followed by a single nonstimulated ventricular depolarization and then sinus rhythm. In C, the coupling interval of the premature impulse is 190 msec (arrow); this is followed by 2 nonstimulated ventricular depolarizations. In D, the coupling interval of the stimulated premature impulse is 175 msec (arrow) and this is followed by 4 nonstimulated depolarizations. (Reproduced from 41.)

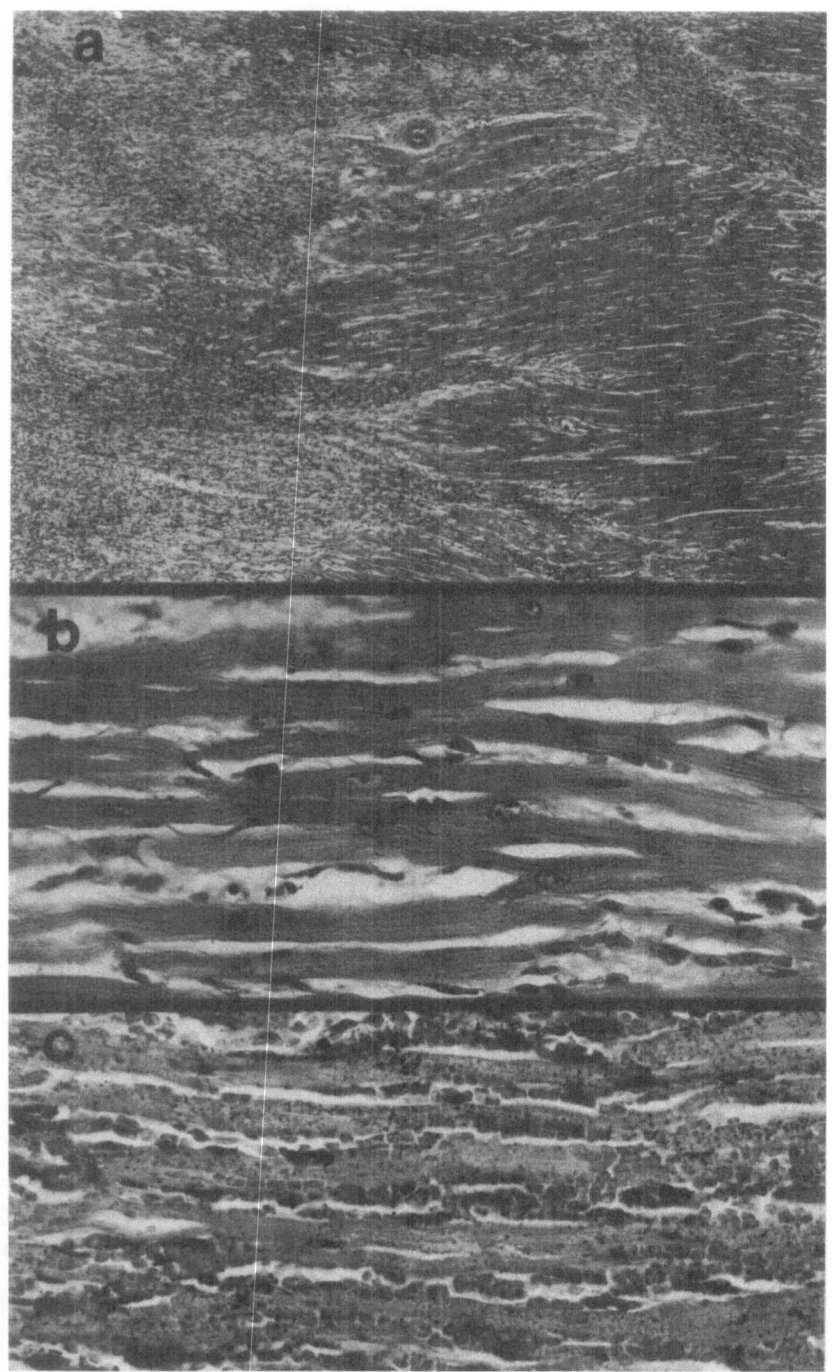

Figure 10. Photomicrographs of infarct caused by a 2 hour period of LAD occlusion followed by reperfusion. In a, (×100) 5 days after occlusion the infarct contains numerous groupings of apparently intact muscle fibers. These muscle fibers surviving in the infarct are shown at higher power (×750) in b. Normal, centrally located nuclei are apparent and cross striations are well defined. Panel c shows at the same magnification (×750) the appearance of necrotic muscle fibers in the infarct. They are hyalinized, nuclei are eccentrically located and cross striations are not plainly evident.

with infarcts caused by permanent occlusion, allowed to recover from surgery and were studied over a 9 day period following surgery while awake and standing in a sling. Ventricular arrhythmias similar to those which occur in dogs after permanent coronary occlusion occurred spontaneously during the first 24 hours after surgery. Beginning on the second day after coronary occlusion (when few arrhythmias appeared spontaneously) premature stimuli were applied to the ventricles as described above for the dogs with permanent occlusion. Premature ventricular stimuli did not induce repetitive responses on the second day. On the third day, as the stimulated premature ventricular depolarizations were induced progressively earlier in the ventricular cycle a coupling interval was reached in most dogs at which one to eight successive non-driven ventricular depolarizations followed the stimulated ventricular depolarization prior to the resumption of sinus rhythm (Figure 11). The longest coupled stimulated premature depolarizations which induced these repetitive responses invariably occurred on the descending limb of the T wave of the preceding regularly driven ventricular depolarization. As the premature stimulus was evoked still earlier in the cycle the number of non-stimulated ventricular depolarizations which followed increased until at a critical coupling interval a protracted ventricular tachycardia was initiated in each dog (Figure 11). Tachycardias had a uniform QRS morphology and a uniform cycle length which ranged from 270 to 160 msec in the different animals. The protracted tachycardias had a mean duration of greater than 15 minutes and could be induced numerous times in each animal. Premature stimuli which induced tachycardia occurred on the apex and the descending limb of the T wave.

Protracted ventricular tachycardia induced by premature stimuli either terminated spontaneously or could be terminated by electrical stimuli applied to the ventricles. Different patterns of spontaneous termination were observed including; 1) termination with no prior change in the tachycardia cycle length or QRS morphology, 2) termination following lengthening of the last several cycles of tachycardia, 3) termination following a spontaneous single premature depolarization with a different QRS morphology than that of the tachycardia, 4) termination following a change in the QRS morphology and lengthening of the last several cycles of tachycardia. We also applied premature stimuli to the ventricles during tachycardia. Fourteen of 17 periods of tachycardia in 5 dogs were terminated by a single stimulus which induced a premature ventricular depolarization early in the tachycardia cycle. Although tachycardia most often terminated abruptly after the stimulus, in 3 instances tachycardia continued after the stimulus for 2–5 impulses but with a different QRS complex and shorter cycle length. Tachycardia then terminated (Figure 12). Induced premature impulses which occurred late in the tachycardia cycle and which did not terminate the tachycardia were followed by a ventricular depolarization with a fully compensatory cycle length. As the premature impulse was induced progressively ealier in the cardiac cycle it was still followed by a compensatory pause if the tachycardia was not terminated. In 4 instances tachycardia could not be terminated by a single premature ventricular depolarization no matter where it occurred in the tachycardia cycle. In these instances, two closely coupled premature impulses applied early in the cardiac cycle successfully terminated the tachycardia (Figure 13) (41).

In most of the dogs studied, tachycardia could also be induced by single premature sti-

84 KARAGUEUZIAN, WIT

REPERFUSED INFARCT

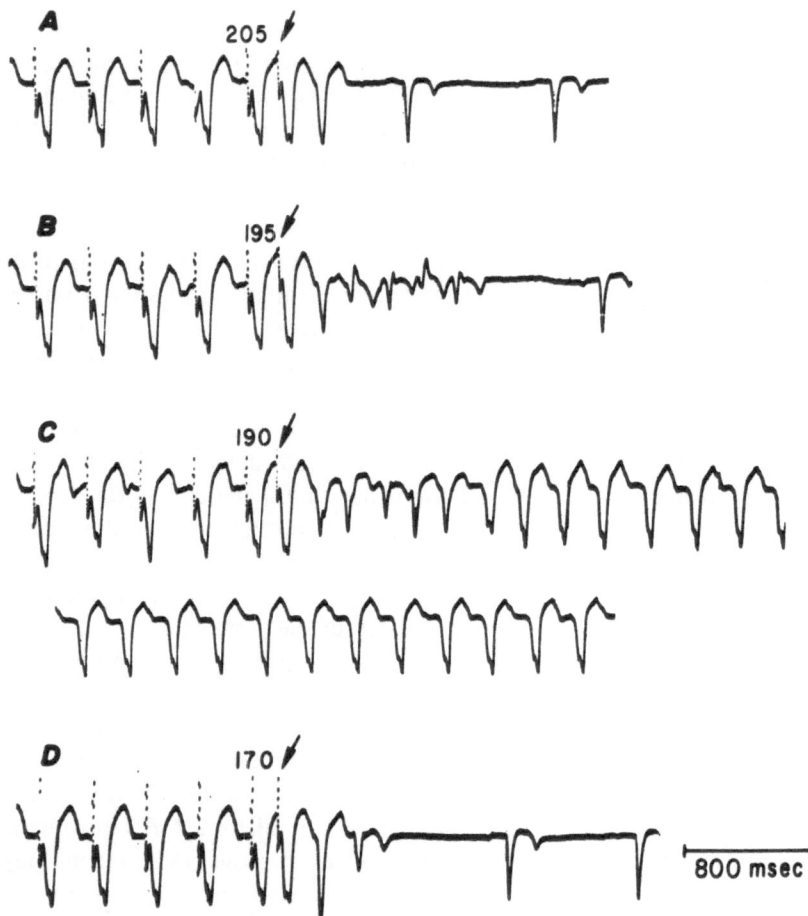

Figure 11. Initiation of protracted ventricular tachycardia in a representative dog on the 3rd day of reperfusion. The ECG is shown in each panel. In panels A-D the ventricles are being driven at a cycle length of 350 msec and a single premature stimulus (arrow) is applied to the ventricle, In Panel A, the coupling interval of the stimulated premature impulse is 205 msec. This is followed by a nondriven impulse. Sinus rhythm resumes after a pause of 390 msec. In Panel B, the coupling interval of the stimulated premature impulse is 195 msec; this is followed by five nondriven impulses. The QRS morphology and the cycle length of the nondriven impulses are variable. After a pause of 720 msec sinus rhythm reoccurs. In Panel C, the coupling interval of the stimulated premature impulse is 190 msec; this is followed by a long period of tachycardia which lasted for 10 min. The lower trace in Panel C shows the electrocardiogram 8 min after initiation of tachycardia. In Panel D, a single stimulated premature impulse induced at a coupling interval of 170 msec is followed by two nondriven impulses. Sinus rhythm occurs after a pause of 760 msec. (Reproduced from 41.)

muli applied to the ventricles on the fourth and fifth days after coronary occlusion. The characteristics of tachycardia were identical to the characteristics on the third day. After the fifth day tachycardia could no longer be induced. This time course of disappearance

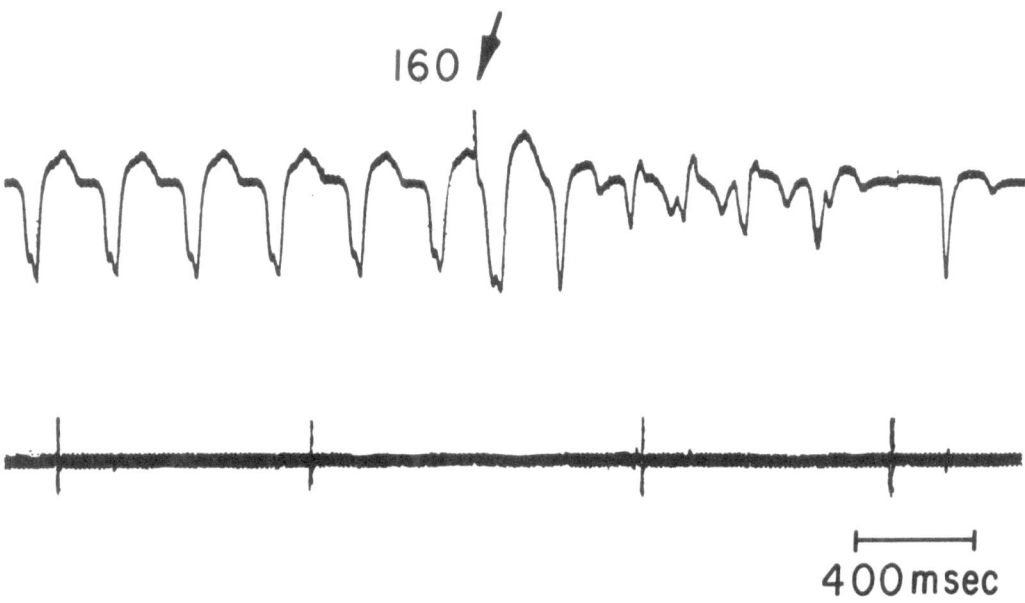

160

400 msec

Figure 12. Effects of ventricular stimulation on ventricular tachycardia induced in a dog 4 days after coronary artery occlusion and reperfusion. The top trace is the ECG and the lower trace is an atrial electrogram. The application of a single ventricular stimulus (arrow) at a coupling interval of 160 msec changes the unifocal tachycardia with a stable cycle length of 275 msec to a multiformed more rapid tachycardia with variable cycle lengths of 186–248 msec. This lasts for one second (5 impulses). Thereafter sinus rhythm ensues.

represents a major difference between the tachycardia in the dog model and some of the tachycardias with similar characteristics in humans since in humans some tachycardias may occur for many months or years. However, it is also likely that in humans some tachycardias initiated by premature ventricular depolarizations do disappear by the end of the first week. Future studies on the canine model of ventricular tachycardia should elucidate the mechanisms responsible for this type of arrhythmia.

3. CONCLUSION

There is no animal model of ischemic heart disease, sudden death or myocardial infarction which is identical to the events occurring in humans. However, the failure to produce such a model for experimental studies in the laboratory should not be discouraging to either the laboratory or clinical investigator. Important information and an improved understanding of the mechanisms of some types of ischemic arrhythmias has resulted from laboratory studies. We have only outlined a few of these, more examples are to be found in other chapters in this book. Many important discoveries can be expected in the future.

REPERFUSED INFARCT

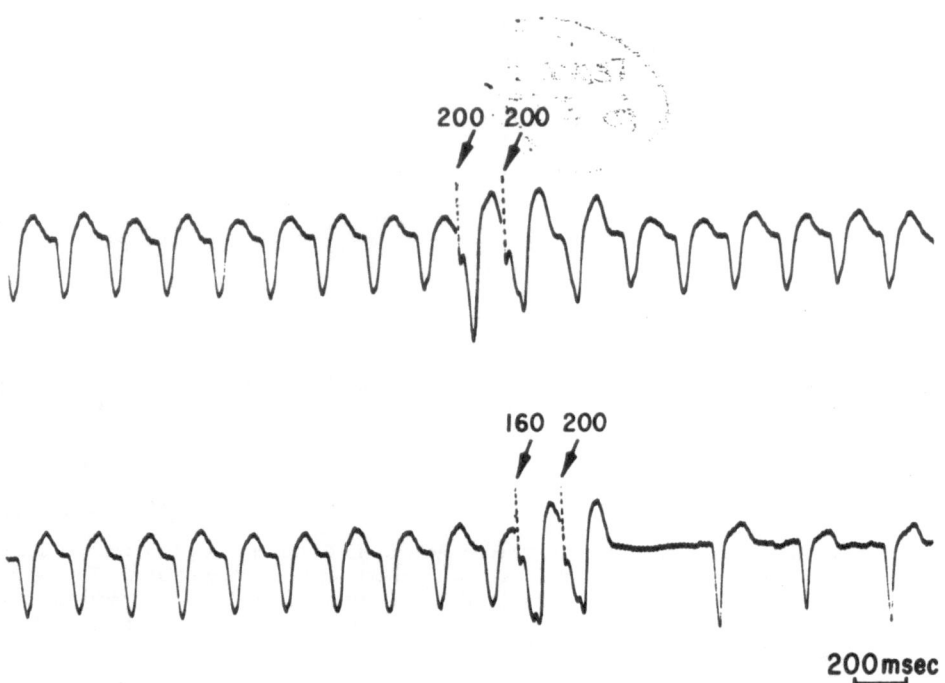

Figure 13. Effects of ventricular stimulation on cardiac rhythm during an established ventricular tachycardia in a dog 4 days after coronary artery occlusion and reperfusion. ECG records are shown in both panels. The upper panels show that application of 2 closely coupled stimuli (200 msec coupling interval) do not interrupt tachycardia when the first stimulated impulse occurs 200 msec after the tachycardia impulse. When the coupling interval of the first premature impulse was made shorter (160 msec) without changing the coupling interval of the second stimulus (lower trace) tachycardia was abruptly terminated. (Modified from 41.)

ACKNOWLEDGMENT

Studies by the authors described in this article were supported by U. S. Public Health Service Grant HL 12738 and NIH Training Grant GM 07182.

REFERENCES

1. Lown B: Sudden cardiac death: The major challenge confronting contemporary cardiology. Amer J. Cardio 43:313–328, 1979.
2. Reichenback DD, Moss NS and Meyer E: Pathology of the heart in sudden cardiac death. Am J Cardiology 39:865, 1977.
3. Fulton M, Julian DG, Oliver MF: Sudden death and myocardial infarction. Circulation 39–40 (suppl IV): IV–182–191, 1969.

4. Pantridge JF, Adgey AAJ: Prehospital coronary care: The mobile coronary care unit. Am J Cardiol 24:666–673, 1969.
5. Friedman M: The pathogenesis of coronary plaques, thromboses, and hemorrhages: An evaluative review. Circulation 51 and 52:III–34–40, 1975.
6. Spain DM: The pathogenesis of sudden cardiac death and the sequelae of myocardial infarction. In: The Heart (IAP Monograph no 15) edited by Edward JE, Lev M, Abell MR Baltimore, Williams and Wilkins 1974, p 67.
7. Harris AS: Delayed development of ventricular ectopic rhythms following experimental coronary occlusion. Circulation 1:1318, 1950.
8. Rosenfeld J, Rosen MR and Hoffman BF: Pharmacologic and behavioral effects of arrhythmias that immediately follow abrupt coronary occlusion: A canine model of sudden death. Am J Cardiol 41:1075–1082, 1978.
9. Schaper W: The collateral circulation of the heart. Amsterdam, North-Holland, 1971.
10. Harris AS and Rojas AG: The initiation of ventricular fibrillation due to coronary occlusion. Expt Med Surg 1:105, 1943.
11. Durrer D, Van Dam RT, Freud GE, Janse MJ: Reentry and ventricular arrhythmias in local ischemia and infarction of the intact dog heart. Proc K Med Acad Wet (Biol Med) 74:321, 1974.
12. Scherlag BJ, Helfant RH, Haft JI, Damato AN: Electrophysiology underlying ventricular arrhythmias due to coronary occlusion. Am J Physiol 219:665, 1970.
13. Waldo AL and Kaiser GA: Study of ventricular arrhythmias associated with acute myocardial infarction in the canine heart. Circulation 47:1222, 1973.
14. Boineau JP, Cox JL: Slow ventricular activation in acute myocardial infarction: A source of reentrant premature ventricular contraction. Circulation 43:702, 1973.
15. El-Sherif N, Scherlag BJ, Lazzara R: Reentrant ventricular arrhythmias in the late myocardial infarction period I. Conduction characteristics in the infarction zone. Circulation 55:686–702, 1977.
16. El-Sherif N, Hope RR, Scherlag BJ, Lazzara R: Reentrant ventricular arrhythmias in the late myocardial infarction period. II. Patterns of initiation and termination of reentry. Circulation 55:702–719, 1977.
17. Fontaine G, Guiraudon G, Frank R, Vedel J, Grosgogeat Y, Cabrol C and Facquet J: Stimulation studies and epicardial mapping in ventricular tachycardia; study of mechanisms and selection for surgery. In: Reentrant arrhythmias, Kulbertus (ed), MTP Press, Lancaster 1977, p 334.
18. Josephson ME, Horowitz LN and Farshidi A: Continuous local electrical activity: A mechanism of recurrent ventricular tachycardia. Circulation 57:659–665, 1978.
19. Bigger JT Jr, Dresdale RJ, Heissenbuttel RH, Weld FM and Wit AL: Ventricular arrhythmias in ischemic heart disease: Mechanism, prevalence, significance and management. Progr Cardiovasc Dis 19: 255–300, 1977.
20. Friedman PL, Stewart JR, Fenoglio JJ Jr and Wit AL: Survival of subendocardial Purkinje fibers after extensive myocardial infarction in dogs: In vitro and in vivo correlations. Circ Res 33:597–611, 1973.
21. Friedman PL, Stewart JR and Wit AL: Spontaneous and induced cardiac arrhythmias in subendocardial Purkinje fibers surviving extensive myocardial infarction in dogs. Circ Res 33:612–626, 1973.
22. Lazzara R, El-Sherif N, Scherlag BJ: Early and late effects of coronary artery occlusion on canine Purkinje fibers. Circ Res 35:391–399, 1974.
23. Scherlag BJ, El-Sherif N, Hope R, Lazzara R: Characterization and localization of ventricular arrhythmias resulting from myocardial ischemia and infarction. Circ Res 35:327–383, 1974.
24. Horrowitz LN, Spear JF, Moore EN: Subendocardial origin of ventricular arrhythmias in 24 hour old experimental myocardial infarction. Circulation 53:56–63, 1976.
25. Friedman PL, Fenoglio JJ Jr, Wit AL: Time course for reversal of electrophysiological and ultrastructural abnormalities in subendocardial Purkinje fibers surviving extensive myocardial infarction in dogs. Circ Res 36:127–144, 1975.
26. Fenoglio JJ Jr, Albala A, Silva FG, Friedman PL and Wit AL: Structural basis of ventricular arrhythmias in human myocardial infarction: A hypothesis. Human Path 7:547–563, 1976.
27. Spear JF, Horowitz LN, Hodess AB, Mac Vaugh H and Moore EN: Cellular electrophysiology of human myocardial infarction. I. Abnormalities of cellular activation. Circulation 59:247–256, 1979.
28. Wittig JH and Boineau JP: Surgical treatment of ventricular arrhythmias using epicardial, transmural and endocardial mapping. Ann Thor Surg. 20:117–126, 1975.
29. Wellens HJJ, Lie KI, Durrer D: Further observations on ventricular tachycardia as studied by electrical stimulation of the heart. Chronic recurrent ventricular tachycardia and ventricular tachycardia during acute myocardial infarction. Circulation 49:647–653, 1974.
30. Chahine RA, Raizner AE, Ishimori T, Luchi R and McIntosh HD: The incidence and clinical implications of coronary artery spasm. Circulation 52:972–978, 1975.

31. Tennant R, Wiggers CJ: The effect of coronary occlusion on myocardial contraction. Am J. Physiol 112:351–361, 1935.
32. Wellens HJJ, Duren DR, Lie KI: Observations on mechanisms of ventricular tachycardia in man. Circulation 54:237–244, 1976.
33. Wellens HJJ, Schuilenburg RM, Durrer D: Electrical stimulation of the heart in patients with ventricular tachycardia. Circulation 46:216–226, 1972.
34. Denes P, Wu D, Dhingra RC, Amat-y-Leon F, Wyndham C, Mautner RK, Rosen KM: Electrophysiological studies in patients with chronic recurrent ventricular tachycardia. Circulation 54: 229–236, 1976.
35. Josephson ME, Horowitz LN, Farshidi A, Spear JF, Kastor JA and Moore EN: Recurrent sustained ventricular tachycardia. 2. Endocardial mapping. Circulation 57:440–447, 1978.
36. Josephson ME, Horowitz LN, Farshidi A, Kastor JA: Recurrent sustained ventricular tachycardia. I. Mechanisms. Circulation 57:431–439, 1978.
37. Mines GR: On circulating excitations in heart muscles and their possible relation to tachycardia and fibrillation. Trans Roy Soc Can Ser 3 Sect IV 8:43–52, 1974.
38. Sasynuk BI and Mendez C: A mechanism for reentry in canine ventricular tissue. Circ Res 28:3–15, 1971.
39. Wit AL, Cranefield PF, Hoffman BF: Slow conduction and reentry in the ventricular conducting system. I. Return extrasystole in canine Purkinje fibers. Circ Res 30:1–10, 1972.
40. Karagueuzian HS, Fenoglio JJ, Hoffman BF, Wit AL: Sustained ventricular tachycardia induced by electrical stimulation after myocardial infarction; relation to infarct structure. Circulation 55 and 56 III–70, (abstract) 1977.
41. Karagueuzian HS, Fenoglio JJ Jr, Weiss MB and Wit AL: Protracted ventricular tachycardia induced by premature stimulation of the canine heart after coronary artery occlusion and reperfusion. Circ Res 44:833, 1979.
42. Maroko PR, Libby P, Ginks WR, Bloor CM, Shell WE, Sobel BE, Ross J Jr: Coronary artery reperfusion. I. Early effects on local myocardial function and the extent of myocardial necrosis. J Clin Invest 51:2710–2716, 1972.
43. Reimer KA, Louie JE, Rasmussen MM and Jennings RB: The wavefront phenomenon in ischemic cell death. I. Myocardial infarct size vs. duration of coronary occlusion in dogs. Circulation 56:786–794, 1977.
44. Fenoglio JJ Jr, Karagueuzian HS, Friedman PL, Albala A and Wit AL: Time course of infarct growth toward the endocardium after coronary occlusion. Am J Physiol 236:H356–H370, 1979.
45. Costantini C, Corday E, Lang T, Meerbaum S, Brasch J, Kaplan L, Rubins S, Gold H, Osher J: Revascularization after 3 hours of coronary arterial occlusion: Effects on regional cardiac metabolic function and infarct size. Am J Cardiol 36:368–384, 1975.
46. Balooki H: Myocardial revascularization after acute infarction. Am. J. Cardiol 36:395–406, 1975.
47. Josephson ME, Horowitz LN: Electrophysiologic approach to therapy of recurrent sustained ventricular tachycardia. Amer J Cardiol 43: 631–642, 1979.

2.2. VENTRICULAR ARRHYTHMIAS IN THE FIRST 15 MINUTES OF ACUTE REGIONAL MYOCARDIAL ISCHEMIA IN THE ISOLATED PIG HEART: POSSIBLE ROLE OF INJURY CURRENTS

M.J. JANSE, H. MORSINK, F.J.L. VAN CAPELLE, A.G. KLÉBER, F. WILMS-SCHOPMAN and D. DURRER

There is a great deal of experimental evidence suggesting that ventricular arrhythmias in myocardial infarction are due to reentry (1–5). Single premature beats, multiple premature beats, ventricular tachycardia and ventricular fibrillation could in principle all be caused by reentrant mechanisms. However, the precise pathways of excitation during such arrhythmias have not been completely delineated. Furthermore, programmed stimulation performed in patients with ventricular tachycardia during the first 24 hours of myocardial infarction revealed that the tachycardia could not be initiated by one, two or even three electrically induced premature beats, and it was suggested that at least some of the early arrhythmias might not be due to reentry but to some sort of automaticity (6).

It has long been known that rhythmic activity in Purkinje fibres can be produced, or, when present, enhanced, by a constant depolarizing current (7). Even in ordinary myocardium depolarizing currents can induce automatic activity (8, 9). Injury currents, flowing across the border between ischemic and non-ischemic cells might induce premature impulses in the non-ischemic tissue (10, 11). Such premature impulses could originate either in the normal myocardium close to the border, or in Purkinje cells which are in proximity to ischemic myocardium. These premature impulses could act as a trigger to set up reentrant activity and thus induce ventricular tachycardia or fibrillation.

The purpose of this paper is to describe experiments in which extracellular DC potentials were measured at multiple epicardial sites on the left ventricle following coronary artery occlusion. We attempted on the one hand to unravel the sequence of activation during spontaneous premature impulses and the initial phases of ventricular fibrillation, and on the other hand to estimate the strength of the injury current flowing across the border zone.

1. METHODS

Isolated hearts of pigs and dogs were perfused according to the Langendorff technique, using as perfusion medium a 1 : 1 mixture of blood and modified Tyrode solution containing dextran (12). Transmembrane potentials were recorded from the subepicardium of the left ventricle, using "floating" microelectrodes; as a reference another floating microelectrode was used, located in the extracellular space as close to the intracellular electrode as possible. Local DC extracellular electrograms were recorded by means of non-polarizable cotton wick electrodes. These potentials were recorded with reference to the DC potential of the aortic root.

For mapping experiments, electrode devices containing 60 of such cotton wick electrodes were used. This multiple electrode consisted of 60 glass microelectrodes, placed in parallel rows and embedded in dental cement. The interelectrode distance was 1.5 mm. The very tips of the microelectrodes were filed off, and a very thin cotton wick was introduced into each microelectrode, which was filled with isotonic saline. The shaft of each microelectrode was attached to a flexible, saline filled polyethylene tube. The saline was in contact with a chlorided silver wire, which was connected to a high impedance, low pass (cut off frequency 40 Hz) 60-channel amplifier, which measured each potential with respect to the reference potential obtained from a wick at the aortic root. The 60 signals, after an initial 20-fold amplification, were led into a high speed multiplexing A to D system. The slew rate of the system was 30 microseconds, and samples were taken every 8 msec and written into a circular buffer. An arbitrary channel was displayed on a Megatek graphic display: when an event (beginning of ventricular fibrillation, or spontaneous premature beat) occurred, a button could be pushed so that the signals of the preceding 2 seconds were transferred to a high speed digital tape recorder. Analysis of the data was performed using the same PDP-11-34 computer by means of an interactive program, where the signals were displayed in groups of 5 on a Megatek graphic display and moments of activation could be indicated using a joy stick. Zero potentials were obtained from control signals, and DC-potential values could be obtained from signals recorded after coronary artery occlusion at any desired moment of the cardiac cycle.

The atrium was paced at cycle lengths varying in the different experiments from 450 to 500 msec; if desired, pacing rate could be increased.

Regional ischemia was produced by clamping the left anterior descending coronary artery (LAD) proximally. Firstly, a 2 min occlusion was performed to localize the border between cyanotic and normal myocardium. The multiple electrode was placed at that border on the epicardial surface, and the occlusion was released. After a suitable reperfusion period, occlusions were made for periods of 10 to 15 min. When no spontaneous ventricular fibrillation occurred within 8 minutes, the driving rate on the atrium was increased.

In a few experiments, intramural multi-electrode needles were inserted into the left ventricular wall, with the aim of recording extracellular activity from Purkinje tissue.

2. DISCUSSION OF RESULTS

2.1. Intracellular recordings

Figure 1 shows transmembrane potentials, and local DC-extracellular electrograms, recorded from an isolated dog heart. The straight line in the extracellular electrogram indicates the DC potential of the aortic root. Following occlusion of the left anterior descending coronary artery, resting membrane potential decreases, resulting in a depression of the TQ-segment in the extracellular electrogram. (If AC-coupled amplifiers had been used, this TQ depression would of course appear as ST segment elevation.) Action potential amplitude decreases, and upstroke velocity diminishes. After 5 min of occlusion, the moment of

dog heart

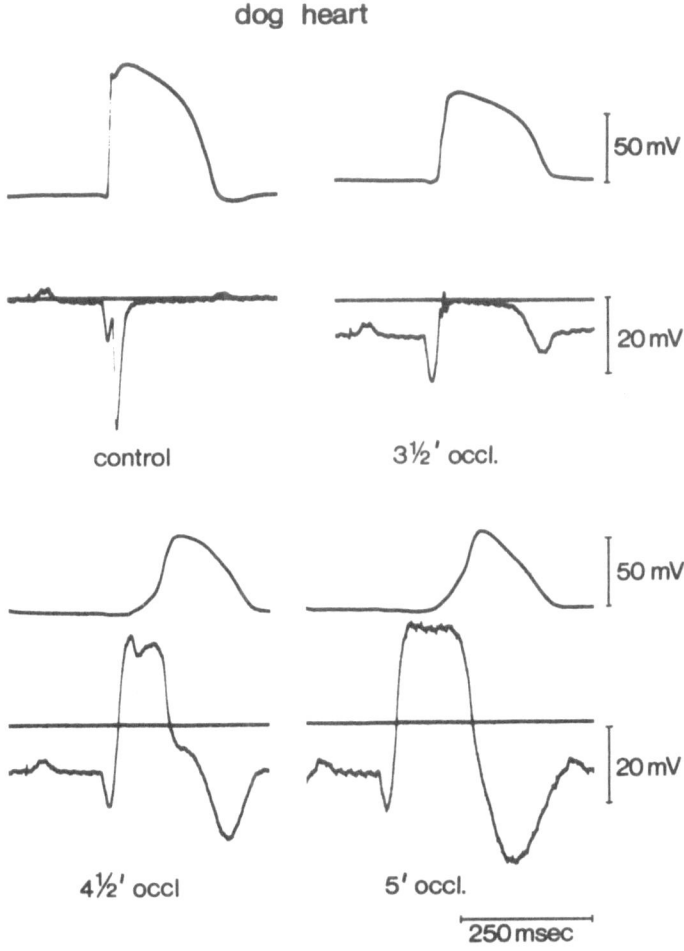

Figure 1. Transmembrane potentials (upper trace) and local DC-extracellular electrograms (lower trace) recorded from the subepicardium of the left ventricle of an isolated perfused dog heart before and after occlusion of the left anterior descending artery. The straight line in the extracellular electrograms is the DC potential level of the aortic root. Note loss of resting potential (resulting in depression of the TQ-segment) and loss of amplitude of action potential and decrease in upstroke velocity following coronary occlusion. The extreme delay in activation, and thus the delayed repolarization of the ischemic cell, causes the negative T wave in the extracellular electrogram (reproduced with permission from reference 13).

activation is extremely delayed (13). The relationship between changes in transmembrane potentials and changes in extracellular potentials becomes clear when the complexes recorded before and after coronary artery occlusion are superimposed, as is done in Figure 2 (14). The potential gradient between the intracellular compartments of ischemic and normal cells, at any moment of the cardiac cycle, determines the flow of current between ischemic and normal cells. For example, in diastole the intracellular potential of the ischemic cells is more positive than that of non-ischemic cells, and thus an intracellular current will flow

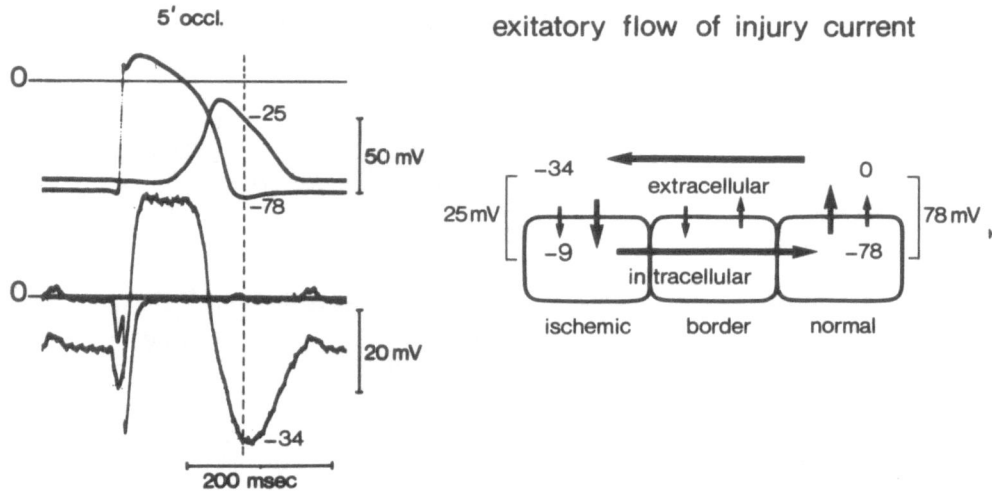

Figure 2. Transmembrane potentials and extracellular complexes from the control situation and after 5 min of coronary artery occlusion are superimposed. Schematic diagram depicts flow of intra-and extracellular currents at the moment indicated by the dotted line. See text for discussion (reproduced with permission from reference 14).

from ischemic towards normal cells. This current crosses the cell membranes, and flows in the extracellular space in the opposite direction, thus resulting in a negative extracellular potential in the ischemic region (depression of the TQ-segment). In one particular situation, illustrated in Figure 2, this injury current may be arrhythmogenic. Because of the extreme delay in activation of the ischemic cell (related to the smaller action potential amplitude and low upstroke velocity), peak depolarization occurs at a time when the normal cells have repolarized and regained their excitability. At that moment (indicated by the dotted line), an intracellular current flows towards the normal cells which will tend to depolarize these cells. When this current is strong enough to depolarize the normal cells in the border zone to threshold, a premature impulse will be elicited. The situation where this may occur can be recognized from the extracellular electrogram from the ischemic area by a pronounced negative T wave.

2.2. Estimation of the strength of the injury current

The principle according to which the strength of the injury current was estimated is outlined in Figure 3. Our mapping experiments provided measurements of the extracellular DC-potential of sites, located in a grid with a distance of 1.5 mm between sampling points. At any desired moment of the cardiac cycle, isopotential maps of the area under the electrode grid could be made. In Figure 3, 5 points of the grid are indicated with their respective potentials. One unit of current flows towards the central point, whereas 3 units of current flow away from this central point. This means that at the central point 2 units of current are

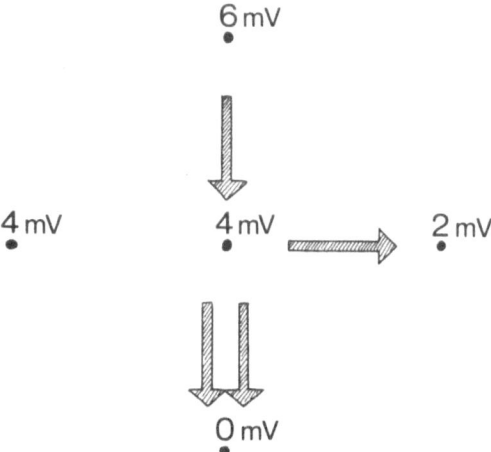

Figure 3. Five points within a grid on the epicardial surface are shown with their DC-potentials, measured with respect to the reference potential of the aortic root. One unit of current flows towards the central point, three units flow away from it. Thus 2 units of current are generated at the central point. See text for the biological significance of such a current source.

generated: the central point is a current source. Two biological explanations can be given for this phenomenon:

1) a transmembrane current flows locally between intra- and extracellular space,
2) an extracellular current flows from deeper intramural layers towards the epicardial surface.

We have shown (11) that in the pig heart no important transmural potential gradients exist during acute ischemia, and therefore this current source represents a site where transmembrane current flows.

To determine the source current (transmembrane current flowing out of the cell) or sink current (transmembrane current flowing into the cell) at a particular site C, we used the potential values of the 8 surrounding sites:

$$
\begin{array}{ccc}
B_1 & A_1 & B_2 \\
A_2 & C & A_3 \\
B_3 & A_4 & B_4
\end{array}
$$

The source current:

$$
i = - \frac{4 \sum_{k=1}^{4} V(A_k) + \sum_{k=1}^{4} V(B_k) - 20V(C)}{6 \rho L^2} \ A/m^3
$$

in which V is the DC potential at each site, ρ is the specific resistance of the tissue, L is the distance between sampling points and 6 is a geometrical factor. When V is given in mV, ρ

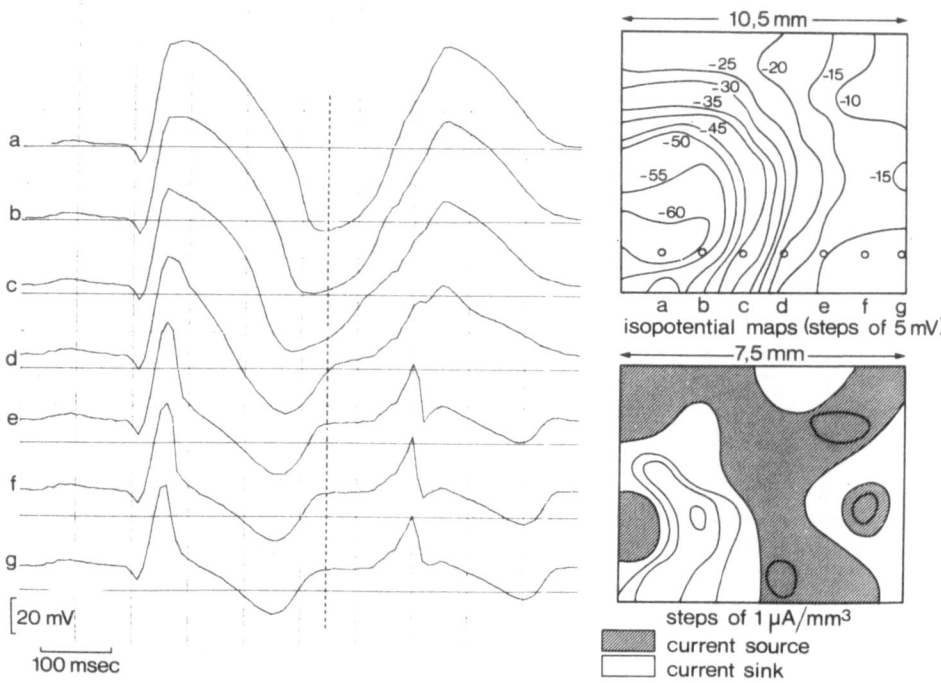

Figure 4. Left panel: 7 DC-extracellular electrograms, as they are printed out by the computer system, recorded from sites a to g 1.5 mm apart, located in a row and extending from central ischemic area (top) towards the ischemic border (bottom) of an isolated pig's heart. A basic beat, propagated from the atrium, and a spontaneous premature beat are shown, which occurred 5 min after coronary artery occlusion.

Right panel, top: Isopotential map of the area under the 60-terminal electrode device at the moment indicated by the dotted line in the extracellular potentials. Lines indicate 5 mV steps. Note large extracellular potential gradients, in the order of 40 mV over distances of 3 mm, present during the negative T wave in the central ischemic zone.

Right panel, bottom: Distribution of current sources and current sinks, representing sites where transmembrane current flows, expressed in $\mu A/mm^3$ tissue. Lines indicated steps of $1\mu A/mm^3$. Since source and sink currents cannot be calculated for sites at the border of the area recorded from, this map is smaller than the isopotential map.

is chosen to be 4Ω m, and L is 1.5 mm, the denominator will be 54, and the current is expressed in microA/mm³.

Spontaneous premature impulses occurred in 15 out of a total of 20 occlusions, between 2.5 and 5 min after LAD occlusion in the isolated pig heart. Most of these premature beats occurred right after a pronounced negative potential recorded from the ischemic area. Figure 4 shows an example. Seven extracellular complexes are shown, recorded from sites 1.5 mm apart in a row which extends from the central ischemic area (top) towards the border zone (bottom). The isopotential map of the area under the 60 electrodes during the negative T wave of the basic beat (dotted line) is shown on the right (top). The map indicating the distribution of current sources and sinks at that moment is shown as well. (The area in this map is smaller than that of the isopotential map because current sources and sinks cannot be calculated for sites which are on the edges of the electrode grid)

The maximal strength of the current sources present during such a negative T wave was in our experiments in the order of 2 to 4 microA/mm^3. The current density in the extracellular space:

$$j = - \frac{\Delta V}{\rho}$$

was for example for a voltage gradient of 39 mV over a distance of 3 mm (such as exists in Figure 4), at a resistivity of 4Ω m:

$$j = \tfrac{13}{4}\,A/m^2, \text{ which is about 3 microA/mm}^2.$$

What do such values mean? A source current of 4 microA/mm^3 tissue could be compared to:

1) stimulation via an intracellular microelectrode, when the space constant of the tissue is in the order of 1 mm, with a current of 4 microA (all current flows through the cell membranes),

2) stimulation with an extracellular electrode with a surface of 1 mm^2 with a current of circa 20 microA, assuming that 1/5th of the current flows through the membrane, and 4/5ths leak away through the extracellular space.

It must be said that the current sources are a second difference quotient of the measured potential values, and are therefore more sensitive to noise. Thus, absolute values should be regarded with some caution. Nevertheless, it would seem that the injury currents can be strong enough to reexcite normal myocardial fibers at the end of their refractory period. Anderson et al. reported in an abstract injury currents of similar magnitude (15).

As already mentioned, injury currents could in principle, by depolarizing either Purkinje cells or myocardial cells, induce repetitive discharges. Trautwein and Kassebaum (7) mentioned that the current needed to produce repetitive discharges in Purkinje fibres was 1.7 to 5 times that necessary for a single response. From Katzung's data (16) it is also evident that the current needed to induce repetitive responses in papillary muscle is more than that required for a single response. It would seem therefore that re-excitation at the end of the refractory period (myocardium) or in the supernormal phase of excitability (Purkinje cells) is more likely to occur as a consequence of the flow of injury current than repetitive responses.

2.3. Site of origin of premature impulses

Activation maps made during spontaneous premature beats showed that the site of origin was the normal tissue in the border zone. In some instances, however, the activation pattern was compatible with a deeper intramural layer being the site of origin (see Figure 5). In the pig's heart it is very difficult to decide from activation maps whether the site of origin is myocardial or Purkinje tissue for the following reason: Contrary to the situation in the human heart or the dog heart, in the pig the Purkinje cells are distributed throughout the ventricular wall and almost reach the epicardium (17, 18). Therefore, an epicardial site of origin of an ectopic beat does not rule out the Purkinje system, as it would in the dog or in the human heart.

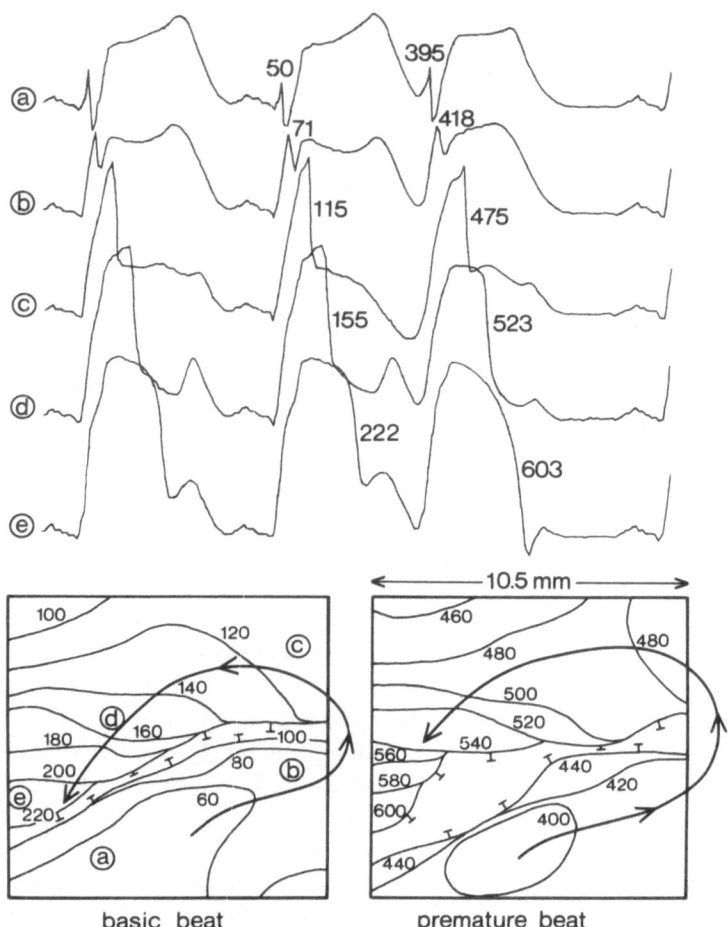

Figure 5. Activation pattern of basic beat and spontaneous premature beat, 6 min after coronary artery occlusion. In the top half, DC electrograms are shown from sites a to e, as indicated in the activation map of the basic beat. Numbers indicate moment of activation in msec relative to an arbitrary time zero. The activation pattern of the basic beat shows an attempt to complete a circus movement. During the premature beat, a circumscript epicardial area is activated earliest, which might indicate a site of origin in deeper intramural layers. Again there is an unsuccessful attempt to complete a reentrant circuit.

Figure 6 shows recordings made with an intramural electrode needle inserted in the left ventricular wall of an isolated pig heart. Extracellular potentials from the Purkinje system were recorded from the subendocardium (arrows). It is evident that in the two premature impulses shown, the Purkinje spike precedes the myocardial deflections, especially in the upper recording. Although no mapping was performed in this experiment, it can be concluded that the Purkinje system can very well be the site of origin of premature impulses in the acute phase of myocardial ischemia.

There are several reasons why injury currents could re-excite Purkinje fibres more easily than myocardial fibres. It is known that stimulation thresholds, both when determined by

circa 5 min occl. 2 different VPB 's

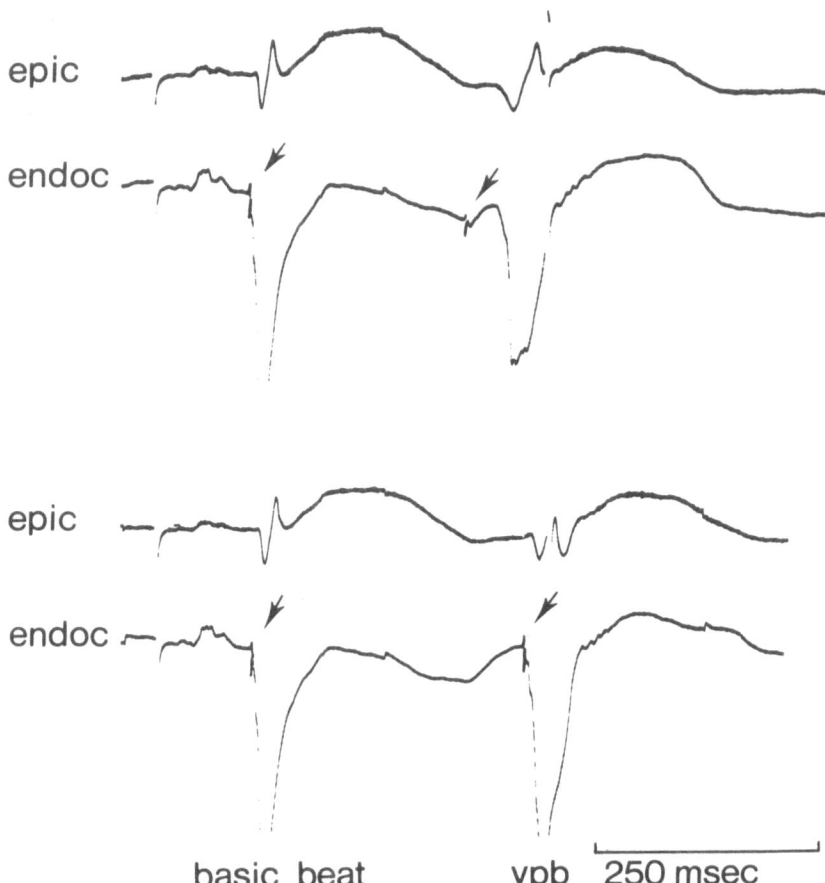

epic

endoc

epic

endoc

basic beat   vpb 250 msec

Figure 6. Recordings from an intramural electrode needle inserted into the left ventricular wall of an isolated pig's heart, 5 min after occlusion of the left anterior descending artery. In the subendocardial recordings, Purkinje spikes are visible. In both premature impulses, recorded 20 seconds apart, the Purkinje activity precedes myocardial activity.

extracellular stimulation (19) and by intracellular stimulation (20), are lower for Purkinje fibres than for myocardial cells. Also, in Purkinje fibres a well defined supernormal phase of excitability exists which is not present in myocardial fibres (21). Finally, the funnel shaped geometry of the Purkinje-muscle junction favours a "concentration" of current flowing between myocardium and Purkinje cells.

2.4. Ventricular fibrillation

Ventricular fibrillation occurred in our experiments in three different ways.

1) In the 15 occlusions where spontaneous premature beats occurred, they initiated ventricular fibrillation in 8.

2) In the 12 occlusions where no ventricular fibrillation had occurred within 7 minutes, the driving rate on the atrium was increased, which in 4 occlusions resulted in VF.

3) In those occlusions where no VF occurred, or when defibrillation was successful, the occlusion was released after 10 to 15 minutes while the heart was following the regular atrial drive. VF occurred in 9 out of 14 reperfusions.

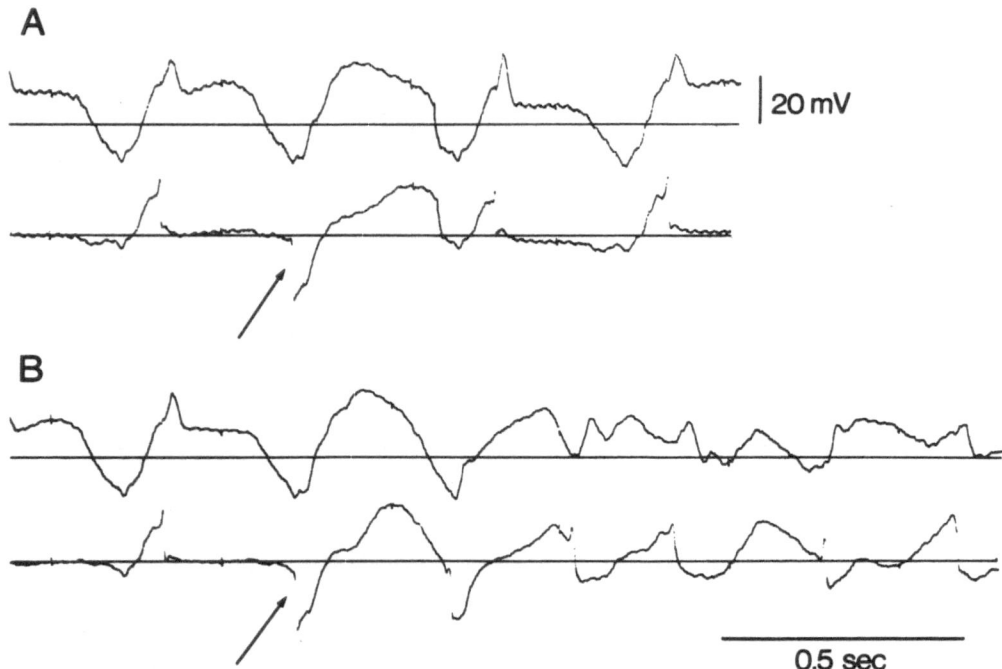

Figure 7. Two DC electrograms from sites 4 mm apart in an isolated pig's heart. As indicated by the shifts in TQ- and ST-segments in the first complexes of panels A and B, representing a propagated impulse from the atrium, the upper signal is from ischemic myocardium. The lower complex has isoelectric TQ and ST segments and represents activity from non-ischemic myocardium. A premature impulse originates from this normal myocardium at the ischemic border zone (arrow) at the time the ischemic complex shows a negative T wave. In panel A, the heart continues to follow the basic atrial drive. In panel B, recorded 10 sec later, a nearly identical premature beat initiates ventricular fibrillation. As discussed in the text, the premature beat may be due to re-excitation by currents of injury across the border zone of the ischemic area, which in its turn triggers reentrant activity resulting in fibrillation (reproduced with permission from reference 22).

In no instance could the activation sequence be mapped in such detail that the site of origin and mechanism of the ectopic activity were unambiguously clear. Yet some pieces of the puzzle emerged.

Figure 7 shows 2 DC extracellular electrograms from sites 4 mm apart (22). The upper complex is from ischemic tissue, as is evident from the TQ segment depression, the elevated ST segment and the small, late intrinsic deflection. The lower complex shows isoelectric

TQ- and ST-segments at the same potential level as the reference potential from the aortic root indicated by the straight line. Its intrinsic deflection is large, fast and early. It represents activity from non-ischemic myocardium. Both in panel A and B, recorded 10 seconds later, a premature impulse occurs in exactly the same way: during the negative T wave of the ischemic complex a large intrinsic deflection without preceding r wave is inscribed at the normal complex. In A, this premature beat is followed by normally driven complexes. In B it initiates ventricular fibrillation. Our working hypothesis is that the premature beat is initiated by injury currents. By its prematurity, this beat increases the differences in conduction velocity and refractory periods of ischemic and non-ischemic tissue in the border zone, and creates the conditions where micro-reentry can become manifest. It is probable that minute differences in the way the premature beat is conducted may decide whether or not reentry succeeds. Very often, we found reentrant patterns of activation where the full circle was not completed (see for example Figure 5).

Wit et al. (23) and El-Sherif and colleagues (3, 24) have emphasized the role of changes in heart rate in eliciting reentrant arrhythmias, particularly in the late infarction period (3, 24). Figure 8 shows that an increase in heart rate increases the inhomogeneity within the acutely

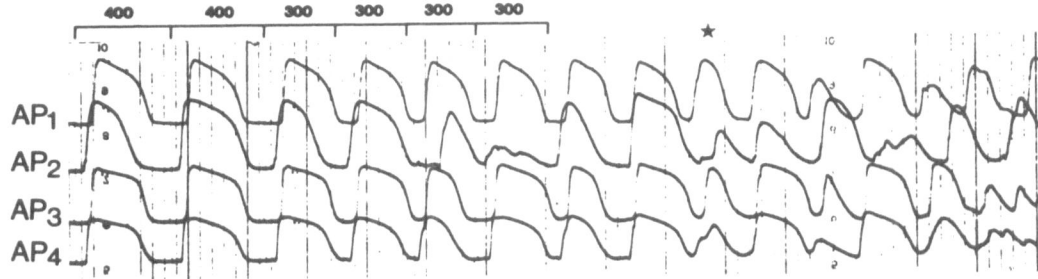

Figure 8. Four simultaneously recorded transmembrane potentials from the ischemic subepicardium of an isolated pig heart. When the atrium is driven at a cycle length of 400 msec, activation of the 4 ischemic cells is fairly synchronous. When cycle length is decreased to 300 msec, this synchronicity is lost. Activation of cell 2 is delayed and even blocked, and eventually the heart is fibrillating (reproduced with permission from reference 13).

ischemic region. Four transmembrane action potentials are shown, simultaneously recorded from the ischemic myocardium in area of about $1\frac{1}{2}$ cm^2. The atrium was driven at a regular rate with a cycle length of 400 msec and the four sites recorded from are fairly synchronously activated. When cycle length is decreased to 300 msec, this synchronicity is lost. Activation of cell 2 is delayed (5th beat) and even blocked (6th beat) and eventually all synchronicity is lost and the heart is fibrillating.

Figure 9 shows activation maps of another experiment in which an increase in heart rate resulted in ventricular fibrillation. Beat a is the last ventricular activation due to normal propagation from the atrium. The 60-fold electrode was placed on the border between ischemic and normal myocardium, and for beats a to f, the activation pattern of the small area of about 1 cm^2 under the electrode is shown. For time zero the P wave of beat a was taken. Isochrones separating areas activated within the same 20 msec interval are drawn

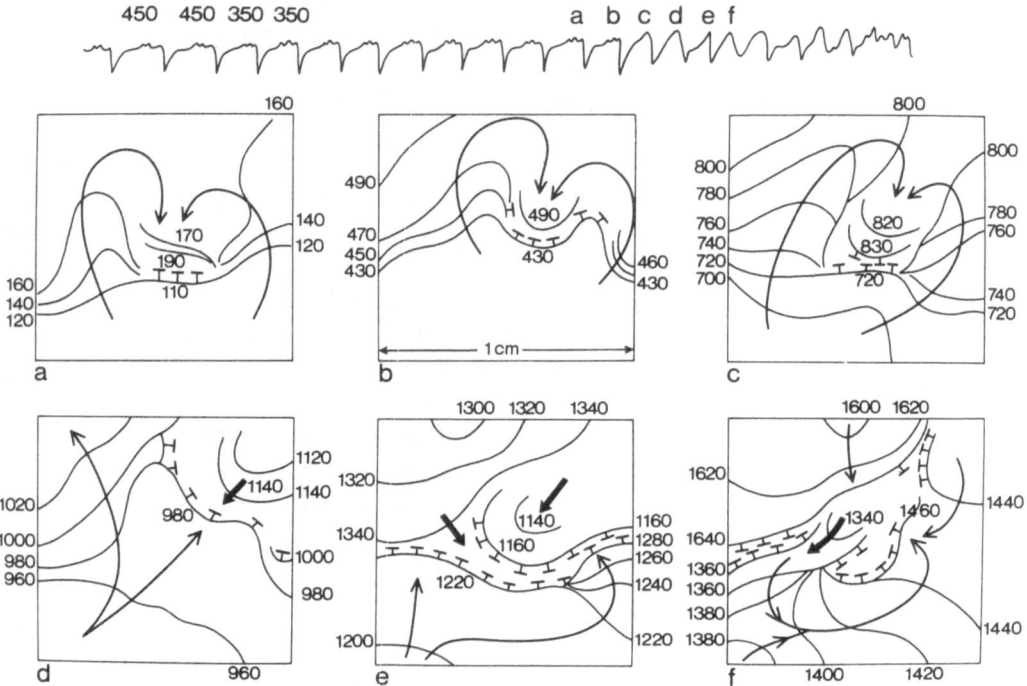

Figure 9. Initiation of ventricular fibrillation by an increase in atrial driving rate. Redrawn extracellular signal shows transition of propagated activity from atrium to ventricular fibrillation. Maps show activation pattern of the area of circa 1 cm² under the 60-fold electrode. Time zero is P wave of beat a. Note similarity in activation pattern between the last propagated beat a, and the first 2 ectopic beats b and c, indicating possibly an origin in the Purkinje system for beats b and c. From beat d on, continuous electrical activity is recorded from the area under the electrode. Reentry is present in the sense that areas of block are re-invaded; complete circus movements are however not present.

and arrows indicate different wave fronts. In beat a, the activation pattern shows already an attempted reentry: a central area of block is bypassed on both sides, and activity turns around the site of block towards the site of origin. However, the interval of 190–110 = 80 msec is evidently too short to overcome the refractory period of the tissue proximal to the site of block. It is in this respect noteworthy that refractory periods of ischemic cells are prolonged, while those of normal cells in the border zone are shortened (2). A similar activation pattern is present in beats b and c, both of which are ectopic activations. Site of origin and nature of these beats is not clear. Reentry could have occurred elsewhere, but it is also possible that the increase in driving rate led to an increased desynchrony between ischemic and normal cells so that repolarization of ischemic cells was delayed and injury currents flowing to already repolarized normal cells (Purkinje or myocardial) re-excited these. The fact that the activation pattern is similar to that of a propagated response from the atrium might be in favour of an origin in the Purkinje system.

From beat d on, continuous activity is recorded from the area under the electrode. This in itself does not prove reentry. Activity entering the ischemic zone at a rapid rate might be so delayed that the interval between successive activations is filled with activity, yet this activity may travel towards the centre of the ischemic zone and be blocked there, without returning to re-excite the border zone. In maps shown, no complete circus movements are seen, yet reentry is present in the sense that areas of conduction block are re-invaded. It is clear that multiple reentrant circuits, which do not have to be complete, must be present. For example, in beat e there are three different wave fronts, all of which may be offshoots from complete, or partly completed circus movements elsewhere. The wave front ending at 1340 msec continues in beat f and nearly completes a full circle before it gets blocked at 1460 msec. Activity propagating centrifugally from this incomplete circus movement may in adjacent areas find tissue where conduction block had occurred and which is now sufficiently recovered to be re-excited. Judging from the activation pattern in beat f, diameters of circus movements may be in the order of 5 mm. This is in the same range as the circus movement described by Allessie et al. in rabbit atrium (25). It must be realized that we only performed mapping at the epicardial surface and that true dimensions of complete circus movements may only be known when intramural activity is recorded as well.

Mapping performed following reperfusion revealed no striking differences between VF during coronary artery occlusion, and VF induced by reperfusion. The return of electrical activity in previously unresponsive cells (Figure 9) was frequently associated with delayed repolarization, and extracellular complexes with deep negative T waves. In the same way as during the first minutes following coronary artery occlusion, the injury currents associated with delayed repolarization could have elicited premature beats, which in their turn set up multiple reentry. The only difference between ventricular fibrillation following reperfusion with that during occlusion was that the interval between successive activations was

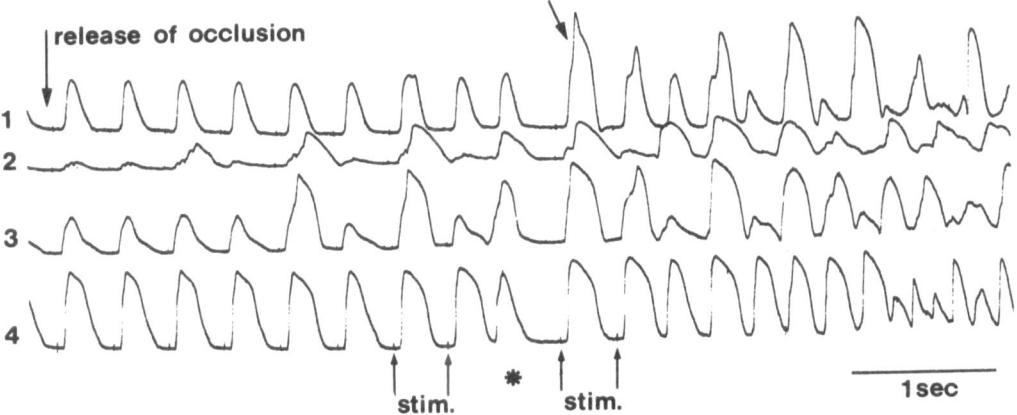

Figure 10. Four simultaneously recorded transmembrane potentials on release of a 6 min LAD occlusion. Within a few beats following reperfusion, cell 2 shows 2 : 1 responses and cell 3 shows alternation between large and small action potentials. Repolarization in cells 2 and 3 is delayed with respect to repolarization of cell 4, which is located in the border. A single premature beat occurs (asterisk) of unknown origin. Responses after the postextrasystolic pause are synchronized, thereafter alternation between cells 2 and 3 gets out of phase, and the activity of cells 1, 2 and 3 may be described as "local fibrillation" since the responses of cell 4 remain fairly regular for 7 beats, before it too participates in the fibrillation (reproduced with permission from reference 12).

much shorter in the reperfusion arrhythmias. Most likely this was related to the rapid recovery in electrical activity following release of the LAD occlusion in the ischemic region, and the shortening of refractory period (2).

In summary, we would like to suggest two mechanisms for ventricular arrhythmias in the acute phase of myocardial ischemia, i.e. the first 15 minutes following coronary artery occlusion. Single premature beats may be elicited by current of injury, re-exciting non-ischemic myocardium in the border zone or even more likely, Purkinje fibres which are in close proximity to ischemic myocardium. This re-excitation would occur when, primarily because of delayed activation within the ischemic zone, repolarization in the ischemic area outlasts repolarization in the normal zone. This situation can be recognized from the local extracellular electrogram from the ischemic area and is represented by a negative T wave (11). The premature impulse in its turn may set the stage for multiple micro reentry in the border zone including both ischemic and normal myocardium, and thus initiate ventricular fibrillation.

Many uncertainties still exist, and further mapping studies, combined with microelectrode recordings from Purkinje cells, will have to be performed before these hypotheses will be proved or disproved. The concept that non-ischemic cells, either Purkinje or myocardial, play an essential role in eliciting the fatal arrhythmias in the hyperacute phase of myocardial infarction is worthy of further study. If true, new possibilities for drug treatment may be opened since obviously non-ischemic cells would be an easier target for drugs than ischemic cells.

Finally, it is by no means to be excluded that reentry itself may be responsible for premature beats. As shown in Figure 5, the pattern of activation of basic beats often show attempted reentry. Certainly, instances may occur, for example when heart rate is increased, when such reentry will be completed and give rise to premature impulses.

REFERENCES

1. Durrer D, van Dam RTh, Freud GE, Janse MJ: Re-entry and ventricular arrhythmias in local ischemia and infarction in the intact dog heart. Proc K Ned Akad Wet (Biol Med) 74:321–334, 1971.
2. Janse MJ, Downar E: The effect of acute ischaemia on transmembrane potentials in the intact heart. Relation to re-entrant mechanisms. In : Re-entrant arrhythmias. Kulbertus HE (ed), MTP Press Lancaster, 1977, p 195–209.
3. El-Sherif N, Scherlag BJ, Lazzara R, Hope RR: Re-entrant ventricular arrhythmias in the late myocardial infarction period: 1. Conduction characteristics in the infarction zone. Circulation 55:686–702, 1977.
4. Boineau JP, Cox JL: Slow ventricular activation in acute myocardial infarction. A source of re-entrant premature ventricular contraction. Circulation 48:702–713, 1973.
5. Waldo AL, Kaiser GA: A study of ventricular arrhythmias associated with acute myocardial infarction in the canine heart. Circulation 47:1222–1228, 1973.
6. Wellens HJJ, Lie KI, Durrer D: Further observation on ventricular tachycardia as studied by electrical stimulation of the heart. Circulation 49:647–653, 1974.
7. Trautwein W, Kassebaum DG: On the mechanism of spontaneous impulse generation in the pacemaker of the heart. J Gen Physiol 45:317–330, 1961.
8. Katzung BG, Hondeghem LM, Grant AO: Cardiac ventricular automaticity induced by current of injury. Pfluegers Arch 360:193–197, 1975.
9. Imanishi S, Surawicz B: Automatic activity in depolarized guinea pig ventricular myocardium. Characteristics

and mechanisms. Circ Res 39:751–759, 1976.

10. Cranefield PF: The conduction of the cardiac impulse. New York, Futura Publishing Company, Mount Kisco, 1975, p 278.

11. Kléber AG, Janse MJ, van Capelle FJL, Durrer D: Mechanisms and time course of S-T- and T-Q-segment changes during acute regional myocardial ischemia in the pig's heart determined by extracellular and intracellular recordings. Circ Res 42:603–613, 1978.

12. Downar E, Janse MJ, Durrer D: The effect of coronary artery occlusion on subepicardial transmembrane potentials in the intact porcine heart. Circulation 56:217–224, 1977.

13. Janse MJ, Kléber AG, Downar E, Durrer D: Changements électrophysiologiques pendant l'ischémie myocardique et mécanisme possible des troubles du rythme ventriculaire. Ann Cardiol Angéiol 26:551–554, 1977.

14. Janse MJ, Moréna H, Cinca J, Kléber AG, Downar E, van Capelle FJL, Durrer D: Role of reentry and currents of injury in early ischemic ventricular tachyarrhythmias: which properties should theoretically make a drug effective in the management of these arrhythmias. In: Management of ventricular tachycardia – role of mexiletine. Sandøe E, Julian DG, Bell JW (eds). Amsterdam, Oxford, Excerpta Medica, 1978, p 183–196.

15. Anderson GJ, Gough WB, Reiser J: Regional current flow across ischemia and thermal boundaries. Am J Cardiol 43:349, (abstract) 1979.

16. Katzung BG. Effects of extracellular calcium and sodium on depolarization-induced automaticity in guinea pig papillary muscle. Circ Res 37:118–127, 1975.

17. Hamlin RL, Burton RR, Leverett SP, Burns JW: Ventricular activation process in minipigs. J Electrocardiol 8:113–116, 1975.

18. Holland RP, Brooks H: The QRS complex during myocardial ischemia. An experimental analysis in the porcine heart. J Clin Invest 57:541–550, 1976.

19. Durrer D, van der Tweel LH: Excitation of the left ventricular wall of the dog and goat. Ann NY Acad Sci 65:779–803, 1956/1957.

20. Merideth J, Mendez C, Mueller WJ, Moe GK: Electrical excitability of atrioventricular nodal cells. Circ Res 23:69–85, 1968.

21. Spear JF, Moore EN: Supernormal excitability and conduction in the His-Purkinje system of the dog. Circ Res 35:782–792, 1974.

22. Janse MJ, Kléber AG, Cinca J, Durrer D: Electrophysiology of early ventricular arrhythmias in acute myocardial ischaemia in the pig's heart. Br Heart J (suppl) 40:44–51, 1978.

23. Wit AL, Hoffman BF, Cranefield PF: Slow conduction and reentry in the ventricular conducting system 1: return extrasystole in canine Purkinje fibers. Circ Res 30:1–10, 1972.

24. El-Sherif N, Hope RP, Scherlag BJ, Lazzara R: Reentrant ventricular arrhythmias in the late myocardial infarction period. 2: patterns of initiation and termination of reentry. Circulation 55:702–719, 1977.

25. Allessie MA, Bonke FIM, Schopman FJG: Circus movements in rabbit atrial muscle as a mechanism of tachycardia III. The 'leading circle' concept: a new model of circus movement in cardiac tissue without the involvement of an anatomical obstacle. Circ Res 41:9–18, 1977.

2.3. ELECTROPHYSIOLOGICAL, BIOCHEMICAL AND PHARMACOLOGICAL ASPECTS OF REENTRANT VENTRICULAR ARRHYTHMIAS IN THE LATE MYOCARDIAL INFARCTION PERIOD

N. EL-SHERIF, J.A.C. GOMES, G.J. KELEN, R.G. KHAN, P.S. KANG and R.H. ZEILER

1. INTRODUCTION

Myocardial infarction represents a highly likely source of reentrant ventricular arrhythmias. Although most studies of the early phase of ventricular arrhythmias that follow acute ligation of a major coronary artery in the dog have shown some of the basic prerequisites for reentry in the form of desynchronized slow conduction in ischemic myocardium (1–8), they all fall short of actually documenting the presence of reentry. This was due, we believe, to the highly dynamic situation following acute ligation of a major coronary artery with constantly changing electrophysiological properties in the ischemic zone. Thus, it is difficult to conduct systematic electrophysiological studies of the possible reentrant mechanism under such dynamic conditions. In addition, the recording techniques usually failed to demonstrate the one unequivocal evidence for reentry, viz: the presence of continuous electrical activity originating from the infarction zone that regularly and predictably bridge the diastolic interval between the reentrant beat and the preceding impulse, as well as between consecutive reentrant beats (9).

In a series of recent studies it was shown that dogs, three to seven days following ligation of the left anterior descending artery, represent a remarkably stable model for reentrant ventricular arrhythmias and one in which systematic electrophysiological and pharmacological studies could be conducted (9–17). Recordings obtained from the epicardial surface of the infarction zone utilizing a new "composite" bipolar electrode (9) were frequently successful in depicting the electrical activity of the reentrant pathway. The experimental model and the recording technique provided new insight into the electrophysiological mechanisms of ischemia-related reentrant ventricular arrhythmias. This report will utilize information obtained from both in vivo and in vitro studies conducted on the canine model to outline in detail the electrophysiological, biochemical and pharmacological aspects of reentrant ventricular arrhythmias in the late myocardial infarction period.

2. THE EXPERIMENTAL MODEL FOR REENTRANT VENTRICULAR ARRHYTHMIAS AND THE RECORDING TECHNIQUE (9)

The model consists of adult mongrel dogs that are studied three to seven days following ligation of the left anterior descending coronary artery just distal to the anterior septal branch. Almost all dogs show evidence of a transmural infarction that involves the subepi-

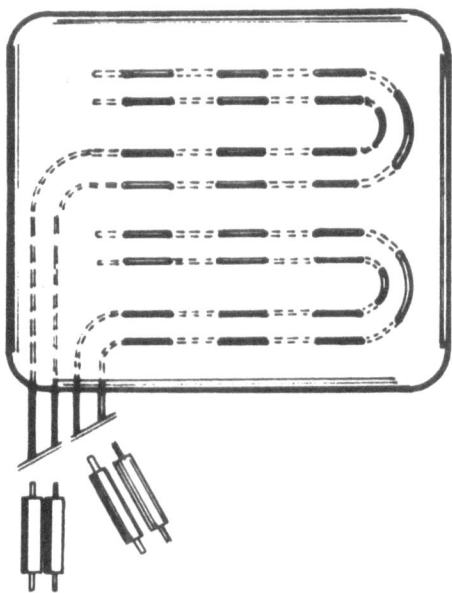

Figure 1. Diagrammatic illustration of the composite electrode. The electrode shown in the figure is made of two separate portions in a single frame; both portions have the same configuration with an exactly similar array of wires. Each portion serves as a bipolar electrode to record from the infarction zone and the adjacent normal zone. Reprinted with permission of The American Heart Association from El-Sherif et al. (9).

cardial layer of muscle. In these dogs, composite electrode recordings from the epicardial surface of the infarction zone (IZ) frequently depict the presence of continuous electrical activity that bridges the entire diastolic interval between the initiating and reentrant beats as well as between consecutive reentrant beats. The composite electrode (Figure 1) has multiple close bipolar contact points that cover a large portion of the IZ and function as multiple individual close bipolar electrodes connected in series. Each contact point will be influenced by the activation wavefront as it approaches its site. The composite electrode recording provides reliable information on the degree of conduction delay in the IZ but is unable to precisely define the anatomic outline of the reentrant pathway.

Figure 2 shows a schematic representation of conduction disorders in the IZ leading to reentry and the type of recordings provided by the composite electrode and individual close bipolar electrodes. The schematic figure is consonant with recent electrophysiological observations (9) including preliminary information on epicardial mapping of reentrant arrhythmias utilizing a multiplexed data recording system (17). It is also corroborated by known anatomic characteristics of the IZ which may show islands of relatively viable muscle alternating with areas of infarction (18). In the figure, the area of straight lines represents normal myocardium. The IZ consists of multiple irregular islands of severely depressed, unexcitable myocardium (the white areas) and intervening portions of less severely depressed myocardium that allows slow conduction of the cardiac impulse (stippled areas). The figure illustrates the area covered by the composite electrode as well as three close bi-

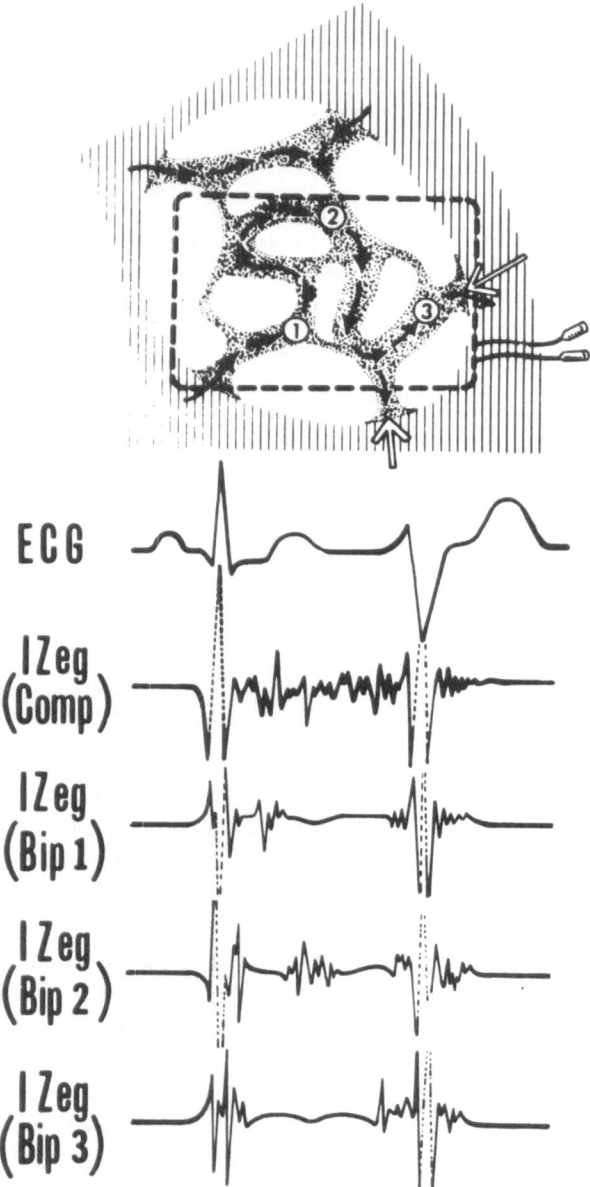

Figure 2. Schematic representation of the conduction disorder in the infarction zone leading to reentry. See text for details. Tracings from top to bottom represent a standard ECG lead, a composite electrode recording (IZeg Comp), and three close bipolar recordings (IZeg Bip. 1–3). Reprinted with permission of The American Heart Association from El-Sherif et al. (9).

polar electrodes. Tracings from top to bottom represent a standard ECG lead, a composite electrode recording, IZeg (Comp.), and three close bipolar recordings, IZeg (Bip.), 1–3. The figure depicts the activation wavefront in the normal zone (NZ) invading the IZ at multiple sites (black arrows) while failing to conduct at other sites (white arrows) creating areas of unidirectional conduction block. The IZ shows more than one pathway. Impulses propagate from opposite directions in the pathway in the upper part of the IZ where they collide and die out. On the other hand, the cardiac impulse enters a potentially reentrant pathway at the lower left side of the IZ and conducts slowly in a highly circuitous pathway. The diagram shows that the impulse reaches the lower part of the IZ but fails to re-excite the NZ, which is still refractory (the white arrow at the bottom of the IZ). The impulse continues propagation to the right border of the IZ; there it succeeds in re-exciting the NZ because of recovery of excitability of the tissues proximal to the unidirectional block, resulting in a reentrant beat.

The schematic diagram illustrates the two prerequisites long considered necessary for reentry (19): 1) unidirectional block of conduction at certain sites; 2) conduction over alternate route(s) at a velocity slow enough to allow recovery of excitability of tissues beyond the block. The composite electrode which covers the entire reentrant pathway records a continuous series of multiple asynchronous spikes that bridge the total diastolic interval between the initiating and reentrant beats. On the other hand, the close bipolar electrodes depict the arrival of the slow activation wavefront as it passes close by. This is reflected in the bipolar electrograms as one or more potentials that only cover part of the diastolic interval.

3. RATE-RELATED CONDUCTION PATTERNS IN THE REENTRANT PATHWAY

Ventricular reentry in the ischemic myocardium is based on characteristic rate-related conduction disorders. Reentry will occur at a critical range of heart rates and will disappear at both slower and faster rates (9–11). The electrophysiologic mechanism underlying these observations is illustrated in Figure 3, which was obtained from a dog in which the left anterior descending artery was ligated for five days. A composite electrode was utilized to obtain recordings from the epicardial surface of the IZ and the adjacent NZ. Panels A and B show that a cardiac cycle length of 390 and 340 msec failed to result in fractionation of the IZ potential. The latter reflects the degree of conduction delay in the IZ. However, a critical range of cardiac cycle lengths (290–310 msec) gave rise to a 3 : 2 Wenckebach-like conduction pattern of the IZ potential and a manifest trigeminal rhythm (panel C). The first beat of the Wenckebach cycle is associated with a relatively more synchronized and sharp IZ potential. During the second beat of a 3 : 2 Wenckebach-like cycle, the IZ potential is replaced by a continuous series of multiple asynchronous spikes that bridge the entire diastolic interval between the supraventricular and reentrant ventricular beats. Panel D shows that further shortening of the cardiac cycle to 285 msec resulted in a 2 : 1 conduction pattern of the IZ potential and disappearance of manifest reentry.

The Wenckebach-like conduction pattern in the IZ is of crucial significance in understanding the electrophysiological basis of certain reentrant rhythms. A schematic representation of conduction in the IZ during three consecutive cycles of a 3 : 2 Wenckebach-like conduction sequence is shown in Figure 4. The schematic illustration of conduction in the

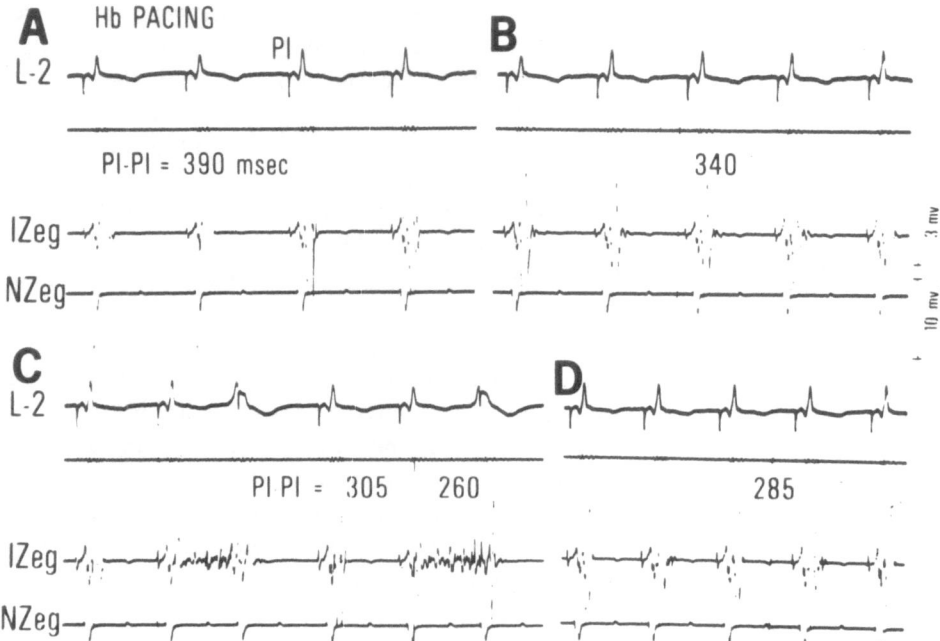

Figure 3. Recordings obtained from a dog in which the left anterior descending artery was ligated for 5 days, that illustrate initiation of a reentrant trigeminal rhythm (panel C) by a critical rate of His bundle pacing. Both slower rates (panels A and B) and faster rates (panel D) failed to induce reentry. See text for details. IZeg = infarction zone composite electrogram; NZeg = normal zone composite electrogram; PI = pacer impulse. Time lines are set at 1 sec intervals. Reprinted with permission of The American Heart Association from El-Sherif and Lazzara (15).

IZ is essentially similar to the one utilized in Figure 2. The three tracings represent from top to bottom: a surface ECG lead, recording of a composite electrode that reflects the entire IZ (IZeg Comp.), and a close bipolar recording from a localized portion of the IZ (IZeg Bip.). Diagram A shows that during the first beat of a 3 : 2 Wenckebach-like cycle, conduction in the IZ is represented by several islands of severely depressed unexcitable myocardium (white areas) with intervening relatively wide pathways of less severely depressed myocardium (stippled areas). The activation wavefront in the NZ invades the IZ at multiple sites (black arrows) where the impulses that propagate from opposite directions collide, and die out. Both the composite and the close bipolar electrograms record an initial multiphasic deflection that represents activation of relatively normal myocardium and a late deflection (marked by arrows) reflecting a delayed but relatively synchronous conduction in the pathway at the lower part of the IZ (the IZ potential).

Diagram B illustrates the changes in conduction in the IZ during the second beat of the 3 : 2 Wenckebach-like cycle. One or more groups of cells in the lower pathway that were showing a slow but synchronized conduction during the first beat develop different degrees of increment of refractoriness resulting in either relatively slower conduction or block of the activation wavefront advancing from the NZ. This is represented by several small white

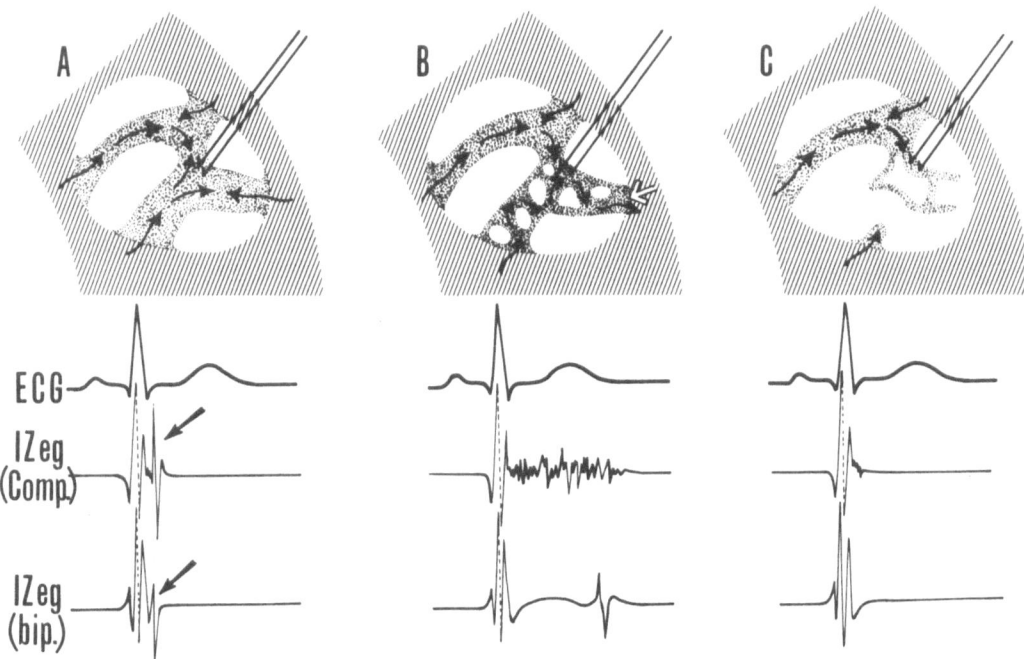

Figure 4. Schematic representation of conduction in the infarction zone during the three beats of a 3 : 2 Wencke-bach-like conduction period (panels A to C). See text for details. Tracings from top to bottom represent a standard ECG lead, a composite electrode recording (IZeg Comp.), and a close bipolar recording (IZeg Bip.). Reprinted with permission of the American Heart Association from El-Sherif et al. (9).

islands in the pathway that was first represented by a homogeneous stippled area in diagram A. Since the myocardium is a free syncytium, the irregular change in refractoriness will force the activation wavefront to take a circuitous and much longer pathway in the IZ. The conduction pattern in the IZ is reflected in the composite electrogram as a series of continuous asynchronous spikes that replace the initial relatively simple IZ potential and extends for a variable distance in diastole. On the other hand, the close bipolar electrode which is positioned relatively distal to the maximum zone of conduction delay will only depict the arrival of activation wavefront as it passes close by. This is reflected in the bipolar electrogram as a marked delay in the inscription of the IZ potential relative to the initial ventricular deflection as well as a varying degree of decrease in amplitude and increase in duration of the potential. An apparently isoelectric interval separates the IZ potential from the rest of the ventricular deflection.

During the third beat of a 3 : 2 Wenckebach-like cycle (diagram C), there is further increment of refractoriness in most of the groups of cells that formed the circuitous pathway in diagram B. This is represented by a significant increase in the portion of the IZ occupied by the white islands which are unable to conduct the cardiac impulse. This will result in complete failure of conduction of the activation wavefront advancing from the NZ through the IZ pathway that was originally conducting slowly in diagram A. Both the composite and the close bipolar electrograms show failure of inscription of the IZ potential. For reentry to take place following the second beat of 3 : 2 Wenckebach-like cycle, two requirements are necessary. These are: 1) unidirectional block of conduction at certain site(s) (white arrow), and 2) sufficient conduction delay of the impulse propagating in the lower pathway to allow recovery of excitability of tissues beyond the block. The reentrant beat will replace the third beat of a 3 : 2 Wenckebach-like cycle that did not result in reentry. (See Figure 3, panel C.) The first reentrant beat can change the refractoriness in several portions of the IZ. This may result in either one or more reentrant beats or change the pathway in the IZ of the next sinus beat.

4. MANIFEST AND CONCEALED EXTRASYSTOLIC GROUPING

The term extrasystolic grouping refers to extrasystoles that occur in repetitive patterns during a basic cardiac rhythm, e.g., sinus rhythm. In this case, one (or more) extrasystole may follow every sinus beat (bigeminy), every other sinus beat (trigeminy), every third sinus beat (quadrigeminy), etc. The majority of these extrasystoles show relatively fixed coupling. However, variable coupling, as well as other characteristic variations in coupling, e.g., gradual lengthening of coupling of successive beats may also be seen. A significant insight into the mechanism of reentrant extrasystolic grouping was recently provided by studies of ventricular reentry in the late myocardial infarction period in the canine heart (11). These studies have shown that extrasystolic grouping of reentrant beats is based on characteristic rate-related conduction disorders in a potentially reentrant pathway in the IZ. (See Figures 5 and 6 which were obtained from the same experiment shown in Figure 3.) A bigeminal rhythm is due to a characteristic 2 : 1 conduction pattern in a potentially reentrant pathway whereby every other sinus beat exhibits a significant degree of conduction delay in the reentrant pathway. If the conduction delay is sufficient to re-excite the bordering normal zone, a reentrant beat will follow every conducted sinus beat in a bigeminal arrangement (Figure 6, C). A trigeminal rhythm is explained by a 3 : 2 Wenckebach-like conduction sequence in the reentrant pathway (Figure 5, A). Quadrigeminy can be due to a 4 : 3 Wenckebach-like conduction pattern (Figure 6, B). However, a quadrigeminal rhythm in the surface ECG is frequently the result of a regular 2 : 1 conduction cycle in a reentrant pathway with manifest reentry only in alternate cycles, i.e., concealed bigeminy. Although longer Wenckebach-like cycles could occasionally be seen, it is rare for a regular pentageminy or hexageminy to be due to successive 5 : 4 or 6 : 5 conduction ratios respectively. However, regular pentageminy is easily explained by the not uncommon alternation of 2 : 1 and 3 : 2 conduction cycles (Figure 5, C). On the other hand, hexageminy can be a manifestation of concealed trigeminy (Figure 5, B).

In the presence of a stable conduction pattern in a reentrant pathway, e.g., regular repetition of a 2 : 1 or 3 : 2 conduction sequence, the reentrant impulse can retrace the same pathway in practically the same span of time and produces extrasystoles with almost constant coupling. On the other hand, different reentrant pathway conduction times, and hence variable coupling intervals of extrasystoles, can occur when there is a change in the

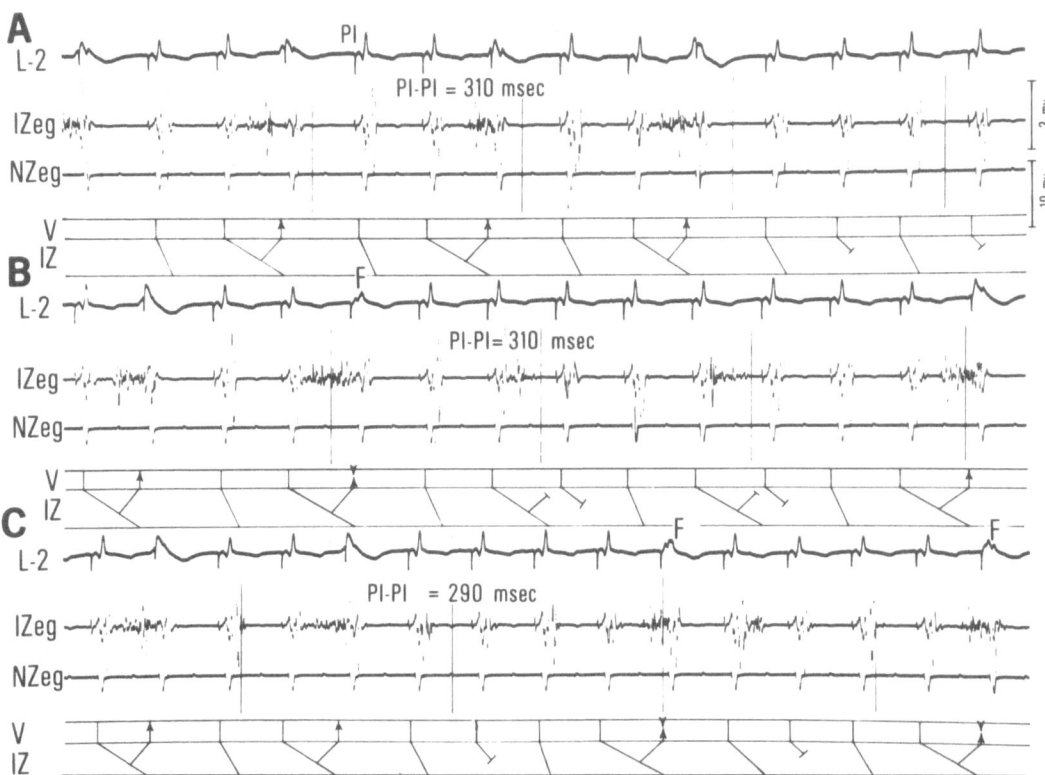

Figure 5. Recordings obtained during His bundle pacing from the same canine experiment shown in Figure 3 that illustrate manifest and concealed extrasystolic grouping. In this and the subsequent figure, the ladder diagrams illustrate the conduction pattern in the reentrant pathway in the infarction zone (IZ). Panel A shows a manifest trigeminal reentrant rhythm explained by a 3 : 2 Wenckebach-like conduction pattern in the reentrant pathway. At the end of the record, the trigeminal rhythm disappeared due to the occurrence of 2 : 1 block in the reentrant pathway associated with relatively less conduction delay during the conducted beat of the 2 : 1 series. Panel B shows concealed trigeminy. Two manifest reentrant beats are interrupted by 8 sinus beats. Analysis of the infarction zone composite electrogram (IZeg) reveals the regular occurrence of 3 : 2 Wenckebach-like cycles. However, the degree of conduction delay during the second beat of a 3 : 2 Wenckebach-like cycle that did not result in a manifest reentrant beat was less marked compared to the same beat during manifest trigeminal rhythm. Panel C illustrates a trigeminal cycle followed by two cycles of pentageminy. The latter is explained by the consecutive occurrence of a 2 : 1 and 3 : 2 Wenckebach-like conduction pattern. NZ = normal zone composite electrogram; V = ventricle; F = fusion beat.

conduction pattern in the pathway (see Figure 6, C). A change of conduction patterns can be easily induced by a minor or major alteration of the cardiac cycle length. However, this change can also occur at remarkably constant cycle lengths (see Figures 5 and 6). In this case, the surface ECG will show sudden "unpredictable" variations in the coupling intervals.

Reentrant beats with extrasystolic grouping can disappear at both relatively slow and fast heart rates. At a slower heart rate, a potentially reentrant pathway will allow conduction of the cardiac impulse in a 1 : 1 pattern with significantly less conduction delay than is necessary for reentry to occur. On the other hand, reentry may disappear on increasing the heart rate due to one of two basic mechanisms: 1) a faster rate may result in a 2 : 1, or higher degree of conduction block in a potentially reentrant pathway with the conducted beat showing less conduction delay thus negating the chance for reentry (see Figure 3, D). 2) At a faster rate, the reentrant pathway conduction time may approach, equal or exceed the basic cardiac cycle length. In this case, reentry may be concealed due to entrapment in the terminal part of the reentrant pathway or a small part of the closely bordering normal zone.

The phenomenon of concealed reentrant extrasystoles has been clearly demonstrated by recent studies of experimental ischemia-related ventricular reentry (11) (see Figures 5 and 6). General laws of conduction of the cardiac impulse reveal that a 3 : 2 conduction pattern can easily convert to a 2 : 1 conduction on slight acceleration of the heart rate and sometimes with no perceptible change in the rate. Alternation of 3 : 2 and 2 : 1 conduction patterns is very commonly observed in ventricular reentrant pathways (9–11). Regular or irregular alternation of concealed 2 : 1 and 3 : 2 conduction patterns in a reentrant pathway can result in varying numbers of intervening sinus beats that may or may not conform to

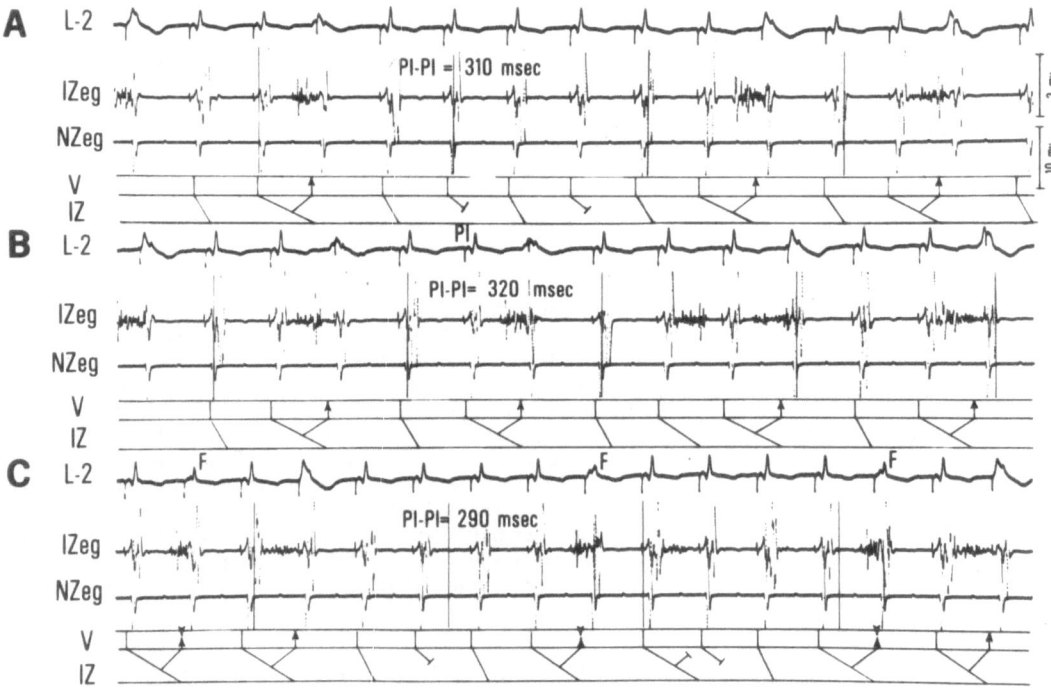

Figure 6. Recordings obtained during His bundle pacing from the same canine experiment shown in Figures 3 and 5 that illustrate manifest and concealed extrasystolic grouping. Panel A shows the occurrence of 6 sinus beats during a regular trigeminal rhythm. This arrangement does not conform to either concealed bigeminy or concealed trigeminy. The infarction zone electrogram (IZeg) shows the occurrence of successive 2 : 1, 2 : 1 and 3 : 2 Wenckebach-like cycles. Panel B shows a quadrigeminal cycle that was not due to a concealed bigeminy but rather to a 4 : 3 Wenckebach-like conduction pattern. Panel C illustrates a manifest bigeminal rhythm at the beginning and end of the record. A concealed bigeminal cycle is seen following the third manifest reentrant beat. Note that the figure shows some variation of the coupling interval of reentrant beats with the occurrence of fusion beats (F) particularly when there is a change in the conduction pattern in the reentrant pathway. NZ = normal zone composite electrogram; V = ventricle.

concealed bigeminy or trigeminy. Alternation of manifest bigeminal and trigeminal extrasystolic rhythms is common in clinical records. Analysis of sufficiently long rhythm strips will almost invariably reveal numbers of intervening sinus beats that do not conform to concealed bigeminy or trigeminy but rather to a varying combination of the two arrangements. One common pattern is pentageminy, which is most probably related to a successive 2 : 1 and 3 : 2 conduction sequence.

Schamroth and Marriott alluded to the practical importance of the recognition of concealed extrasystoles in a clinical record since it implies a state of greater ectopic irritability than is apparent (20). Concealed extrasystoles, as were originally described and diagnosed using rigid mathematical formulas (20, 21), are very uncommon. With the recent understanding of conduction patterns in ventricular reentrant pathways, specifically the common alternation of 2 : 1 and 3 : 2 conduction sequences, concealed extrasystoles may be an extremely common occurrence. The prognostic significance of concealed versus manifest reentrant extrasystoles is not fully elucidated. However, the possible common occurrence of concealed extrasystoles casts some doubt on the commonly established practice of using the frequency of manifest VPCs in clinical records both as a prognostic marker and as a guide to the efficacy of antiarrhythmic therapy.

5. INITIATION OF REENTRANT VENTRICULAR TACHYCARDIA

A reentrant ventricular tachycardia can be initiated by one or more of three electrical stimulation procedures that consistently entail shortening of the cardiac cycle length (10). These are: 1) rapid cardiac pacing, 2) abrupt termination of rapid cardiac pacing, and 3) premature beats with a critical coupling interval.

5.1. Rapid cardiac pacing

This can be obtained through atrial, His bundle or ventricular pacing. However, sufficient increase of the heart rate through rapid atrial pacing is frequently limited by the AV nodal refractoriness. A reentrant ventricular arrhythmia could be induced during rapid cardiac pacing at a critically fast rate that varies from one case to the other. The rate of the reentrant tachycardia is usually faster than the critical pacing rate that induces the arrhythmia. Figure 7 illustrates the initiation of reentrant ventricular tachycardia by rapid His bundle pacing. Panel A shows the recording during normal sinus rhythm. The normal zone composite electrogram (NZeg) records a sharp multiphasic deflection with a duration approximately equal to the QRS complex in ECG leads. On the other hand, the IZeg records a relatively wide multiphasic deflection, the initial part of which corresponds to activation of relatively normal myocardium while the late terminal deflection represents the IZ potential. Panel B illustrates His pacing at a cycle length of 245 msec that failed to result in fractionation of the IZ potential. However, further shortening of the pacing cycle length to 175 msec in panel C resulted in periodic fractionation of the IZ potential into a series of multiple asynchronous spikes that extended for the entire diastolic interval. A reentrant ventricular tachycardia

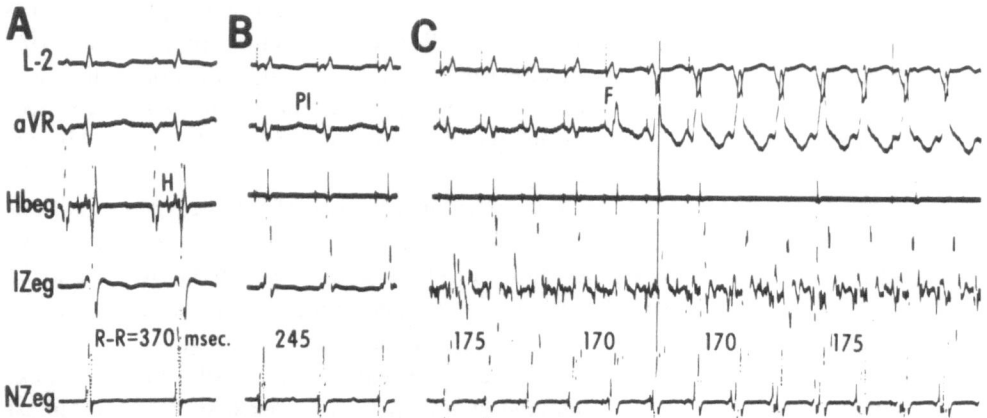

Figure 7. Initiation of reentrant ventricular tachycardia by a critical rate of rapid cardiac (His bundle) pacing. See text for details. In this and subsequent figures: Hbeg = His bundle electrogram; IZeg = infarction zone composite electrogram; NZeg = normal zone composite electrogram; PI = pacer impulse; H = His bundle deflection; F = fusion beat. The timelines are set at one second intervals. Reprinted with permission of The American Heart Association from El-Sherif et al. (10).

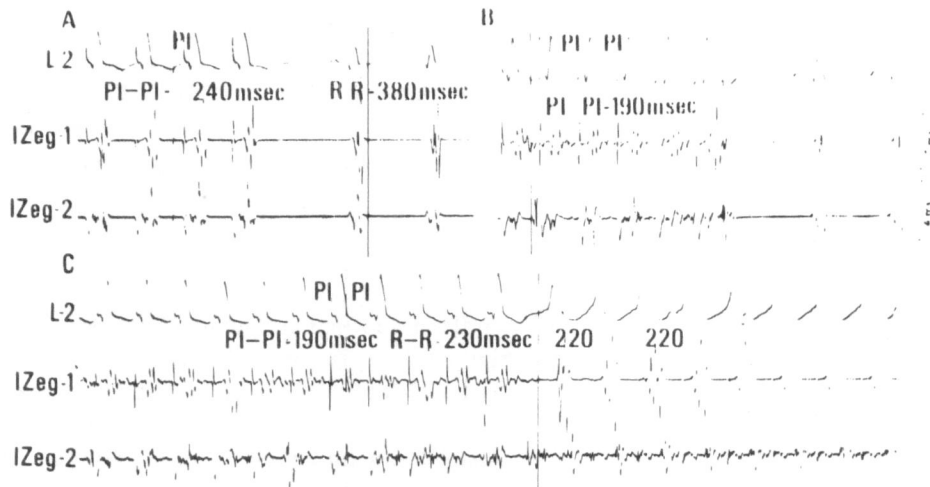

Figure 8. Initiation of reentrant ventricular tachycardia upon abrupt termination of a critical rate of rapid cardiac (His bundle) pacing. See text for details. IZeg-1 and IZeg-2 represent two composite electrograms from the infarction zone.

broke through regular His pacing starting with a ventricular fusion beat (marked F). The rate of the tachycardia was almost equal to or only slightly faster than that of His pacing. Continuous electrical activity was present preceding the onset of the tachycardia as well as between consecutive beats of the arrhythmia. The electrogram recorded from the NZ closely adjacent to the IZ failed to show this continuous electrical activity.

5.2. Abrupt termination of rapid cardiac pacing

Abrupt termination of cardiac pacing at rates associated with periodic fractionation of the IZ potential is usually more successful in initiating a reentrant ventricular tachycardia than when regular pacing is maintained. However, reentry would only occur if and when cardiac pacing is abruptly terminated during those cardiac beats associated with prolonged fractionation of the IZ potential that extends beyond the T wave of the surface electrocardiogram (ECG). This is illustrated in Figure 8. Panel A shows that His pacing at a cycle length of 240 msec did not result in significant fractionation of the IZ potential compared to normal sinus beats. On the other hand, pacing at a cycle length of 190 msec in panels B and C resulted in periodic marked fractionation of the IZ potential that bridged the entire diastolic interval. In panel B, pacing was abruptly terminated after a beat that was not followed by prolonged fractionation of the IZ potential and failed to initiate a reentrant rhythm. By contrast, in panel C, pacing was abruptly terminated following a beat that was associated with prolonged fractionation of the IZ potential extending beyond the ST-T segment of the surface ECG. This was followed by a reentrant ventricular tachycardia. It is noted that the coupling interval of the first reentrant beat which reflects the reentrant pathway conduction time (230 msec) and the cycle length of the reentrant tachycardia (220 msec) are both longer than the pacing cycle length that was necessary to initiate the arrhythmia (190 msec).

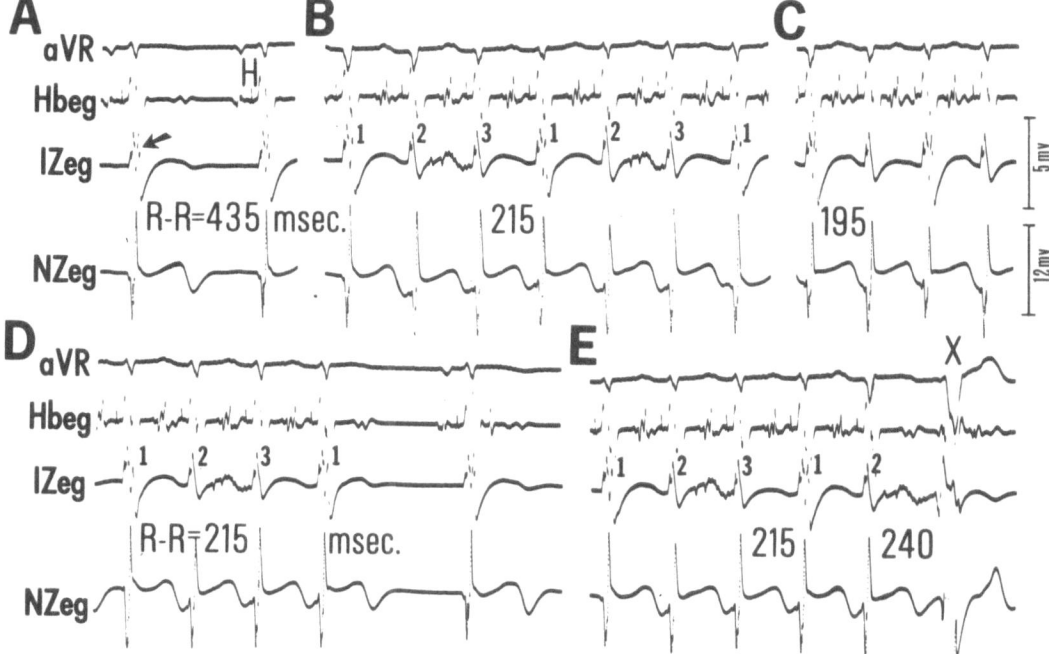

Figure 9. Initiation of reentrant ventricular rhythm (X) upon abrupt termination of a critical rate of rapid atrial pacing. See text for details. Panels B, D and E illustrate 3 : 2 Wenckebach-like conduction pattern of the IZ potential. The three beats of the Wenckebach cycle are labelled 1 to 3. The arrow refers to the IZ potential during normal sinus rhythm.

The electrophysiologic mechanism by which abrupt termination of a critical rate of cardiac pacing can occasionally – but not consistently – initiate a reentrant ventricular tachycardia is illustrated in Figure 9. Panel A shows the control recording during normal sinus
rhythm. The IZ potential (marked by an arrow) is a relatively sharp deflection. Atrial pacing
at a cycle length of 215 msec in panel B resulted in a 3 : 2 Wenckebach-like conduction pattern
of the IZ potential as was previously illustrated in Figure 4. The opening beat of the Wenckebach-like cycle associated with a relatively sharp IZ potential is marked 1. The second beat
of the cycle associated with marked fractionation of the IZ potential bridging the entire
diastolic interval is marked 2. The third beat of the cycle associated with block of the IZ
potential is labelled 3. Further shortening of the cardiac cycle length to 195 msec in panel C
resulted in 2 : 1 block of the IZ potential. Panels D and E illustrate that abrupt termination
of atrial pacing at the rate associated with 3 : 2 Wenckebach-like conduction of the IZ
potential can initiate a reentrant ventricular rhythm (marked X) only if pacing is terminated
following beat 2 of the cycle (panel E) and not beat 1 of the cycle (panel D). Failure to initiate
reentry would also occur if pacing is terminated following beat 3 of a 3 : 2 Wenckebach-like
cycle. Further, abrupt termination of a faster pacing rate that results in 2 : 1 block of the
IZ potential would fail to initiate reentry. Although during beat 2 of a 3 : 2 Wenckebach-
like cycle the fractionated IZ potential spanned the entire diastolic interval, manifest
or concealed reentry failed to occur so long as regular pacing was maintained. Only following termination of pacing was reentry possible. This is explained as follows: The coupling
interval of the first reentrant beat (marked X), which reflects the reentrant pathway conduction time, was 240 msec. This was 25 msec longer than the pacing cycle length associated
with the Wenckebach-like conduction pattern (215 msec). Thus, so long as regular pacing is
maintained, the very terminal part of the reentrant parthway will be regularly pre-excited
by the activation wavefront advancing from the normal zone.

5.3. Premature beats with a critical range of coupling intervals

A reentrant ventricular tachycardia can be initiated by a single critically timed premature
impulse. Only premature beats within a critical range of coupling intervals that result in
sufficient conduction delay in the reentrant pathway can induce reentry. This range of
coupling intervals is called "the reentry zone". Premature beats with longer coupling intervals would result in an insufficient degree of conduction delay in the reentrant pathway and
fail to induce reentry. On the other hand, premature beats with coupling intervals shorter
than the reentry zone that succeed in capturing the normal myocardium would fail to conduct in the reentrant pathway in the IZ which usually has a relatively long refractory period.
These beats would also fail to induce reentry. Figure 10 illustrates the initiation of a reentrant ventricular tachycardia by a critically-timed atrial premature beat coupled to regular
sinus rhythm. Coupling intervals of 235 msec (panel A) and 225 msec (panel B) resulted in
only a limited degree of conduction delay of the IZ potential (marked by an arrow) and
failed to induce reentry. In panel C, a critical coupling interval of 220 msec resulted in
marked fractionation and delay of the IZ potential initiating a reentrant ventricular tachycardia. The width of the reentry zone in this case measured 15 msec (coupling intervals of 250–

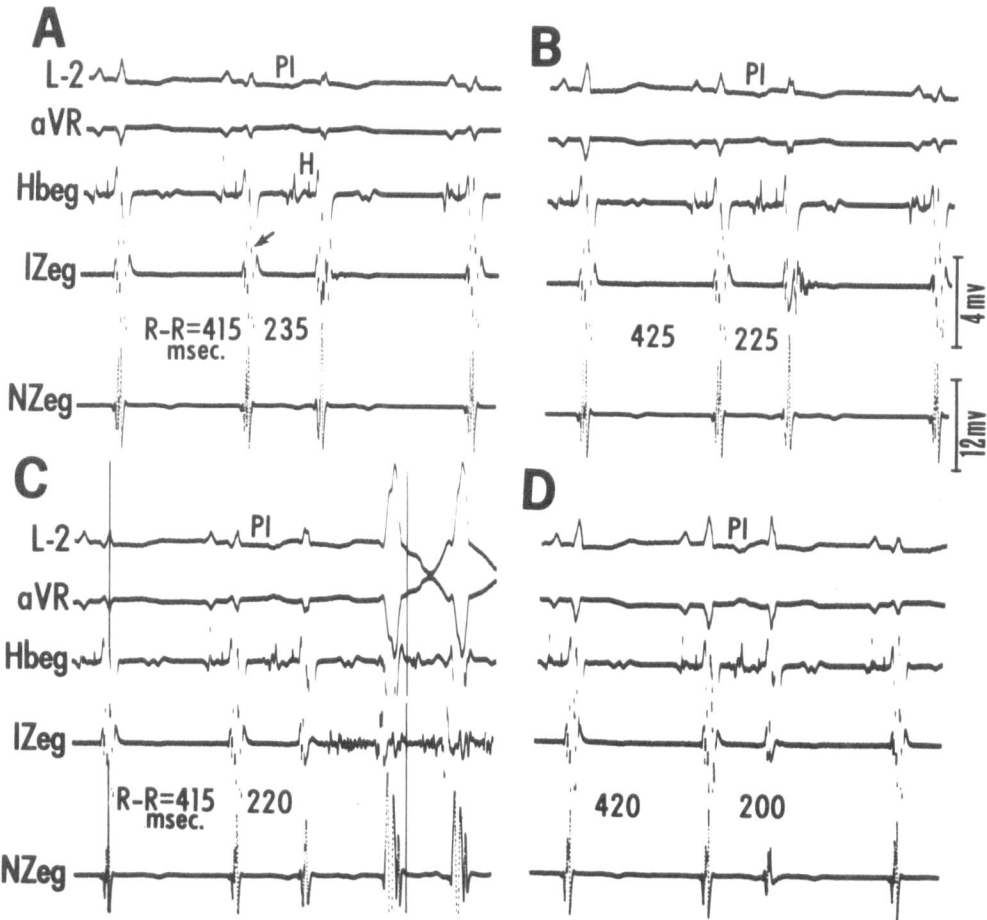

Figure 10. Initiation of reentrant ventricular tachycardia by programmed premature atrial stimulation. See text for details. The arrow refers to the IZ potential during normal sinus beats. Reprinted with permission of The American Heart Association from El-Sherif et al. (10).

220 msec). A premature beat with a coupling interval of 200 msec (panel D) resulted in block of the IZ potential and failed to initiate the arrhythmia.

Although the critical range of coupling intervals of a premature beat that would result in reentry may differ slightly according to the basic cardiac cycle length, it is usually comparable to the range of cycle lengths at which Wenckebach-like conduction in the reentrant pathway may occur. This is illustrated in Figure 11. Panel A illustrates the initiation of a reentrant ventricular tachycardia by a premature atrial beat (PI) with a coupling interval of 235 msec. Panel B shows that atrial pacing at a cycle length of 220 msec resulted in a 3 : 2 Wenckebach-like conduction of the IZ potential (marked by arrows). Slight further shortening of the cycle length in panel C induced 2 : 1 block of the IZ potential. Although the fractionated IZ potential during beat 2 of the 3 : 2 Wenckebach-like sequence bridged the entire diastolic interval, it failed to induce reentry as long as atrial pacing was maintained.

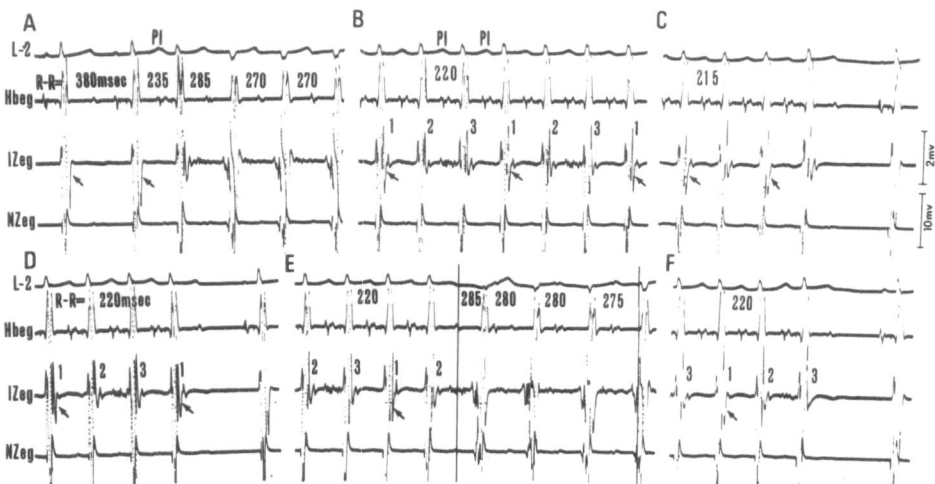

Figure 11. Initiation of reentrant ventricular tachycardia by either a premature atrial beat with a critical coupling interval (panel A) or upon abrupt termination of a critical rate of atrial pacing (panel E). See text for details. 1, 2 and 3 represent the three beats of a 3 : 2 Wenckebach-like sequence of the IZ potential. The latter is marked by arrows.

Panels D to F illustrate that abrupt termination of atrial pacing could induce a reentrant ventricular tachycardia only if pacing is interrupted following beat 2 of the 3 : 2 Wenckebach-like cycle (panel E) and not beats 1 or 3 of the cycles (panels D and F respectively).

There are two other considerations besides a critical range of coupling intervals for successful initiation of reentrant ventricular tachycardia by a single premature beat. These are: 1) the basic pacing rate and 2) the site of stimulation. The basic pacing rate influences the duration of the refractory period of both normal myocardium and the reentrant pathway. It is usually easier to initiate reentry by critically-timed premature beats applied during a relatively slow basic heart rate. On the other hand, the premature beat may have to be applied close to the site of the reentrant pathway in the IZ to facilitate the induction of reentry. In some cases with a relatively slight prolongation of the refractory period of the reentrant pathway relative to surrounding myocardium, a single premature stimulus may fail to induce reentry while two or more stimuli may succeed. This is explained by shortening of the refractory period at the site of stimulation allowing one of the stimuli to conduct to the reentrant pathway during its relative refractory period thus setting the stage for reentry.

6. TERMINATION OF REENTRANT VENTRICULAR TACHYCARDIA

A reentrant ventricular tachycardia could be terminated by either a single properly timed premature beat applied to the atria, His bundle or the ventricles, or by a series of two or more premature beats in close succession. Usually tachycardias with relatively slow rates could be terminated by a single premature beat. On the other hand, tachycardias with relatively fast rates usually require a short run (three or more beats) of rapid cardiac pacing at a rate faster than the spontaneous rate of the tachycardia. Figure 12 illustrates the effect of a single premature beat of variable coupling applied during a reentrant ventricular tachycardia. The cycle length of the tachycardia was remarkably constant at 225 msec. Panel A shows that an induced His bundle premature beat with a coupling interval of 210 msec succeeded in completely capturing the NZ but failed to change the regular sequence of the tachycardia since the following cardiac cycle was fully compensatory. This suggests that the premature beat did not engage any part of the regular reentrant circuit. In panel B, a more premature His bundle ectopic beat resulted in a change of the reentrant pathway as revealed by change in configuration of the QRS complexes in the surface ECG as well as the configuration of the IZeg. The cardiac cycle following the premature beat was less than compensatory. This suggests that the premature beat did in fact activate part of the original reentrant circuit and forced the reentrant wavefront to change its pathway. The new reentrant ventricular tachycardia was, however, self limited and lasted for only three beats. It also showed lengthening of the last cycle prior to spontaneous termination.

Panel C shows that the tachycardia could be terminated by a slightly more premature His

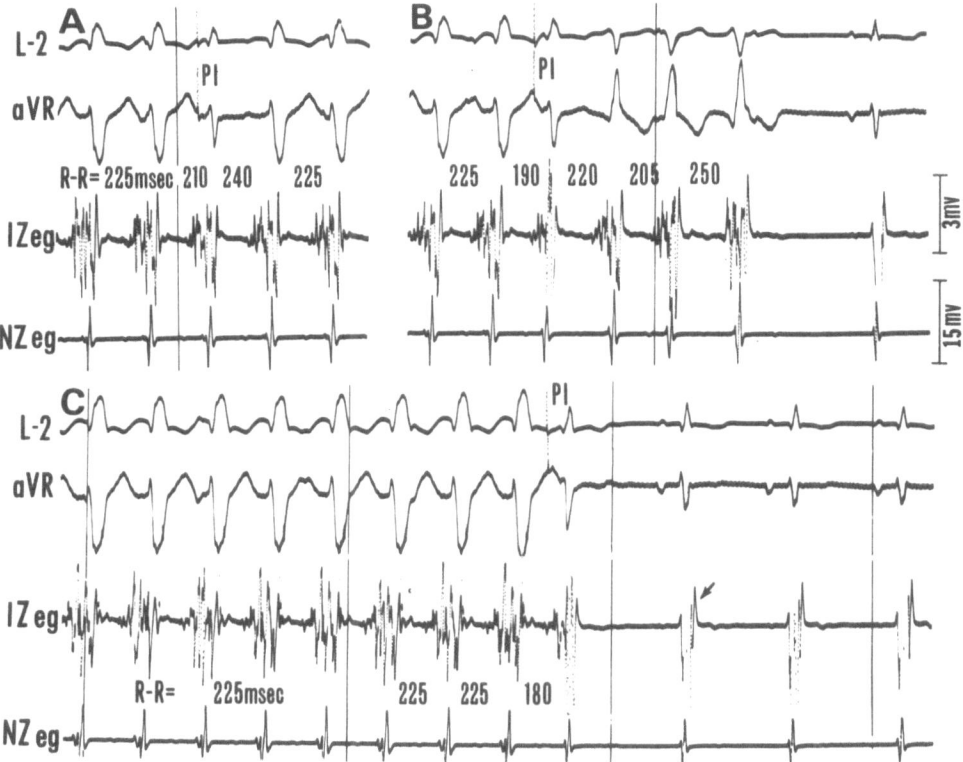

Figure 12. Termination of reentrant ventricular tachycardia by an induced His bundle premature beat (PI) with a critical coupling interval (panel C). Premature beats with longer coupling intervals either failed to interrupt the reentrant pathway (panel A) or forced a change in the reentrant pathway (panel B). See text for details. Reprinted with permission of The American Heart Association from El-Sherif et al. (10).

bundle beat. The IZeg of this beat showed failure of inscription of a part of the IZ potential (marked by an arrow during a sinus beat). There was also no evidence of the multiple asynchronous spikes that occupied the diastolic interval between consecutive reentrant beats. It is suggested that the premature beat advancing from the NZ activated a relatively large part of the reentrant pathway (evidence for this activation could not be detected by analysis of the IZeg) and collided in the IZ with the reentrant wavefront. In contrast to the situation in panel B, the reentrant wavefront failed to find an excitable alternate pathway and reentry was abruptly terminated.

Figure 13 illustrates the termination of a reentrant ventricular tachycardia by a short run of rapid His bundle pacing (PI) at a rate faster than the tachycardia rate. The relatively wide QRS during His pacing is explained by the fact that pacing was applied a few minutes following the intravenous administration of 10 mg/Kg of procainamide. During the reentrant tachycardia only one of the two IZ electrograms (IZeg-2) clearly illustrated continuous fractionation of the IZ potential bridging the entire diastolic interval. Faster His pacing resulted in additional fractionation of the other electrogram (IZeg-1). In panel A, termination of rapid His pacing was followed by prolonged fractionation of the IZ potential and resumption of the reentrant tachycardia. On the other hand, in panel B, following termination of His pacing, the fractionated IZ potential failed to be inscribed suggesting block in the reentry pathway and resulting in the resumption of sinus rhythm. The figure suggests that faster cardiac pacing during a reentrant tachycardia may result in periodic conduction block in the reentrant pathway. Only termination of pacing following the beat associated with conduction block in the reentrant pathway can result in interruption of reentry. Otherwise, termination of pacing will be followed by resumption of the tachycardia. Not uncommonly,

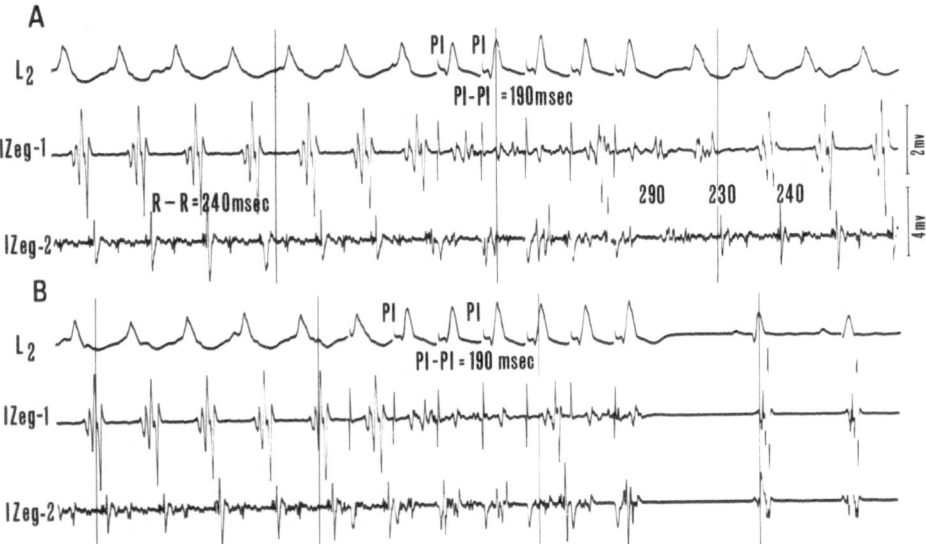

Figure 13. Termination of reentrant ventricular tachycardia following a short run of rapid cardiac (His bundle) pacing. See text for details.

pacing will be followed by one or more reentrant beats with a different configuration of the IZeg and the QRS in surface ECG suggesting the induction of a different reentrant pathway. Frequently, however, the new reentrant pathway is unable to sustain continuous reentry resulting in the resumption of sinus rhythm. A similar situation may also follow a single critically-timed premature beat as was illustrated in Figure 12, panel B.

7. ACTION POTENTIAL CHARACTERISTICS IN THE IZ

Recent in vitro studies (15, 16) have shown that cells in the IZ are heterogeneously abnormal showing variable degrees of partial depolarization (resting potentials from -85 to $-50\,\mathrm{mV}$), reduced action potential amplitude and decreased upstroke velocity. The slow upstrokes are sometimes fractionated into one or more segments of negative slope or show low amplitude slow step potentials. The inhomogeneity of action potentials is betrayed by the finding of relatively good intracellular responses in cells only a few millimeters from other cells which are practically unresponsive. Conduction in the IZ is heterogeneously slowed to values less than 0.01 m/sec resulting in irregular wavefronts. Further evidence of inhomogeneity is the presence of widely disparate refractory periods in cells in close proximity to one another. Full recovery of responsiveness frequently outlasts the action potential duration reflecting the presence of "post-repolarization refractoriness" (22–24). In these cells, premature stimuli would elicit graded responses over a wide range of coupling intervals. Critically coupled premature stimuli could frequently result in one or more spontaneous beats. Conduction in myocardial cells is invariably greatly slowed and irregular when abnormal spontaneous beats occur suggesting that the mechanism of the spontaneous beats is reentry involving depressed ischemic cells. On the other hand, there is no evidence of abnormal automaticity in the ischemic zone. In some cells, full recovery of responsiveness is not complete up to 1000–2000 msec. For these cells, regular pacing at relatively short cycles would result either in a 2 : 1 response or a Wenckebach-like pattern of conduction block. A Wenckebach-like conduction pattern could be commonly elicited in ischemic cells (15). This is illustrated in Figure 14. Intracellular recordings were obtained from two myocardial cells 5 mm apart in the infarction zone. The two cells had widely different resting potentials. The cell at site Y was only slightly depolarized (resting potential of $-80\,\mathrm{mV}$), but it still showed a poor action potential. This observation suggests that responses of ischemic cells might be depressed by factors other than the decrease of resting potential. Pacing at a cycle length of 290 msec resulted in a synchronous Wenckebach-like conduction pattern at the sites of both intra-cellular recordings and the extracellular electrogram. The action potentials of the opening beat of the Wenckebach-like cycle showed a relatively rapid but still abnormally slow upstroke. The second and third beats of the cycle showed a slow initial step followed by a more rapid but still abnormally slow upstroke. In the last beat of the Wenckebach cycle (illustrated at the beginning of the record), the rapid upstroke failed to be inscribed and only a long slow step was recorded. The extracellular bipolar electrogram (marked by arrows) coincided with the relatively rapid upstrokes and illustrated the occurrence of grad-ual conduction delay before failure of conduction during the last beat of the Wenckebach-

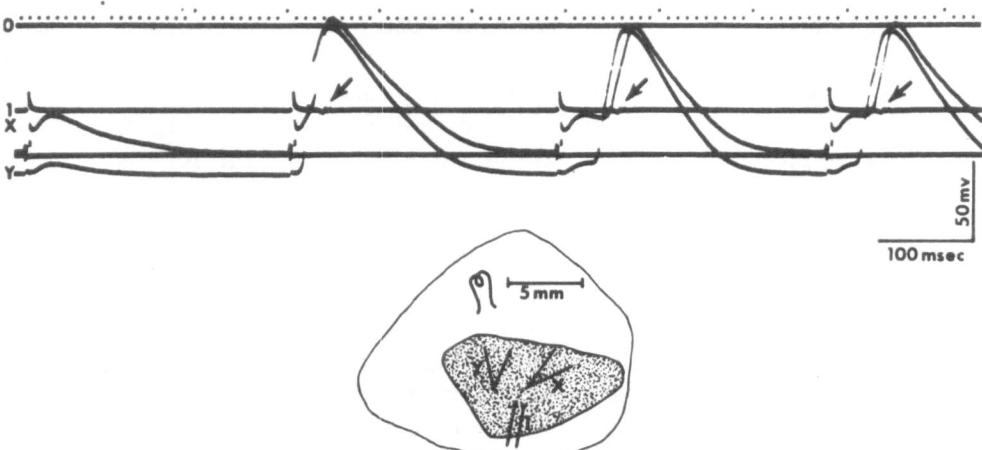

Figure 14. Recordings from an in vitro experiment illustrating action potential characteristics in ischemic epicardium. The sketch of the preparation shows two intracellular recordings (X and Y) and a close bipolar recording (1) from the infarction zone (the hatched area). Ischemic cells had decreased upstroke velocity, reduced action potential amplitude, and a variable degree of partial depolarization. The two cells were recorded 5 mm apart in the infarction zone but showed significant difference in their resting potential. The resting potential of the Y cell was only slightly reduced (− 80 mV) but it still had a poor action potential. The preparation was stimulated at a cycle length of 290 msec which resulted in a Wenckebach-like conduction pattern. Note that the pacing cycle length exceeded the action potential duration of the two cells suggesting that refractoriness extended beyond the completion of the action potential, i.e., post-repolarization refractoriness. Reprinted with permission of The American Heart Association from El-Sherif and Lazzara (15).

like cycle. In Figure 14, the pacing cycle length that resulted in a Wenckebach-like conduction pattern exceeded the action potential duration of the two cells in the IZ. This suggests that full recovery of responsiveness extended beyond the action potential duration, reflecting the presence of "post-repolarization refractoriness".

8. IONIC CONDUCTANCE ABNORMALITIES IN ISCHEMIC MYOCARDIUM

The slow response action potentials were implicated in the genesis of reentrant arrhythmias because of their propensity for very slow propagation with a low safety factor for conduction (25–27). Slow response action potentials could be artificially produced by depolarizing normal Purkinje fibers by high extracellular potassium (K^+) to levels of membrane potential where the rapid Na^+ channel would be inactivated and by enhancing the slow channel by the addition of catecholamine (26, 28–30). This model of slow response action potentials was found to satisfy the necessary requisite for the occurrence of reentrant ventricular arrhythmias (27, 31). The contrived slow response action potential was also readily depressed by verapamil and D-600 (32). The analogy has been drawn between the K^+ depolarized catecholamines-stimulated Purkinje fiber model for slow response action potential and ionic conductance abnormalities in acute ischemia (33). It has been postulated that in the ischemic zone, high concentrations of extracellular K^+ may depolarize the cells to the extent that the rapid Na$^+$ channel is inactivated and high concentrations of catecholamines may stimulate the slow channel resulting in slow response action potentials. The latter would explain slowed conduction and reentrant ventricular arrhythmias associated with ischemia. Although a high K$^+$, high catecholamines environment is plausible in the early states of ischemia (34–36), the postulate is perturbed by several considerations. The principal role of high extracellular K$^+$ in electrophysiologic abnormalities of acute ischemia was questioned in a recent study by Downar et al. (37). Cardiac cells superfused in vitro by coronary venous blood draining an ischemic region developed abnormal electrophysiologic properties. The effects of ischemic blood could not be attributed to increased K$^+$ concentrations even in combination with acidosis, hypoxia and hypoglycemia. The authors suggested that during ischemia, unidentified factors are released which have potent depressant effects on the excitability of myocardial cells.

Furthermore, the effects of verapamil on conduction delays in ischemic myocardium during the early states of ischemia are controversial. In a study by Kuppersmith et al. (38), verapamil administered following coronary occlusion was found to prolong conduction time in the ischemic zone but failed to have an antiarrhythmic effect on the frequency of ventricular beats. The study suggested that slow channel action potentials play a role in the transmission of impulses in the ischemic zone. On the other hand, in a study by Elharrar et al. (39), verapamil administered prior to coronary ligation was found to reduce the extent of conduction delay in ischemic myocardium and decrease the incidence of ventricular arrhythmias. Because the authors still believed in the slow response action potentials as responsible for ischemia-induced conduction delays, they tried to explain their unexpected results on the basis of favorable hemodynamic and metabolic effects of the drug, particularly in limiting the extent of ischemic injury (40, 41).

The K$^+$ depolarized, catecholamines-stimulated Purkinje fiber model and the slow response action potential concept loses much of its plausibility in the later stage of myocardial infarction as in the case of the present model. The extracellular K$^+$ concentration at this stage is not exactly known but is probably not as high as in the early stage of ischemia. Besides, total catecholamines decline in the ischemic region to a very low level on the day after coronary occlusion (36). However, ischemic myocardium still shows markedly depressed action potentials, slow conduction, and a high propensity for reentrant rhythms. In vitro observations show that ischemic myocardial cells are usually partially depolarized. However, other cells with depressed responses may only exhibit a slightly reduced resting potential. This suggests that responses of ischemic cells might be depressed by factors other than the decrease in resting potential.

Depressed ischemic cells were found to be exquisitely sensitive to the depressant effect of tetrodotoxin (15, 16), a specific blocker of the fast Na$^+$ channel (42) (Figure 15, B). In a vivid contradiction to what would be expected from the effect of verapamil and D-600 on a slow response action potential, these two drugs do not depress but rather slightly improve poor membrane responses of ischemic myocardial cells (15) (Figure 15, D). On a purely theoretical note, it is possible to explain the effect of D-600 by suggesting that ischemia results in a host of responses including depressed fast responses and slow responses and that D-600 would abolish the later responses. Because of electrotonic interaction, this effect of D-600

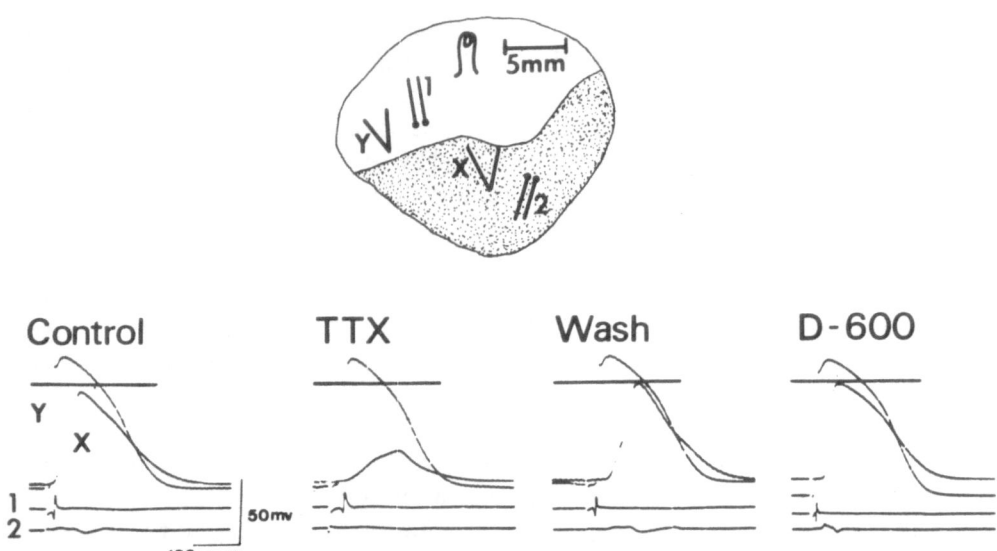

Figure 15. Recordings from an in vitro experiment comparing the effect of tetrodotoxin (TTX) and D-600 on ischemic myocardial cells. The sketch of the preparation shows an intracellular and extracellular recording from both the infarction zone (the hatched area) and the normal zone. The resting potential of the ischemic cell (X) was only slightly different from the normal cell (Y) but the cell had a markedly decreased upstroke velocity and a reduced action potential amplitude. TTX slightly reduced the upstroke velocity of the normal cell but markedly attenuated the ischemic cell action potential and abolished the ischemic zone electrogram 2. In contrast, D-600 slightly improved the upstroke velocity of the ischemic cell with noticeable improvement of the ischemic zone electrogram. Reprinted with permission of The American Heart Association from El-Sherif and Lazzara (15).

could result in improvement of upstroke velocity of depressed fast responses. These assumptions are, however, refuted because of the consistent failure to demonstrate slow responses that were further depressed or abolished by D-600 in the subacute IZ (15). On the contrary, recent observations strongly suggest that the slow inward current does not play a role in the transmission of the cardiac impulse in ischemic myocardium, at least in the late myocardial infarction period (15). Also significant is the failure to demonstrate spontaneous or triggered abnormal automaticy in ischemic myocardium at this stage (15). Poor membrane responses of ischemic myocardial cells appear to be related to depression of the fast Na^+ channel (15). It may be pointed out that contrary to Purkinje fibers, which are specialized for rapid conduction, ventricular myocardium has normally slower conduction with slow recovery from inactivation of inward currents (43). Myocardial cells may be particularly susceptible to partial depression of the fast channel with further impairment of recovery from inactivation of the Na^+ current. The latter would explain the marked prolongation of post-repolarization refractoriness of ischemic myocardial cells.

The exact mechanism(s) for ischemia-induced depression of the fast channel is unknown. A clear formulation of the effects of ischemia on membrane currents and ionic conductance will require further studies, as well as better understanding of the biochemical processes governing ion movements in normal cells.

9. PHARMACOLOGICAL ASPECTS OF REENTRANT VENTRICULAR ARRHYTHMIAS IN THE LATE MYOCARDIAL INFARCTION PERIOD

Antiarrhythmic drugs can have significant effects on the electrophysiologic determinants of ventricular reentrant pathways. Studies of the effects of drugs on reentrant ventricular arrhythmias in the late myocardial infarction period help not only to elucidate the mechanism of action of antiarrhythmic drugs but also to unravel some of the ionic conductance abnormalities in ischemia. The majority of clinically available antiarrhythmic drugs (e.g., procainamide, quinidine, lidocaine and diphenylhydantoin) owe their antiarrhythmic effect on ischemic reentrant ventricular arrhythmias to prolongation of refractoriness and further depression or block of conduction in the reentrant pathway (12, 13, 44). The difference between lidocaine and diphenylhydantoin on one hand and procainamide and quinidine on the other hand is that the former drugs result in a selective further impairment of depressed myocardial cells forming part of the reentrant pathway at a concentration that has little or no effect on electrophysiologic properties of normal myocardium (12, 13).

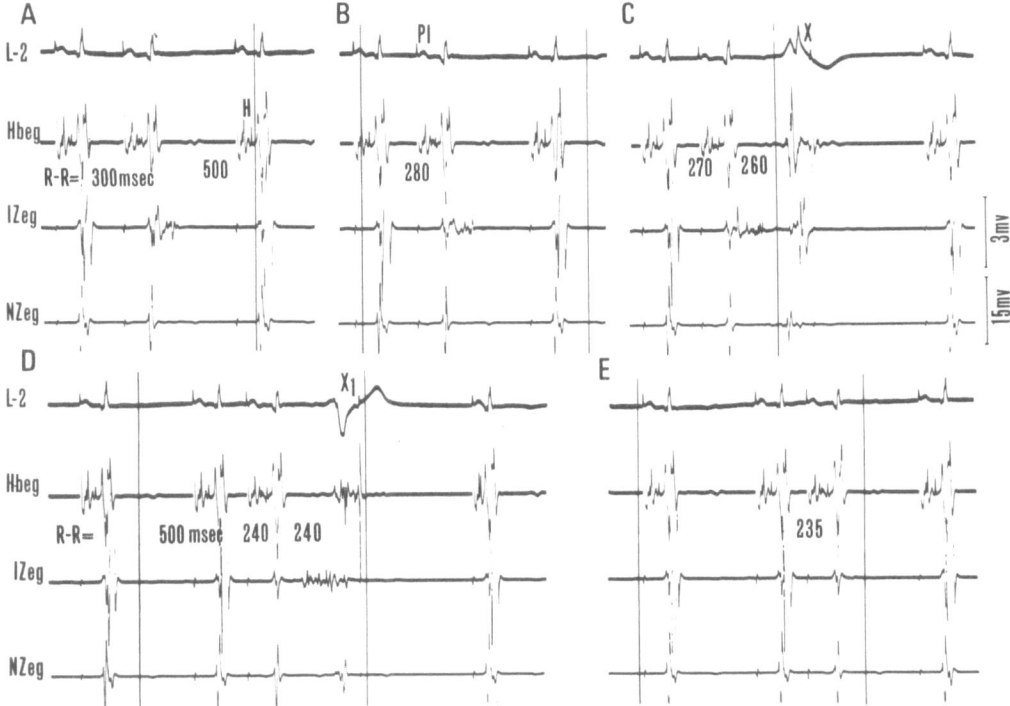

Figure 16. Programmed atrial premature stimulation inducing two different reentrant ventricular beats (X and X$_1$) at different critical coupling intervals. The width of the reentrant zone is 35 msec. See text for details. In this and subsequent figures: Hbeg = His bundle electrogram; IZeg = infarction zone electrogram; NZeg = normal zone electrogram; PI = pacer impulse; H = His bundle deflection; X and X$_1$ = two different reentrant beats. Timelines are set at one second intervals.

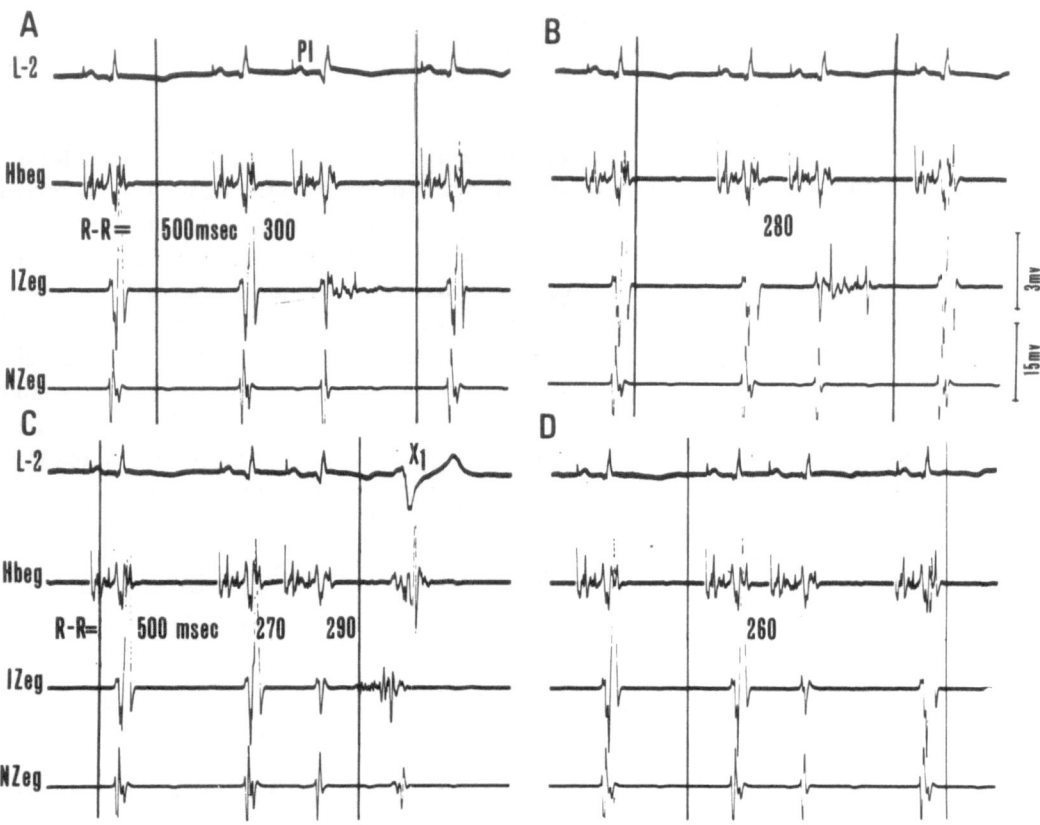

Figure 17. Effect of lidocaine on reentrant ventricular arrhythmia induced by programmed premature stimulation. Recordings were obtained from the same experiment shown in Figure 16 one minute following intravenous injection of 2 mg/Kg of lidocaine. See text for details.

Figures 16–18 illustrate the effect of lidocaine on electrophysiologic parameters of an ischemia-related reentrant ventricular rhythm induced by programmed premature stimulation. Figure 16 shows control recordings. Panels A to E illustrate atrial pacing at a basic cycle length of 500 msec with programmed atrial premature stimulation at gradually shorter coupling intervals. Premature beats with a coupling intervals of 300 msec (panel A) and 280 msec (panel B) resulted in a limited degree of fractionation and delay of the IZ potential. A critical range of coupling intervals (240 to 275 msec) resulted in sufficient fractionation and delay of the IZ potential and initiated one or more reentrant beats. The "reentry zone" measured 35 msec. Two reentrant pathways could be identified by different configuration of the fractionated IZ potential and the reentrant QRS in surface ECG and are labelled X (panel C) and X_1 (panel D). Panel E shows that a premature beat with a coupling interval of 235 msec resulted in block of the IZ potential and failed to induce reentry.

Figure 17 was obtained one minute following intravenous bolus administration of 2 mg/Kg of lidocaine. Panels A and B show that premature beats with coupling intervals

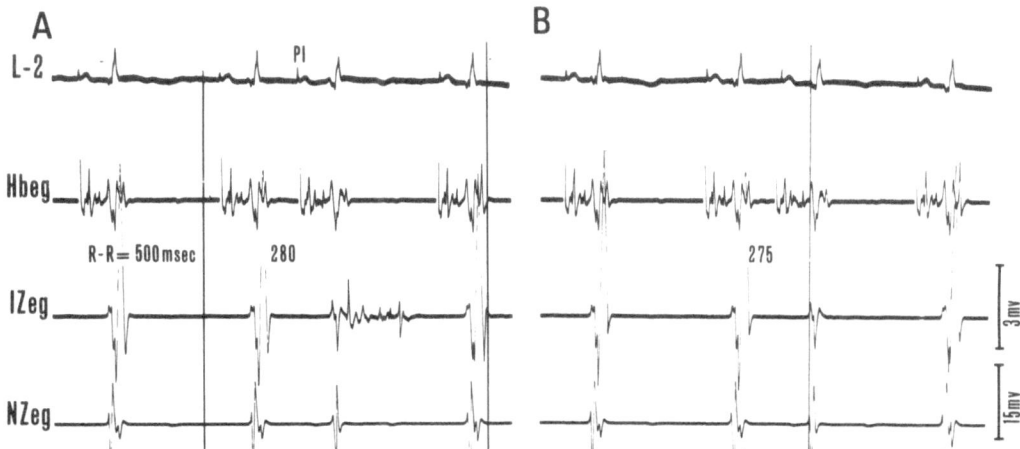

Figure 18. Recordings obtained from the same experiment shown in Figures 16 and 17, two minutes following lidocaine administration. Note abolition of the reentry zone. See text for details.

of 300 and 280 msec, respectively, resulted in relatively more fractionation and delay of the IZ potential compared to control recordings in Figure 16. The reentrant beat marked X could no longer be produced by premature stimulation suggesting block of conduction in this reentrant pathway. On the other hand, the reentrant beat marked X_1 could be induced by a premature beat with a longer coupling interval compared to control (270 msec in Figure 17, panel C, compared to 240 msec in Figure 16, panel D). Also the coupling interval of the reentrant beat which reflects the reentrant pathway conduction time was longer (290 msec) compared to control (240 msec). Panel D shows that a premature beat with a longer coupling interval of 260 msec resulted in block of the IZ potential compared to a control interval of 235 msec in Figure 16, panel E. The reentry zone following lidocaine administration was thus reduced to 10 msec compared to a control value of 35 msec.

Figure 18 was obtained two minutes following lidocaine administration and illustrates complete obliteration of the reentry zone. Panel A shows that a premature beat with a coupling interval of 280 msec resulted in marked fractionation and delay of the IZ potential but failed to induce reentry. Shortening of the coupling interval by 5 msec in panel B resulted in complete block of the IZ potential.

A classical response of ischemia-related reentrant ventricular tachycardia induced by programmed premature stimulation to antiarrhythmic drugs that act by prolonging refractoriness and depressing conduction in the reentrant pathway can be summarized as follows (12, 13, 44): 1) narrowing of and/or abolition of the reentry zone, 2) shift of the narrowed reentry zone to longer cardiac cycle lengths. This means that premature beats with longer coupling intervals may be required to induce the arrhythmia, 3) lengthening of the coupling interval of the first reentrant beat as well as slowing of the rate of reentrant tachycardia.

In individual cases, a depressant antiarrhythmic drug may fail to abolish reentry or may even paradoxically lengthen the reentry zone (13, 44). Since these drugs act by further impairment of the already slow conduction in a reentrant pathway, they may have the potential

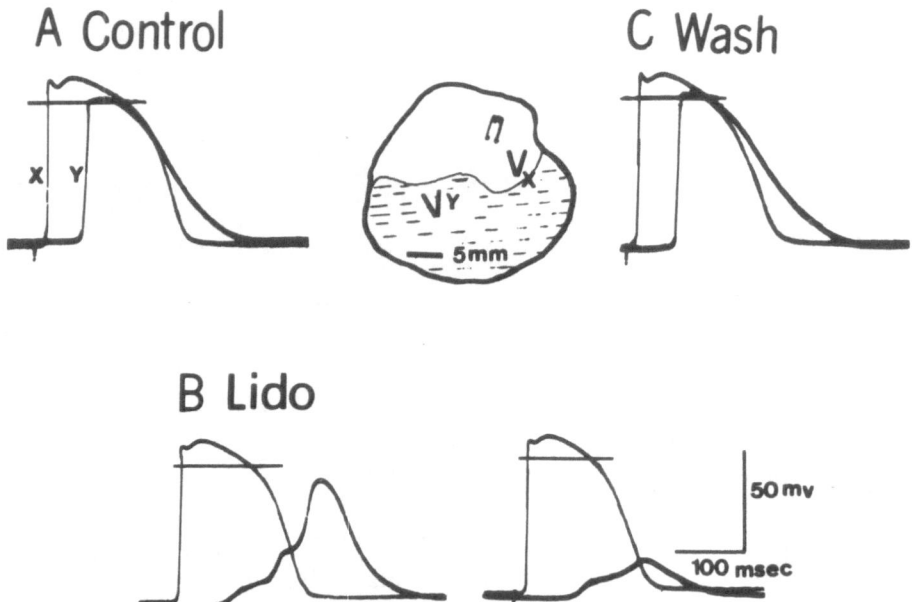

Figure 19. Differential effects of lidocaine, 1.1×10^{-5} molar, on ischemic (Y) and normal (X) myocardial cells with similar resting potentials. The resting potential of the cell in the ischemic zone was -75 mv but it had a poor action potential compared with the cell in the normal zone near the border. The $\dot{V}max$ of the cell at site Y was 18 v/sec, whereas at site X it was 110 v/sec. The "normal" cell may have been mildly depressed by virtue of being near the border of the infarct. The ischemic zone is at the bottom of the sketch. Lidocaine markedly depressed the ischemic Y cell but had little effect on the normal X cell. Reprinted with permission of The American Journal of Cardiology from Lazzara et al. (16).

to create successful reentrant circuits by critically slowing conduction in moderately depressed cells (44). Similar observations on the effect of procainamide on clinical examples of reentrant ventricular tachycardias have been recently reported (45).

Recent in vitro studies of ischemic muscle cells have shown that lidocaine in therapeutic concentrations nearly abolished propagated action potentials in severely affected cells while it modestly depressed membrane responsiveness in cells which were nearly normal (16) (Figure 19). The recovery of responsiveness of abnormal cells was also greatly prolonged by lidocaine. Observations in both in vivo and in vitro studies help to formulate a "selectivity hypothesis" for the antiarrhythmic action of lidocaine (12, 16). Thus, lidocaine further depresses in a selective way, severely depressed cells forming part of the reentrant pathway while it had little or no effect on normal or moderately depressed cells. The ionic mechanisms for the selective depressant effect of lidocaine in ischemic cells are still largely conjectural. However, the effect of lidocaine on depressed ischemic cells is remarkably similar to that of tetrodotoxin, a specific blocker of the fast channel (see Figure 15, B). This would suggest that ischemia may result in depression of the fast Na channel and that lidocaine may act by further depressing this channel.

It is generally assumed that the two mechanisms by which an antiarrhythmic agent can exert its effect on reentrant rhythms are either further depression and block of the reentrant pathway or improvement of conduction in the pathway (46). Recent observations suggest that one group of antiarrhythmic drugs (verapamil and D-600) owe their antiarrhythmic effect on ischemic reentrant ventricular arrhythmias to improvement of conduction in the reentrant pathway (15). Both verapamil and D-600 are thought to act by blocking the slow inward current carried by calcium (47–49) and possibly by sodium (32). These drugs were shown to be effective on reentrant rhythms that depend on slow response action potentials, e.g., AV nodal reentrant tachycardia (50). In this case, the drugs act by further depression and block of conduction in the reentrant pathway. However, the mechanism of action of the two drugs on ischemic reentrant ventricular arrhythmias is diametrically opposite to their effect on AV nodal reentrant rhythms.

Figures 20 and 21 illustrate the effect of verapamil on ischemia-related reentrant ventricular tachycardia induced by programmed premature stimulation. Figure 20 shows control recordings during His bundle pacing at a basic cycle length of 450 msec and the effect of premature beats introduced at gradually shorter coupling intervals. Panel A shows that a

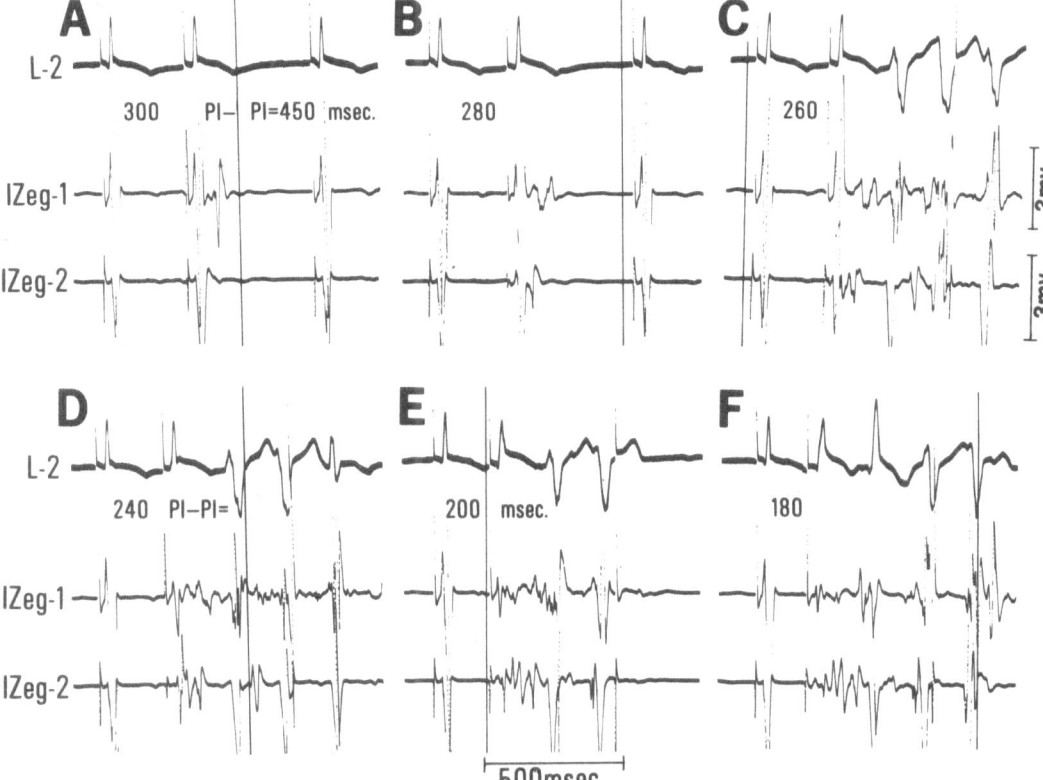

Figure 20. Initiation of reentrant ventricular tachycardia by programmed premature cardiac (His bundle) stimulation. See text for details. IZeg-1 and IZeg-2 represent two composite electrograms from the infarction zone. Reprinted with permission of The American Heart Association from El-Sherif and Lazzara (15).

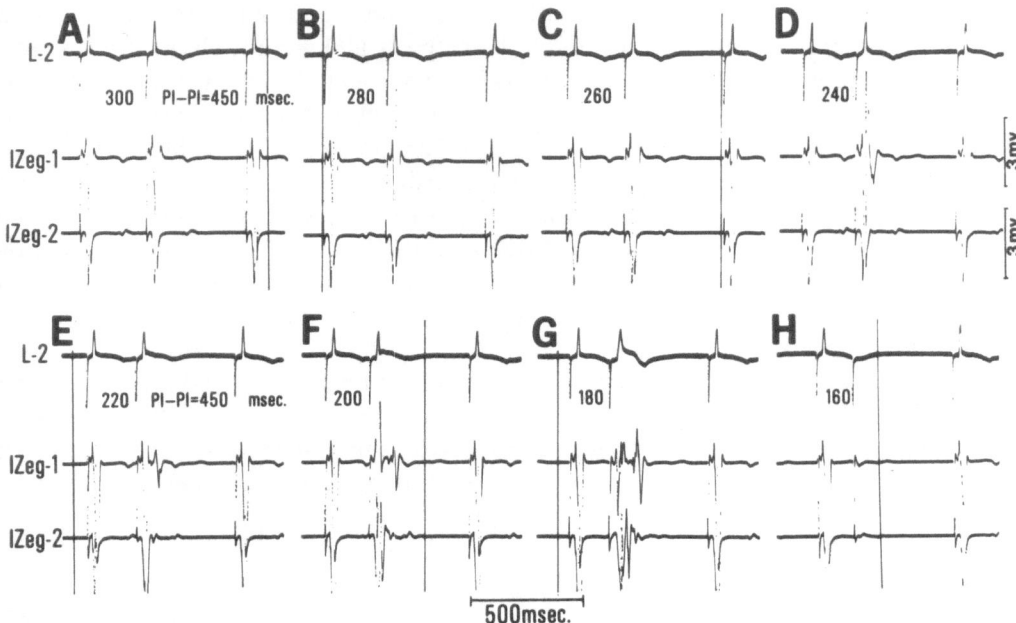

Figure 21. Recordings from the same experiment shown in Figure 20 that illustrate the effect of verapamil on ischemic reentrant ventricular arrhythmias initiated by programmed premature stimulation. Note failure to initiate reentry following verapamil due to limited fractionation of the IZ potential. See text for details. Reprinted with permission of The American Heart Association from El-Sherif and Lazzara (15).

premature beat with a coupling interval of 300 msec resulted in more fractionation and delay of the IZ potential compared to the regular paced beat at a cycle length of 450 msec. Shortening of the coupling interval to 280 msec in panel B resulted in further fractionation and delay of the IZ potential. At a critical coupling interval of 260 msec in panel C, the fractionated and delayed IZ potential extended beyond the T wave of the surface ECG and resulted in a manifest reentrant ventricular tachycardia. Coupling intervals between 180 and 260 msec resulted in manifest reentry (panels D to F). Coupling intervals shorter than 180 msec blocked in the His-Purkinje system and did not excite the ventricular myocardium.

Figure 21 was obtained two minutes following an intravenous bolus injection of 0.5 mg/Kg of verapamil. Following verapamil injection, coupling intervals of 260–300 msec failed to result in any noticeable change in the configuration and duration of the IZeg compared to regular paced beats (panels A to C). On the other hand, coupling intervals of 180–240 msec resulted in a limited degree of fractionation and delay of the IZ potential that did not extend beyond the T wave of the surface ECG (panels D to G). Consequently, these premature beats failed to induce manifest reentrant rhythms. A coupling interval of 160 msec blocked in the His-Purkinje system (panel H). Figures 20 and 21 suggest that the antiarrhythmic effect of verapamil on ischemia-related reentrant ventricular tachycardias initiated by premature beats is most probably related to shortening of post-repolarization refractoriness in ischemic myocardium with the resultant improvement of conduction of premature beats. It should be emphasized, however, that verapamil was found to have no significant effect on chronic recurrent reentrant ventricular tachycardia (45).

Improvement of depressed membrane responses of ischemic myocardial cells by verapamil and D-600 can be possibly related to either hemodynamic and metabolic effects of the drugs or to a direct electrophysiologic action. Verapamil has been shown to reduce the extent of ischemic injury following coronary artery ligation (40). It is doubtful, however, that it will have a similar effect when administered 3–7 days following myocardial infarction. Verapamil in a dose of 0.1 mg/Kg or less was found to cause peripheral vasodilatation which leads to reflex increase of the sympathetic tone (51). A recent study has shown that verapamil induced catecholamine release may enhance electrophysiologic properties of depressed Purkinje fibers (52). Recent in vivo and in vitro observations have shown, however, that verapamil and D-600 improve depressed responses of ischemic myocardial cells in doses of 0.5 mg/Kg in vivo and 0.5-mg/liter in vitro (15). These doses were not shown to be associated with reflex catecholamine release (51). Furthermore, pretreatment with propranolol did not prevent the enhancing effect of a smaller dose of verapamil in vivo (0.2 mg/Kg) (15). The possibility that verapamil and D-600 would increase myocardial blood flow to the epicardial ischemic zone and that this effect would improve membrane responses of ischemic myocardial cells has not been investigated but seems unlikely to be a major contributing factor. On the other hand, recent in vitro observations clearly illustrate that at least part of the D-600 induced improvement of depressed ischemic cells is due to a direct electrophysiologic action on altered membrane responses (15) (see Figure 15, D). The exact mechanism by which verapamil or D-600 would improve the kinetics of ischemia-induced depressed fast channel as well as the abnormally delayed recovery of inactivation of the Na^+ current is largely unknown. Some studies have shown the action of D-600 to be complex involving not only reduction of the maximal Ca^{++} conductance but also a change in both the kinetics of the Ca^{++}-carrying system and the amplitude of the steady state outward current (53). An interesting possibility is that verapamil or D-600 may improve the depressed Na^+ channel by a sparing effect on endogenous energy resources. This possibility is, however, perturbed by incomplete understanding of the energy requirement of both normal and depressed Na^+ channel (54).

The effect of verapamil and D-600 on ischemia-related reentrant ventricular arrhythmias raises the interesting question of whether it is desirable and/or practical for an ideal antiarrhythmic drug to act by selectively depressing or by improving conduction of depressed cells forming part of the reentrant pathway. In this regard, recent observations suggest that verapamil is probably a weaker antiarrhythmic drug compared to lidocaine in reentrant ventricular arrhythmias in the late myocardial infarction period (15). This may suggest that an ideal antiarrhythmic drug in ischemia-related reentrant ventricular arrhythmias should probably selectively depress rather than improve membrane responses of depressed cells critically involved in the establishment of successful reentrant circuits.

REFERENCES

1. Gambetta M, Childers RW: The initial electrophysiologic disturbance in experimental myocardial infarction. Ann Intern Med 70:1076, (abstr) 1969.
2. Han J: Mechanisms of ventricular arrhythmias associated with myocardial infarction. Am J Cardiol 24:800–813, 1969.
3. Durrer D, Van Dam RTH, Freud GE, Janse MJ: Reentry and ventricular arrhythmias in local ischemia and infarction of the intact dog heart. Proc Kon Ned Akad Van Wetensch Amsterdam C73: no 4, 1971.
4. Waldo AL, Kaiser GA: A study of ventricular arrhythmias associated with acute myocardial infarction in the canine heart. Circulation 47:1222–1288, 1973.
5. Boineau JP, Cox JL: Slow ventricular activation in acute myocardial infarction. A source of re-entrant premature ventricular contractions. Circulation 48: 702–713, 1973.
6. Scherlag BJ, El-Sherif N, Hope R. Lazzara R: Characterization and localization of ventricular arrhythmias due to myocardial ischemia and infarction. Circ Res 35:372–383, 1974.
7. Williams DO, Scherlag BJ, Hope R, El-Sherif N. Lazzara R: The pathophysiology of malignant ventricular arrhythmias during acute myocardial ischemia. Circulation 50:1163–1172, 1974.
8. El-Sherif N, Scherlag BJ, Lazzara R: Electrode catheter recordings during malignant ventricular arrhythmias following experimental acute myocardial ischemia. Circulation 51:1003–1014, 1975.
9. El-Sherif N, Scherlag BJ, Lazzara R, Hope RR: Reentrant ventricular arrhythmias in the late myocardial period. 1. Conduction characteristics in the infarction zone. Circulation 55:686–702, 1977.
10. El-Sherif N, Hope RR, Scherlag BJ, Lazzara R: Reentrant ventricular arrhythmias in the late myocardial infarction period. 2. Pattern of initiation and termination of reentry. Circulation 55:702–719, 1977.
11. El-Sherif N, Lazzara R, Hope RR, Scherlag BJ: Reentrant ventricular arrhythmias in the late myocardial infarction period. 3. Manifest and concealed extrasystolic grouping. Circulation 56:225–234, 1977.
12. El-Sherif N, Scherlag BJ, Lazzara R, Hope RR: Reentrant ventricular arrhythmias in the late myocardial infarction period. 4. Mechanism of action of lidocaine. Circulation 56:395–402, 1977.
13. El-Sherif N, Lazzara R: Reentrant ventricular arrhythmias in the late myocardial infarction period. 5. Mechanism of action of diphenylhydantoin. Circulation 57:465–472, 1978.
14. El-Sherif N: Reentrant ventricular arrhythmias in the late myocardial infarction period. 6. Effect of the autonomic system. Circulation 58:103–110, 1978.
15. El-Sherif N, Lazzara R: Reentrant ventricular arrhythmias in the late myocardial infarction period. 7. Effect of verapamil and D-600 and role of the "slow channel". Circulation 60: 605–615, 1979.
16. Lazzara R, Hope RR, El-Sherif N, Scherlag BJ: Effects of lidocaine on hypoxic and ischemic cardiac cells. Am J Cardiology 41:872–879, 1978.
17. Smith RA, El-Sherif N, Evans AK: Epicardial mapping of ventricular reentrant pathways in the late myocardial infarction period. (abstr) Am J Cardiol 41:427, 1978.
18. Edwards JE: What is myocardial infarction? Circulation 39, 40 (suppl IV): IV-5–12, 1969.
19. Schmitt FO, Erlanger J: Directional differences in the conduction of the impulse through heart muscle and their possible relation to extrasystolic and fibrillary contractions. Am J Physiol 87:326, 1928.
20. Schamroth L, Marriott HJL: Concealed ventricular extrasystoles. Circulation 27:1043–1049, 1963.
21. Schamroth L: The physiological basis of ectopic ventricular rhythm: A unifying concept. So Afr Med J (suppl) 3–26:1971.
22. El-Sherif N, Scherlag BJ, Lazzara R, Samet P: Pathophysiology of tachycardia and bradycardia-dependent block in the canine proximal His-Purkinje system after acute ischemia. Am J Cardiol 33: 529–540, 1974.
23. Lazzara R, El-Sherif N, Scherlag BJ: Disorders of cellular electrophysiology produced by ischemia of the canine His bundle. Circ Res 36:444–454, 1975.
24. Lazzara R, El-Sherif N, Hope RR, Scherlag BJ: Ventricular arrhythmias and electrophysiologic consequences of ischemia and infarction. Cir Res 42:740–749, 1978.
25. Cranefield PF, Klein HO, Hoffman BF: Conduction of the cardiac impulse: 1. Delay, blocks and one-way block in depressed Purkinje fibers. Circ Res 28:199–219, 1971.
26. Cranefield PF, Wit AL, Hoffman BF: Conduction of the cardiac impulse. II. Characteristics of very slow conduction. J Gen Physiol 59:227–246, 1972.
27. Cranefield PF: The conduction of the cardiac impulse. Mount Kisco, New York, Futura Pub Co, 1975.
28. Carmeliet E, Vereeke S: Adrenaline and the plateau phase of the cardiac action potential: Importance of Ca^{++}, Na^+, and K^+ conductance. Pflueger Arch 313:300–315, 1969.
29. Pappano AJ: Calcium-dependent action potentials produced by catecholamines in guinea pig atrial muscle

fibers depolarized by potassium. Circ Res 27:379–390, 1970.

30. Shigenobu K, Sperelakis N: Calcium current channels induced by catecholamines in chick embryonic hearts whose fast sodium channels are blocked by tetrodotoxin or elevated potassium. Circ Res 31:932–952, 1972.

31. Wit AL, Hoffman BF, Cranefield PF: Slow conduction and reentry in the ventricular conducting system. Return extrasystole in canine Purkinje fibers. Circ Res 30:11–22, 1972.

32. Shigenobu K, Schneider JA, Sperelakis N: Verapamil blockade of slow Na$^+$ and Ca^{++} responses in myocardial cells. J Pharmacol Exp Ther 190:280–288, 1974.

33. Wit AL, Bigger JT Jr: Possible electrophysiological mechanisms for lethal arrhythmias accompanying myocardial ischemia and infarction. Circulation 51 (suppl 3): 96–115, 1975.

34. Thomas M, Shulman G, Opie L: Arteriovenous potassium changes and ventricular arrhythmias after coronary artery occlusion. Cardiovasc Res 4:327–333, 1970.

35. Cherry G, Myers MB: The relationship to ventricular fibrillation of early tissue sodium and potassium shifts and coronary vein potassium levels in experimental myocardial infarction. J Thorac Cardiovasc Surg 61: 587–598, 1971.

36. Griffith J, Leung F: The sequential estimation of plasma catecholamines and whole blood histamine in myocardial infarction. Am Heart J 82:171–179, 1971.

37. Downar E, Janse MJ, Durrer D: The effect of "ischemic" blood on transmembrane potentials of normal porcine ventricular myocardium. Circulation 55:455–462, 1977.

38. Kuppersmith J. Shiang H, Litwak RS, Herman MV: Electrophysiologic effects of verapamil in canine myocardial ischemia. Am J Cardiol 37:149, 1976 (abstr).

39. Elharrar J, Gaum WE, Zipes DP: Effect of drugs on conduction delay and incidence of ventricular arrhythmias induced by acute coronary occlusion in dogs. Am J Cardiol 39:544–549, 1977.

40. Smith HJ, Singh BN, Nisbet HD, et al: Effect of verapamil on infarct size following experimental coronary occlusion. Cardiovasc Res 9:569–578, 1975.

41. Nayler W, Grau A, Slade A: A protective effect of verapamil on hypoxic heart muscle. Cardiovasc Res 10: 650–662, 1976.

42. Dudel J, Peper K, Rudel R: Effect of tetrodotoxin on the membrane current in cardiac muscle (Purkinje fibers). Pfluegers Arch 295:213–226, 1967.

43. Gettes LS, Reuter H: Slow recovery from inactivation of inward currents in mamalian myocardial fibers. J Physiol 240:703–724, 1974.

44. El-Sherif, N: Electrophysiologic basis of procainamide therapeutic and toxic effects on ischemia-related reentrant ventricular arrhythmias. Am J. Cardiology 43:429, 1979 (abstr).

45. Wellens HJJ, Bär FWHM, Lie KI, Düren DR, Dohmen KJ: Effect of procainamide, propranolol and verapamil on mechanism of tachycardia in patients with chronic recurrent ventricular tachycardia. Am J Cardiol 40:579–585, 1977.

46. Rosen MR, Hoffman BF: Mechanisms of action of antiarrhythmic drugs. Circ Res 32:1–8, 1973.

47. Kohlhardt M, Bauer B, Kranse H, Fleckenstein A: Differentiation of the transmembrane Na and Ca channels in mammalian cardiac fibers by use of specific inhibitors. Pfluegers Arch 335:309–322, 1972.

48. Cranefield PF, Aronson RS, Wit AL: Effect of verapamil on the normal action potential and on a calcium-dependent slow response of canine Purkinje fibers. Circ Res 34:204–216, 1974.

49. Watanabe AM, Besch HR Jr: Subcellular myocardial effects of verapamil and D-600: Comparison with propranolol. J Pharmacol Exp Ther 191:241–251, 1974.

50. Wit AL, Cranefield PF: The effects of verapamil on the sino-atrial and atrioventricular nodes of the rabbit and the mechanism by which it arrests reentrant AV nodal tachycardia. Circ Res 35:413–425, 1974.

51. Angus JA, Richmond DR, Dhumma-Upakorn P, Cobbin LB, Goodman AH: Cardiovascular action of verapamil in the dog with particular reference to myocardial contractility and atrioventricular conduction. Cardiovasc Res 10:623–632, 1976.

52. Danile P, Hordoff AJ, Delphin Es, Rosen MR: Verapamil effects on blood superfused Purkinje fibers: Evidence for direct and catecholamine-mediated actions. Am J Cardiol 41:417, 1978 (abstr).

53. Nawrath H, Ten Eick RE, McDonald TF, Trautwein W: On the mechanism underlying the action of D-600 on slow inward current and tension in mamalian myocardium. Circ Res 40:408–414, 1977.

54. Carmeliet E: Cardiac transmembrane potentials and metabolism. Circ Res 42:577–587, 1978.

SECTION 2
THE ELECTROPHYSIOLOGY OF LETHAL ARRHYTHMIAS

SECTION 2B
THE NERVOUS SYSTEM AND CARDIAC ARRHYTHMIAS

2.4. NEURAL FACTORS AND VENTRICULAR ELECTRICAL INSTABILITY

R.L. VERRIER

1. INTRODUCTION

Coronary care unit and out-of-hospital resuscitation experience have made it clear that ventricular fibrillation (VF) is the main mechanism for sudden cardiac death. Since prolonged survival is possible after resuscitation, this lethal arrhythmia represents an electrical accident rather than the end-product of far advanced, irreversible structural disease of the heart (1). In most cases of sudden death, acute pathologic lesions either in the coronary arteries or in the myocardium are absent or inadequate to account for the fatal event. How, then, is the derangement in electrical activity of the heart precipitated?

Two hypotheses relating to the genesis of VF have guided our work during the past decade: 1) the patient susceptible to sudden death has electrical instability of the myocardium, and 2) transient risk factors, due primarily to altered neural activity, can trigger VF in the electrically unstable heart. These formulations have been extended in the past few years to include a third conception, namely, that prevention of sudden death requires restraining of neurophysiologic triggers in addition to protecting the cardiac target (2). This presentation will deal with our current studies aimed at prevention of sudden death by modifying neural activity which predisposes to VF.

2. EXPOSURE OF ELECTRICAL INSTABILITY

2.1. Cardiac electrical testing by inducing VF

Our search for a technique to expose the presence of electrical instability which could be employed clinically has been ongoing for more than a decade. The first method consisted of administering suprathreshold electrical energies to the intact chest during the vulnerable period. The emergence of ventricular tachycardia of the vulnerable period with energies subthreshold for VF was deemed to indicate the presence of electrical instability (3). A second technique was sequential R/T pulsing. This latter method represents a significant advance since threshold currents are sufficient to provoke VF. The time course of VF threshold exposed using this method closely paralleled the susceptibility to VF during both coronary artery occlusion and reperfusion (4, 5). While the induction of VF by sequential pulsing provided a valuable approach for modelling the problem of electrical instability in the animal, it obviously had no relevance in man.

2.2. The repetitive extrasystole (RE) threshold as an index of vulnerability to VF

Recently we found that the evocation of a repetitive extrasystole (RE) in response to a single stimulus discharged in the ventricular vulnerable period is a sensitive index of susceptibility to VF (6). Repetitive extrasystoles are elicited when approximately two thirds of the fibrillatory current is delivered (Figure 1). The nadir of the RE threshold is coincident in the cardiac cycle with the vulnerable period for VF under diverse experimental interventions which alter cardiac vulnerability in the conscious as well as the anesthetized animal (2, 6, 7). Thus, RE and VF phenomena appear to share a common electrophysiologic basis and the RE threshold can be used as an index of ventricular susceptibility to fibrillation. The relation between RE and VF also obtains when the sequential R/T pulsing technique is employed. The close coupling of the sequential R/T stimuli results in corresponding reductions in the currents required to elicit RE and VF. Thus, when the sequential R/T pulsing method is employed to measure the RE threshold, electrical instability can be exposed using relatively low stimulus intensities. These techniques are currently being utilized to assess ventricular electrical instability in man. Green and coworkers (8) and Farshidi et al. (9) have shown a close correlation between the elicitation of multiple ventricular responses with threshold electrical stimuli and the subsequent risk for sudden death. Pharmacologic suppression of repetitive ventricular response appears to be associated with a reduction in recurrent ventricular arrhythmias (10).

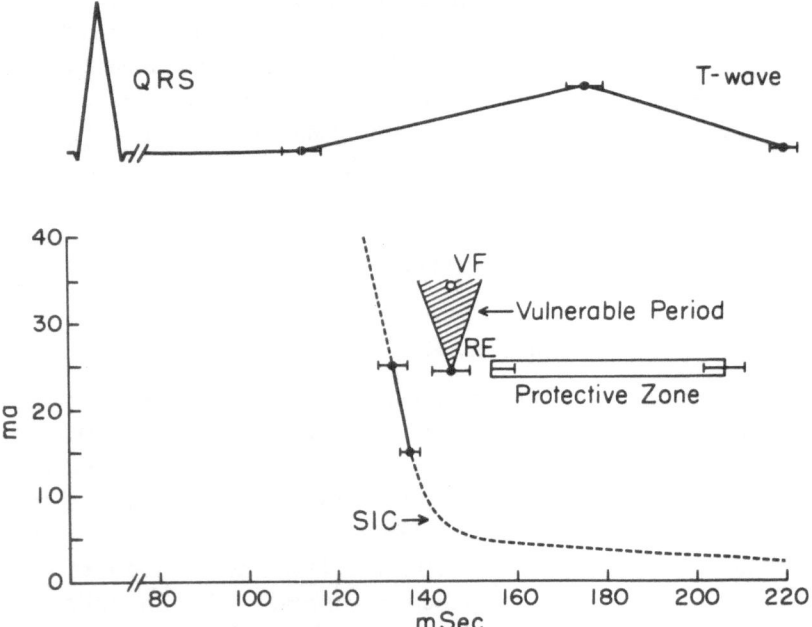

Figure 1. Temporal relationships between T wave, vulnerable period (VP), strength-interval curve (SIC), and protective zone (PZ). The vulnerable period curve for repetitive extrasystoles (RE) has a characteristic V shape, the nadir of which coincides temporally with that for provoking ventricular fibrillation (VF). The PZ is a relatively broad zone which occurs 10–20 msec after the VP nadir and is approximately 50 msec in duration (7).

2.3. Precordial mechanical stimulation for exposing electrical instability

Conventional techniques for assessing ventricular instability require cardiac catheterization and therefore are impractical for large scale screening of patients with ischemic heart disease. We examined the possibility of utilizing precordial mechanical thumping to assess electrical instability in the canine heart (11). Myocardial fibers were depolarized by transduction of the mechanical thump to an electrically propagated response. By delivering synchronized sequential R/T pulses, the provocation of RE can be used as a marker of ventricular electrical instability (Figure 2). It remains to be shown whether this approach will prove effective in man. Whatever the outcome with this technique, the principle of employing direct and preferably noninvasive approaches for uncovering electrical instability of the heart deserves intensive investigation.

3. CENTRAL NERVOUS SYSTEM STIMULATION AND VENTRICULAR ELECTRICAL INSTABILITY

The evidence implicating central and peripheral nervous system activity in the genesis of VF has been recently published (2, 12, 13), and will be only briefly reviewed. The emphasis in this presentation will be on our current neurophysiologic and neuropharmacologic studies aimed at combating neural triggers for VF.

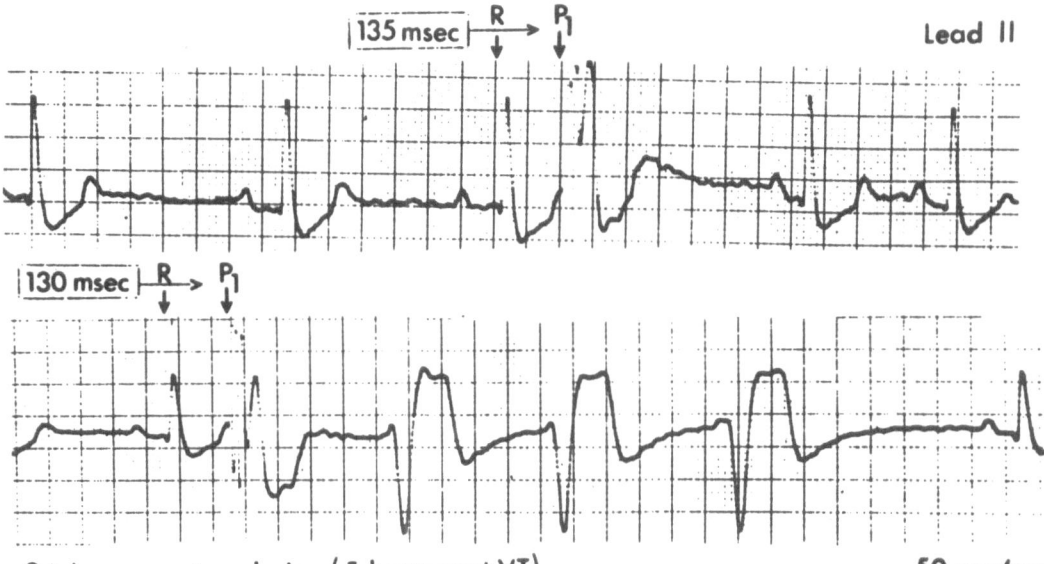

Figure 2. A single mechanical pulse (P_1) of chest wall in an awake dog 135 msec after the preceding QRS complex evoked only a single response (upper tracing). However, when the mechanical pulse was delivered 5 msec earlier (130 msec), ventricular tachycardia was consistently induced. When the thump was administered even earlier, ventricular fibrillation occurred in this animal, which had recovered 5 hours earlier from ventricular tachycardia (VT), resulting from occlusion of the left anterior descending coronary artery that had been induced in the preceding 24 hours (11).

Electrical stimulation of various sites in the central nervous system can profoundly alter ventricular electrical instability and elicit a diversity of arrhythmias (14, 15). Excitation of the posterior hypothalamus, for example, substantially lowers the VF threshold in the normal canine heart and results in a tenfold increase in the incidence of spontaneous VF during acute left anterior descending coronary artery occlusion (15, 16, 17). The susceptibility to VF during central nervous system stimulation can be prevented by cardiac sympathectomy or beta-adrenergic blockade (15, 17, 18). The arrhythmogenic effect of higher nervous system stimulation is not altered by vagotomy (15, 19). The ventricular arrhythmias which follow cessation of diencephalic or hypothalamic stimulation require intact parasympathetic neural pathways (19, 20).

These findings indicate that stimulation of certain areas in the brain can increase ventricular electrical instability in the normal heart and provoke VF during acute myocardial ischemia. The profibrillatory effect appears to be largely mediated by the sympathetic nervous system.

4. PERIPHERAL SYMPATHETIC NERVOUS SYSTEM INFLUENCE

The direct effects of sympathetic neural influence on ventricular vulnerability can be examined by electrical stimulation of the stellate ganglia. In normal animals, stimulation of cardiac sympathetic efferent fibers markedly lowers the vulnerable period threshold (21–23) and increases the incidence of VF during myocardial ischemia (24). Left- and right-sided stellate activation exert reciprocal effects on the S-T segment and T wave, as recorded by local electrograms. Stimulation of the left or removal of the right stellate ganglion in dogs results in prolongation of the QT interval. No such change occurs when the left stellate ganglion is ablated or the right ganglion is stimulated (25). However, stimulation of either ganglion results in a significant lowering of the vulnerable period threshold. Left-sided stimulation is nearly twice as effective as right-sided stimulation in lowering the vulnerability threshold (23, 26) (Figure 3). These observations are consistent with those of Schwartz et al. (27, 28), who maintain that the left stellate ganglion is dominant in enhancing cardiac vulnerability to fibrillation. The effects of sympathetic stimulation on vulnerability occur independently of concomitant changes in heart rate and arterial blood pressure and appear to result from the direct action of norepinephrine at localized myocardial sites (22).

The influence on vulnerable period threshold of catecholamines released from the adrenal medulla appears to be substantially less than that exerted by neural activation (22). Recently, however, we have demonstrated that when subpressor doses of norepinephrine are given or when the pressor response to the drug is controlled, norepinephrine produces a significant and persistent decrease in the vulnerable period threshold (29).

4.1. Role of alpha- and beta-adrenergic receptors in ventricular vulnerability

Already in 1906 Sir Henry Dale speculated that the physiologic effects of catecholamines were related to their interactions with receptor sites on effector organs (30). The classical studies of Ahlquist demonstrated the existence of at least two adrenergic receptors (31).

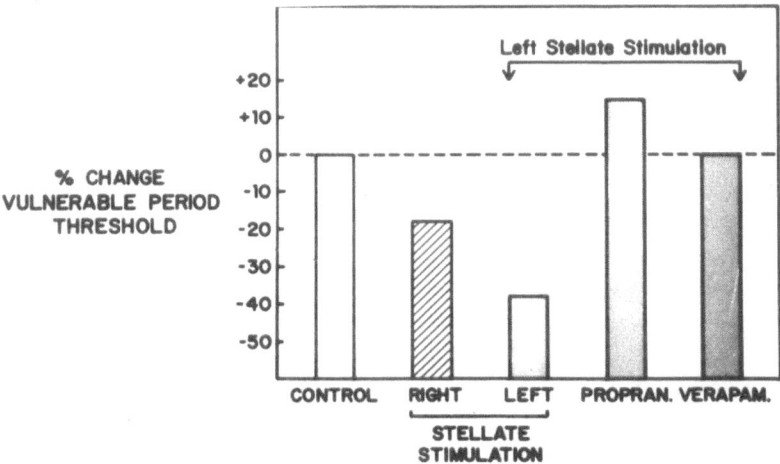

Figure 3. Effect of stellate ganglion stimulation on ventricular vulnerability before and after pharmacologic block-ade. Left stellate ganglion stimulation exerted a predominant effect on the vulnerable period threshold, but a substantial effect was also produced by right stellate stimulation. The decrease in threshold induced by sympathetic stimulation was abolished by beta-adrenergic blockade with propranolol (0.25 mg/kg) or verapamil infusion (0.01 mg/kg/min for 15 min) (26).

The electrophysiologic effects of beta-adrenergic stimulation on the myocardium are complex, varying from site to site as a function of nonuniformity of innervation (21). The essential properties of beta-adrenergic stimulation and blockade on the specialized conducting system and myocardium have been widely studied (32). There is considerable evidence ascribing a role to beta-receptors in accounting for the effects of sympathetic stimulation on the ventricular threshold for VF. This view is supported by the findings that enhanced vulnerability to VF associated with adrenergic stimulation, whether induced by posterior hypothalamic stimulation, stellate ganglion excitation, infusion of catecholamines, or exposure of animals to psychologic stress, is completely prevented by beta-adrenergic blockade (2, 12). This protective action can be achieved by cardioselective agents, free of membrane stabilizing actions such as practolol or tolamolol, thus indicating specific involvement of beta-adrenergic receptors.

Less attention has been directed to the role of alpha-adrenergic receptors in the genesis of cardiac arrhythmias. However, a number of clinical and experimental observations indicate that participation of alpha-receptors in modulation of vulnerability to VF deserves study. For example, Gould et al. (33, 34) reported that the oral administration of the alpha-adrenergic drug, phentolamine, in small, well-tolerated doses abolished ventricular premature beats (VPBs) elicited by digitalis toxicity and chronic ischemic heart disease and reduced the number of VPBs in patients during the first 24 hours of acute myocardial infarction (35). In experimental animals, DiMicco et al. (36) found that ventricular tachycardia provoked in the feline heart by the central nervous stimulant, picrotoxin, could be prevented by stellectomy plus adrenalectomy, or by the alpha-blockers, phentolamine or tolazoline, but not by propranolol, atropine or vagotomy. Zipes and coworkers (37) noted that in dogs predisposed to arrhythmias by the hypocholesterolemic agent probucol, the induction of VF by adrenergic stimulation was prevented by phentolamine, consistent with earlier findings that a variety of alpha-blocking agents prevented or abolished ventricular tachycardia produced by epinephrine in human and animal hearts which were sensitized by hydrocarbons, such as chloroform and cyclopropane (38, 39). If alpha-adrenergic receptors are involved in altering vulnerability to VF in man as well, this might account for the fact that some patients with the long QT syndrome are not protected against recurrent VF by beta-adrenergic blocking drugs, yet respond to left stellectomy (27, 28) – a procedure which diminishes tonic alpha- as well as beta-adrenergic inputs to the heart (28, 68).

The influence of alpha-adrenergic blockade on vulnerability to VF has recently been investigated by Cassells et al. (40) in our laboratory. Alpha-blockade in cats resulted in a substantial increase in VF threshold and prompted spontaneous defibrillation (Figure 4). However, these results could not be replicated with an equipotent alpha-adrenergic blocking dose of phenoxybenzamine. In this context, it is pertinent that administration of the alpha-agonist phenylephrine does not alter vulnerability to VF when the drug's pressor activity is prevented. These findings suggest that the antifibrillatory effects of phentolamine may be due to extra-adrenergic effects. For example, phentolamine has a direct cardiac membrane stabilizing action (41), stimulates insulin secretion (42, 43), inhibits platelet aggregation and opposes coronary vasospasm (44). *Thus, current studies indicate that in the normal heart alpha-adrenergic receptors do not affect ventricular vulnerability to fibrillation.*

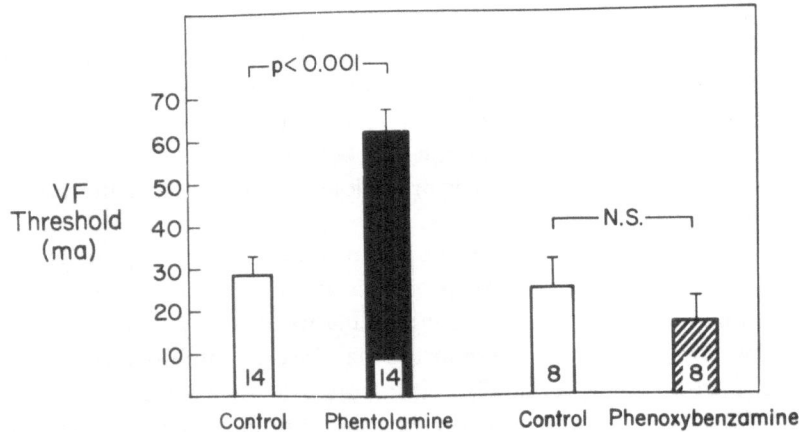

Figure 4. Comparative effect of alpha-adrenergic blockade with phentolamine and phenoxybenzamine on the ventricular fibrillation threshold in normal cats. Whereas phentolamine resulted in a substantial elevation in threshold, the latter produced a moderate but not statistically significant reduction in threshold. Evidence discussed in the text suggests that the phentolamine-induced increase in threshold was due to extra-adrenergic actions of the drug.

4.2. Slow channel blockade and vulnerability

The vulnerable period threshold can be significantly altered by blocking agents which act at a locus distal to the adrenergic receptor. For example, the slow channel blocking drug verapamil has been shown to exert potent anti-adrenergic actions (45–50). It reduces the occurrence of VF in the chloroform-epinephrine treated animal (45) and decreases the precipitation of ventricular arrhythmias by norepinephrine infusion during coronary artery occlusion (46). Furthermore, arrhythmias induced by lateral hypothalamic stimulation during coronary artery ligation are markedly suppressed by prior verapamil administration (48). Recently, we have found that the reduction in VF threshold produced by stellate ganglion stimulation or norepinephrine infusion is completely prevented by verapamil (51). The precise mechanism for the drugs' protective effect, however, remains to be defined. It is clear though that beta-adrenergic receptors are not involved, since blockade of these sites does not inhibit the action of verapamil in altering the effects of sympathetic stimulation on myocardial function (52). Verapamil thus exerts its action at a locus distal to the beta-adrenergic receptor and permits, for example, catecholamine elevation of cyclic AMP levels without resulting increase in calcium influx (53). Furthermore, verapamil does not influence the calcium-dependent release of norepinephrine from nerve endings (54).

4.3. Adrenergic factors during myocardial ischemia and reperfusion

There is evidence to suggest that reflex activation of the sympathetic nervous system may play a major role in the genesis of VF during acute coronary occlusion. Malliani, Schwartz and Zanchetti (55) have shown that within one minute of coronary occlusion in the cat, potent cardio-cardiac reflexes are elicited which result in a surge in firing rate of cardiac-bound sympathetic nerve fibers. Kelliher et al. (56) noted that the secretion rate of epinephrine increases up to eightfold within the first two minutes following coronary artery ligation. The time course of changes in adrenergic input to the heart appears to correspond closely both with the spontaneous occurrence of VF, as well as with the reduction in vulnerable period threshold during coronary occlusion (5).

Beta-adrenergic blocking drugs such as propranolol (57, 58) and practolol (59, 60) afford significant protection against VF during acute coronary artery occlusion in the experimental animal. The salutary influence of these agents appears to be due primarily to their adrenoreceptor-blocking properties rather than to their membrane-stabilizing actions (59, 60). Recently, practolol has been shown to be superior to propranolol in protecting against VF during coronary ligation (61). The authors suggested that part of the beneficial effect of beta-adrenergic blockade of a noncardioselective agent such as propranolol may be negated by its potential vasoconstrictor effect due to inhibition of beta$_2$-receptor mediated vascular smooth muscle relaxation. Indeed, there have been a number of patients with Prinzmetal's variant of angina in whom aggravation of symptoms resulted from the use of propranolol (62). Presumably the propranolol prompted vasoconstriction; such an effect would not be anticipated in response to cardioselective agents. This is quite problematic since it is uncertain whether sudden death in man is due to acute myocardial ischemia or to reperfusion. In the latter case, beta-adrenergic blockade might prove without avail since it has proved ineffectual in preventing VF following release of coronary artery occlusion (57, 60).

The influence of alpha-adrenergic blockade on vulnerability to VF is of particular interest in the setting of acute coronary occlusion. Recent clinical evidence suggests that coronary vasospasm may be present during the early phases of acute myocardial infarction (64–66). Thus, following coronary artery obstruction, alpha-adrenergic blockade may influence vulnerability not only through a possible effect on myocardial receptors but also through an action on vascular receptors as well. Indeed, it has been demonstrated that coronary vascular diameter depends on tonic alpha-adrenergically mediated vasoconstriction as well as upon metabolic regulation (65–69). Alpha-adrenergic blockade with phentolamine (0.1 mg/kg) in low doses decreases susceptibility to VF during myocardial ischemia (57) and in high doses (3–7 mg/kg) is also effective against reperfusion-induced fibrillation (70–72). It remains uncertain, however, whether the drug exerts its antifibrillatory influence through an action on myocardial alpha-receptors or by an indirect effect of blocking coronary artery vasospasm. As mentioned earlier, other extraadrenergic actions of the drug may also be implicated.

4.4. Coronary dilators and vulnerability

We have found that three drugs with potent dilatory properties, namely prenylamine (73), verapamil (51) and nitroglycerin (74) decrease significantly susceptibility to VF during both myocardial ischemia and reperfusion. Whereas prenylamine increased the vulnerable period threshold in the nonischemic heart, indicating a direct myocardial effect of the drug, verapamil or nitroglycerin were without effect on vulnerability in the absence of coronary artery obstruction (74) (Figure 5). The finding that nitroglycerin or verapamil altered the vulnerable period threshold only in the presence of impaired flow indicates that their beneficial effect on the VF threshold relates to an influence on the extent of ischemia rather than to a nonspecific cardiac stabilizing action (75–77) (Figure 5). Our current hypothesis is that coronary dilation can exert a beneficial effect on vulnerability by improving perfusion of ischemic sites and thereby reducing the accumulation of metabolic by-products of cellular ischemia. The reduced accumulation of ischemic by-products may also protect against reperfusion VF, since a reduced quantity of washout products would be liberated upon restoration of coronary blood flow. Further studies involving coronary flow measurements, sizing of ischemic area and sampling of coronary venous effluent will be required to verify or refute these speculations.

Increased adrenergic input to the heart may be largely responsible for susceptibility to VF during myocardial ischemia. Whereas beta-adrenergic blocking drugs are effective in decreasing vulnerability during coronary artery occlusion, they are ineffective against induction of VF during reperfusion. This observation may account, in part, for failure of these drugs to protect against sudden death in some patients with recurring ventricular tachycardia and VF. Coronary dilators may be of potential value in combating reperfusion-induced VF.

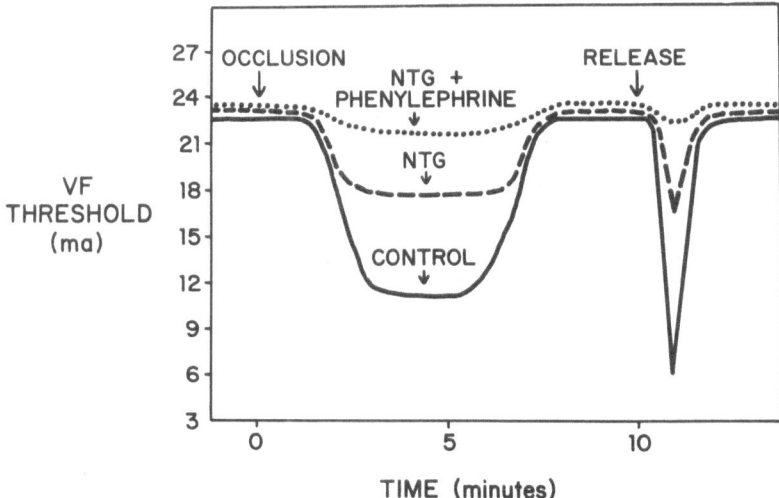

Figure 5. Schematic representation of the time course of change in the ventricular fibrillation threshold during coronary occlusion and release. Infusion of nitroglycerin alone provided partial protection during coronary occlusion and release. Combined infusion of nitroglycerin plus phenylephrine provided nearly complete protection against the decrease in threshold during myocardial ischemia and reperfusion (74).

5. VAGUS NERVE INFLUENCE

The prevailing view has been that vagal innervation does not extend to the ventricular myocardium. Clinical teaching was in accord with this perception. If a tachycardia responded to cholinergic measures, the site of impulse formation was judged to be supraventricular. However, considerable evidence has now been amassed indicating that parasympathetic neural influences directly affect the inotropic and chronotropic properties of the ventricles (78). Cogent evidence that vagal influences also alter ventricular electrical properties in the intact heart was provided by Kent, Epstein and coworkers (79, 80). They demonstrated that vagus nerve stimulation increased the VF threshold in both the normal and ischemic canine ventricle. They demonstrated, moreover, the cholinergic innervation of the specialized conducting system through which antifibrillatory action of the vagus is thought to occur.

5.1. Sympathetic-parasympathetic interactions

Our view has been that the effect of the vagus on ventricular vulnerability is contingent on the level of preexisting cardiac sympathetic tone (2, 6, 29, 81). This viewpoint is based on the observation that when sympathetic tone to the heart is augmented by thoracotomy (81), sympathetic nerve stimulation (81), or catecholamine infusion (6, 29), simultaneous vagal activation exerts a protective effect on ventricular vulnerability. Vagus nerve stimulation is without effect on vulnerability when adrenergic input to the heart is ablated by beta-adrenergic blockade (81).

The influence of the vagus on ventricular vulnerability appears to be due to activation of muscarinic receptors because vagally mediated changes in vulnerability are prevented by atropine administration (29). The diminution of adrenergic effects by muscarinic activation has a physiologic and cellular basis. Muscarinic agents have been shown both to inhibit the release of norepinephrine from sympathetic nerve endings (82) and to attenuate the response to norepinephrine at receptor sites by cyclic nucleotide interactions (83).

5.2. Direct vagal influences

Muscarinic stimulation may also decrease susceptibility to ventricular arrhythmias by a direct action of acetylcholine on automaticity of conducting tissue. Tse et al. (84) have demonstrated that in isolated Purkinje fiber preparations injection of acetylcholine suppresses automaticity and increases maximum diastolic potential. These actions of muscarinic stimulation on ventricular vulnerability are believed to be mainly mediated by an increase in K^+ conductance (84). This mechanism differs from that of catecholamines, which alter automaticity by a change in slow, inward current (85).

These direct actions of the vagus may explain certain clinical observations. For example, it has been found that increasing cardiac vagal drive by phenylephrine administration (86, 87) or by carotid massage may terminate ventricular tachycardia. These maneuvers are more effective when the patients are pretreated with the cholinesterase inhibitor edrophonium and are ineffective following prior atropine administration. Since these arrhythmias were not prevented by propranolol administration, a direct effect on the ventricles may be the mechanism of such vagal action rather than through muscarinic antagonism of beta-adrenergic influences. Another possibility is that vagal influences on ventricular arrhythmias may be mediated by the attendant changes in heart rate (88).

Direct actions of the vagus on ventricular electrophysiologic properties may, in part, explain why in certain patients sleep suppresses ventricular arrhythmias which are not controlled by propanolol therapy (89). It is, indeed, established that certain stages of sleep are accompanied by substantial augmentation of cardiac vagal drive (90).

5.3. Vagus nerve activity in the ischemic and infarcted heart

The issue is as yet unresolved as to whether enhanced vagal activity alters cardiac predisposition to VF during acute coronary artery occlusion. Kent and Epstein (79, 80) found that vagus nerve stimulation significantly increased the VF threshold and decreased susceptibility to fibrillation in the ischemic canine heart. Subsequently, Corr, Gillis and coworkers (91, 92) observed that the presence of intact vagi protected against VF in chloralose-anesthetized cats during left anterior descending coronary artery ligation, but was not beneficial during right coronary artery obstruction. Yoon et al. (93) and James et al. (94) were unable to demonstrate any effect of vagus nerve stimulation on VF threshold during left anterior descending coronary artery occlusion in the canine heart. Corr and coworkers

(95) have even found that cholinergic stimulation may exacerbate rather than ameliorate the arrhythmias which ensue upon release of occlusion, with attendant reperfusion of the ischemic myocardium.

We have found that intense cholinergic stimulation by electrical stimulation of the decentralized vagi or by direct muscarinic enhancement with methacholine, affords only partial protection during myocardial ischemia in dogs in which heart rate was maintained constant by pacing (96, 97). No salutary influence of cholinergic stimulation, however, was noted during reperfusion (97) (Figure 6). However, additional countervailing factors come into play when myocardial perfusion is impaired. Thus, vagal stimulation does not completely suppress the arrhythmias which result from myocardial infarction (98). In fact, it has been found that enhanced vagus activity or acetylcholine infusion consistently elicited ventricular tachycardia during the quiescent arrhythmia-free phase of myocardial infarction in dogs. This effect was completely rate-dependent since preventing the vagally induced bradycardia abolished the arrhythmias. Thus, the antiarrhythmic effects of the vagus may be augmented or reversed by its profound influence on heart rate in the setting of acute myocardial infarction (98, 99).

Vagal tone enhancement may be beneficial in preventing excessive elevations in heart rate associated with increased sympathetic drive to the heart and thereby conserve malperfused tissue from advancing ischemia. On the other hand, if profound bradycardia ensues, this may expose rate-sensitive ventricular ectopy, produce hypotension and reduced coronary flow to jeopardized myocardial segments, which may in turn precipitate VF.

Clinical experience indicates that at the onset of acute myocardial infarction there is a

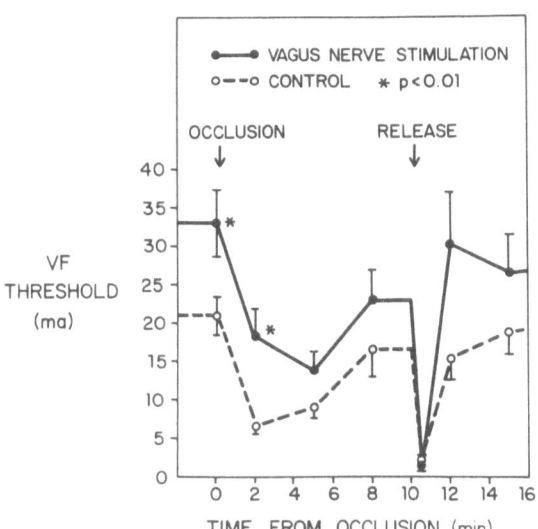

Figure 6. Influence of vagal stimulation on VF threshold during a 10 minute period of left anterior descending coronary artery occlusion followed by abrupt release. Partial protection against vulnerability to VF occurred during occlusion with vagal stimulation. No protection was afforded by vagal stimulation, however, during reperfusion. The results were obtained from 8 dogs with and 10 dogs without vagal stimulation (97).

tendency to bradycardia, believed to be mediated by enhanced vagal activity. This was first brought to light by the Belfast group who popularized the mobile coronary care unit (100). Among 400 patients who came under intensive care within four hours of onset of the attack, bradycardia was found to be a remarkably frequent manifestation. With diaphragmatic infarction, 61 % of patients who were seen within one hour of onset exhibited some bradycardia. These arrhythmias were transient. When patients were seen within 30 minutes of acute myocardial infarction, signs of autonomic imbalance were detected in 92 % of 68 patients (101). In 41 of these (55 %) there was excessive vagal activity, while in 27 (36 %) there was sympathetic overactivity. Augmented parasympathetic activity was judged by heart rates of 60 beats per minute or less, presence of atrioventricular block, or transient hypotension not caused by undue bradycardia.

There is little if any information on the level of vagal tone at the very inception of a heart attack, at the very time when the heart is most susceptible to VF. The case report by Biorck and Erhardt (102) is pertinent. They monitored a woman while she developed a heart attack. Within one minute of onset of symptoms, her heart rate receded from 65 to 40 beats per minute, with progression to AV dissociation and nodal rhythm over the ensuing few minutes. Ventricular premature beats made their appearance only 41 minutes later at a time when vagotonia was no longer in evidence.

The full clinical implication of vagal modulation of sympathetic tone during myocardial ischemia, especially as it relates to sudden cardiac death, is largely an unexplored area.

6. PSYCHOLOGIC FACTORS AND VF

An essential question is whether psychophysiologic stimuli can significantly affect cardiac vulnerability. More specifically, do behavioral stresses alter susceptibility to VF? To study this question, we examined the influence of mild aversive conditioning stimuli on ventricular vulnerability using the RE threshold method (103). We compared the influence of two different environments on the vulnerable period threshold in conscious dogs. The first setting was a cage in which the animals were left undisturbed, whereas the second was a Pavlovian sling in which the animals received a mild transthoracic shock at the end of each conditioning session. The influence of the two environments were compared on days 4 and 5, at which time no shocks were administered. In the stressful environment, the dogs were restless, exhibited somatic tremor and had elevated heart rate and arterial blood pressure. The RE threshold was reduced by 40 % in the stressful environment. When acute left anterior descending coronary artery occlusion and release was carried out in the stressful setting, the incidence of VF was more than 3 times greater (14 % versus 46 %) than that observed in the nonstressful environment (26) (Figure 7). Elevation in plasma catecholamine levels, particularly of epinephrine, closely correlate with the alteration in the vulnerable period threshold (104) (Figure 8).

The type of stress is not critical to the effects on vulnerability since aversive instrumental conditioning also substantially lowers the vulnerable period threshold (105). Moreover, beta-adrenergic blockade completely prevented stress-induced alterations in cardiac

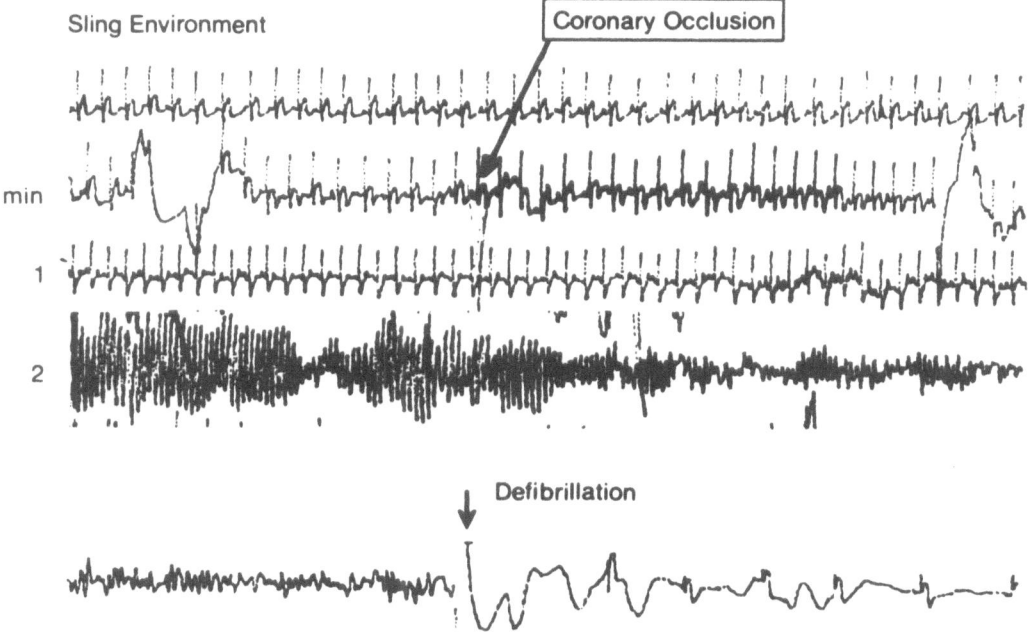

Figure 7. Coronary occlusion while the animal was in a sling environment resulted within 2 minutes in ventricular fibrillation. Note the instability of the baseline due to restlessness when the animal was merely standing quietly. When coronary occlusion was carried out while the animal was in the nonaversive cage environment, ventricular fibrillation did not occur.

vulnerability, indicating that the decrease in threshold was mediated by the sympathetic limb of the autonomic nervous system (26, 105, 106). Left or right stellectomy, however, did not prevent the reduction in vulnerable period threshold during psychologic stress and only partial protection was conferred by bilateral stellectomy (107). These results suggest that adrenergic inputs in addition to those derived from the stellate ganglia impinge upon the heart during stress to alter vulnerability. These inputs appear to derive mainly from the adrenal medulla. Plasma epinephrine levels are markedly elevated in stellectomized animals exposed to behavioral stress (107).

6.1. Effect of vagal stimulation during stress

Vagal influences also appear to play a role in modulating vulnerability during psychological stress. This view is based on the observations of DeSilva et al. (108) that enhancing cardiac vagal tone by administration of morphine to dogs in a stressful environment increases the vulnerable period threshold to the value observed in a nonstressful setting. When vagal efferent activity was blocked by atropine, a major portion of morphine's protective effect was abolished. Administration of morphine in the nonstressful setting, where cardiac adrenergic input was presumed to be low, failed to alter the vulnerable period threshold. These findings indicate that central activation of the vagi by morphine protects against

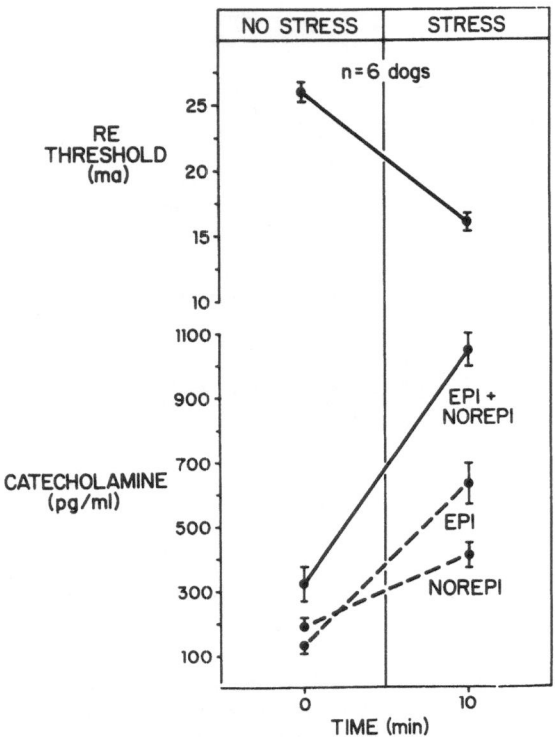

Figure 8. Effect of aversive sling environment on repetitive extrasystole (RE) threshold and circulating plasma catecholamine level. The RE threshold decreased 41 % within 10 minutes of placing the animals in the sling after removal from the cage. The reduction in threshold was accompanied by substantial increases in both norepinephrine and epinephrine. Values are means ±S.E.M. (104).

vulnerability during stress and that this beneficial action is due to antagonism of the fibrillatory influence of enhanced adrenergic input to the heart.

7. FINAL COMMENT

Current investigations indicate that diminution of sympathetic tone and enhancement of vagal input to the heart are capable of conferring significant protections against vulnerability to VF. Protection against VF by antagonism of sympathetic influences can be achieved by pharmacologic blockade of myocardial beta-adrenergic receptors or by blocking slow channels. Alpha-adrenergic blockade or administration of coronary dilators reduce susceptibility to VF during both myocardial ischemia and reperfusion. This beneficial action, however, appears to be due to opposition of coronary vasospasm rather than through a direct myocardial effect. Increasing cardiac vagal drive may decrease vulnerability by antagonizing the fibrillatory influence of sympathetic input to the heart and by direct effects of acetylcholine on automaticity of cardiac tissue.

These findings indicate the feasibility of decreasing susceptibility to VF by neurochemical and neuropharmacologic means. But more important than the particular findings is the emerging concept that containment of neurophysiologic triggers may provide a powerful therapeutic tool in the management of malignant cardiac arrhythmias.

ACKNOWLEDGEMENT

This work was supported in part by Grants no. MH-21384 from the National Institute of Mental Health and no. HL-07776 and no. HL-05242 from the National Heart, Lung and Blood Institute, National Institutes of Health, U.S. Public Health Service, Bethesda, Maryland.

REFERENCES

1. Lown B: Sudden death from coronary heart disease. In: Early phases of coronary heart disease, Waldenström, Larsson, Ljungstedt (eds), Stockholm, Nordiska Bokhandelns Forlag, 1973, p 255–277.
2. Lown B, Verrier RL: Neural activity and ventricular fibrillation. N Engl J Med 294:1165–1170, 1976.
3. Wolff GA, Veith F, Lown B: A vulnerable period for ventricular tachycardia following myocardial infarction. Cardiovasc Res 2:111–121, 1968.
4. Thompson PL, Lown B: Sequential R/T pacing to expose electrical instability in the ischemic ventricle. Clin Res 20:401, 1972.
5. Axelrod PJ, Verrier RL, Lown B: Vulnerability to ventricular fibrillation during acute coronary arterial occlusion and release. Am J Cardiol 36:776–782, 1976.
6. Matta, RJ, Verrier RL, Lown B: The repetitive extrasystole as an index of vulnerability to ventricular fibrillation. Am J Physiol 230:1469–1473, 1976.
7. Verrier RL, Brooks WW, Lown B: Protective zone and the determination of vulnerability to ventricular fibrillation. Am J Physiol 234:H592–H596, 1978.
8. Greene HL, Reid PR, Schaeffer AH: The repetitive ventricular response in man: A predictor of sudden death. N Engl J Med 299:729–734, 1978.
9. Farshidi A, Michelson EL, Greenspan AM, Spielman SR, Kastor JA, Horowitz LN, Josephson ME: Repetitive responses to ventricular extrastimuli – incidence, mechanism and significance. Am J Cardiol 43:390, 1979.
10. Greene HL, Reid PR, Schaeffer AH: The repetitive ventricular response in man – a new predictor of sudden death and symptomatic ventricular tachycardia. In: Management of ventricular tachycardia – role of mexiletine, Sandøe E, Julian DG, Bell JW (eds), Amsterdam, Excerpta Medica (International Congress Series no 458) 1978, p 513–526.
11. Lown B, Verrier RL, Blatt CM: Precordial mechanical stimulation for exposing electrical instability of the heart. Am J Cardiol 42:425–428, 1978.
12. Lown B, Verrier RL, Rabinowitz SH: Neural and psychologic mechanisms and the problem of sudden cardiac death. Am J Cardiol 39:890–902, 1977.
13. Hoff EC, Kell JF, Carroll MN: Effects of cortical stimulation and lesions on cardiovascular function. Physiol Rev 43:68–114, 1963.
14. Korteweg GCJ, Boeles TF, Tencate J: Influence of stimulation of some subcortical areas on electrocardiogram. J Neurophysiol 20:100–107, 1957.
15. Verrier RL, Calvert A, Lown B: Effect of posterior hypothalamic stimulation on the ventricular fibrillation threshold. Am J Physiol 228:923–927, 1975.
16. Satinsky J, Kosowsky B, Lown B, Kerzner J: Ventricular fibrillation induced by hypothalamic stimulation during coronary occlusion. Circulation 44:II–60, 1971.
17. Manning JW, Cotten MD: Mechanism of cardiac arrhythmias induced by diencephalic stimulation. Am J Physiol 203:1120–1124, 1962.
18. Hockman CH, Mauck HP, Hoff EC: ECG changes resulting from cerebral stimulation: II. A spectrum of ventricular arrhythmias of sympathetic origin. Am Heart J 71:695–700, 1966.

19. Korteweg GCJ, Boeles TF, Tencate J: Influence of stimulation of some subcortical areas on electrocardiogram. J Neurophysiol 20:100–107, 1957.
20. Evans DE, Gillis RA: Reflex mechanisms involved in cardiac arrhythmias induced by hypothalamic stimulation. Am J Physiol 234:H199–H209, 1978.
21. Han J, Garcia de Jalon P, Moe GK: Adrenergic effects on ventricular vulnerability. Circ Res 14:516–524, 1964.
22. Verrier RL, Thompson P, Lown B: Ventricular vulnerability during sympathetic stimulation: Role of heart rate and blood pressure. Cardiovasc Res 8:602–610, 1974.
23. Brooks WW, Verrier RL, Lown B: Influence of vagal tone on stellectomy-induced changes in ventricular electrical stability. Am J Physiol 234:H503–H507, 1978.
24. Harris AS, Otero H, Bocage A: The induction of arrhythmias by sympathetic activity before and after occlusion of a coronary artery in the canine heart. J Electrocardiol 4:34–43, 1971.
25. Yanowitz F, Preston JB, Abildskov JA: Functional distribution of right and left stellate innervation to the ventricles: production of neurogenic electrocardiographic changes by unilateral alteration of sympathetic tone. Circ Res 18:416–428, 1966.
26. Verrier RL, Lown B: Influence of neural activity on ventricular electrical instability during acute myocardial ischemia and infarction. In: Management of ventricular tachycardia – role of mexiletine, Sandøe E, Julian DG, Bell JW (eds), Amsterdam, Excerpta Medica (International Congress Series no 458), 1978, p 133–150.
27. Schwartz PJ, Periti M, Malliani A: The long Q-T syndrome. Am Heart J 89:378–390, 1975.
28. Moss A., Schwartz PJ, Sudden death and the idiopathic long Q-T syndrome. Am J 66:6–7, 1979.
29. Rabinowitz SH, Verrier RL, Lown B: Muscarinic effects of vagosympathetic trunk stimulation on the repetitive extrasystole threshold. Circulation 53:622–627, 1976.
30. Dale HH: On some physiologic actions of ergot. J Physiol (London) 34:163–206, 1906.
31. Ahlquist RP: A study of the adrenotropic receptors. Am J Physiol 153:586–600, 1948.
32. Wit AL, Hoffman BF, Rosen MR: Electrophysiology and pharmacology of cardiac arrhythmias: IX. Parts A, B, C. Cardiac electrophysiologic effects of beta adrenergic receptor stimulation and blockade. Am Heart J 90:521–533, 665–675, 795–803, 1975.
33. Gould L, Reddy CVR, Weinstein T, et al: Antiarrhythmic prophylaxis with phentolamine in acute myocardial infarction. J Clin Pharmacol 15:191–197, 1975.
34. Gould L, Gomprecht RF, Zahir M: Oral phentolamine for treatment of ventricular premature contractions. Br Heart J 33:101–104, 1971.
35. Gould L, Zahir M, Shariff M: Treatment of cardiac arrhythmias with phentolamine. Am Heart J 78:189–193, 1969.
36. DiMicco JA, Prestel T, Pearle DL, Gillis RA: Mechanism of cardiovascular changes produced in cats by activation of the central nervous system with picrotoxin. Circ Res 41:446–451, 1977.
37. Zipes D. Elharrar V, Watanabe AM, et al: Induction of ventricular fibrillation in probucol-treated dogs. Clin Res 25:459A, 1977.
38. Nickerson M, Collier B: Drugs inhibiting adrenergic nerves and structures innervated by them. In: The pharmacologic basis of therapeutics, Goodman LS, Gilman A (eds), New York City, The Macmillan Company, 1968, p 546–577.
39. Nickerson M, Brown HO: Protection by dibenamine against "spontaneous" arrhythmias occurring during cycloproprane anesthesia. Anesthesiol 12: 216–224, 1949.
40. Casscells W, Verrier RL, Lown B: Influence of phentolamine on ventricular vulnerability and spontaneous defibrillation in the cat (abstract). Am J Cardiol 43: 375, 1979.
41. Rosen MR, Gelband H, Hoffman BF: Effects of phentolamine on electrophysiologic properties of isolated canine Purkinje fibers. J Pharmacol Exp Ther 170:586–593, 1971.
42. Majid PA, Saxton C, Dykes JRW, Galvin MC, Taylor SH: Autonomic control of insulin secretion and the treatment of heart failure. Br Med J 4:320–333, 1970.
43. Pfister B, Imhof PR: Inhibition of adrenalin-induced platelet aggregation by the orally administered alpha-adrenergic receptor blocker phentolamine (Regitine®). Europ J Clin Pharmacol 11:7–10, 1977.
44. Levene DL, Freeman MR: Alpha-adrenoreceptor-mediated coronary artery spasm. JAMA 236:1018–1022, 1976.
45. Fondacro JD, Han J, Yoon MS: Effects of verapamil on ventricular rhythm during acute coronary occlusion. Am Heart J 96:81–86, 1978.
46. Melville KI, Shister HE, Huq S: Iproveratril: Experimental data on coronary dilatation and antiarrhythmic action. Can Med Assoc J 90:761–769, 1964.
47. Melville KI, Bewfey BG: Coronary vasodilatory and cardiac adrenergic blocking effects of iproveratril.

Can J Physiol Pharmacol 43:339–342, 1965.

48. Garvey HL, Melville KI: Effect of verapamil on cardiovascular responses to lateral hypothalamic stimulation in normal and coronary-ligated dogs. Can J Physiol Pharmacol 47:675–684, 1969.

49. Melville KI, Garvey HL, Shister HE: On the cardiac adrenergic blocking action of iproveratril in normal and coronary-ligated dogs. Rev Can Biol 27:225–235, 1968.

50. Huang TF, Peng YI: Effect of verapamil on experimental arrhythmias. Europ J Pharmacol 42:363–370, 1977.

51. Brooks WW, Verrier RL, Lown B: Protective effect of verapamil on ventricular vulnerability during coronary artery occlusion and reperfusion (abstract). Am J Cardiol. 41:426, 1978.

52. Naylor WG. Szeto J: Effect of verapamil on contractility, oxygen utilization and calcium exchangeability in mammalian heart muscle. Cardiovasc Res 6:120–128, 1972.

53. Watanabe AM, Besch HR: Subcellular myocardial effects of verapamil and D600: Comparison with propranolol. J Pharmacol Exp Ther 191:241–251, 1974.

54. Haeusler G: Differential effect of verapamil on excitation-contraction coupling in smooth muscle and on excitation-secretion coupling in adrenergic nerve terminals. J Pharmacol Exp Ther 180:672–682, 1972.

55. Malliani A, Schwartz PJ, Zanchetti A: A sympathetic reflex elicited by experimental coronary occlusion. Am J Physiol 217:703–709, 1969.

56. Kelliher GJ, Widmer C, Roberts J: Influence of the adrenal medulla on cardiac rhythm disturbances following acute coronary artery occlusion. Recent Adv Stud Cardiac Struct Metab 10:387–400, 1975.

57. Corbalan R, Verrier RL, Lown B: Differing mechanisms for ventricular vulnerability during coronary artery occlusion and release. Am Heart J 92:223–230, 1976.

58. Khan MI, Hamilton JT, Manning GW: Protective effect of beta-adrenoceptor blockade in experimental occlusion in conscious dogs. Am J Cardiol 30:832–837, 1972.

59. Fitzgerald JD: Role of adrenergic blockade. In: Effect of acute ischaemia on myocardial function. Oliver MF, Julian DG, Donald KW (eds), Baltimore, Williams and Wilkins Co, 1972, p 321–351.

60. Hai HA, Temte JV, Lown B: Changes in ventricular fibrillation threshold during coronary artery occlusion and release induced by beta-adrenergic blockade (abstract). Am J Cardiol 37:140, 1976.

61. Pearle DL, Williford D, Gillis RA: Superiority of practolol versus propranolol in protection against ventricular fibrillation induced by coronary occlusion. Am J Cardiol 42:960–964, 1978.

62. Yasue H: Beta-adrenergic blockade and coronary arterial spasm. In: Management of ventricular tachycardia – role of mexiletine, Sandøe E, Julian DG, Bell JW (eds), Amsterdam, Excerpta Medica (International Congress Series no 458), 1978, p 305–310.

63. Norris RM, Congbey DE, Scott PJ: A trial of propranolol in acute myocardial infarction. Br Med J 2: 398–400, 1968.

64. Oliva PB, Breckinridge JC: Arteriographic evidence of coronary arterial spasm in acute myocardial infarction. Circulation 56:366–374, 1977.

65. Maseri A, L'Abbate A, Baroldi G, Chierchia S, Marzilli M, Ballestra AM, Severi S, Parodi O, Biazini A, Distante A, Pesola A: Coronary vasospasm: A possible cause of myocardial infarction: A conclusion derived from the study of "Preinfarction Angina." N Engl J Med 299:1221–1277, 1978.

66. Braunwald E: Coronary spasm and acute myocardial infarction – new possibility for treatment and prevention. N Engl J Med 299:1301–1303, 1978.

67. Mudge GH, Goldberg S, Gunther S: Comparison of metabolic and vasoconstrictor stimuli on coronary vascular resistance in man. Circulation 59:544–550, 1979.

68. Mohrman DE, Feigl EO: Competition between sympathetic vasoconstriction and metabolic vasodilation in the canine coronary circulation. Circ Res 42:79–86, 1978.

69. Schwartz PJ, Stone HL: Tonic influence of the sympathetic nervous system on myocardial reactive hyperemia and on coronary blood flow distribution in dogs. Circ Res 41: 51–58, 1977.

70. Penkoske PA, Sobel BE, Corr PB: Inhibition by alpha-adrenergic blockade of the ventricular dysrhythmias induced by reperfusion. Clin Res 26:259A, 1978.

71. Sheridan DJ, Penkoske PA, Corr PB: Specific antiarrhythmic effectiveness of alpha-adrenergic blockade during coronary reperfusion. Am J Cardiol 43:372, 1979.

72. Stewart JR, Burmeister WE, Burmeister JL, Lucchesi BR: Electrophysiologic and antiarrhythmic effects of phentolamine in experimental coronary artery occlusion and reperfusion in the dog. Am J Cardiol 43:359, 1979.

73. Schoeneberger A, Verrier RL, Lown B: Protective effect of prenylamine on ventricular vulnerability in the normal and ischemic canine myocardium. Proc Soc Exp Biol Med, 161:56–59, 1979.

74. Stockman MB, Verrier RL, Lown B: Effect of nitroglycerin on vulnerability to ventricular fibrillation during myocardial ischemia and reperfusion. Am J Cardiol 43:233–238, 1979.

75. Elharrar V, Gaum WE, Zipes D: Effect of drugs on conduction delay and incidence of ventricular arrhythmias induced by acute coronary occlusion in dogs. Am J Cardiol 39:544–549, 1977.
76. Kent KM, Smith ER, Redwood DR, Epstein SE: Beneficial electrophysiologic effects of nitroglycerin during acute myocardial infarction. Am J Cardiol 33:513–516, 1974.
77. Levites R, Boderheimer MM, Helfant RHL: Electrophysiologic effects of NTG during experimental coronary occlusion. Circulation 52:1050–1055, 1975.
78. Higgins CB, Vatner SF, Braunwald E: Parasympathetic control of the heart. Pharmacol Rev 25:119–155, 1973.
79. Kent KM, Smith ER, Redwood DR, Epstein SE: Electrical stability of acutely ischemic myocardium: Influences of heart rate and vagal stimulation. Circulation 47:291–298, 1973.
80. Kent KM, Epstein SE, Cooper T, Jacobowitz DM: Cholinergic innervation of the canine and human ventricular conducting system: Anatomic and electrophysiologic correlation. Circulation 50:948–955, 1974.
81. Kolman BS, Verrier RL, Lown B: The effect of vagus nerve stimulation upon vulnerability of the canine ventricle. Role of sympathetic-parasympathetic interactions. Circulation 52:578–585, 1975.
82. Levy MN, Blattberg B: Effect of vagal stimulation on the overflow of norepinephrine into the coronary sinus during cardiac sympathetic nerve stimulation in the dog. Circ Res 38:81–85, 1976.
83. Watanabe AM, Besch HR: Interaction between cyclic adenosine monophosphate and cyclic guanosine monophosphate in guinea pig ventricular myocardium. Circ Res 37:309–317, 1975.
84. Tse WW, Han J, Yoon MS: Effect of acetylcholine on automaticity of canine Purkinje fibers. Am J Physiol 203:116–119, 1976.
85. Vassalle M: Cardiac automaticity and its control. Am J Physiol 2:H625–H634, 1977.
86. Weiss T, Lattin GM, Engelman K: Vagally mediated suppression of premature ventricular contractions in man. Am Heart J 89:700–707, 1975.
87. Waxman MB, Wald RW: Termination of ventricular tachycardia by an increase in cardiac vagal drive. Circulation 56:385–391, 1977.
88. Weiss T, Mancia G, Delbo A, Cavoretto D, Grazi S, Preti J, Schwartz PJ. The role of heart rate in the phenylephrine-induced suppression of premature ventricular beats. (Abstract). Eur. J Clin. Invest 9:39, 1979.
89. Lown B, Tykocinski M, Garfein A, Brooks P: Sleep and ventricular premature beats. Circulation 48:691–701, 1973.
90. Baust W, Bohnert B: The regulation of heart rate during sleep. Exp Brain Res 7:169–180, 1969.
91. Corr PB, Gillis RA: Role of the vagus in the cardiovascular changes induced by coronary occlusion. Circulation 49:86–97, 1974.
92. Corr PB, Pearle DL, Gillis RA: Coronary occlusion site as a determinant of the cardiac rhythm effects of atropine and vagotomy. Am Heart J 92:741–749, 1976.
93. Yoon MS, Han J, Tse WW, Rogers R: Effects of vagal stimulation, atropine, and propranolol on fibrillation threshold of normal and ischemic ventricles. Am Heart J 93:60–65, 1977.
94. James RGG, Arnold JMO, Allen JD, Pantridge JF, Shanks RG: The effects of heart rate, myocardial ischemia and vagal stimulation on the threshold for ventricular fibrillation. Circulation 55:311–317, 1977.
95. Corr PB, Penkoske PA, Sobel BE: Adrenergic influences on arrhythmias due to coronary occlusion and reperfusion. Br Heart J 40 (suppl):62–70, 1978.
96. Verrier RL, Brooks WW, Lown B: Effect of cholinergic stimulation on vulnerability to ventricular fibrillation during myocardial ischemia and reperfusion (abstract). Am J Cardiol 41:366, 1978.
97. Verrier RL, Lown B: Sympathetic-parasympathetic interactions and ventricular electrical stability. In: Neural mechanisms in cardiac arrhythmias, Schwartz PJ, Brown AM, Malliani A, Zanchetti A (eds), New York City, Raven Press, 1978, p 75–85.
98. Kerzner J, Wolf M, Kosowsky BD, Lown B: Ventricular ectopic rhythms following vagal stimulation in dogs with acute myocardial infarction. Circulation 47:44–50, 1973.
99. El-Sherif N: Reentrant ventricular arrhythmias in the late myocardial infarction period: VI. Effect of the autonomic system. Circulation 58:103–110, 1978.
100. Pantridge JF, Adgey AAJ, Geddes JS, Webb SW: The acute coronary attack, New York City, Grune & Stratton, 1975.
101. Webb SW, Adgey AAJ, Pantridge JF: Autonomic disturbance at onset of myocardial infarction. Br Med J 3:89–92, 1972.
102. Biorck G, Erhardt LR: The earliest phase of acute myocardial infarction in man. Acta Med Scand 193:251–255, 1973.
103. Lown B, Verrier RL, Corbalan R: Psychologic stress and threshold for repetitive ventricular response. Science 182:834–836, 1973.

104. Liang B, Verrier RL, Lown B, Melman J: Correlation between circulating catecholamine levels and ventricular vulnerability during psychological stress in conscious dogs. Proc Soc Exptl. Biol Med. 161:266–269, 1979.

105. Matta RJ, Lawler JE, Lown B: Ventricular electrical instability in the conscious dog: effects of psychologic stress and beta adrenergic blockade. Am J Cardiol 38:594–598, 1976.

106. Verrier RL, Lown B: Effect of left stellectomy on enhanced cardiac vulnerability induced by psychologic stress (abstract). Circulation 56:III–80, 1977.

107. Verrier RL, Lown B: Influence of stellectomy and beta-adrenergic blockade on ventricular vulnerability during psychologic stress in the canine model. In preparation.

108. DeSilva RA, Verrier RL, Lown B: Effect of psychologic stress and sedation with morphine sulfate on ventricular vulnerability. Am Heart J 95:197–203, 1978.

2.5. AUTONOMIC NERVOUS SYSTEM AND SUDDEN DEATH

D.P. ZIPES, R.F. GILMOUR Jr., J.B. MARTINS and R. RUFFY

1. INTRODUCTION

A great deal of information exists regarding the influence of the autonomic nervous system on the electrical properties of the myocardium and on the genesis of a variety of cardiac arrhythmias. The purpose of this presentation is not to review this vast literature, but to present new information we have developed over the past several years. Specifically, in this manuscript, we will discuss the effects of the autonomic nervous system on recovery properties in the endocardium and the epicardium of the canine left ventricle (1, 2); the effects of the autonomic nervous system on myocardial activation during acute myocardial ischemia in the dog (3); and new models in which to study the effects of ischemia, including vascularized hamster cardiac allographs (4); and rodent myocardium damaged by epinephrine (5).

2. EFFECTS OF SYMPATHETIC AND VAGAL NERVE INTERVENTIONS ON RECOVERY PROPERTIES OF THE ENDOCARDIUM AND EPICARDIUM OF THE CANINE LEFT VENTRICLE (1, 2).

It is well established that sympathetic stimulation shortens the duration of the ventricular refractory period (6). Recent information suggests that parasympathetic stimulation prolongs the duration of refractoriness, presumably by modulating concurrent sympathetic tone (7, 8). However, it is not known whether either sympathetic or parasympathetic nerves influence endocardial recovery differently than epicardial recovery. Histologic information suggests that transmural differences in innervation may exist. For example, the endocardium may be less well innervated with sympathetic nerves (9), and be better innervated with parasympathetic nerves (10), compared to the epicardium.

The purpose of this study was to measure the effective refractory period (ERP) of the anterior left ventricular epicardium and underlying endocardium to determine whether the autonomic nervous system exerts a differential effect on recovery of excitability. Studies were performed in open-chest dogs anesthetized with alpha-chloralose (60 mg/kg). The cervical vagi were isolated, doubly ligated and cut. The region of the sinus node was crushed and the atria and ventricles were paced simultaneously at a fixed cycle length. The left ventricle was stimulated with unipolar cathodal stimuli delivered through one pole of a multipolar plunge needle electrode placed perpendicular to the epicardium. ERP was measured by the extrastimulus technique (11), employing a programmable stimulator that delivered pulses 11/2 to 2 times the late diastolic threshold. The train of 8 basic stimuli (S_1) was followed by a late premature stimulus (S_2) that initially produced a propagated ventricular response. The $S_1 - S_2$ interval was shortened until S_2 failed to produce ventricular depolarization. The longest $S_1 - S_2$ interval at which S_2 failed to produce depolarization was taken as the ERP. Strength interval curves were performed in six experiments at current intensities of 200, 400, 800, and 1600 μA. ERP was determined from the endocardial surface of the upper half of the left septum and in the anterior left ventricular epicardium and underlying endocardium. The sites of all electrodes were confirmed at necropsy.

Sympathetic interventions were produced by occlusion of both common carotid arteries, surgical interruption of both stellate ganglia, and electrical stimulation of right and left sympathetic nerves with 4 msec pulses, at 1–8 Hz, ranging from 1–7mA. The electrode nearest the heart was always the cathode. The distal end of the cervical vagus was stimulated with rectangular pulses 4 msec in duration at a frequency of 20 Hz and current between 0.2–1.5 mA. Vagal stimulation was performed alone and during concomitant adrenergic manipulations and after administration of the following drugs: physostigmine (0.5, 5.0, and 50 μg/kg), propranolol (0.7 mg/kg) and atropine (0.4 mg/kg IV).

We found that bilateral carotid occlusion shortened both epicardial and endocardial ERP significantly, by a mean of 4 msec. Bilateral surgical sympathectomy prolonged both epicardial and endocardial ERP by a mean of 10 msec. Electrical stimulation of both right and left sympathetic nerves decreased endocardial ERP by 19 msec and epicardial ERP by 18 msec. No difference in the percent change of ERP in endocardium or epicardium occurred with these three interventions. In addition, no differences resulted in the extent of shortening of endocardial compared to epicardial ERP during right or left unilateral or bilateral sympathetic stimulation.

Vagal stimulation at a cycle length of 300 msec lengthened epicardial and endocardial ERP by 4 msec (2.4 %) and left septal ERP by 2 msec (1.6 %). Vagal stimulation during bilateral carotid occlusion reversed the 2–5 msec shortening produced by the latter and increased ERP by 2–4 msec. Thus, vagal stimulation during augmented sympathetic tone prolonged ERP by 6.2 % in epicardium, 4.3 % in endocardium and 3.8 % in left septum.

The magnitude of vagal-induced prolongation of ERP was also influenced by heart rate and various drugs. At slower heart rates (cycle length 500 msec) the extent of ERP prolongation produced by vagal stimulation was significantly increased, in epicardium to 3.9 % and in endocardium to 3.2 %. However, no significant difference was found between the percent change in endocardium compared with the percent change in epicardium. Similarly, physostigmine administration potentiated the effects of vagal stimulation on ERP, to a maximum of 3.6 % prolongation in the epicardium and 3.9 % in the endocardium, but at each dose level no significant difference in percent change was found between epicardium and endocardium. Both atropine and propranolol administration prevented vagal-induced prolongation of ERP.

Vagal stimulation shifted epicardial and endocardial strength-interval curves to the right. The percent change at each level of current intensity in the epicardium was not different from that in the endocardium.

In summary, the results of this study indicate that sympathetic nerves to the left ventricle exerted equivalent effects on the duration of epicardial and underlying endocardial ERP during reflex augmentation, denervation and unilateral or bilateral electrical stimulation of the stellate ganglia. Electrical stimulation of the vagal nerves prolonged ERP similarly in the epicardium and left septum. By activating muscarinic, cholinergic receptors, vagal stimulation prolonged ventricular ERP directly in relation to the level of sympathetic activity. These data in normal animals do not exclude the possibility that the autonomic nervous system may exert unequal effects on recovery of endocardium and epicardium in various disease states.

The results of this study have important clinical implications and provide a possible mechanism to explain the observation that activation of muscarinic, cholinergic receptors by vagal maneuvers, may terminate ventricular tachycardia in man (12). Vagal-induced prolongation of ERP might be more accentuated in clinical states characterized by heightened sympathetic tone, such as during ventricular tachycardia. In addition, it is clear from the present study that the vagus can act on arrhythmias involving ventricular muscle and that termination of a ventricular arrhythmia by vagal intervention does not necessarily implicate the specialized conduction system in the maintenance of the ventricular arrhythmia (10).

3. EFFECTS OF VAGAL AND SYMPATHETIC NEURAL INTERRUPTION ON ELECTROGRAM CHANGES IN ISCHEMIC EPICARDIUM AND ENDOCARDIUM OF THE DOG LEFT VENTRICLE (3)

The purpose of this study was to determine the role played by the tonic influence of vagal and sympathetic nerves on ischemia-induced electrogram alterations in the canine left ventricle. Studies were performed in open-chest dogs anesthetized with alpha-chloralose (60 mg/kg). Electrogram recordings were obtained with decapolar plunge needle electrodes placed in the ischemic and nonischemic myocardium. Heart rate was kept constant by right ventricular pacing. The left anterior descending coronary artery was isolated and, following heparin administration, intermittently occluded distal to the origin of the anterior septal artery for durations of less than 5 minutes. At least 30 minutes recovery was allowed between repeated occlusions. Following the first two control occlusions in one series of dogs, bilateral cervical vagotomy was performed and the left anterior descending coronary artery was occluded for a third time. After a 30 minute recovery period, the stellate ganglia were decentralized and the coronary artery occluded once more. The duration of each occlusion was kept constant. In a separate series of dogs, the order of autonomic intervention was reversed: the stellate ganglia were decentralized after the second occlusion, while the vagal nerves were interrupted after the third occlusion. The changes in amplitude, time-to-onset, time-to-end (total time), and duration in each electrogram were measured prior to, and during the occlusion, using a computerized data acquisition system.

We found that stellate ganglia decentralization, with intact vagal nerves, significantly reduced the increase in epicardial electrogram duration and the decrease in electrogram amplitude induced by ischemia. Stellate ganglia interruption did not significantly affect time-to-onset or total electrogram time. Vagal interruption after stellate ganglia decentralization slightly decreased total electrogram time. Vagal nerve interruption, preceding stellate ganglia decentralization, resulted in a significant increase in total electrogram time and electrogram duration during ischemia, but did not significantly affect electrogram amplitude or time-to-onset. Stellate ganglia decentralization following vagal interruption resulted in a significant decrease in total electrogram time and electrogram duration induced by ischemia but did not significantly affect changes in electrogram amplitude.

The extent of endocardial electrogram changes following left anterior descending coronary artery occlusion were significantly less than those that occurred at the epicardium (13). Stellate ganglia decentralization and vagal nerve interruption minimally affected ischemia-induced changes at the endocardium.

In summary, these data indicate that in the open-chest dog subjected to left anterior descending coronary artery occlusion, stellate sympathetic activity when unopposed by vagal influence accentuated the conduction delay that occurs in epicardial ischemic zones. Stellate ganglia interruption reversed these changes. These observations may provide at least a partial explanation for the known arrhythmogenic effect of sympathetic activity in acute myocardial ischemia.

4. TRANSMEMBRANE ELECTROPHYSIOLOGIC PROPERTIES OF VASCULARIZED HAMSTER ALLOGRAPHS (4)

The purpose of this study was to develop a model in which transmembrane electrophysiologic properties of blood *perfused* mammalian heart cells could be studied. To accomplish this goal, 1–2 mm cubes of neonatal atrial and ventricular muscle were transplanted to the adult female hamster cheek pouch and studied 5–7 days later, when vascularization was complete and spontaneous contractions occurred. The cheek pouch chamber was opened and superfused with oxygenated Tyrode's solution. Standard microelectrode techniques were employed.

Both atrial and ventricular allographs were easily stimulated electrically. They displayed spontaneous pacemaker potentials and superfusion with isoproterenol (1×10^{-7} M) sped the spontaneous discharge rate. Reducing the temperature of the Tyrode's solution from 37 °C to 30 °C prolonged action potential duration and slowed the spontaneous discharge rate. Interrupting blood flow resulted in reduced resting membrane potential, shortened action potential duration, and slowing of the spontaneous discharge rate. Although these data are preliminary, we expect that studies in this model will provide a means to evaluate effects of ischemia on transmembrane electrical properties recorded from Purkinje fibers, subendocardial ventricular muscle, subepicardial ventricular muscle, and atrium. In addition, studies can be performed to separate the effects of superfusion from perfusion with various antiarrhythmic agents. An important feature of the transplants is that they do not appear to be innervated by the autonomic nervous system. Thus, it may be possible to sharply separate the role played by the autonomic nervous system during acute ischemia by investigating the effects of various cholinergic and adrenergic agonists and antagonists.

5. ELECTROPHYSIOLOGIC PROPERTIES OF RODENT MYOCARDIUM DAMAGED BY EPINEPHRINE (5)

The administration of large doses of norepinephrine and epinephrine or certain sympathomimetic amines has been shown to produce cardiac lesions in a variety of experimental animals. The injury consists of focal myocytolysis. Similar lesions have been reported in patients with pheochromocytoma, following prolonged catecholamine infusion and in patients who experienced sudden death. Although the electrophysiologic alterations following coronary artery occlusion have been extensively studied, both in vivo and in vitro, the possible electrophysiological alterations resulting from catecholamine-induced myocardial injury have not yet been investigated. The purpose of this study was to characterize such abnormalities and to attempt to relate them to the genesis of ventricular arrhythmias.

Male Sprague-Dawley rats and guinea pigs of either sex were injected subcutaneously with one dose of epinephrine (base, 3.0 mg/kg body weight), as a 5 % ascorbate saline solution of 1-epinephrine bitartrate. Twenty-four to seventy-two hours following the injection, the rodents were anesthetized with sodium secobarbital (30 mg/kg, intraperitoneally) and a standard lead II electrocardiogram was recorded. The hearts were subsequently removed, and a portion of the left ventricle and interventricular septum containing normal and necrotic myocardium was excised, and studied with standard microelectrode techniques during superfusion with oxygenated Tyrode's solution. Preparations were stimulated and also allowed to discharge spontaneously. In some preparations, current was passed between poles of a bipolar stimulating electrode, with one pole placed on either side of a necrotic zone. Current was delivered by means of a custom built high current stimulus isolator as rectangular pulses of 2 seconds duration at 7 second intervals.

In these preparations, we found no significant differences in any of the action potential characteristics recorded in hearts of untreated control animals compared to recordings obtained from normal zones of treated animals, for either species, with the exception of action potential duration at 100 % repolarization (APD_{100}). The latter was significantly prolonged in the normal zones of treated rats and guinea pigs. The injured zones in the hearts from treated rats and guinea pigs displayed reduced action potential amplitude, duration, resting membrane potential and maximum rate of rise of phase 0, compared to normal zones from both groups.

Conduction disturbances, such as unidirectional block, were common findings in these preparations. Stimulus site, stimulus intensity, stimulus duration and frequency all modified the degree of propagation. As stimulus duration, intensity, or cycle length was increased, propagation improved. Superfusion with isoproterenol (1×10^{-7} M) for 10 minutes facilitated conduction and reduced the minimum stimulus duration, intensity, and cycle length at which 1 : 1 conduction occurred. Summation was a common finding, while inhibition was produced less often. In addition to "all or none" summation which resulted in propagation of a response, graded increases in summated action potential amplitudes could also be produced.

Spontaneous activity was frequent, often consisting of two or more independently competing foci, with variable entrance and exit block. Both overdrive suppression and overdrive acceleration was noted. Passage of depolarizing current pulses increased the spontaneous discharge rate of the automatic focus, and the increase was proportional to the magnitude of the current passed. Hyperpolarizing pulses completely suppressed spontaneous automaticity for the duration of the pulse and tended to retard spontaneous activity following termination of the pulse. Automaticity in a previously quiescent preparation could often be triggered by a single stimulus, stretch, trauma from impalement, superfusion with isoproterenol or depolarizing current pulses. In addition, automatic discharge often started and terminated spontaneously, without obvious interventions. Automatic activity that occurred early in the experiment was often characterized by very irregular discharge, during which some action potentials failed to repolarize, and generated voltage oscillations at greatly reduced resting potentials, resembling those produced by current passage.

Lead II electrocardiograms recorded 24 hours after epinephrine injection in rats prior to sacrifice showed no arrhythmias, although slight ST elevation was present in some tracings. Nevertheless, these animals had varying degrees of myocardial necrosis and animals with more severely injured myocardium exhibited many of the electrical abnormalities described above. In a separate series of rats examined 72 hours following epinephrine injection, premature ventricular complexes were noted in lead II, prior to sacrifice.

Many of the abnormalities of impulse information and conduction present in the rodent myocardium injured by epinephrine are similar to those observed previously in a variety of experimental preparations. An important facet of these observations is that the electrical aberrations occurred in a setting of naturally evolving injury, rather than in an artificially manipulated environment, such as elevated potassium, sucrose gaps and other ionic manipulations. The method of producing this particular environment, i.e., epinephrine injection, was not physiologic, but once produced, areas of damaged myocardium electrophysiologically resembled cardiac tissue injured by coronary artery occlusion. In addition, anatomical abnormalities similar to those produced in this model do occur clinically and therefore, the electrophysiologic data obtained may be relevant to some clinically occurring states characterized by prolonged adrenergic stimulation.

ACKNOWLEDGMENT

This work was supported in part by the Herman C. Krannert Fund, by Grants HL-06308, HL-07182 and HL-18795 from the National Heart, Lung and Blood Institute of the National Institutes of Health, Bethesda, Maryland, and by the American Heart Association, Indiana Affiliate, Inc.

REFERENCES

1. Martins JB, Zipes DP: Vagal nerve stimulation prolongs refractory period of epicardium and endocardium in the canine left ventricle. Am J Cardiol 43:373, (abstract) 1979.
2. Martins JB, Zipes DP: Sympathetic nerves affect endocardial and epicardial refractory periods equivalently

in the canine left ventricle. Clin Res 27: 186A, (Abstract) 1979.

3. Ruffy R, Lovelace DE, Zipes DP: Study of vagal and sympathetic influence on conduction in canine ventricular myocardium following coronary artery occlusion. Clin Res 26:267A, (abstract) 1978.

4. Gilmour RF, Zipes DP: Transmembrane electrophysiologic properties of vascularized hamster cardiac allographs. Fed Proc 38(3):1117, (abstract) 1979.

5. Gilmour RF Jr, Zipes DP: Electrophysiologic properties of epinephrine-induced necrotic myocardium. Am J Cardiol 43:350, (abstract) 1979.

6. Yanowitz F, Preston JB, Abildskov JA: Functional distribution of right and left stellate innervation of the ventricles. Circ Res 18:416–428, 1966.

7. Kolman BS, Verrier RL, Lown B: Effect of vagus nerve stimulation upon excitability of the canine ventricle. Am J Cardiol 37:1041–1045, 1976.

8. Bailey JC, Watanabe AM, Besch HR Jr, Lathrop DA: Acetylcholine antagonism of the electrophysiologic effects of isoproterenol on canine cardiac Purkinje fibers. Circ Res 44:378–383, 1979.

9. Dahlstrom A, Fuxe F, Mya-Tu M, Zetterstrom BEM: Observations on adrenergic innervation of the dog heart. Am J Physiol 209:689–692, 1965.

10. Kent KM, Epstein SE, Cooper T, Jacobowitz DM: Cholinergic innervation of the canine and human ventricular conducting system. Circulation 50:948–955, 1974.

11. Krayer O, Mandoki JJ, Mendez C: Studies on veratrum alkaloids XVI. The action of epinephrine and veratramine on the functional refractory period of the auriculo-ventricular transmission in the heart-lung preparation of the dog. Am J Physiol 103:412–419, 1951.

12. Waxman MB, Wald R: Termination of ventricular tachycardia by an increase in cardiac vagal drive. Circulation 56:385–391, 1977.

13. Ruffy R, Lovelace DE, Knoebel SB, Elharrar V, Zipes DP: Relationship between left ventricular electrogram and regional blood flow in acute myocardial ischemia with and without stellate stimulation. Circ Res. 45: 764–770, 1979.

SECTION 2

THE ELECTROPHYSIOLOGY OF LETHAL ARRHYTHMIAS

SECTION 2C

ELECTROPHYSIOLOGIC MECHANISMS INVOLVED IN VENTRICULAR TACHYCARDIA-FIBRILLATION

2.6. EPICARDIAL ACTIVATION SEQUENCES DURING THE ONSET OF VENTRICULAR TACHYCARDIA AND VENTRICULAR FIBRILLATION

R.E. IDEKER, G.J. KLEIN, W.M. SMITH, L. HARRISON, J. KASELL, A.G. WALLACE and J.J. GALLAGHER

Much has been learned about the activation sequence of stable arrhythmias by recording directly from the epicardium with a single electrode (1). By recording from numerous epicardial sites in sequence with a single, hand-held electrode, the global sequence of epicardial activation can be determined when activation occurs in repeating, identical cycles as during a stable arrhythmia. The importance of the information gained with the hand-held electrode has been demonstrated by the successful surgical treatment of over one-hundred patients with recurrent, drug-resistant arrhythmias secondary to the Wolff-Parkinson-White syndrome (2).

Since recordings are made sequentially with the hand-held electrode, each epicardial site is recorded during a different cycle. The construction of a composite map of global epicardial activation for an arrhythmic cycle requires that the arrhythmia remain unchanged over the several minutes required to record from all of the epicardial sites. Unfortunately, many episodes of arrhythmia are not stable and will revert to sinus rhythm or degenerate into fibrillation before all epicardial recordings can be made with the hand-held electrode. Such unstable arrhythmias would have to be reinduced a number of times until all epicardial sites were recorded. If the arrhythmia could not be successfully reinduced, or if the activation sequence was not the same every time the arrhythmia was induced, then global epicardial activation could not be determined with the hand-held electrode. In addition, even long lasting, stable arrhythmias may change from cycle to cycle for the first few cycles following their initiation. These first cycles may contain information about the genesis of the arrhythmia that is not present in the stable, repeating cycles that follow (3).

These difficulties can be overcome if a large number of electrodes is used, and if all recordings are made simultaneously (4–8). In this manner global epicardial activation can be determined in a single cycle, and can be followed cycle by cycle if the activation sequence is changing. The utility of simultaneous recording from many electrodes has already been demonstrated for both atrial and ventricular arrhythmias (3–6, 9).

1. RECORDING AND DISPLAYING EPICARDIAL ELECTRICAL ACTIVITY

We have developed a method to apply 27 electrodes rapidly and atraumatically to the epicardium, to record simultaneously from all electrodes, and to display global epicardial activation rapidly by means of a computer (7, 8). Although not discussed here, the method can also utilize both a small grid of 25 electrodes to determine in detail the activation can also utilize both a small grid of 25 electrodes to determine in detail the activation sequence of a 3 by 3 cm square of epicardium, and five plunge needles each containing multiple electrodes to determine transmural activation in a small region of myocardium (8).

1.1. Recording the electrograms

Each electrode consists of two poles embedded 1.5 mm apart in a Teflon button, permitting unipolar or bipolar recording (Figure 1). A circumferential groove at the perimeter of the button allows it to be secured within the meshwork of a nylon sock. Twenty-five such electrodes are evenly distributed within the flexible nylon mesh sock (Figure 2). The sock is made in the shape of the heart and can be slipped rapidly over the ventricles. The elasticity of the sock helps to maintain the position of the electrodes on the epicardium but does not hinder cardiac function.

Two additional electrodes are sutured directly to the epicardium and serve as reference electrodes in conjunction with the grid and needle electrode arrays (8). These two electrodes

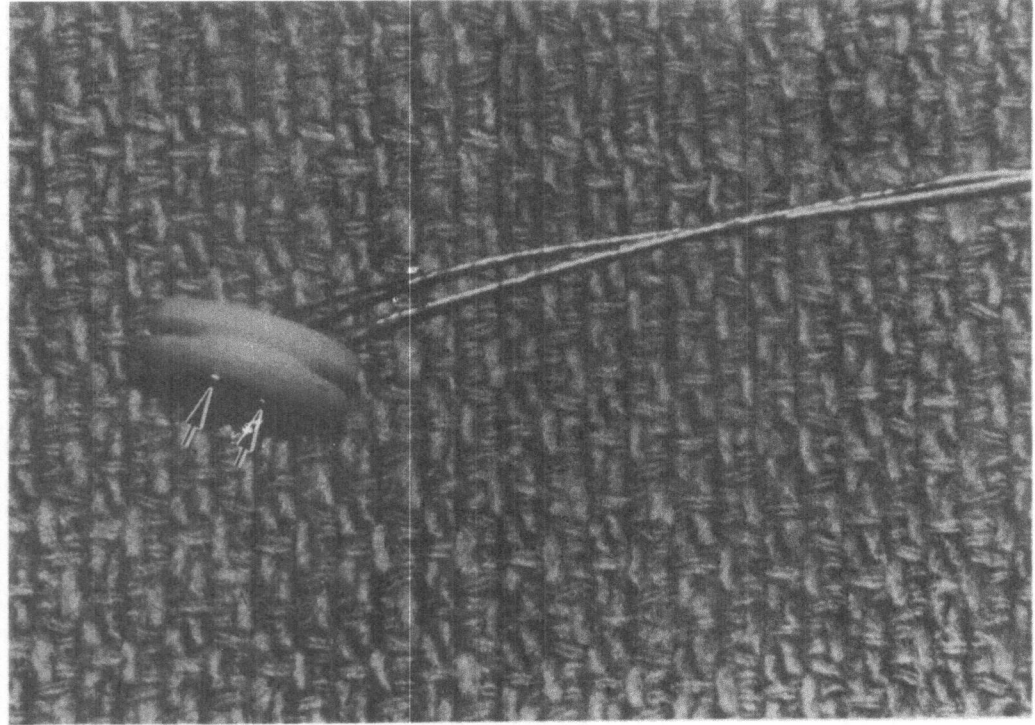

Figure 1. A button electrode used for epicardial recording. Twenty-five such electrodes are held in place within a nylon mesh sock as shown in Figure 2. Arrows indicate the two poles of the electrode. The groove at the periphery allows the button to be secured within the mesh sock.

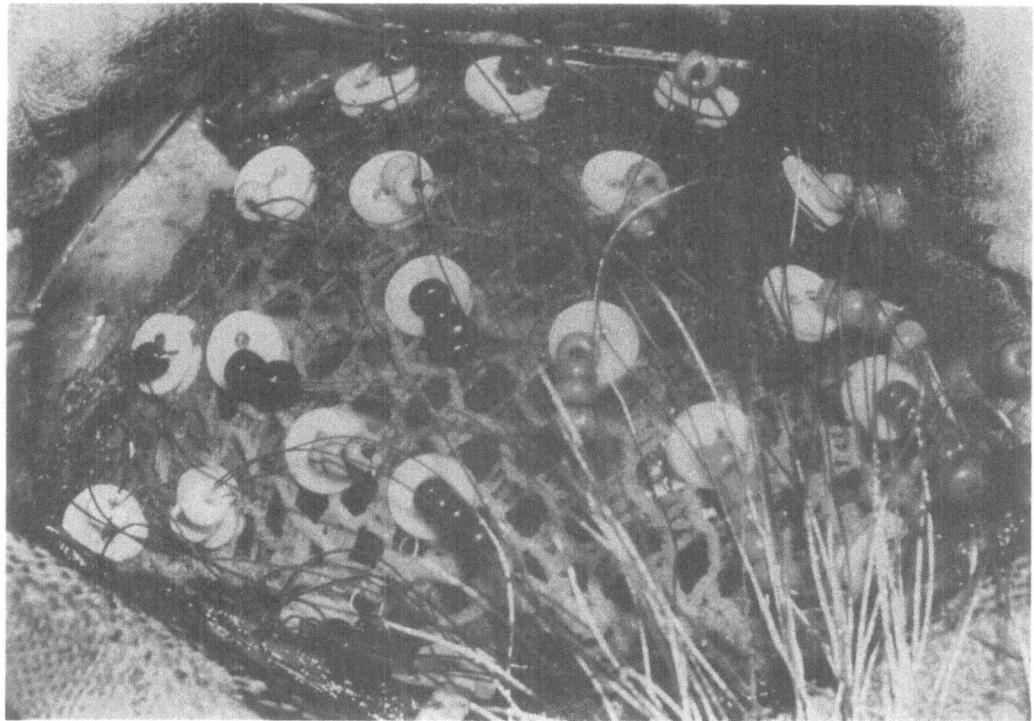

Figure 2. The sock array of electrodes in place on the epicardium. The elastic sock with its enmeshed electrodes has been pulled over the ventricles. The electrodes are identified by color-coded beads.

are sutured to the centers of the two largest regions of epicardium that do not contain sock electrodes. Thus, 27 electrodes are approximately evenly distributed over the epicardium of both ventricles.

Potentials from the 27 epicardial electrodes are recorded simultaneously on a 32 channel FM analog tape recorder (Ampex PR 2200). Three electrocardiographic leads, a voice log, and a time code are also recorded (8).

1.2. Digitizing the potentials

The potentials from each electrode are digitized at 1000 samples per second, multiplexed, and stored on the disk of a computer (Digital Equipment Corporation PDP 11/34). The potentials can be digitized during real time while they are being simultaneously recorded on tape or they can be digitized later by playing back the tape recorder (8). Thus, potentials can still be recorded while the computer is occupied analyzing a previously occurring event. The computer disk holds up to 38.4 seconds of data. After the disk is filled, the earliest data are overwritten so that the last 38.4 seconds of potentials are always present on the disk (8).

1.3. Verifying the potentials and activation times

After digitization is halted, the time interval is selected during which epicardial activation is to be displayed. This time interval is determined from a display on the screen of a graphic computer terminal (Tektronix 4014). The potentials from any two of the epicardial electrodes or electrocardiographic leads are shown for all 38.4 seconds of data stored on the disk (8). An eight-second portion of this display is shown in Figure 3. Figures 3–8 were all obtained from the same experiment in which ventricular tachycardia was induced by programmed premature stimulation in a dog with a one-month-old myocardial infarct. A vertical cursor line, which can be positioned on the screen of the terminal by the operator, is used to indicate to the computer the onset and offset (lines I and II in Figure 3) of the time interval for which epicardial activation is to be displayed. The interval in Figure 3 includes the last three paced cycles, the ensuing episode of ventricular tachycardia, and the next normal sinus cycle.

The potentials for all electrodes recorded throughout the selected time interval are shown in a series of displays on the computer terminal (8). Each display shows one second of data for five electrodes at a time (Figure 4). The points on each tracing which the computer identifies as local activation times are shown on these same displays as vertical lines (Figure 4). For unipolar recordings, local activation times are selected at those points of fastest downslope that are decreasing at least 5 mV in 2 msec (10). Activation times can be modified manually from the keyboard of the computer terminal.

1.4. Displaying the activation sequences

The activation times are shown for all the epicardial electrodes in a single display (Figure 5). The activations are numbered sequentially for each electrode so that the activation

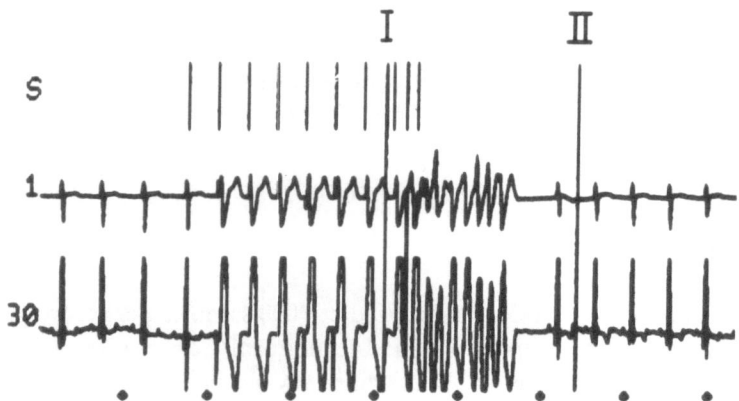

Figure 3. A portion of the display used to select cycles for mapping from the 38.4 seconds of digitized potentials stored on the computer disk. Potentials can be shown for any two of the electrodes (in this example, channels 1 and 30). To the right of the letter S are vertical lines representing the times of programmed stimulation. The diamonds below the potentials are spaced one second apart. The long vertical lines labeled I and II were entered from the terminal by the operator to inform the computer of the onset (I) and offset (II) of the window that is to be mapped. In this example the window encompasses an episode of ventricular tachycardia.

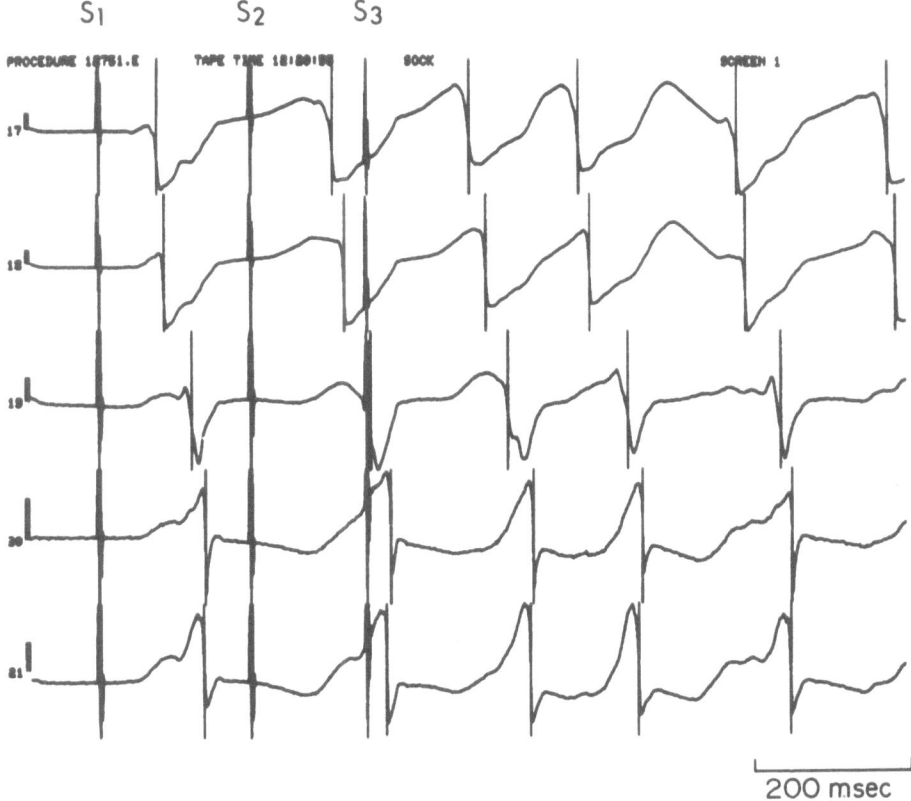

Figure 4. Display of one second of potentials and activation times for five of the electrodes for the window shown in Figure 3. The vertical bar adjacent to each electrode number on the left side of the display represents 10 mv as determined from calibration signals. Activation times selected by the computer are shown as vertical lines. The stimulus artifacts are labeled S1, S2, and S3.

times are grouped for displaying isochronous activation maps, even if consecutive cycles overlap partially in time (8). If any cycles were blocked at one or more electrodes, the operator informs the computer which cycles were blocked at which electrodes. These blocked cycles are represented by asterisks.

The epicardial activation sequence for each cycle is displayed by an isochronous map (Figure 6). The location of each epicardial electrode on a computer display of the ventricles is entered by the operator from the terminal using the intersection of vertical and horizontal cursor lines. Isochronous maps (Figure 6) are drawn based on the algorithms of Barr et al. (11), and Davidow and Brown (12).

2. EPICARDIAL MAPPING OF THE ONSET OF VENTRICULAR TACHYCARDIA

Before a constant QRS morphology is established, ventricular tachycardia induced by

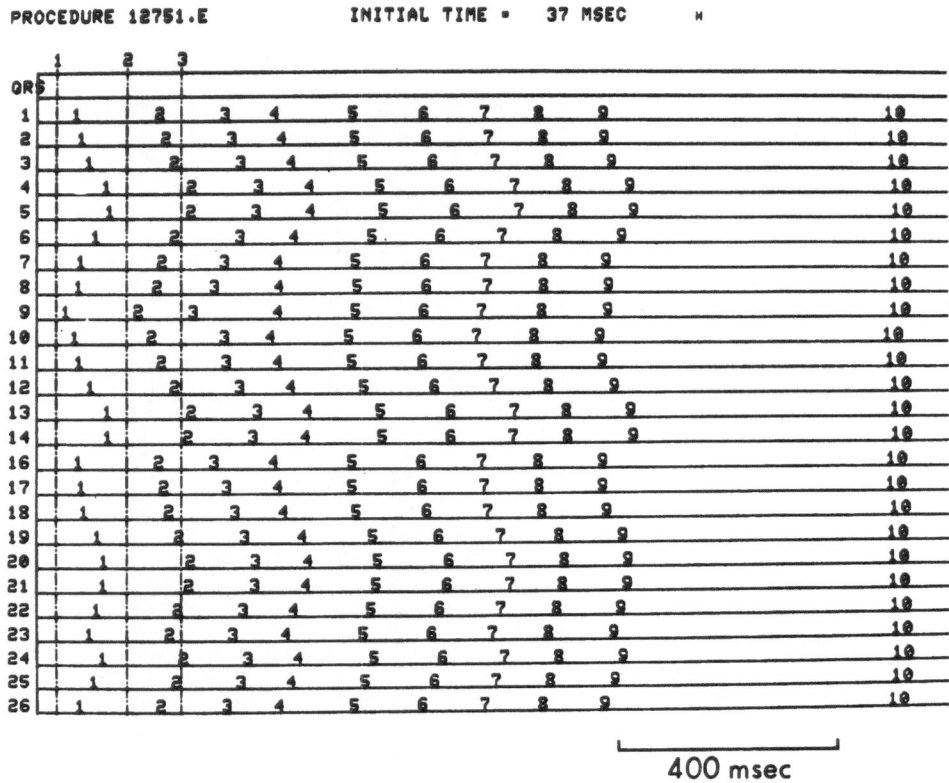

Figure 5. Display of the electrode activation times for the window shown in Figure 3 with time plotted horizontally. The electrodes are numbered on the left side of the display. The local activations at each electrode are numbered consecutively to the right of the electrode number. The long vertical lines are the times of programmed stimulation and are numbered consecutively at the top of the display.

programmed stimulation of the ventricular myocardium may begin with cycles of variable morphology after the last stimulus (13–16). We have recently used the computerized system described above to study global epicardial activation during the initiation of ventricular tachycardia induced by programmed stimulation in a canine model of chronic myocardial infarction (3). Ventricular tachycardia was usually produced by 2 consecutive ventricular extrastimuli programmed during ventricular pacing. The stable phase of ventricular tachycardia was most frequently associated with earliest recorded epicardial activation occurring in the infarction zone, that is overlying the infarct or within 3 cm of its border. In approximately one half of the experiments, the initial 1–5 cycles of tachycardia were of different QRS morphology than the subsequent stable cycles. Three patterns of initiation were observed: 1) The initial cycles broke through to the epicardium over the right ventricle in a pattern similar to that in normal sinus rhythm: 2) The initial cycles broke through to the epicardium at the stimulation site: 3) The initial cycles broke through to the epicardium at variable sites in the infarction zone. In addition, combinations of the above patterns were observed.

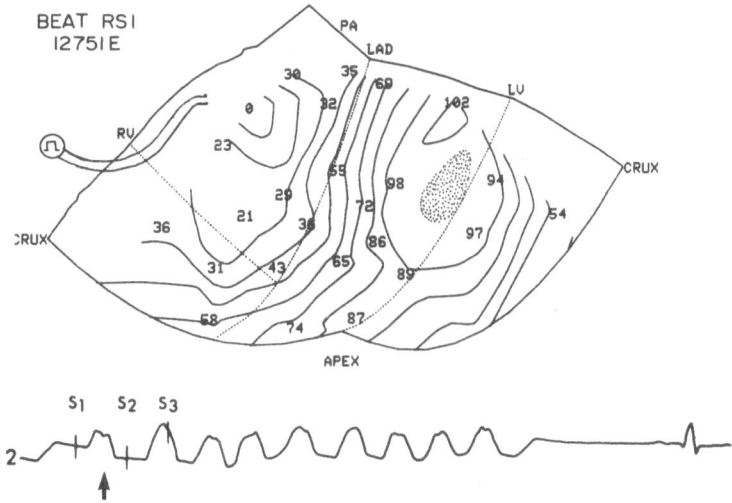

Figure 6. Isochronous map of the first cycle shown in Figure 5 (S1). The total epicardial surface is depicted as if the ventricles were folded out after a cut was made from the crux to the apex. The numbers indicate the locations of the electrodes and give the electrode activation times in msec. Activations are timed with respect to the first epicardial electrode to register activation. The computer-estimated sequence of epicardial activation is shown by isochrone lines spaced 10 msec apart. The stimulus site at the base of the right ventricle is indicated by the ends of the two wires arising from the square wave symbol. The location of an infarct determined by gross examination at the end of the experiment is indicated by stippling. Limb lead 2 is below the map with the stimulus times labeled S1, S2, and S3. The arrow points to the complex for which the epicardial activation sequence is displayed. RV = acute margin of the right ventricle. LV = obtuse margin of the left ventricle. LAD = course of the left anterior descending coronary artery. PA = pulmonary artery.

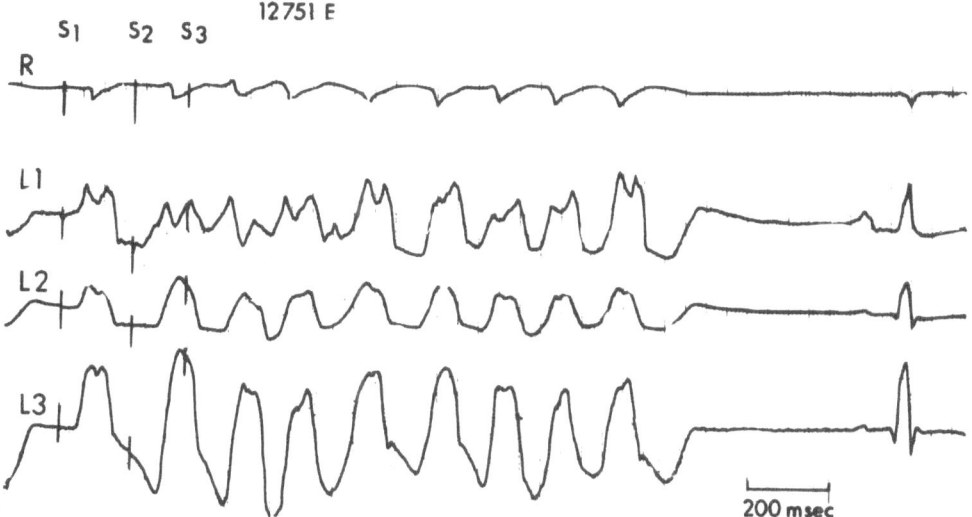

Figure 7. Initial cycles of ventricular tachycardia surfacing near the terminus of the right bundle branch. The induction of tachycardia by two consecutive premature stimuli, S2 and S3, is shown preceded by the last beat of a drive of eight ventricular beats (S1). The limb leads 1, 2, 3 and a reference epicardial electrogram (R) are shown.

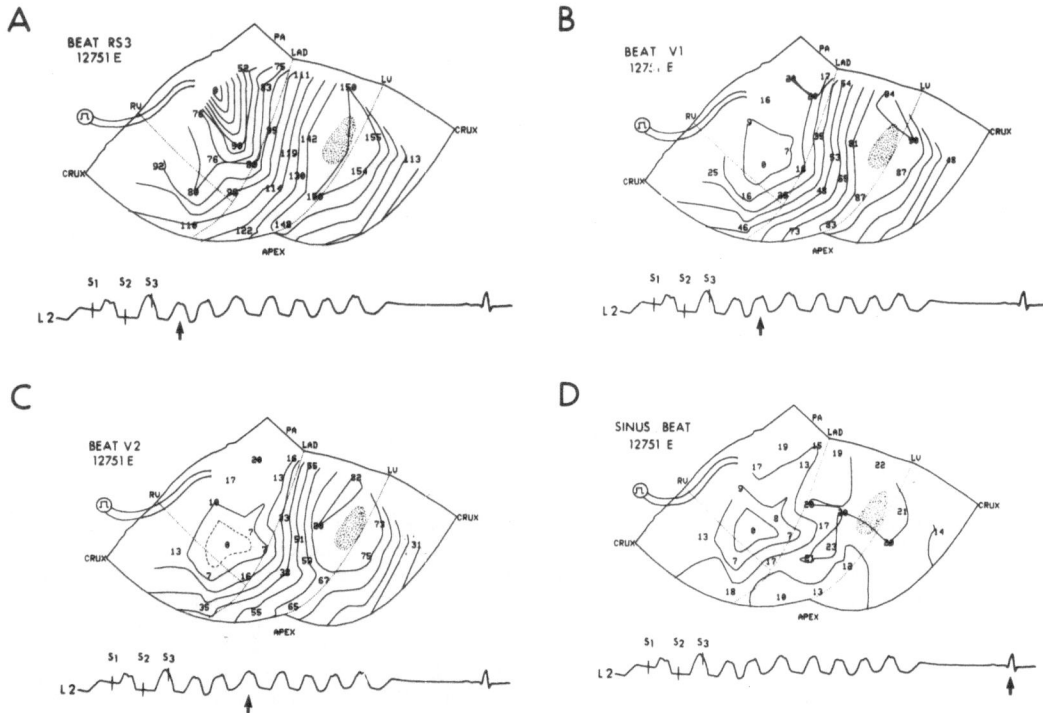

Figure 8. Isochronous maps of epicardial activation for the arrhythmia shown in Figure 7. Cycle RS3 (the second consecutive premature cycle) shows earliest recorded epicardial activity near the pacing electrode. The cycles during tachycardia (only V1 and V2 are shown) demonstrate right ventricular epicardial activation similar to that seen for the sinus beat shown in panel D. Isochrones are shown at 10 msec intervals for panels A-C and 5 msec intervals for panel D. The dotted line in panel C represents the 5 msec isochrone.

2.1. Epicardial breakthrough over the right ventricle with early right ventricular activation pattern similar to sinus rhythm

In some cases, the initial cycles of ventricular tachycardia showed a single area of epicardial breakthrough in the right ventricular paraseptal area, with right ventricular activation similar to that seen during normal sinus rhythm (Figures 7 and 8). This sequence of activation during tachycardia strongly suggests that activation is propagated initially by means of the right bundle branch terminus. The most probable mechanism is bundle branch reentry with utilization of the left bundle branch as the retrograde limb and the right bundle branch as the antegrade limb of the circuit (3). After several such cycles, earliest recorded epicardial activation moved to a stable location in the infarction zone or the tachycardia terminated spontaneously (Figure 7). On one occasion, a prolonged episode of "bundle branch" tachycardia was observed.

2.2. Epicardial breakthrough at the site of the pacing electrode

Most commonly, the initial cycles of tachycardia showed epicardial breakthrough at the stimulation site, before a stable pattern was established with breakthrough at a constant site in the infarction zone. This was observed with both right and left ventricular pacing sites. Brief runs of tachycardia with epicardial breakthrough entirely in the region of the pacing electrode were also observed (Figures 9 and 10). Possible explanations for the mechanism of this phenomenon include mechanical stimulation by the pacing electrode, effects of local injury caused by the pacing electrode, triggered "automaticity", or reentry occurring in local circuits around the stimulation site. Several points favor local rentry: 1) Conduction around the pacing electrode always slowed during the immediately pre- ceding prematurely paced cycles. This was indicated by progressive crowding or closer spacing of isochrone lines around the site of the pacing electrode (Figure 10 B, C). 2) When several cycles were induced near the stimulation site, variation in the activation sequence for each cycle was not uncommon, although all cycles broke through to the epicardium in the vicinity of the pacing electrode. 3) When four to five such cycles were observed (Figure 10), there was a tendency for the cycles to lengthen progressively before spontaneous termination of the arrhythmias. This was associated with early activation of more and more of the electrodes around the stimulation site. By the last cycle, a large area surrounding the pacing electrode showed early, nearly simultaneous epicardial activation. Nonuniform slowing of conduction and dispersion of refractoriness induced by premature stimulation (17–19) could result in the occurrence of unstable local reentrant circuits that would explain these observations. Reentry induced by stimulation in normal myocardial tissues has been described by others (20, 21).

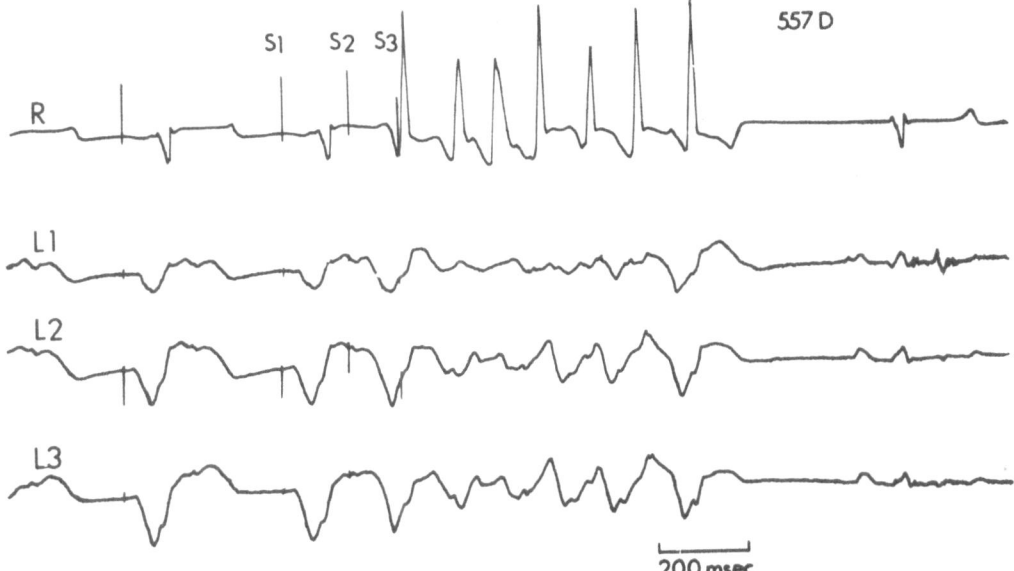

Figure 9. Initial beats of tachycardia surfacing near the pacing electrode. The format of Figure 7 is followed.

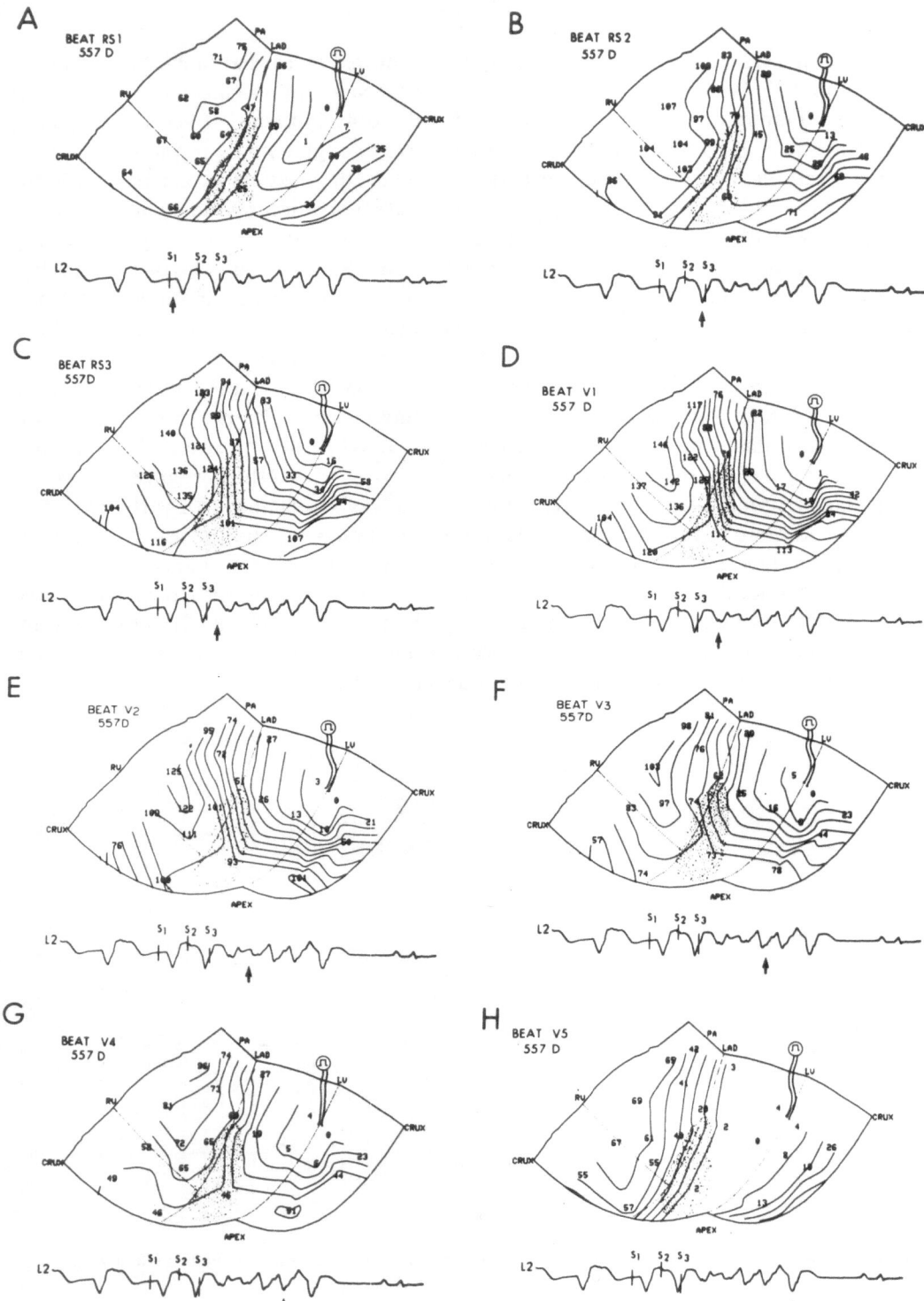

2.3. Epicardial breakthrough at variable sites in the infarction zone

In some experiments, the initial cycles of ventricular tachycardia showed cycle by cycle change in the site of epicardial breakthrough within and around the infarct at regions different from the stimulation site or from the termini of the bundle branches. The tachycardia then stabilized with epicardial breakthrough at a constant location in the infarction zone (Figures 11 and 12). Greater electrode density, including intramyocardial and subendocardial electrodes, would be required in the infarction zone to determine whether the variability in breakthrough location is caused by a changing reentrant circuit or by changing routes of exit at the onset of tachycardia (3). Clearly, further work is required to test these hypotheses.

2.4. Two patterns of epicardial breakthrough during initiation of a single episode of tachycardia

Occasionally, more than one of the above patterns occurred during the initiation phase of ventricular tachycardia. The short run of repetitive firing illustrated (Figures 13 and 14)

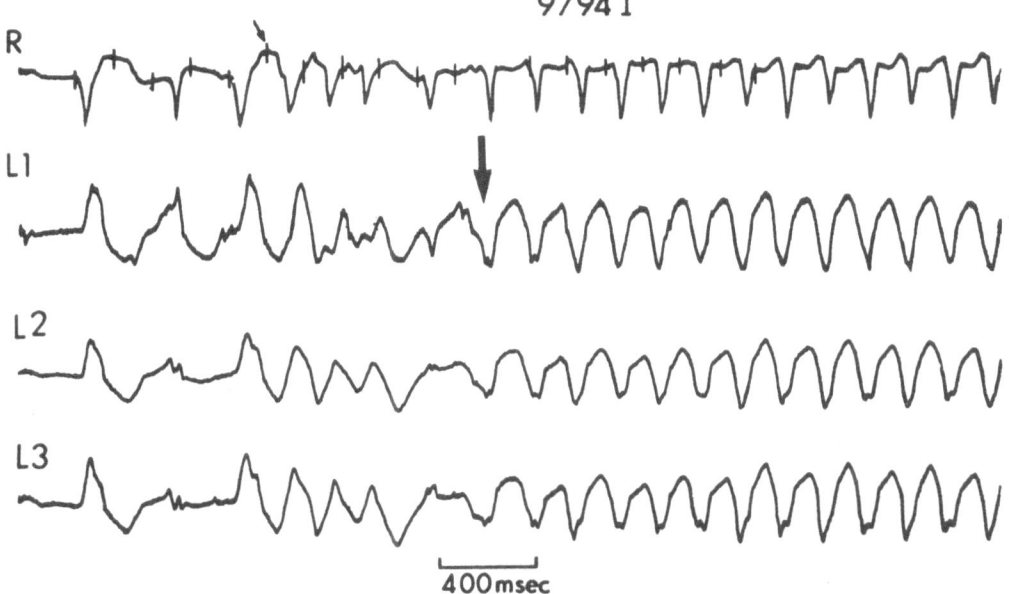

Figure 11. Initial cycles of ventricular tachycardia with variable epicardial breakthrough in the infarction zone. The small arrow points to one of the stimulus artifacts. The large arrow indicates the first cycle of ventricular tachycardia that was induced during a burst of rapid ventricular pacing.

Figure 10. Isochronous maps of epicardial activation for the arrhythmia shown in Figure 9. RS1 represents the response to S1 (last of eight regularly paced cycles). RS2 and RS3 represent the response to the two premature stimuli, S2 and S3. The non-driven cycles of tachycardia (V1-V5) break through to the epicardium near the pacing electrode. Isochrones are shown at 10 msec intervals.

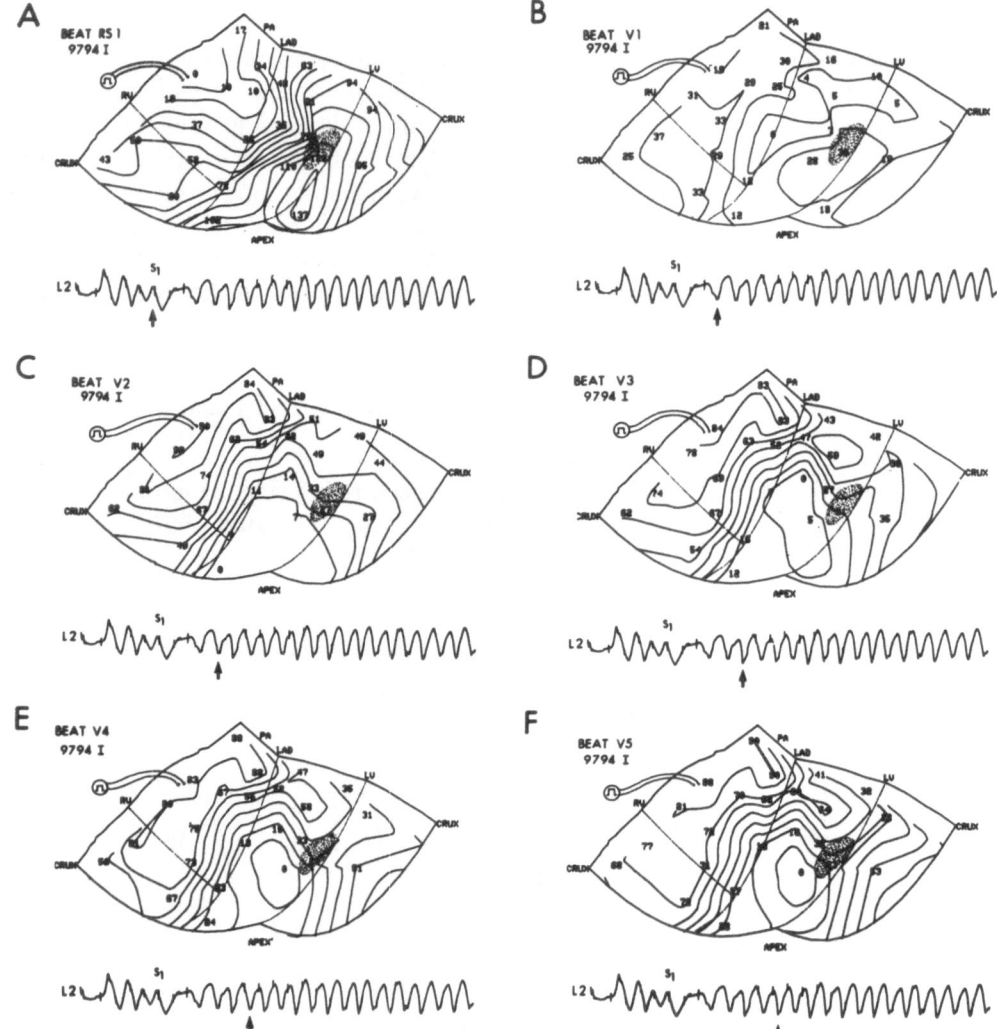

Figure 12. Isochronous maps of epicardial activation for the arrhythmia shown in Figure 11. RS1 is the last stimulated cycle and shows early epicardial activation near the pacing electrode. The first cycle of tachycardia (V1) breaks
through to the epicardium over a large area between the infarct and the left anterior descending coronary artery.
The second cycle (V2) breaks through over a large area between the infarct and the apex. The third cycle (V3) breaks
through at a still different area adjacent to the infarct. Cycles V4, V5, and the remainder of the cycles of this tachycardia break through consistently at the lower border of the infarct. Isochrones are shown at 10 msec intervals.

shows the first cycle breaking through to the epicardium at the stimulation site while
subsequent cycles broke through over the right bundle branch terminus.

12751 H

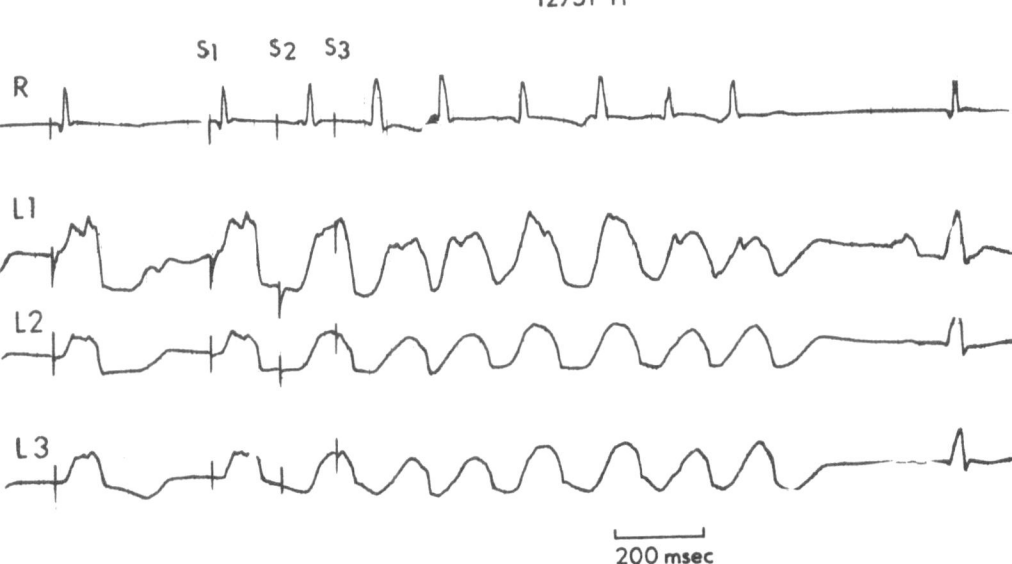

Figure 13. Initial cycles of tachycardia with epicardial breakthrough initially at the pacing electrode and subsequently moving to the right bundle branch terminus.

2.5. Role of initiating cycles in ventricular tachycardia

In some patients with recurrent ventricular tachycardia, clinical electrophysiological studies have shown that stable ventricular tachycardia can be induced with or without initial unstable cycles (13). This was true in most of our experiments. In some cases, however, stable tachycardia was induced only when unstable initial beats were present while in others, it was induced only when they were absent. This would suggest that, in some instances, the initial beats act like "premature stimulus equivalents" either aiding or impeding the emergence of stable ventricular tachycardia.

In summary, we have described three distinct phenomena occurring at the initiation of ventricular tachycardia induced by electrical stimulation. Mechanisms to explain these phenomena include: 1) reentry involving the infarction zone (Figure 15A); 2) reentry involving local circuits near the stimulation site (Figure 15B); and 3) reentry involving the main bundle branches (Figure 15C).

3. EPICARDIAL MAPPING OF THE TRANSITION TO VENTRICULAR FIBRILLATION

Simultaneous recording from numerous epicardial sites can supply information about other unstable arrhythmias besides ventricular tachycardia. We have used the sock electrode array to map the sequence of epicardial activation during the transition to ventricular fibrillation from normal sinus rhythm or ventricular tachycardia in the dog (9). Ventricular

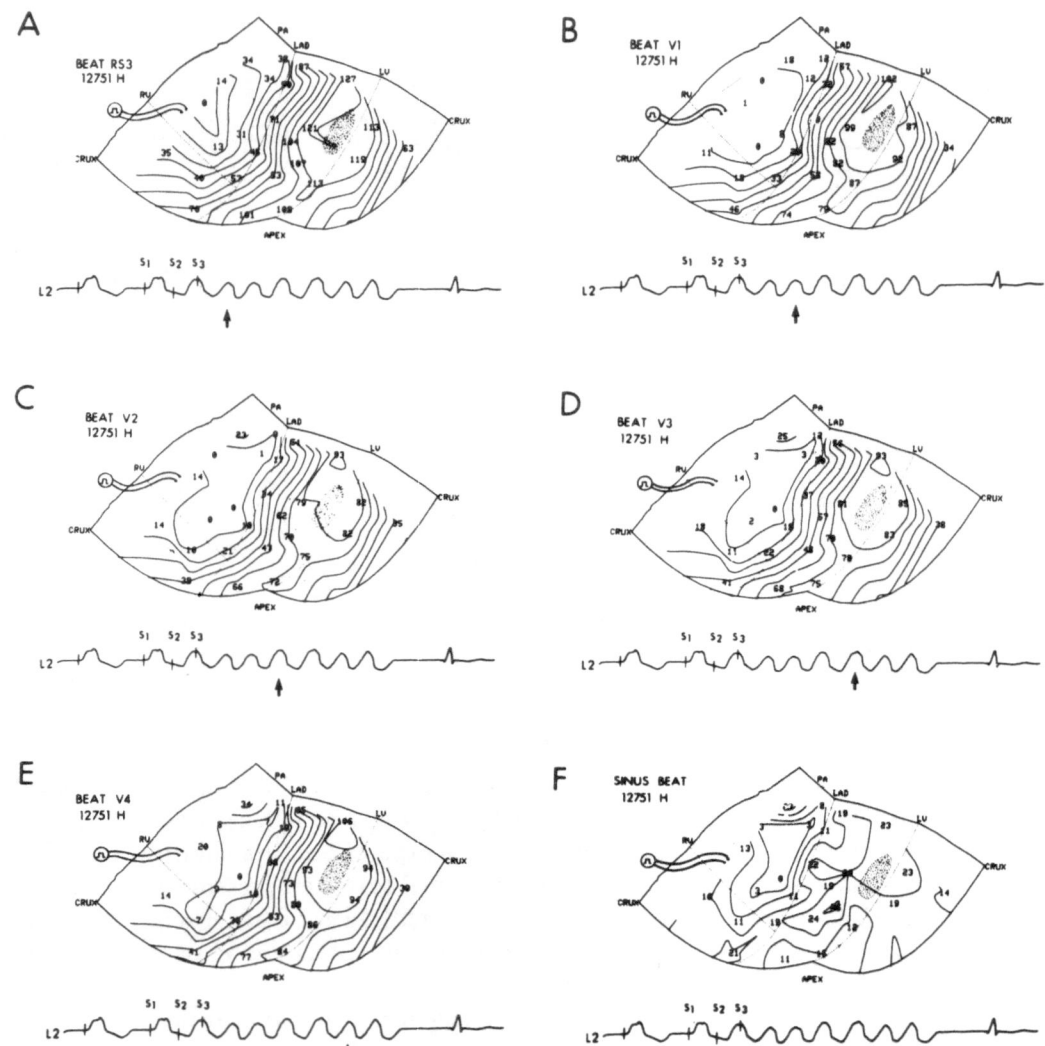

Figure 14. Isochronous maps of epicardial activation for the arrhythmia shown in Figure 13. Cycle RS3 is the last driven cycle and breaks through to the epicardium near the pacing electrode. Cycle VI is the first cycle of ventricular tachycardia and breaks through at the stimulation site. The subsequent cycles of tachycardia (V2 to V4 shown) demonstrate epicardial breakthrough over the right bundle branch terminus similar to that seen in normal sinus rhythm (panel F). Isochrones are shown at 10 msec intervals for panels A-E and at 5 msec intervals for panel F.

fibrillation was induced by reperfusion after a 15 minute occlusion of the proximal left circumflex coronary artery.

Analysis of the first 1.5–2.5 seconds of the transition period revealed that ventricular activation occurred in an orderly, rapidly-repeating sequence (Figure 16 and 17). The activation rate at each epicardial electrode was very fast, seven or eight cycles per second. Numbering activations consecutively (Figure 17) demonstrated that the successive cycles appeared so rapidly that before one cycle ended the next had already broken through to

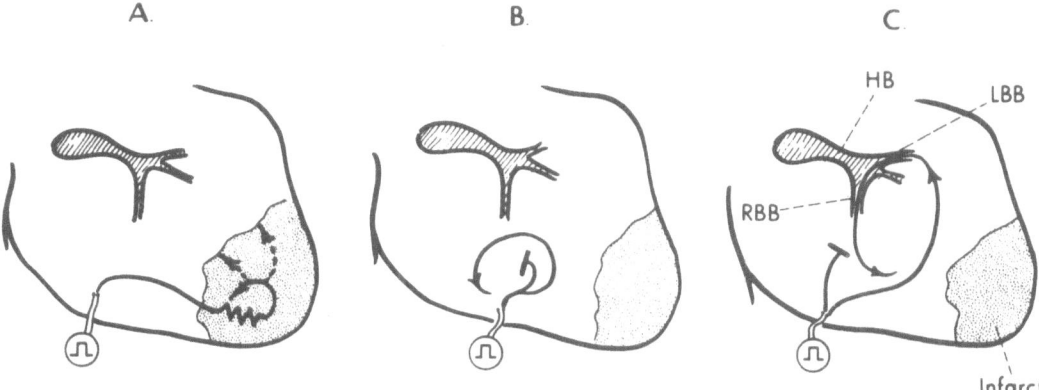

Figure 15. Schematic representation of proposed mechanisms to explain the phenomena at the initiation of ventricular tachycardia induced by programmed stimulation. Panel A shows variation in epicardial breakthrough near an infarct due to changing reentrant circuits or variable routes of exit of a single reentrant circuit from the infarction zone. Panel B shows reentry occuring in local circuits around the stimulation site. Panel C shows bundle branch reentry with the premature cycle encountering retrograde block in the right bundle branch. Conduction occurs retrogradely over the left bundle branch and subsequently antegradely over the right bundle branch to complete the circuit. **HB** = His bundle. **LBB** = left bundle branch. **RBB** = right bundle branch.

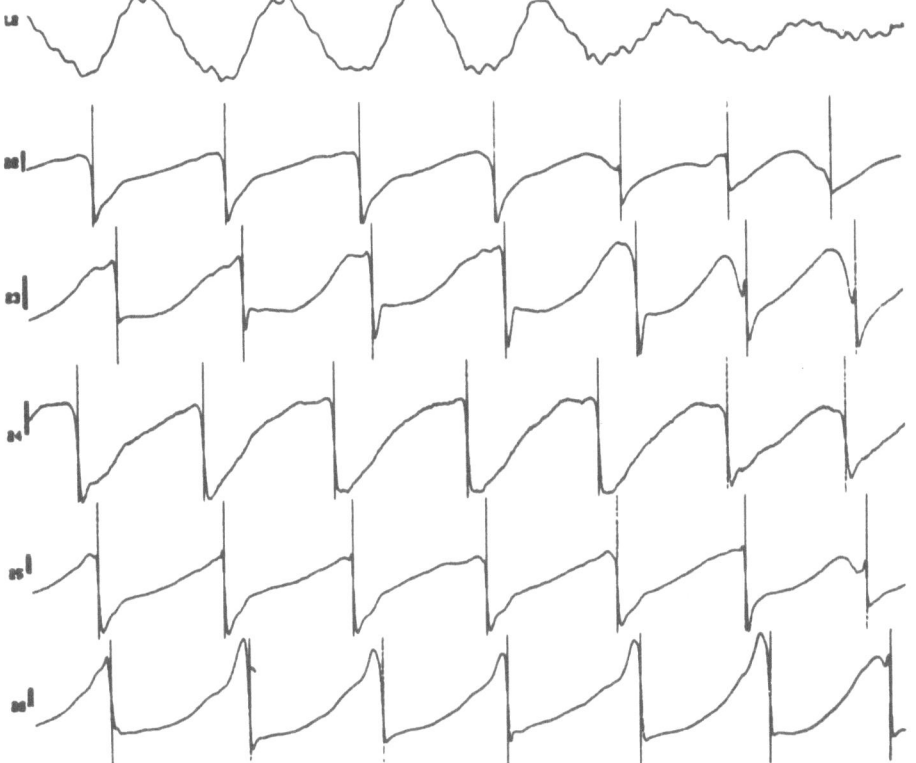

Figure 16. Limb lead 2 and unipolar potential with local activation times for five epicardial electrodes during the initiation of ventricular fibrillation. A 10 mV calibration bar is at the left of each tracing next to the electrode number. The vertical lines superimposed on each tracing indicate the points of most rapid downslope in the potentials identified by the computer and represent the times of local activation of tissue around the electrode. Figures 16–19 are from the same experiment.

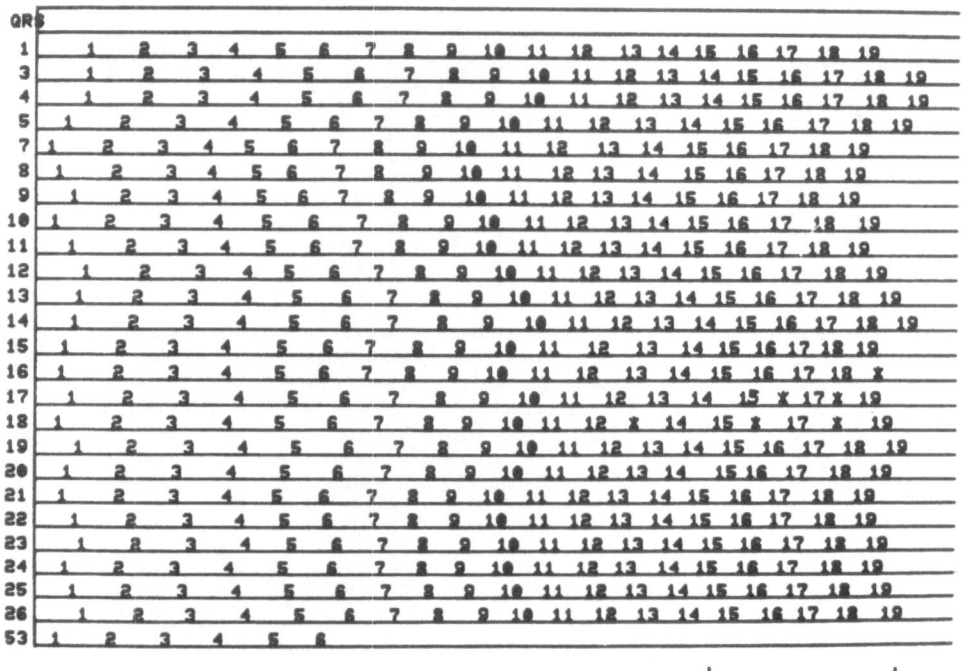

Figure 17. Local activation times for all epicardial electrodes demonstrating that activation is occurring in repeating, overlapping cycles. The electrodes are numbered at the left. The horizontal axis represents time. The times of local activation at each electrode are numbered consecutively. Asterisks indicate cycles for which no activation was detected in the electrode tracing.

the epicardium. For example, cycle nine reached electrode seven before cycle eight reached electrodes three and four (Figure 17).

Epicardial isochronous maps reveal that each cycle consisted of a single, organized activation front (Figure 18). Activation for each cycle broke through to the epicardium within or near the ischemic-reperfused region, passed across the heart as an organized wavefront, and terminated on the opposite side of the heart at the base of the right ventricle (Figure 18). This simple activation sequence is similar to that for a premature ventricular

Figure18. Isochronous maps of epicardial activation for selected cycles of Figure 17 demonstrating that activation during the transition to fibrillation is occurring in organized, repeating cycles. Panels A-H show the first eight even-numbered cycles of Figure 17. Limb lead III is at the bottom of each panel with an arrow indicating the center of the time interval during which the cycle was present on the epicardium. Asterisks (panel H) indicate electrode locations at which no activation was detected for that cycle. Isochrones are shown at 20 msec intervals. The ischemic-reperfused region is stippled.

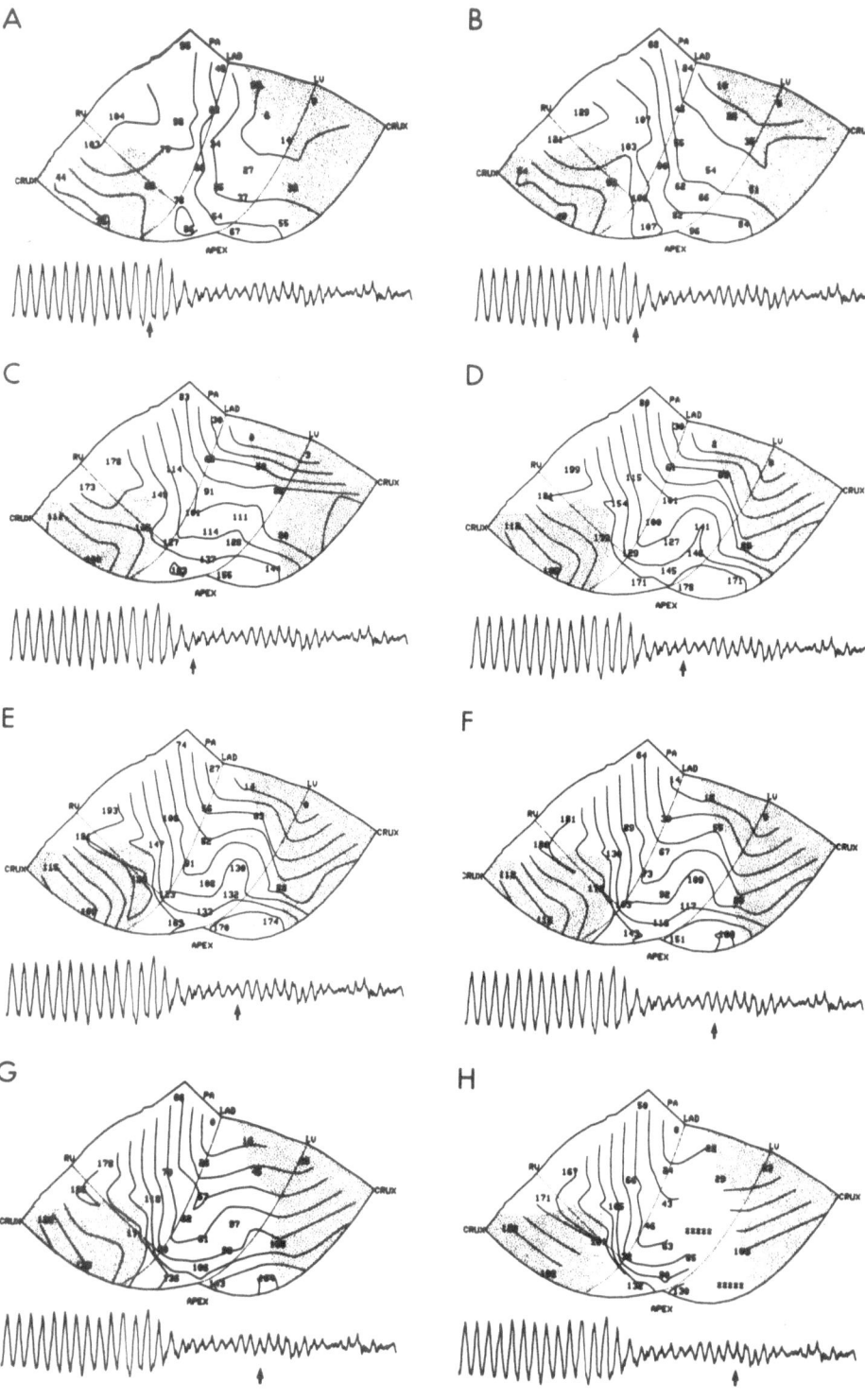

depolarization (9) or an ectopically paced complex (22). Ventricular muscle remote from the ischemic-reperfused region appeared to play no active role during the transition to fibrillation; rather it responded in an orderly fashion to activation fronts originating rapidly from the ischemic-reperfused region.

The overlap between consecutive cycles can be demonstrated by showing the location of all activation fronts on the epicardium at successive points in time (Figure 19). Cycle 14 is shown at 25 msec intervals throughout its passage across the ventricles. Note that cycle 14 broke through to the epicardium near the ischemic-reperfused border (Figure 19A) before cycle 13 ended at the base of the right ventricle (Figure 19C). Similarly, cycle 15 appeared (Figure 19F) before cycle 14 terminated (Figure 19H).

Although fibrillation is defined as chaotic, random, asynchronous electrical activity of the ventricles (19, 23), it is usually identified from the electrocardiogram, not from the ventricles themselves. Our results show that a disorganized tracing in the electrocardiogram does not always mean that ventricular electrical activity is disorganized (Figure 19). We have referred to this period in which the electrocardiogram appears disorganized while ventricular activation is still organized as the "transition" phase of fibrillation since the classic criterion for fibrillation is not present during this period (9).

The duration of the transition phase is not known. After 1.5–2.5 seconds, local epicardial excitation can no longer be reliably identified because the rapid deflection signaling activation in the electrogram greatly slows. Determination of the duration of the transition phase awaits the development of improved techniques and quantitative criteria for the detection of local myocardial activation. These improved techniques are also needed to determine whether the change in electrical activity from organization to chaos is gradual or sudden.

We have not yet been able to determine the mechanism by which activation is initiated during the transition phase because of the wide spacing between epicardial electrodes and the lack of intramyocardial and endocardial electrodes. Macro-reentry involving the bundle branches is unlikely because the site of earliest recorded epicardial activation during the transition phase was generally not the same as the sites of epicardial breakthrough overlying the termination of the fascicles of the left bundle branch or the right bundle branch during the normal sinus complexes immediately preceding fibrillation. The presence of an R wave of sizable duration before the rapid deflection in the electrogram that registered earliest epicardial activation during the transition cycles suggests that the activation fronts do not originate directly from the epicardium, but arise from subjacent myocardium or endocardium (9).

Figure 19. Passage of a single cycle (cycle 14 of the experiment displayed in Figures 16–18) across the ventricles demonstrating the presence of overlapping cycles. The activation fronts for each cycle are identified by the same numbers as in Figure 17. Panels A-H show the location of the activation fronts at 25 msec intervals. Limb lead III is at the bottom of each panel with an arrow indicating the point in time represented by the panel.

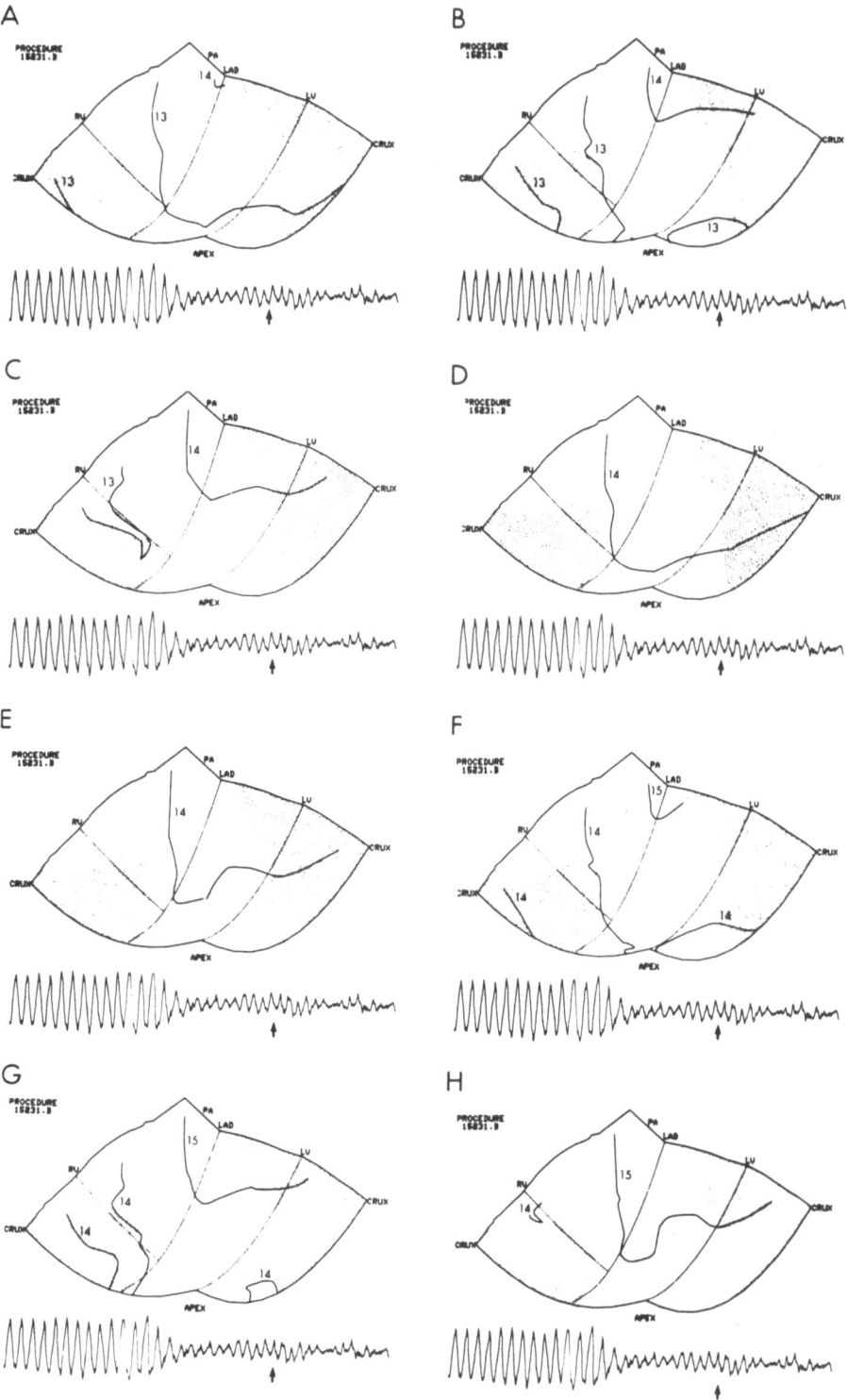

4. CONCLUSIONS

Our results (3, 9), as well as those of others (4–6), demonstrate the usefulness of simultaneous recording from numerous electrodes for the study of unstable arrhythmias. Simultaneous recording allows the mapping of ventricular tachycardia even when the arrhythmia is short lived or when activation changes from cycle to cycle during initiation (3). Simultaneous recording from the epicardium, followed by simultaneous recording from the myocardium and endocardium, may allow identification of a small myocardial region that is responsible for the tachycardia. If so, the arrhythmia could be prevented by surgical ablation or modification of the region.

Our studies provide a basis for postulating that in some cases ventricular fibrillation can also originate from a localized, identifiable region of myocardium (9). The fact that organized activity persists for a series of repeating cycles during the transition to fibrillation suggests that intramural activation studies might contribute to a better understanding of the mechanism of the initiation of fibrillation. Fibrillation, in some cases, may also be preventable by local ablation of a region of myocardium responsible for its onset.

ACKNOWLEDGEMENTS

The authors wish to express their gratitude to Ms. Jo Ann Horan, Mr. Don Powell and Mr. David Huggett who prepared the illustrations, Mr. Jimmy Manley who assisted in the animal laboratory and to Ms. Hilda Smith and Ms. Frances Slocum who typed the manuscript.

This work was supported in part by Research Grants HL-17670 and HL-15190 from the National Heart, Lung and Blood Institute. While this work was performed, Dr. Ideker was recipient of Training Grant Award HL-07101 from the National Heart, Lung and Blood Institute, Dr. Klein was a Research Fellow of the Medical Research Council of Canada and Dr. Gallagher was an Established Investigator of the American Heart Association.

REFERENCES

1. Gallagher JJ, Kasell J, Sealy WC, Pritchett ELC, Wallace AG: Epicardial mapping in the Wolff-Parkinson-White syndrome. Circulation 57:854–866, 1978.
2. Gallagher JJ, Gilbert M, Svenson RH, Sealy WC, Kasell J, Wallace AG: Wolff-Parkinson-White syndrome: The problem, evaluation, and surgical correction. Circulation 51:767–785, 1975.
3. Klein GJ, Ideker RE, Smith WM, Harrison LA, Kasell J, Wallace AG, Gallagher JJ: Epicardial mapping of the onset of ventricular tachycardia initiated by programmed stimulation in the canine heart with chronic infarction. Circulation 60: 1375–1384, 1979.
4. Sano T, Scher AM: Multiple recording during electrically induced atrial fibrillation. Circ Res 14:117–125, 1964.
5. Smith RA, El-Sherif N, Evans AK: Epicardial mapping of ventricular reentrant pathways in the late myocardial infarction period (abstract). Am J Cardiol 41:427, 1978.
6. Harumi K, Wyatt R, Lux R, Abildskov JA, Smith CR: Initiating mechanisms of ventricular fibrillation (abstract). Am J Cardiol 43:374, 1979.
7. Smith WM, Ideker RE, Kinicki RE, Harrison LA, Wallace AG, Gallagher JJ: A computer system for the on-line study of ventricular arrhythmias. Computers in Cardiology. Long Beach, IEEE, 1977, p 311–316.

8. Ideker RE, Smith WM, Wallace AG, Kasell J, Harrison LA, Klein GJ, Kinicki RE, Gallagher JJ. A computerized method for the rapid display of ventricular activation during the intraoperative study of arrhythmias. Circulation 59:449–458, 1979.

9. Ideker RE, Klein GJ, Harrison L, Smith WM, Kasell J, Reimer KA, Wallace AG, Gallagher JJ: Epicardial mapping of the transition to ventricular fibrillation induced by reperfusion following acute ischemia in the dog (submitted for publication).

10. Durrer D, van der Twell LH: Excitation of the left ventricular wall of the dog and goat. Ann NY Acad Sci 65:779–803, 1957.

11. Barr RC, Gallie TM, Spach MS: Automated construction and display of spatial maps of cardiac electrophysiological events for heart or body surfaces. II. Construction of contour maps Comp Biomed Rev (in press).

12. Davidow LS, Brown PB: A contour mapping algorithm suitable for small computers. In Computer Technology in Neuroscience, Brown PB (ed), New York, John Wiley and Sons, 1975, p 321–335.

13. Josephson ME, Horowitz LN, Farshidi A, Kastor JA: Recurrent sustained ventricular tachycardia. 1. Mechanisms. Circulation 57:431–440, 1978.

14. Denes P, Wu D, Dhingra RC, Amat-Y-Leon F, Wyndham C, Mautner RK, Rosen KM: Electrophysiological studies in patients with chronic recurrent ventricular tachycardia. Circulation 54:229–236, 1976.

15. Wellens HJJ, Durrer DR, Lie KI: Observations on mechanisms of ventricular tachycardia in man. Circulation 54:237–244, 1976.

16. Drew TM, Josephson ME, Horowitz LM, Kastor JA, Herling I: The significance of the repetitive ventricular response to programmed ventricular stimulation (abstract). Clin Res 25:218A, 1977.

17. Han J, DeJabon PDG, Moe GK: Fibrillation threshold of premature ventricular responses. Circ Res 18:18–25, 1966.

18. Sugimoto T, Schaal SF, Wallace AG: Factors determining vulnerability to ventricular fibrillation induced by 60-CPS alternating current. Circ Res 21:601–608, 1967.

19. Surawicz B: Ventricular fibrillation. Am J Cardiol 28:268–287, 1971.

20. Allessie MA, Bonke FIM, Schopman FJG: Circus movement in rabbit atrial muscle as a mechanism of tachycardia. 3. The "leading circle" concept: a new model of circus movement in cardiac tissue without the involvement of an anatomical obstacle. Circ Res 41:9–18, 1977.

21. Sasyniuk BI, Mendez C: A mechanism for reentry in canine ventricular tissue. Circ Res 28:3–15, 1971.

22. Spach MS, Barr RC: Analysis of ventricular activation and repolarization from intramural and epicardial potential distributions for ectopic beats in the intact dog. Circ Res 37:830–843. 1975

23. Zipes DP: Electrophysiological mechanisms involved in ventricular fibrillation. Circulation 52 (III) 120–130, 1975.

2.7. ELECTROPHYSIOLOGICAL OBSERVATIONS ON VENTRICULAR FIBRILLATION IN THE HUMAN HEART

M.E. JOSEPHSON, S.R. SPIELMAN, A.M. GREENSPAN and L.N. HOROWITZ

The mechanism of ventricular fibrillation induced by either ischemia or electric impulses has been considered by most investigators to result from multiple reentrant wavelets creating sustained rapid and irregular excitation of the heart (1–6). However, some investigators maintain that one or more rapidly firing foci initiate and maintain ventricular fibrillation (7, 8). The present report details our observations on the initiation (spontaneous or induced) and spontaneous termination of ventricular fibrillation in man using endocardial electrode catheter recordings and the relationship of the surface ECG and intracardiac electrograms.

1. METHODS AND MATERIALS

Twenty-two of 529 consecutive patients studied at the Hospital of the University of Pennsylvania from June 1974 to April 1979 developed ventricular fibrillation during electrophysiologic study (Table 1). In 15 patients ventricular fibrillation was induced by programmed ventricular stimulation, and in 7 patients ventricular fibrillation occurred spontaneously either by degeneration from ventricular tachycardia (6 patients) or from spontaneous ventricular depolarizations (1 patient). In all 22 patients the electrophysiologic study was undertaken to evaluate suspected malignant ventricular arrhythmias after informed consent was obtained. There were 15 males and 7 females ranging in age from 18 to 73 years (Table 1). Nineteen patients had a history of documented syncope and/or cardiac arrest, in each of whom ventricular tachycardia or ventricular fibrillation had been documented. Three patients were studied because of near-syncopal episodes, in one of whom spontaneously converting ventricular fibrillation had been documented. Fourteen patients had coronary artery disease (3 of whom also had hypertensive cardiovascular disease, and one of whom had concomitant rheumatic heart disease), one had cardiomyopathy, one had rheumatic heart disease, and 6 had no heart disease as documented by cardiac catheterization.

Standard multipolar (2 to 6 electrodes) electrode catheters (1 cm interelectrode distance) were inserted percutaneously via the femoral and/or brachial veins and arteries and positioned in the heart under fluoroscopic guidance. In each patient two to five simultaneous ventricular electrograms were recorded at the onset and/or termination of ventricular fibrillation. These always included electrograms recorded at the atrioventricular junction (His bundle electrogram) and right ventricular apex. In addition, coronary sinus electro-

Table 1. Clinical data.

Patient	Age	Sex	Cardiac Diagnosis	ECG	History of Syncope or Cardiac Arrest	Spontaneously Documented Arrhythmias
1	73	F	HCVD, ASHD	LVH	+	VF, VPDs
2	67	M	NHD	normal	+	VF, VT
3	54	F	ASHD	NTMI	+	VF, VT, SB
4	24	M	CM	IVCD	+	VF, VT, AFl, SVT
5	52	M	ASHD	ASMI	+	VF, VT
6	53	F	RHD, ASHD	ASMI, RBBB	+	VF, VT
7	72	F	ASHD	LBBB, 1°AVB	+	VF, VPDs
8	18	M	NHD	normal	+	VT
9	67	F	NHD	RBBB, LAH, 1°AVB	– *	none
10	64	M	ASHD	AMI, LAH, 1°AVB	+	VF, VT
11	46	M	NHD	normal	– *	SB
12	62	M	ASHD	ASMI	+	VF, VT
13	66	M	ASHD	ASMI	+	VF, VT
14	52	M	ASHD, HCVD	LVH, IVCD	+	VF, VT
15	52	M	RHD	AF, marked prolonged QT (.70 sec)	+	VF, VT
16	55	M	NHD	Normal	– *	VF
17	57	M	ASHD	RBBB, LAH	+	VF, VT
18	58	F	NHD	LBBB	+	VPDS, couplets
19	66	F	ASHD, HCVD	LBBB	+	VPDS, couplets, TDP
20	58	M	ASHD	IVCD, ASMI	+	VF, VT
21	67	M	ASHD	IMI, LAH	+	TDP
22	52	M	ASHD	IMI, LAH	+	TDP

AF	– atrial fibrillation	
AFL	– atrial flutter	
ASHD	– atherosclerotic heart disease	
ASMI	– anteroseptal myocardial infarction	
AVB	– atrioventricular block	
CM	– cardiomyopathy	
IVCD	– intraventricular conduction defect	
HCVD	– hypertensive cardiovascular disease	
LAH	– left anterior hemiblock	
LBBB	– left bundle branch block	

LVH	– left ventricular hypertrophy
NHD	– no heart disease
NTMI	– nontransmural myocardial infarction
RBBB	– right bundle branch block
RHD	– rheumatic heart disease
SB	– sinus bradycardia
SVT	– supraventricular tachycardia
TDP	– torsade de pointes
VF	– ventricular fibrillation
VPD	– ventricular premature depolarization
VT	– ventricular tachycardia

*– recurrent near-syncopal episodes

gram recording posterobasal left ventricular activity was recorded in 17 patients, and one or two bipolar left ventricular electrograms were obtained from catheters positioned in the left ventricle. The intracardiac electrograms were filtered at 40 and 500 Hz and simultaneously displayed with two or three surface electrograms. The data were recorded on a Honeywell 5600C tape recorder and later retrieved on photographic paper at speeds of 100 to 400 mm/second. In patients in whom ventricular fibrillation did not spontaneously convert to normal sinus rhythm DC shock was utilized to reestablish sinus rhythm as soon as loss of consciousness occurred.

Stimulation was performed using a custom-designed programmable stimulator (Bloom Associates Inc., Narberth, Pa.) with optically isolated constant current sources. Stimuli were 1 msec in duration and twice diastolic threshold, ranging from 0.6 to 2.5 mA. All equipment was isolated from the patients and leakage current ranged from 2 to 6 μA. The stimulation protocol included the introduction of single and double ventricular extrastimuli during sinus rhythm, ventricular pacing and ventricular tachycardia as previously published (9).

Ventricular fibrillation was defined using standard electrocardiographic criteria as a rapid ventricular arrhythmia with irregular polymorphic complexes. The diagnosis of ventricular fibrillation based on surface electrocardiographic criteria did not take into account electrical activity recorded in local ventricular electrograms. Rapid, irregular, and frequently continuous electrical activity observed in an intracardiac electrogram was called "local fibrillation" although the exact mechanism of such activity is not yet established.

2. RESULTS

2.1. Mode of initiation

Ventricular fibrillation was initiated by the introduction of two ventricular extrastimuli during ventricular pacing (14 patients) or sinus rhythm (1 patient). In 13 patients these were delivered from the right ventricle, and in 2 from the left ventricle. Left ventricular stimulation was performed only after completion of the right ventricular stimulation protocol and no ventricular arrhythmia had occurred. In each of the patients in whom ventricular fibrillation was initiated by double ventricular extrastimuli, single ventricular extrastimuli scanning diastole had failed to induce the arrhythmia. Typically one or more intraventricular reentrant complexes were observed at longer coupling intervals than those initiating ventricular fibrillation (Figure 1). In each case in which double stimuli produced ventricular fibrillation the second ventricular extrastimulus was introduced at shorter coupling intervals than the first.

"Local fibrillation" developed in at least one intracardiac recording immediately following the second extrastimulus in 3 patients, but more commonly (12 of 15 patients) one or more discrete repetitive ventricular responses were observed before fragmentation developed in any individual electrogram. In the patients in whom one or more additional spontaneous ventricular responses occurred prior to degeneration to local fibrillation in any intracardiac recording, the coupling intervals of those ventricular complexes shortened. Thus, at the onset of ventricular fibrillation, there was an acceleration of ventricular responses in any local electrogram which preceded fragmentation and fractionation of that electrogram to local fibrillation. This acceleration was coincident with an acceleration of ventricular complexes on the surface electrocardiogram prior to the appearance of electrocardiographic ventricular fibrillation (Figure 2). The most common pattern of degeneration to local fibrillation was that of splintering of the local electrogram as shown in Figure 2. In no instance did all of the intracardiac ventricular electrograms degenerate into local fibrillation simultaneously. Occasionally two ventricular electrograms de-

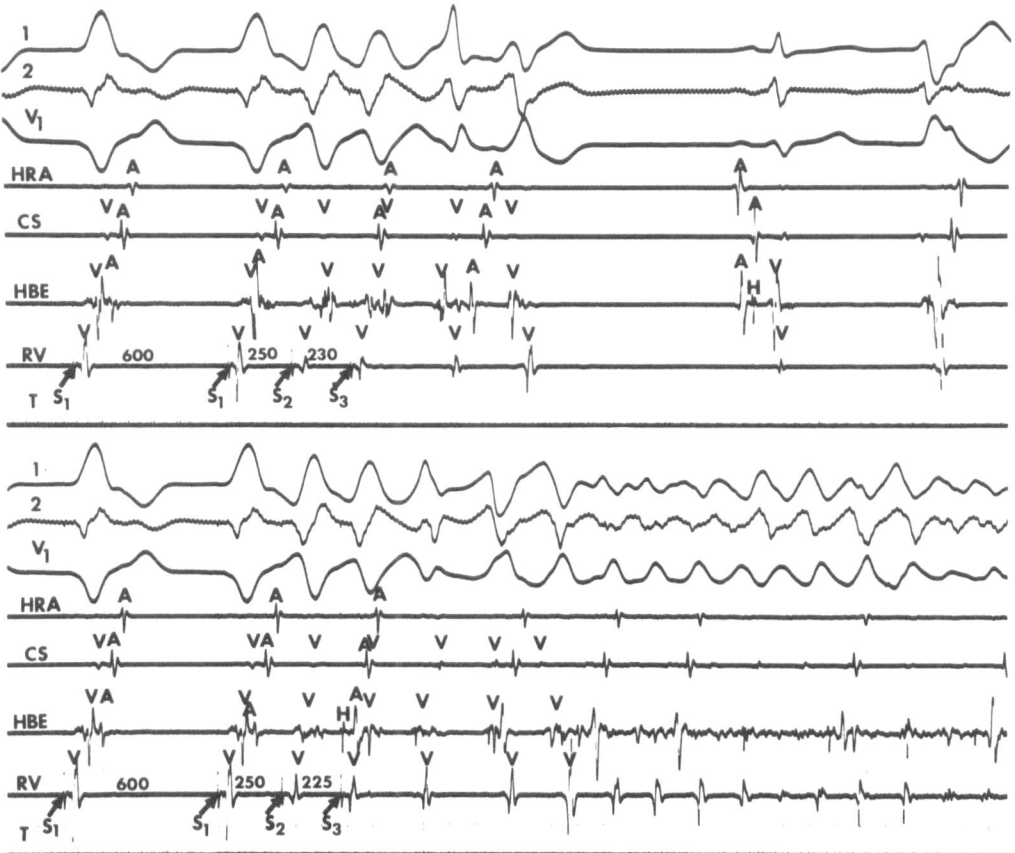

Figure 1. Initiation of ventricular fibrillation by ventricular extrastimuli. Both panels are organized from top to bottom as ECG leads 1, 2 and V$_1$ and electrograms from the high right atrium (HRA), coronary sinus (CS), AV junction at the His bundle recording site (HBE), and low right ventricular septum (RV). In both panels ventricular extrastimuli (S$_2$, S$_3$) are introduced following the eighth complex of a paced drive cycle (S$_1$ − S$_1$) of 600 msec. In the top panel, two ventricular extrastimuli (S$_2$, S$_3$) delivered at coupling intervals of 250 and 230 msec respectively result in two intraventricular reentrant complexes (IVR). In the bottom panel, when S$_3$ is delivered slightly earlier (S$_2$ − S$_3$ of 225 msec), ventricular fibrillation is initiated. The first two complexes resemble the IVR in the top panel. Note the development of local fibrillation in the HBE while the electrograms from the CS and RV remain relatively discrete.

generated simultaneously, but the electrograms from the remaining areas of the ventricles degenerated in varying periods of time. There was no pattern or sequence of development in local fibrillation; i.e., fibrillation did not appear to spread from right to left ventricle, or vice versa.

Ventricular fibrillation spontaneously developed by degeneration of a sustained ventricular tachycardia in 5 patients (Figure 3). In each of these cases there was acceleration of the ventricular tachycardia prior to degeneration to ventricular fibrillation. The fragmentation in local ventricular electrograms did not spread between contiguous areas, but occurred randomly (Figure 3). The acceleration of the surface and local electrograms prior to the development of fibrillation was analogous to that during fibrillation induced by ventricular extrastimuli. In the remaining patient ventricular fibrillation developed from a spontaneous ventricular premature depolarization in a patient with a long QT syndrome (QT 0.65–0.70 sec) secondary to procainamide. Five to 10 beat runs of poly-morphic ventricular tachycardia (torsade de pointes) occurred following late (> 600 msec) coupled ventricular premature depolarizations. When the ventricular premature de-polarizations occurred at the peak of the T wave (approximately 480 msec) a prolonged episode of ventricular fibrillation developed.

2.2. Mode of termination

Ventricular fibrillation spontaneously converted to sinus rhythm in 7 patients. In 5 cases spontaneous termination was preceded by reorganization of the electrograms with the

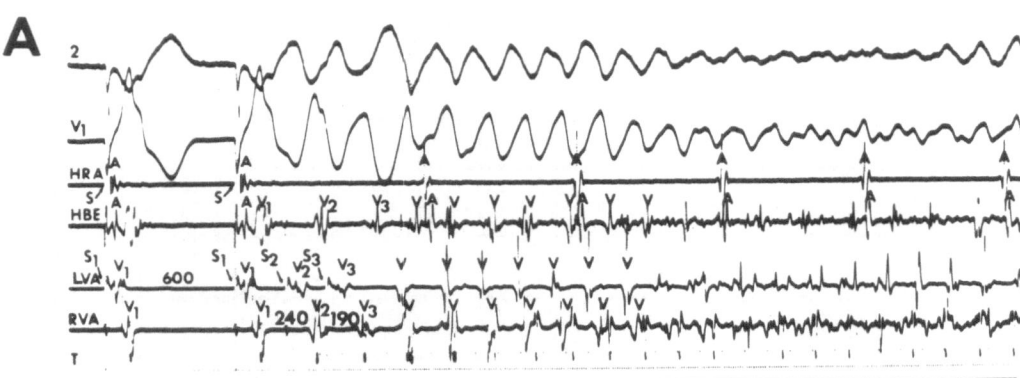

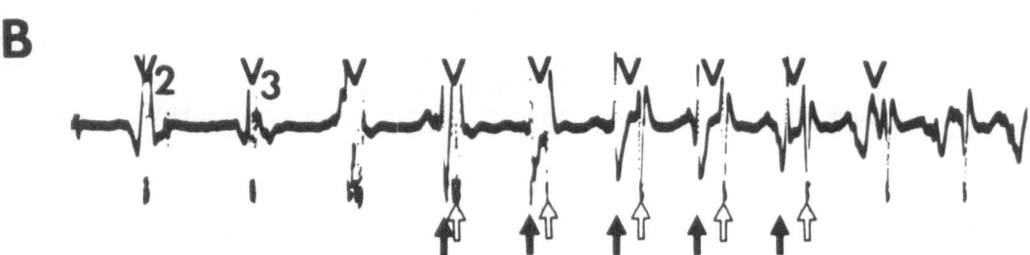

Figure 2. Pattern of development of local fibrillation. Panel A is arranged with ECG leads 2 and V$_1$ displayed with electrograms from the high right atrium (HRA), His bundle (HBE), left ventricular apex (LVA), and right ventric-ular apex (RVA). Two ventricular extrastimuli (S$_2$, S$_3$) are delivered during a basic drive cycle (S$_1$ − S$_1$) of 600 msec from the LVA resulting in ventricular fibrillation. The onset of ventricular fibrillation is heralded by acceleration of the ECG complexes. This acceleration is associated with the development of local fibrillation in the HBE and RVA. Local fibrillation develops first in the HBE, followed by the RVA, and finally the LVA. Characteristically local fibrillation develops with acceleration of the local ventricular electrograms which splinter and fragment into two or more discrete electrograms before degeneration into local fibrillation (panel B, a blowup of the RVA).

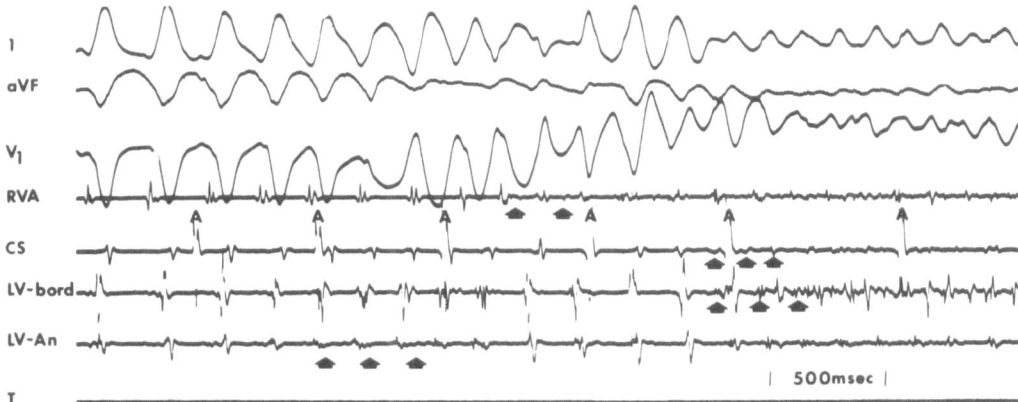

Figure 3. Initiation of ventricular fibrillation by spontaneous degeneration from ventricular tachycardia. ECG leads 1, aVF and V₁ are shown with electrograms from the right ventricular apex (RVA), coronary sinus (CS), and from the border and within a left ventricular aneurysm (LV-bord, LV-An). Ventricular tachycardia is present on the left. The onset of ventricular fibrillation (right-hand part of the panel) is heralded by progressive acceleration of the surface ECG complexes. This is associated with a random development of local fibrillation in the intracardiac recordings (broad arrows). Local fibrillation begins first in the LV-An and is followed by degeneration in the RVA. Finally, local fibrillation occurs in the LV-bord and CS. When all four intracardiac electrograms manifest local fibrillation, the surface electrocardiogram has become totally chaotic. (With permission of Josephson et al. Am. J. Cardiol. 44:623–631, 1979.)

appearance of discrete recordings (Figure 4). Usually this was accompanied by synchronization of the electrograms following which abrupt termination was observed. In 2 cases multiple short-lived episodes of ventricular fibrillation spontaneously terminated when the chaotic electrograms demonstrating local fibrillation suddenly coalesced and fused into broad, but discrete synchronized electrograms (Figure 5). In the remaining patients electric shock was required to terminate ventricular fibrillation. This was accomplished without neurologic or cardiac sequelae in all cases.

2.3. Relationship of QRS morphology to local ventricular electrograms

It was not possible to predict the nature of activity in the intracardiac recordings by analysis of the QRS morphology during ventricular fibrillation. While a totally disorganized QRS morphology demonstrating a grossly irregular, disorganized and continuously undulating waveform was usually associated with a larger number of intraventricular electrograms demonstrating local fibrillation (Figure 6), the number and type of fragmented electrograms at any point in time could not be predicted. Similar QRS morphologies were also associated with one or more organized and regular intracardiac electrograms (Figure 7).

3. DISCUSSION

Ventricular fibrillation has generally been considered to represent the result of chaotic,

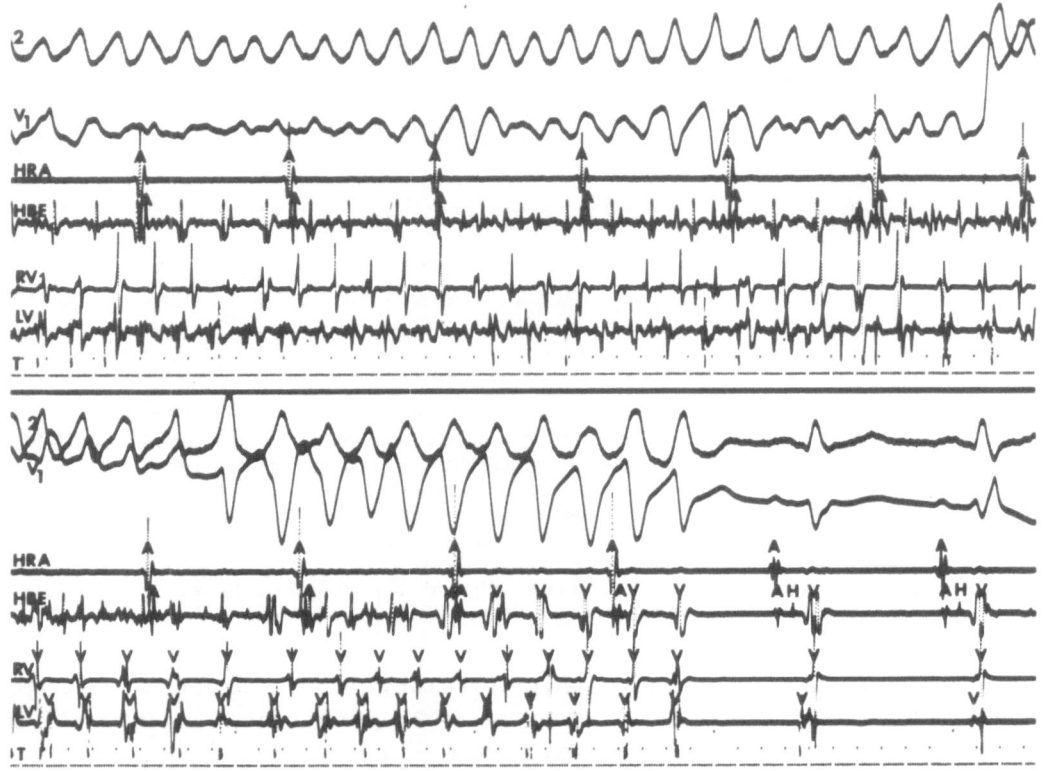

Figure 4. Spontaneous termination of ventricular fibrillation by progressive organization. Both panels are continuous and are arranged with surface leads 2 and V_1 and electrograms from the HRA, HBE, RV and LV. Ventricular
fibrillation is present as surface ECG in the top panel and is associated with local fibrillation in the HBE and LV
and intermittently in the RV. In the bottom panel, progressive reorganization of electrograms to discrete electrograms appears first in the RV, then in the LV, and finally in the HBE. When all three electrograms become discrete and synchronous, ventricular fibrillation abruptly terminates to sinus rhythm.

random, and asynchronous electrical activation of the ventricles. The mechanism of
ventricular fibrillation – either multiple repetitive reentrant wavelets, or rapid focal
discharges – is not yet established and it is likely that both play a role. Using intracardiac
recordings and programmed stimulation we have been able to analyze the characteristics
of onset and spontaneous termination of ventricular fibrillation and relate the surface
ECG morphology to intracardiac recordings.

3.1. Mode of initiation

Our data suggest that factors tending to shorten ventricular refractoriness are required
for the initiation of ventricular fibrillation. In all instances of ventricular fibrillation
induced by programmed stimulation, two ventricular extrastimuli were required, with the
second always at a shorter coupling interval than the first. Moreover, one or more ad-

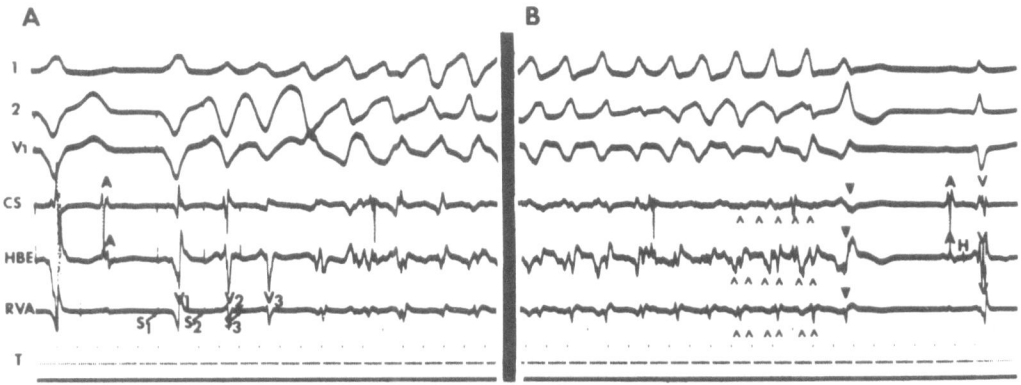

Figure 5. Spontaneous termination by abrupt synchronization. Panels A and B are arranged with surface leads 1, 2 and V_1 and electrograms from the coronary sinus (CS), His bundle (HBE), and right ventricular apex (RVA). In panel A, ventricular fibrillation is initiated by two ventricular extrastimuli (S_2, S_3). In panel B, spontaneous termination is shown. Note that spontaneous termination occurs when the chaotic electrograms (open arrowheads) abruptly coalesce to broad but discrete and synchronous electrograms. (With permission of Josephson et al. Am. J. Cardiol. 44:623–631, 1979.)

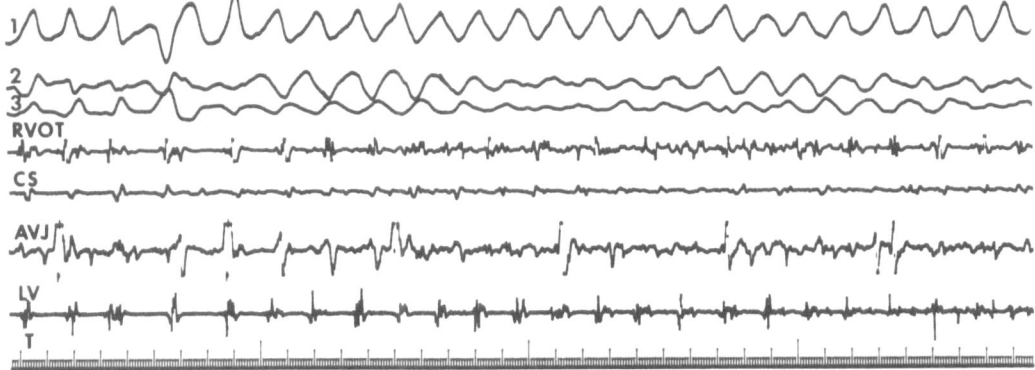

Figure 6. Relationship of surface ECG to intracardiac recordings. Leads 1, 2 and 3 are shown with electrograms from the right ventricular outflow tract (RVOT), coronary sinus (CS), atrioventricular junction (AVJ), and the left ventricle (LV). During ventricular fibrillation on the surface ECG, local fibrillation is present in all electrograms, although intermittent discrete recordings are observed in the RVOT, CS and LV.

ditional repetitive ventricular responses were frequently observed before degeneration to ventricular fibrillation in both the local ventricular electrograms and the surface electrocardiogram.

Our observations are consonant with experimental studies in animals and man which demonstrate that both ventricular premature depolarizations and ventricular pacing shorten ventricular refractoriness (13, 14) and that this was requisite for the development of fibrillation. Since at least two ventricular extrastimuli of increasing prematurity were always required to initiate ventricular fibrillation and since acceleration of local ventricular responses was required in the majority of instances, we believe that each sequential ventric-

Table 2. Mode of initiation and termination of ventricular fibrillation.

Patient	Mode of Initiation			Mode of Termination	
	2 VPD	Spontaneous VPD	Spontaneous Degeneration from VT	Spontaneous	DC Shock
1	+			+	
2	+				+
3	+				+
4	+				+
5	+*				+
6			+**		+
7	+			+	+
8	+			+	
9	+			+	
10	+				+
11	+				+
12			+		+
13			+		+
14			+**		+
15		+		+	
16	+			+	
17			+		+
18	+			+	+
19	+				+
20	+				+
21			+		+
22	+				+

VPD– ventricular premature depolarization
VT   – ventricular tachycardia
*   – 2 VPDs delivered during VT
**   – VF also induced by 2 VPDs delivered during VT

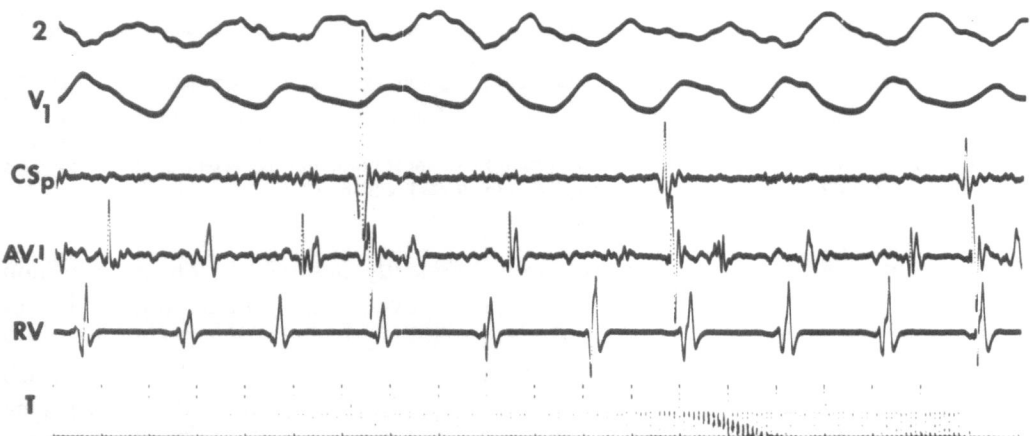

Figure 7. Discrete intracardiac recordings associated with ventricular fibrillation. Leads 2 and V_1 are shown with proximal coronary sinus (CS_p), atrioventricular junction (AVJ), and right ventricle (RV) electrograms. During ventricular fibrillation, local fibrillation is seen in the CS_p and AVJ. However, the electrogram in the RV remains discrete and orderly throughout. T = time lines.

ular depolarization produced progressive shortening of ventricular refractoriness and increased the inhomogeneity of recovery until fibrillation ensued.

Moreover, the development of local fibrillation was characterized by fractionation in the local electrogram during acceleration. Experimental studies suggest that such fragmentation represents slowing and fractionation of activation wavefronts (15, 16) which together with shortened refractoriness would predispose to reentry. Combined shortened refractoriness and slowed conduction are the hallmarks of reentry.

The second mode of initiation of ventricular fibrillation was spontaneous degeneration of ventricular tachycardia. Analogous to ventricular fibrillation induced by premature stimuli, acceleration of the ventricular tachycardia always preceded disorganization to ventricular fibrillation. This pattern is analogous to Type B pattern described by Watanabe and Dreifus (17) as well as by Harris (4). Ventricular fibrillation induced in this manner was usually preceded by a change in the relationship of electrograms to each other with progressive fractionation in one or more areas until fibrillation ensued. Local fibrillation did not occur simultaneously in all areas and did not appear to spread from one fibrillating area to the remainder of the heart, but appeared to arise in different areas of the heart in random sequence and then gradually enveloped the entire heart. This differs from experimental ventricular fibrillation induced by a strong current (3) or ischemia (4) during which the acceleration of responses to ventricular fibrillation began at either the site of stimulation or ischemia and spread from there to the remainder of the heart. These phenomena were also observed during fibrillation induced by double ventricular stimuli during which local fibrillation appeared to spread randomly and in all but two instances initially occurred at a site distant to the site of stimulation.

These data do suggest that a generalized state of ventricular fibrillation throughout the heart results from independent areas degenerating into ventricular fibrillation which eventually engulf the entire heart in the fibrillatory process. A recent experimental model of fibrillation using over 100 simultaneous mapping electrogram sites also demonstrated that fibrillation can in fact develop in areas on the periphery of the initial wavefront (18). These data are to be distinguished from the spread of fibrillation from the initially fibrillating area to the adjacent areas, the mechanism observed by Moe (3) and Harris (4) in their experimental models. The apparent requirement of shortened ventricular refractoriness, fractionation, and desynchronization of local electrograms prior to the development of local fibrillation is most consistent with the reentrant wavelet theory of its genesis (19).

3.2. Maintenance and termination of ventricular fibrillation

Prior workers have demonstrated that the maintenance of ventricular fibrillation requires a large mass of tissue with an irregularly shortened ventricular refractory period and areas of slow conduction and local block which allow continued reexcitation (18, 19, 20). According to the multiple wavelet theory of continued reexcitation (18, 19) the more wavelets present the more likely the persistence of fibrillation and the less likely for collision and fusion resulting in extinguishing of the arrhythmia. Progressive block in large areas or marked prolongation of ventricular refractoriness caused by pharmacologic agents or metabolic alterations can result in progressive organization of these fragmented electrograms and termination of the arryhthmia (5, 6, 19, 20). In 5 of the 7 cases in which we observed spontaneous termination of ventricular fibrillation reorganization to discrete electrograms occurred prior to termination. This observation is most compatible with the multiple wavelet theory of ventricular fibrillation and suggests that the maintenance of the arrhythmia is not dependent upon a rapidly firing focus. Progressive organization results from the inability of multiple areas to be sequentially reexcited, therefore reducing the number of wavelets. When the number of wavelets is reduced below a critical number, they can collide and extinguish the arrhythmia. Despite the fact that large areas of fibrillation (i.e., electrograms from both right and left ventricles) were observed in 5 of the 7 patients in whom spontaneous defibrillation occurred, reorganization was always observed prior to termination. In the remaining 2 patients in whom spontaneous conversion occurred, sudden fusion and apparent coalescence of fractionated electrograms resulted in synchronization and sudden termination. Of the 7 patients in whom spontaneous defibrillation occurred, 5 had organic heart disease and 2 had no heart disease documented by catheterization. These observations suggest that the mass of muscle required to maintain fibrillation is dependent upon the electrophysiologic properties; i.e., a larger mass is required if conduction is not slow enough and/or refractoriness is not short enough to allow reexcitation. Thus, in man we believe the cardiac mass is not a primary prerequisite to the development of ventricular fibrillation. In experimental models using small animal hearts mass may play a more critical role than it does in the larger human heart. It is the ability to be continually reexcited that will determine how much mass is required. These data are most consistent with reentry and are much less compatible with enhanced automaticity as the mechanism for sustained ventricular fibrillation.

3.3. Relationship of QRS morphology of ventricular electrograms to ventricular fibrillation

Our data suggest that the pattern of excitation of the heart during ventricular fibrillation cannot be determined from the surface electrocardiogram. Several areas of the heart could demonstrate organized rapid excitation during ventricular fibrillation while in other cases the entire heart may be fibrillating and irregularly activated. The continuous undulating baseline characteristic of ventricular fibrillation is merely the expression of activation of some part of the ventricles throughout the cardiac cycle. Thus, the greater the degree of desynchronization of activation, the more irregular and undulating the QRS morphology, despite the fact that each of the areas activated could be activated by regular activity. This situation is analogous to that of impure atrial flutter during which parts of the atrium manifest organized activity while other areas demonstrate localized atrial fibrillation.

An explanation of this phenomenon could be that areas with more organized activity had longer refractory periods which prevented reexcitation despite slowed conduction, thereby preventing the formation of small wavelets. Further slowing of conduction with shortening refractoriness in these areas could result in the development of fibrillation, but unless these two electrophysiologic properties were appropriate, regular activity will continue. The regular or discrete activity in these areas could be the result of activation from isolated areas of fibrillation with only those areas with shortened refractoriness manifesting continuous fractionated activity. Supporting this concept is the fact that factors which lengthen refractoriness, such as antiarrhythmic agents or potassium chloride, tend to regularize local fibrillation into discrete activity.

4. CONCLUSIONS

The use of intracardiac recordings has allowed us to describe patterns in the development and termination of ventricular fibrillation and relate these intracardiac recordings to the surface electrocardiogram. Although our observations are limited by the number of recording sites, they are most compatible with the multiple reentrant wavelet theory of ventricular fibrillation. The development of local fibrillation appears dependent upon factors which shorten refractoriness and slow conduction, an observation which argues against automaticity and favors reentry as the method for sustaining arrhythmia. Our data do not exclude the role of triggered automaticity as the cause for the early initiating complexes, although reentry has been demonstrated to cause even these responses in the chronically infarcted canine model (15, 16). Although more recording sites would be necessary to more accurately delineate the mechanism responsible for initiation, maintenance and termination of ventricular fibrillation, it is unlikely that this can be accomplished in man due to the limitation of catheters that can be positioned in the heart without risk to the patient. These data will have to come from experimental models or intraoperative human studies which record multiple simultaneous electrograms as currently being developed by Harumi et al. (18).

ACKNOWLEDGMENTS

This work was supported in part by grants from the American Heart Association, South-eastern Pennsylvania Chapter and National Heart, Lung and Blood Institute.

While the work was performed Dr. Josephson was recipient of a Research Carter Development Award, National Heart, Lung and Blood Institute (1 KO4 H L00361-01), Dr. Spielman was recipient of NIH Institutional Training Grant IT 32, HL 07346-01, Dr. Greenspan was recipient of NIH Grant 1 F 32 HL05816.01 and Dr. Horowitz recipient of a Career Development Investigatorship, American Heart Association, Southeastern Pennsylvania Chapter and Young Investigator Award, National Heart, Lung and Blood Institute Number 1 R 23 HL 21291-01.

REFERENCES

1. Wiggers CJ: The mechanism and nature of ventricular fibrillation. Am Heart J 20:399–412, 1940.
2. Wiggers CJ, Wegria R: Ventricular fibrillation due to single, localized induction and condenser shocks applied during the vulnerable phase of ventricular systole. Am J Physiol 128:500–505, 1940.
3. Moe GK, Harris AS, Wiggers CJ: Analysis of the initiation of fibrillation by electrographic studies. Am J Physiol 134:473–492, 1941.
4. Harris AS, Rojas AG: The initiation of ventricular fibrillation due to coronary occlusion. Exper Med Surg 1:105–122, 1943.
5. Zipes DP: Electrophysiological mechanisms involved in ventricular fibrillation. Circulation 52 (suppl III): 120–130, 1975.
6. Surawicz B: Ventricular fibrillation. Am J Cardiol 28:268–287, 1971.
7. Scherf D: The mechanism of flutter and fibrillation. Am Heart J 71:273–280, 1966.
8. Sano T, Sawanobori T: Mechanism initiating ventricular fibrillation demonstrated in cultured ventricular muscle tissue. Circ Res 26:201–210, 1970.
9. Josephson ME, Horowitz LN, Farshidi A, Kastor JA: Recurrent sustained ventricular tachycardia. 1. Mechanisms. Circulation 57:431–439, 1978.
10. Spielman SR, Farshidi A, Horowitz LN, Josephson ME: Ventricular fibrillation during programmed ventricular stimulation – Incidence and significance. Am J Cardiol 42:913–918, 1978.
11. Roberts R, Ambos HD, Loh CW, Sobel BE: Initiation of repetitive ventricular depolarizations by relatively late premature complexes in patients with acute myocardial infarction. Am J Cardiol 41:678–683, 1978.
12. El-Sherif N, Myerburg RJ, Scherlag BJ, Befeler B, Aranda JM, Castellanos A, Lazzara R: Electrocardiographic antecedents of primary ventricular fibrillation. Value of the R on T phenomenon in myocardial infarction. Br Heart J 38:415–422, 1976.
13. Guss SB, Kastor JA, Josephson ME, Scharf DL: Human ventricular refractoriness. Effects of cycle length, pacing site and atropine. Circulation 53:450–455, 1976.
14. Spear JF, Moore EN, Horowitz LN: Effect of current pulses delivered during the ventricular vulnerable period upon the ventricular fibrillation threshold. Am J Cardiol 32:814–822, 1973.
15. El-Sherif N, Scherlag BJ, Lazzara R, Hope RR: Reentrant ventricular arrhythmias in the late myocardial infarction period. 1. Conduction characteristics in the infarction zone. Circulation 55:686–702, 1977.
16. El-Sherif N, Hope RR, Scherlag BJ, Lazzara R: Reentrant ventricular arrhythmias in the last myocardial infarction period. 2. Patterns of initiation and termination of reentry. Circulation 55:702–719, 1977.
17. Watanabe Y, Dreifus LS: Mechanisms of ventricular fibrillation. Jap Heart J 7:110–120, 1966.
18. Harumi K, Wyatt R, Lux R, Abildskov JA, Smith CR: Initiating mechanisms of ventricular fibrillation. Am J Cardiol 43:374, 1979.
19. Moe GK: On the multiple wavelet hypotheses of atrial fibrillation. Arch Int Pharmacodyn 140:183–188, 1962.
20. Garrey WE: The nature of fibrillatory contraction of the heart. Its relation to tissue mass and form. Am J Physiol 33:397, 1914.

2.8. UNUSUAL FORMS OF SEVERE VENTRICULAR TACHYARRHYTHMIAS: THEIR RELATIONSHIPS WITH THE QT INTERVAL AND THE VAGO-SYMPATHETIC BALANCE

PH. COUMEL, J.F. LECLERCQ, M. ROSENGARTEN, P. ATTUEL and D. MILOSEVIC

1. DEFINITION

In this paper, we shall designate as "unusual", some ventricular tachyarrhythmias which are rare, are not related to any definite cardiac disease, show bizarre electrocardiographic patterns, have an unpredictable evolution (including the risk of sudden death) and have no clear therapy. They represent a difficult problem.

One of the major difficulties we face is the lack of a precise definition (1). The term "ventricular tachyarrhythmias" covers all aspects of rapid heart action originating from the ventricle. The distinction between ventricular tachycardia and fibrillation is based upon the apparently synchronized or desynchronized pattern of ventricular activity in the surface electrocardiogram. However, in many tracings the distinction between ventricular tachycardia or fibrillation can be difficult. Let us consider the 6 examples of the right panel of Figure 1. The term ventricular tachycardia is applicable to strips 3 and 4 if we accept the possibility for a ventricular tachycardia to be slightly irregular. The diagnosis of ventricular fibrillation should be rejected for the others, because, although multiform and irregular activity is present, there is no electrical desynchronisation or complete loss of mechanical activity of the heart leading to death. In addition, self termination of the arrhythmia is usually not included in the definition of ventricular fibrillation. The term ventricular flutter does not apply either because the tracing is not sinusoidal. The denomination "torsade de pointes" (2, 3) is acceptable for tracings 5 and 6 since the two main characteristics are clearly present: there is a progressive QRS axis shift during the paroxysm, and the first beat of the tachycardia has a long coupling interval. Tracing 1 also shows a changing QRS axis but the coupling interval of the first beat is extremely short: this rhythm disorder does not belong to any of the classical categories of ventricular tachyarrhythmias. As to strip 2, it may be labelled as an irregular and multiform ventricular tachycardia.

Clear definition of phenomena often represents the first step in the progress of our knowledge. The lack of precision we have underlined is apparent in many publications related to ventricular tachyarrhythmias which did not help our understanding of their mechanisms.

Our challenge is to examine whether the very different patterns of ventricular tachyarrhythmias shown in the right panel of Figure 1 as well as the variable coupling interval of the corresponding isolated extrasystoles (seen on the left panel) might in fact correspond to different expressions of an unique electrophysiological mechanism. This pos-

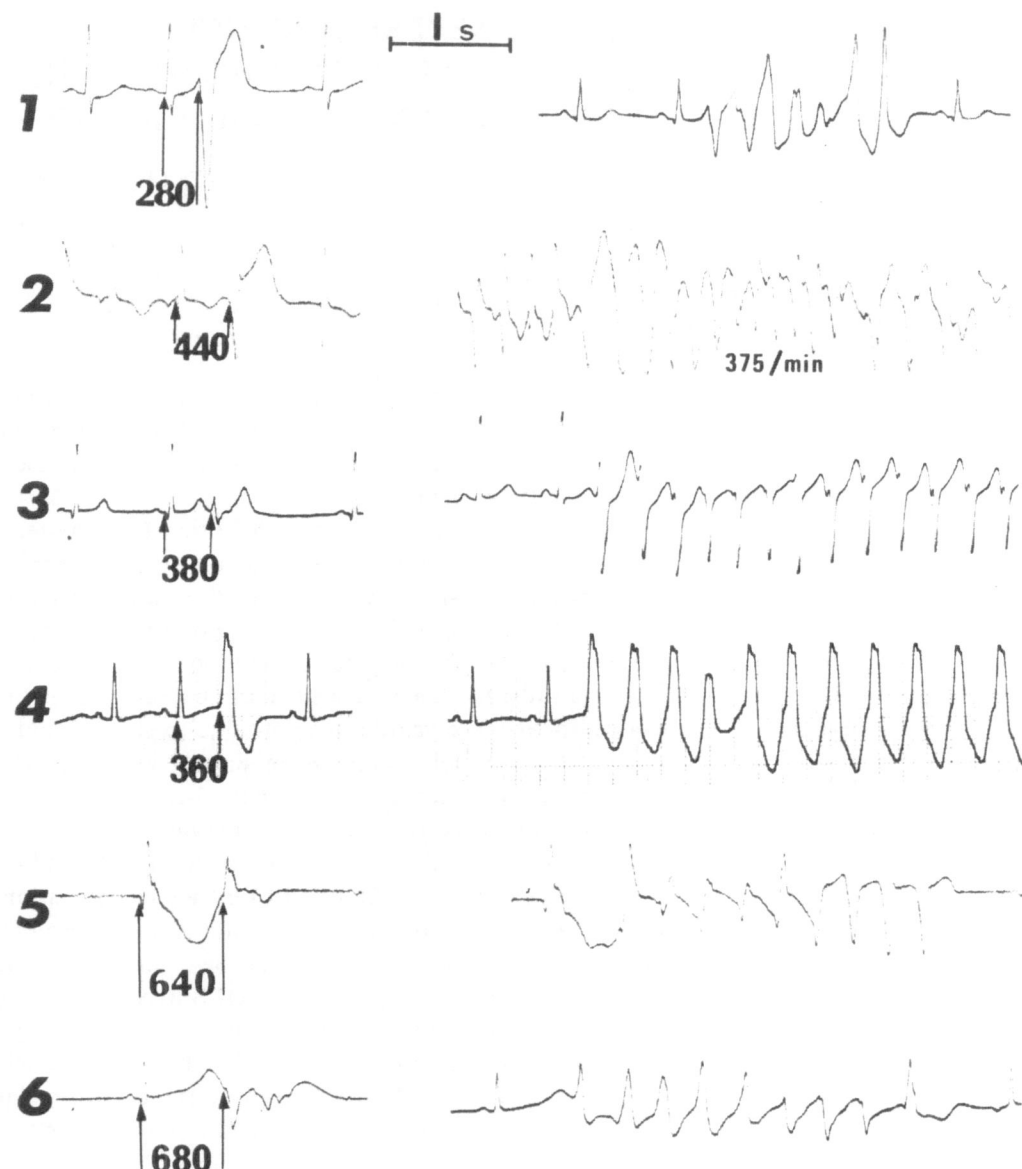

Figure 1. Electrocardiographic tracings of the 6 reported cases of unusual ventricular tachycardia. Numbers 1 to 6 refer to the cases described in the text. On the left, are shown, for each case, examples of isolated extrasystoles, with the most frequently observed coupling interval (in milliseconds); on the right, electrocardiographic tracings during tachycardia.

sibility will be discussed below. Two characteristics common to these cases should be noted from the start. In all instances, the arrhythmia was apparently idiopathic and most probably congenital, and was predominantly if not exclusively under the influence of the autonomic nervous system.

It has been accepted for a long time that, at ventricular level, the electrophysiological properties of the myocardium are influenced by the sympathetic drive only. Recently, however, the possible role of the vagus nerve provoked an increasing interest (4) because of its indirect action on cardiac vulnerability by antagonizing augmented sympathetic tone. Muscarinic stimulation inhibits the release of norepinephrine from sympathetic nerve endings and attenuates the response to catecholamines at receptor sites. Afferent vagal activity also exerts a tonic inhibition of sympathetic neural discharge. The presence at ventricular level of parasympathetic as well as sympathetic nerves seems well established; they form a "network" around the Purkinje cells (5). There is presently no doubt that the autonomic nervous system influence on the ventricles is not exclusively sympathetic but depends on a vagosympathetic balance as well. Clinicians are increasingly concerned by these problems which may have practical diagnostic and therapeutical implications in the interpretation of the Holter monitoring and of the action of stimulating and blocking agents of the vagal and sympathetic systems.

2. REPORT OF CASES

2.1. Case 1

This 45-year-old patient, whose history was previously reported (6) suffered three syncopal attacks within two weeks. He had runs of tachycardia which were characterized by a "torsade de pointes"-like pattern and especially by the unusually short coupling interval of the first beat of tachycardia (no. 1, Figure 1; Figure 2). The arrhythmia was particularly

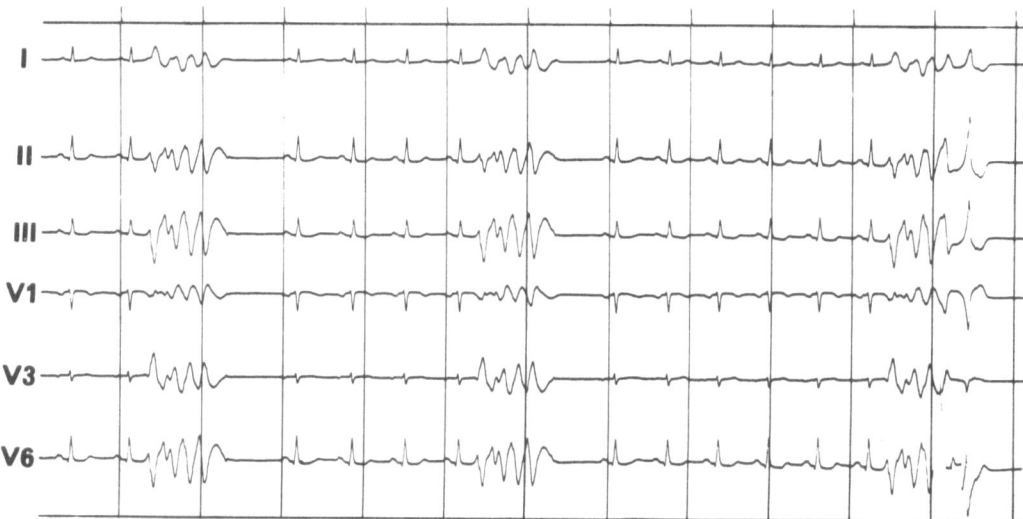

Figure 2. Case 1. Torsade de pointes-like tachyarrhythmia with a short coupling interval of the first beat, which makes it quite different from what is seen in Cases 5 and 6.

refractory to usual antiarrhythmic agents, including propranolol and pindolol. Yet a sympathetic influence was suggested by the longer duration of the episodes during the day as compared to the night. During sleep, only isolated ectopic beats or couplets were recorded. Awaking the patient was a good way to reinitiate the paroxysms.

Attempts to influence the vago-sympathetic balance gave rather paradoxical results (7). An isoprenaline infusion was followed by the disappearance of all extrasystolic activity even though the cardiac rate remained constant. On the other hand, the injection of

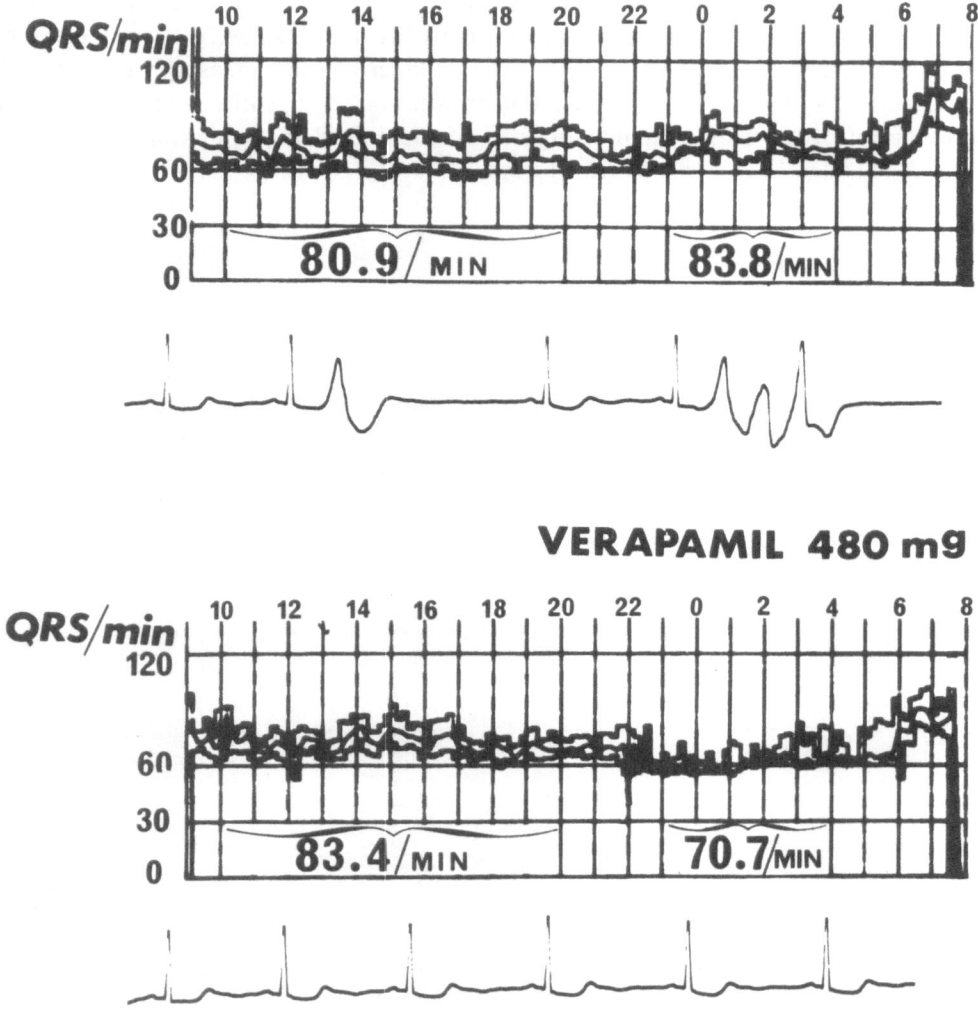

Figure 3. Case 1. Day and night variations in sinus rate. The mean cardiac rate (middle curve) is shown together with the curves of maximal and minimal rates (calculated from 16 consecutive beats during every 10 minute period). The diurnal rate is averaged from 10 consecutive hours, and the nocturnal rate from 5 consecutive hours. Surprisingly, the former is lower than the latter, in the control Holter monitoring (upper diagram). The day to night relationship is normalised by verapamil (lower diagram).

atropine (1) lengthened the duration of the paroxysms up to 8 or 10 beats instead of 2 at the time of the electrophysiologic study.

Surprisingly, verapamil administered intravenously resulted in perfect control of the arrhythmia. This was also obtained by the long term oral treatment during a follow-up of 3 years: this observation is certainly more than coincidental because it was indirectly confirmed by sudden death in an identical patient shortly after discontinuing the same treatment. The mechanism of action of verapamil in this case deserves to be discussed. It suggests, of course, a role of the slow calcium channel in the mechanism of the arrhythmia. However, the reversibility by atropin of the effects of verapamil on the sinus and A-V nodes suggests that verapamil has a vagotonic effect. Figure 3 indicates that the sinus rate of our patient showed a very strange behaviour in the control Holter monitoring (upper panel): the daytime cardiac rate (calculated from 10 consecutive hours: 80.9 min) was lower than the night-time rate (calculated from 5 consecutive hours: 83.8 min). In addition to controlling the ventricular arrhythmia, verapamil was also responsible for the inversion of this abnormal day to night variation (lower panel).

We have investigated (Figure 4) the effect of verapamil on sinus rate in 24 normal subjects. During the control period, they showed a mean rate of 84.04/min $\pm$ 2.58 (S.E.M.) during the day and of 68.04 $\pm$ 2.26 during the night as compared to 78.99 $\pm$ 2.49 ($p < 0.05$) and 62.24 $\pm$ 1.99 ($p < 0.01$) respectively after verapamil treatment. The cardiac rate of our patient was clearly influenced by the treatment, particularly during the night, but it still remained outside the range of treated normal subjects.

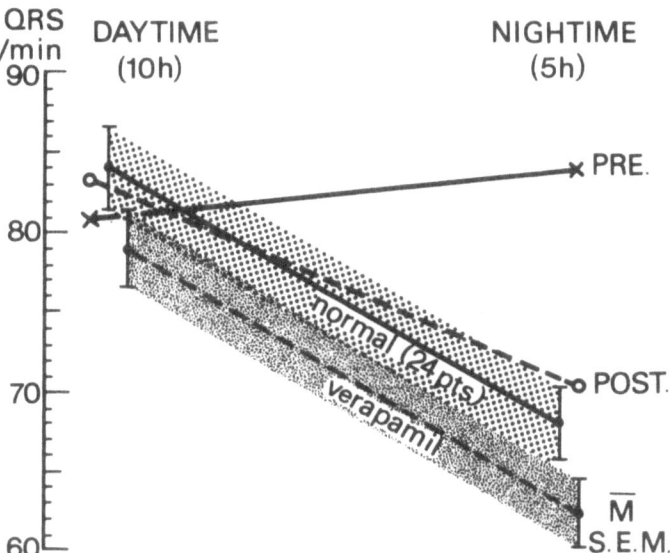

Figure 4. Effects of verapamil on diurnal and nocturnal sinus rate in 24 normal patients as compared to Case 1. The effect of verapamil is much less marked in Case 1 than in control patients. In Case 1, verapamil treatment does not affect the rate during day time, but lowers it during the night without bringing it within the range of the verapamil treated normal patients.

These observations support the hypothesis that the arrhythmia, instead of being related to an increased sympathetic drive, might be due to a low parasympathetic drive. Enforcement of the latter could explain the role of verapamil and also why beta-blocking agents had no effect.

2.2. Case 2

Panel 2 of Figure 1 and Figure 5 were obtained in a 9 year old girl whose history was previously reported as Case 3 of reference (8). The latter study reported four cases of severe catecholamine-induced ventricular arrhythmias in children. The characteristics of this syndrome are remarkably constant in the 14 cases published in the literature. The family history is the only inconstant feature of this syndrome which predominates in girls who have otherwise normal hearts. According to the severity of the disease, the first syncopal attack occurs between the age of 3 to 14 and the evolution is apparently fatal before the age of 20. The arrhythmia is generally misdiagnosed as a neurological disease for months

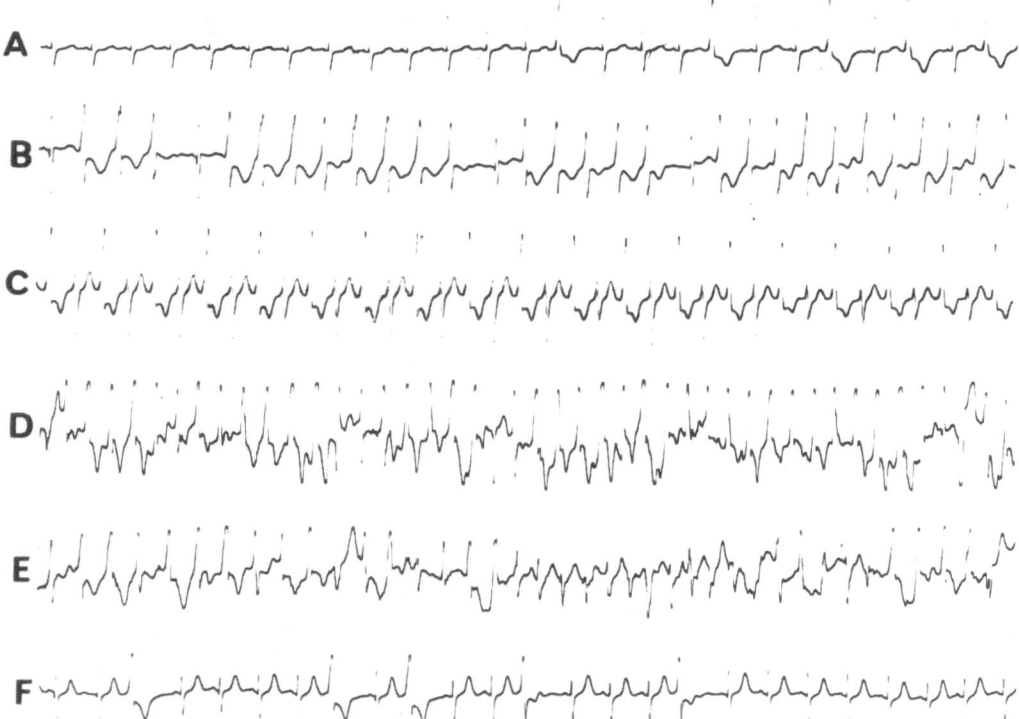

Figure 5. Case 2. Catecholamine-induced ventricular tachycardia in a child. Strips A to F are recorded by the Holter monitoring technique during normal activity including moderate exercise. In panel A, the sinus rate increases progressively followed by an increase in isolated ventricular extrasystoles. In B, salvos of tachycardia appear, followed in C by a typical bidirectional tachycardia. In D and F, the tachycardia is faster and becomes multiform. The ectopic activity progressively disappears in F when the effort is discontinued.

or years until a clear relationship with effort or emotion, or stress is established. Then, it is easy to record many attacks of varying severity during normal daytime activity or following the administration of small amounts of isoprenaline. These episodes are surprisingly well tolerated unless they culminate into an arrhythmia which looks like ventricular fibrillation, without ever becoming totally chaotic and completely disorganised. A typical and constant sequence is observed during the attacks and consists of 1) sinus tachycardia, 2) AV junctional tachycardia, 3) ventricular extrasystoles arranged in quadri, tri and bigeminy with progressive shortening of coupling intervals, 4) bidirectional tachycardia, multiform irregular ventricular tachycardia, and 5) the progressive disappearance of these phenomena in the reverse order, with inconstant changes of repolarisation at the end of the episodes.

A particular sensitivity of junctional and ventricular pacemakers, rather than an increased release of catecholamines seems to be the cause of these rhythm disorders. This is in agreement with a favourable effect of treatment with beta-blocking agents. Amiodarone which has a beta-adrenergic lessening action is also known to be effective and can be added in refractory cases. The resistance to all other antiarrhythmic drugs is not surprising.

2.3. Case 3

Panel 3 of Figure 1, and Figures 6 and 7 were recorded in a 35-year-old woman. She had had short runs of palpitations for several years with or without dizziness related to the magnitude of stress she was undergoing. Exercise was well tolerated if it was not excessive, but psychological stresses were more likely triggering circumstances. Most antiarrhythmic drugs had been given without any beneficial effects; but intensive beta-blocking treatment has not been tried. Tracings A and B, Figure 6, recorded at rest show isolated ventricular extrasystoles, couplets or a maximum of three successive ectopic beats. During normal activity, numerous attacks of slightly irregular and multiform ventricular tachycardia at rates up to 250/min were recorded during Holter monitoring (tracings C to F, Figure 6). Figure 7 shows the quantitative analysis of the 24-hour tapes recorded during the first two days of hospitalization. During the first day (on the left), the patient was not accustomed to the hospital premises; she had to undergo several examinations (X-ray, laboratory, etc.) and numerous attacks were present during the day, with a mean number of extrasystoles of 16/min. In contrast, at night, their number decreased dramatically with no runs of tachycardia. The second day of Holter monitoring is analyzed on the right panel: the patient was completely at rest; there was no tachycardia and curiously the mean number of extrasystoles was lowered to about 8/min, equally distributed over the whole day. Propranolol treatment at a daily dosage of 240 mg resulted in good control of the tachycardia, with lowering of the number of extrasystoles to an average of 4/min.

It was not possible to determine whether the arrhythmia had been present for a long time, and particularly since childhood. Our impression is that it was possibly the case. Mild forms of catecholamine-induced ventricular tachycardia similar to those we have described in children can very well remain undetected for long periods of time if they do not produce syncope. Indeed, the younger the patient, the better the tolerance. Apparently

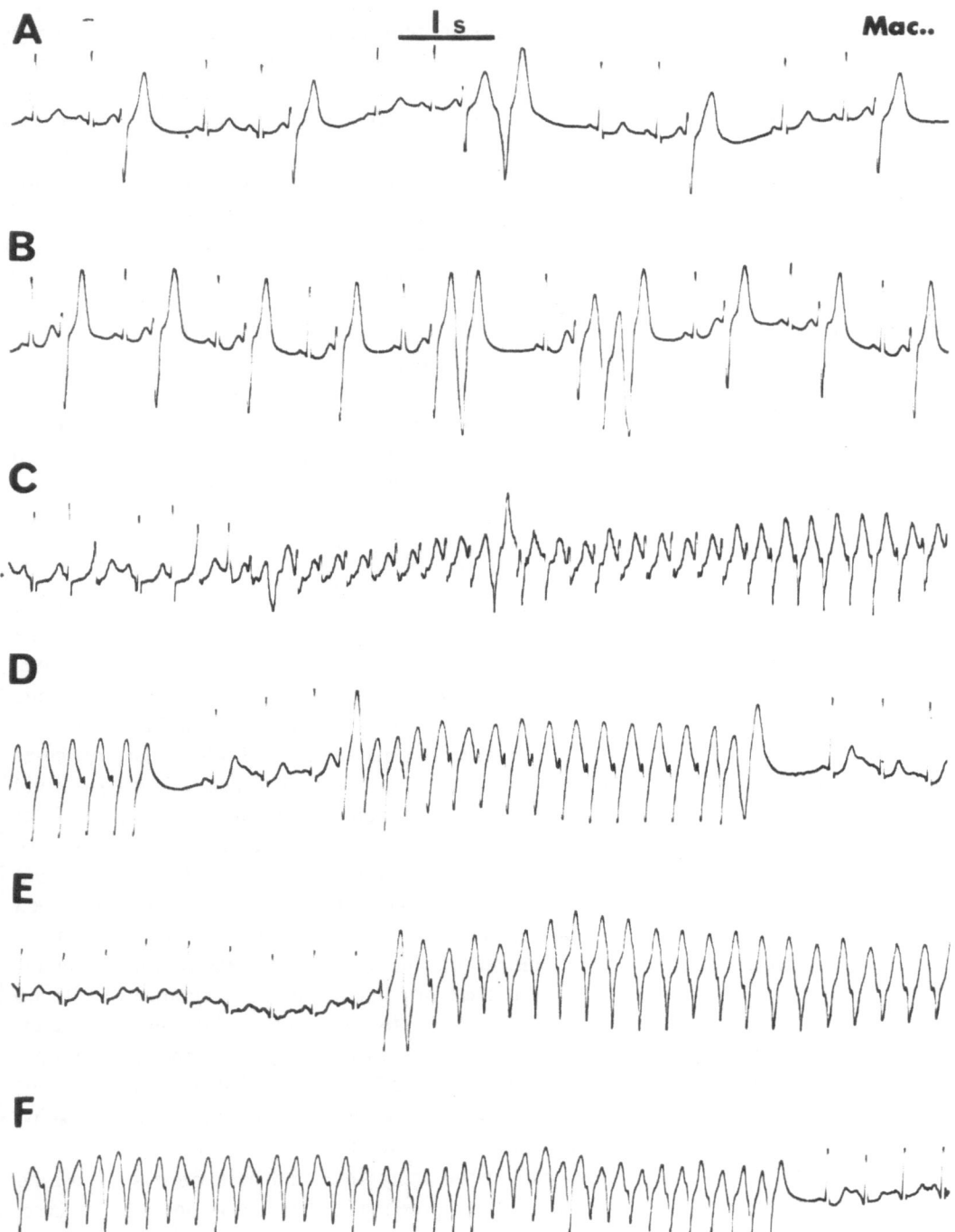

Figure 6. Case 3. Catecholamine-related tachyarrhythmia in an adult. Tracings A and B are recorded at rest; tracings C to F are recorded during normal activity. Although the rate sometimes exceeds 250/min, the tachycardia is only responsible for palpitations and dizziness. Note, in C, the tendency to irregularity and a multiform pattern of the ventricular activity making this case resemble Case 2.

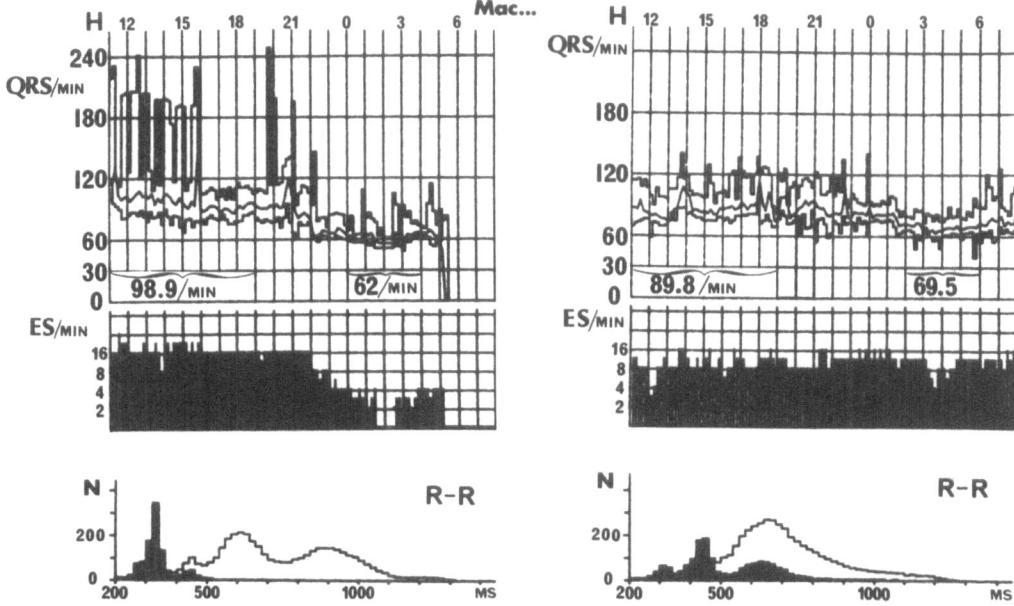

Figure 7. Case 3. Computerized analysis of two days of Holter monitoring. The left panel corresponds to the first day of hospitalization during which the patient underwent the various medical examinations. The right panel corresponds to the second day without treatment, but during which the patient was left completely at rest. The upper diagram in each panel represents the mean cardiac frequency curve accompanied by the curves of maximal and minimal rates (calculated from 16 consecutive beats) during each of the six periods of 10 minutes analyzed every hour. The middle diagram shows the number of isolated extrasystoles or couplets per minute, and their distribution at day time and at night. The lower diagram is the R–R interval histogram where the cycle length is indicated in milliseconds, and the number of enlarged (solid) or narrow (open) beats is averaged to one hour for the entire tracing (see text for discussion)

severe tachycardias may induce no symptoms of palpitations, especially if the rhythm is only slightly irregular.

An asymptomatic form of mitral valve prolapse was detected in this patient by echocardiographic examination. We will not discuss here the causal or coincidental relationship between the arrhythmia and the valvular abnormality: let us mention that a hyperadrenergic state has recently been demonstrated (9) in symptomatic patients with mitral valve prolapse.

In the three preceding cases, the ventricular arrhythmias were exclusively under the influence of the vago-sympathetic balance, but apparently there was no relationship between the tachycardia and the length of the QT interval. The repolarisation phase is clearly involved in cases 5 and 6. Patient 4 is an example where this relationship was not obvious at first glance.

2.4. Case 4

This 16-year-old patient had a 2 year history of paroxysmal ventricular tachycardia occurring at a rate of about one attack per month. In Figure 8, the basic tracing is normal,

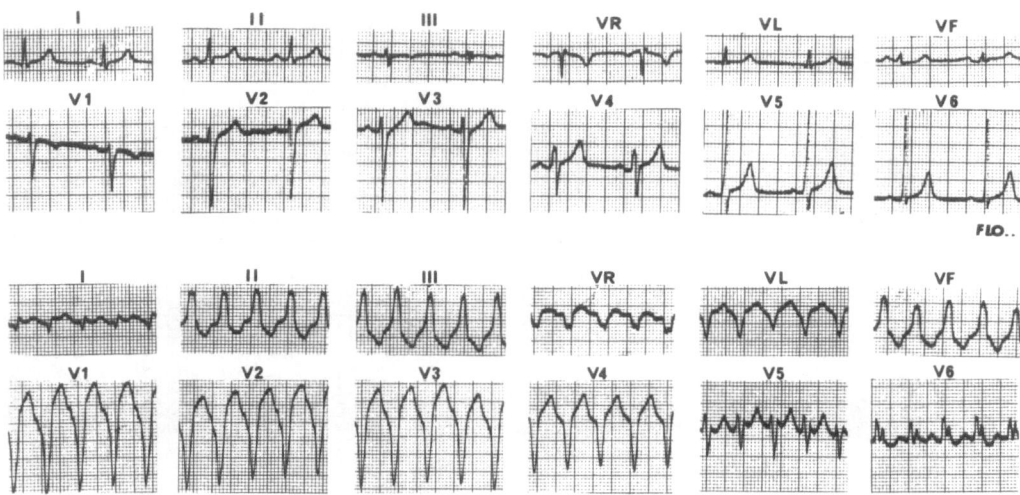

Figure 8. Case 4. "Benign" paroxysmal ventricular tachycardia. The upper panel shows the normal basic tracing, and the lower panel, the ventricular tachycardia.

particularly as far as the QT interval is concerned. Otherwise, the ventricular tachycardia shows a vertical axis, a left bundle branch block pattern and a regular rate of 170/min. What is important in this patient is the recording of the mode of onset of tachycardia (Figure 9). Although the patient's activity was limited because he was hospitalized, unusual variations in sinus rate were present, ranging from 60 to 140/min. The most surprising phenomenon was the absence of adaptation of the QT interval during these variations. In strip A, recorded shortly after 12.30 a.m., the QT interval is normal for the rate. In strips B to D, while the rate progressively increases (without extrasystoles), the QT interval remains unchanged so that the T wave progressively collides with the subsequent P. This phenomenon was never present during numerous previous recordings. After 1.30 p.m., the sinus rate decreases; the onset of tachycardia is immediately preceded by a rapid sinus acceleration from 70 to 100/min during a short period of about 30 seconds; at that very moment, the patient was moving in his bed without significant effort.

We have no explanation for the absence of adaptation of the QT interval to changes in heart rate. This is known to be one of the main characteristics of the long QT syndrome. In our patient, the peculiar feature is that the discrepancy between rate and QT duration was transient and immediately preceded the onset of tachycardia. This was obviously not a coincidence and most probably resulted from some imbalance in the autonomic nervous activity. It is not possible however to precisely establish whether this was an increased sympathetic drive or a decreased parasympathetic tone, or both. A partial improvement as evidenced by a reduction of the number of recurrences could be obtained by either beta-blocking drugs or verapamil, but complete control of the arrhythmia could only be achieved by amiodarone, which, because of its complex action does not permit definite conclusion as to the most likely mechanism of the arrhythmia.

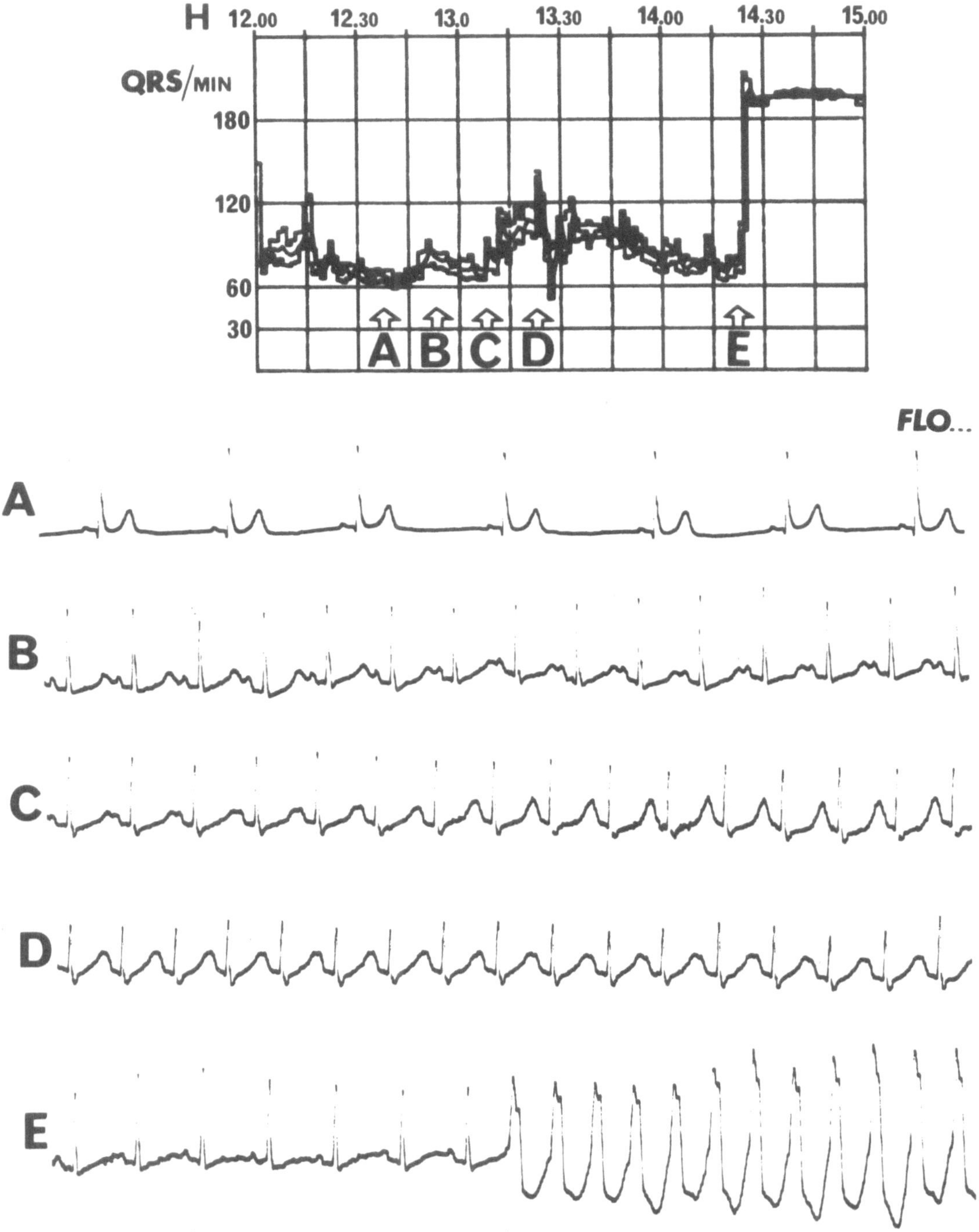

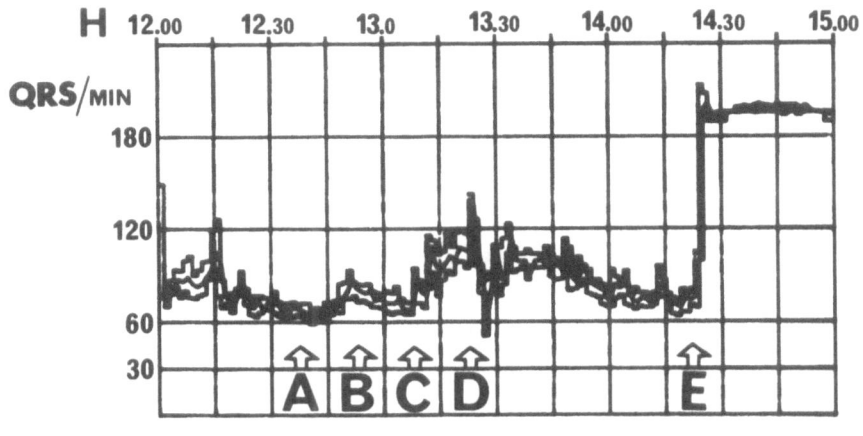

Figure 9. Case 4. Absence of adaptation of the QT interval to sinus rate before the tachycardia. The upper diagram shows the computerized analysis of the 3-hour tracing between 12.00 and 15.00. Tracings A to E refer to the corresponding times indicated in the diagram. Adaptation of the QT interval to cardiac rate was absent; this was not observed during the Holter monitoring carried out on days where no ventricular tachycardia occurred. The onset of tachycardia is not preceded by any ventricular extrasystole and progressive slowing of the sinus rate occurs between 13.30 and 14.25. The initiation of tachycardia is preceded by reacceleration of sinus rate during a few seconds.

2.5. Case 5

This case (Figure 1, panel 5 and Figure 10) is in fact much more common than the preceding ones, and is only reported for comparison with Case 6. It is an example of "torsades de pointes" of a well-known aetiology, i.e. complete A-V block. The paroxysmal intra-hisian A-V block which in the present case was the determinant of the "torsades de pointes" is probably not the causal but the triggering factor. It is well known that only some 10 % of the patients having some kind of bradycardia can develop this type of tachyarrhythmia. In our opinion, it must be considered as related to a congenital tendency in some patients, unmasked in various circumstances (10). The huge T waves which usually precede the runs of tachycardia (terminating in some cases in true and irreversible ventricular fibrillation) are closely related to the bradycardia itself, and usually disappear when a ventricular pacing is undertaken. The other way to treat this life-threatening arrhythmia is to give large doses of intravenous isoprenaline, thereby demonstrating that the abnormality is not only due to bradycardia but to an imbalance of the autonomic nervous influence at the ventricular level.

2.6. Case 6

A number of patients with the Jervell and Lange-Nielsen or Romano-Ward syndrome have been previously reported (11), but in relatively few of them was a three channel electrocardiogram recorded during tachycardia (12) (Figure 11). The general pattern is exactly the same as in Figure 10, so that there is no doubt that those arrhythmias have something in common, even though clinical data and treatment are clearly different. In the present case, the clinical setting was very classical. She was a 21-year-old woman with a personal history of syncope, and a family history of sudden death. She was treated 4 years previously by left stellate ganglionectomy, with an initially good result (12) followed by a recurrence of syncopal attacks after 3 years (Figure 11). She is now under acebutolol (a beta-blocker) with persistence of the long QT interval but without any loss of consciousness during the last year.

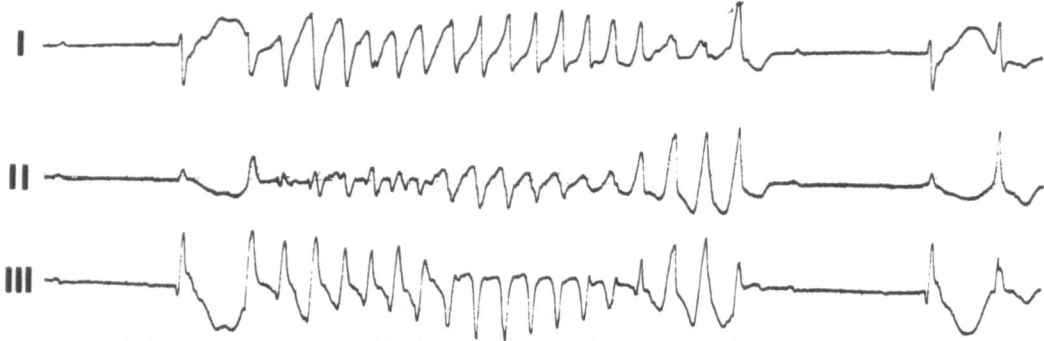

Figure 10. Case 5. Typical torsade de pointes during paroxysmal atrioventricular block. Note the long coupling interval of the first beat of the tachycardia, and the progressively changing QRS axis in all three leads.

The asymmetrical and focal distribution of the cardio-neural lesions as recently reported by James (13) suggests to him that "although it is uncertain how many of the observed neural lesions were in sympathetic as compared to vagal nerves, it is the adrenergic neural control of the heart which may be the more functionally important derangement in these patients, even though vagal neuropathy could contribute to this imbalance". Such a philosophy is in accordance with the unpredictable results of the various treatments which have been proposed in this type of arrhythmia, ranging from phenobarbital to diphenyl-hydantoin, guanethidine and even digitalis. We fully agree with James about the focal distribution of the neural imbalance which should make us cautious in using either agonists or antagonists of the autonomic nervous system; their effect is unpredictable.

This statement is illustrated by comparing the obvious benefit of isoprenaline treatment in the "torsade de pointes" of Case 5, whereas this same treatment, cautiously undertaken in the acute stage of Case 6, made the condition worse. On the other hand large doses of atropine in the latter case did produce a transient improvement while verapamil seemed to increase the number of episodes. Finally, we could demonstrate a beneficial effect of acebutolol.

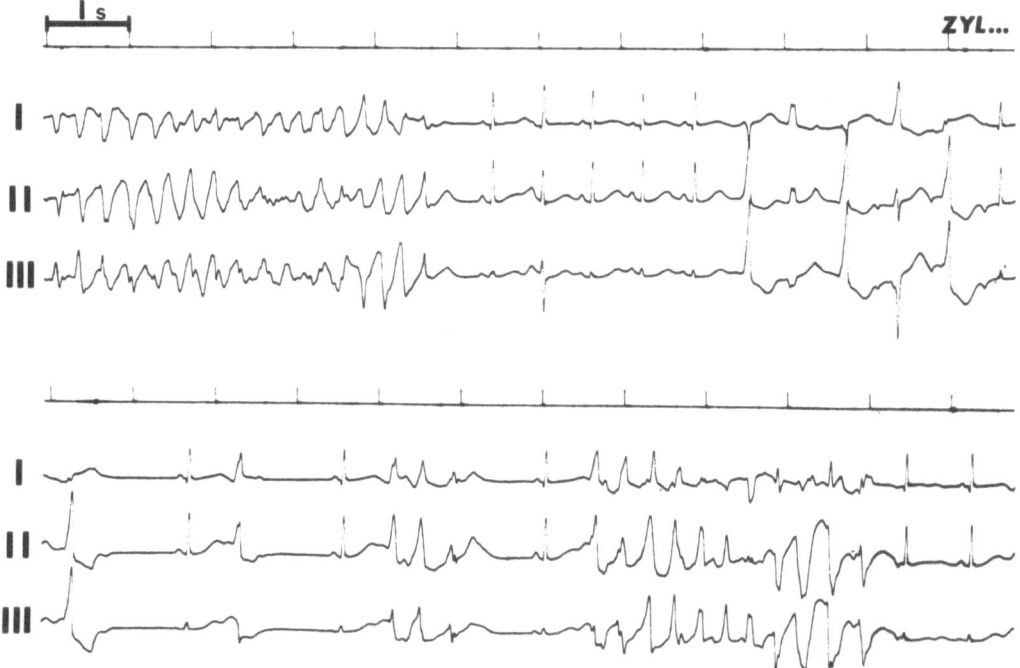

Figure 11. Case 6. Romano-Ward syndrome. The tracings meet all the criteria for the electrocardiographic syn-drome of torsade de pointes: long QT interval of sinus beats, long coupling interval of the isolated extrasystoles grouped in begiminy, and typical pattern of attacks of spontaneously terminating tachycardia.

3. DISCUSSION

We have collected six cases of unusual and life-threatening ventricular tachyarrhythmias in an effort to determine whether they had a common causal factor related to some "disease" of the autonomic nervous system which was responsible for the various electrocardiographic patterns. Many findings show these cases to be different in appearance, but possibly common in aetiology.

These arrhythmias occur in patients having no detectable myocardial disease. Of course, the patients had no coronary angiography or myocardial biopsy. However, all of them were under 45 years of age and none had a clinical history other than syncope (Case 1, 2, 5 and 6) or dizziness (case 3) or palpitations (case 4). There were no abnormalities of myocardial function on clinical, radiological, mechanographic and echocardiographic examination. This does not mean that in Cases 3 and 5, we consider that the mild form of mitral valve prolapse or the paroxysmal A-V block had no relation whatsoever with the ventricular tachyarrhythmia: they were probably related, but not in a cause-to-effect relationship. In addition, in most cases, the 12-lead electrocardiogram was basically normal. The problem of the long QT will be discussed below, but in any case, it is well known that the long QT may be intermittent or even absent in true cases of the Jervell and Lange-Nielsen syndrome.

These apparently idiopathic arrhythmias occur in young or middle-aged patients; one has to assume that they are congenital even though they may become apparent at different ages. A family history exists in a number of cases, at least in identical patients reported although not in the patients that we have described; family history was present in one case quite similar to Case 1 and in published cases similar to Case 2 (8). Familial cases are not uncommon in ventricular tachycardia (Case 4) and in paroxysmal A-V block; the hereditary character of the long QT syndrome is well known.

Most of these patients have in common the risk of sudden death. This is unquestionable as far as Cases 1, 2, 5 and 6 are concerned. It is also most likely in Case 3 who had a tachycardia with a rate sometimes exceeding 250/min. Case 4 is the only one in whom this type of ventricular tachycardia is sometimes labelled as "benign" because it can be well tolerated for many years. But we know that some of these idiopathic and so-called benign tachycardias end with unexpected sudden death (14). The predominant, if not exclusive, role of an autonomic nervous system imbalance is clearly demonstrated in all patients, either by the nycthemeral variations of the arrhythmia or by the triggering effect of exertion, or, more importantly, psychological stress. That the latter is always much more effective than the former has recently been shown by Lown (4).

The study of the effects of drugs further allows us to analyze the role of the vago-sympathetic balance, but the results may often be surprising, if not paradoxical. Figure 12 is an attempt to summarize our observations. We have already underlined the opposite effects of beta-adrenergic blockade and stimulation in Cases 5 and 6; there was a beneficial effect of isoprenaline in Case 5 and of beta-blockers in Case 6 where left stellate ganglion-ectomy had failed to improve the patient. However, the effect of parasympathetic blockade was similar in both cases: atropine was beneficial which seems logical in the presence of

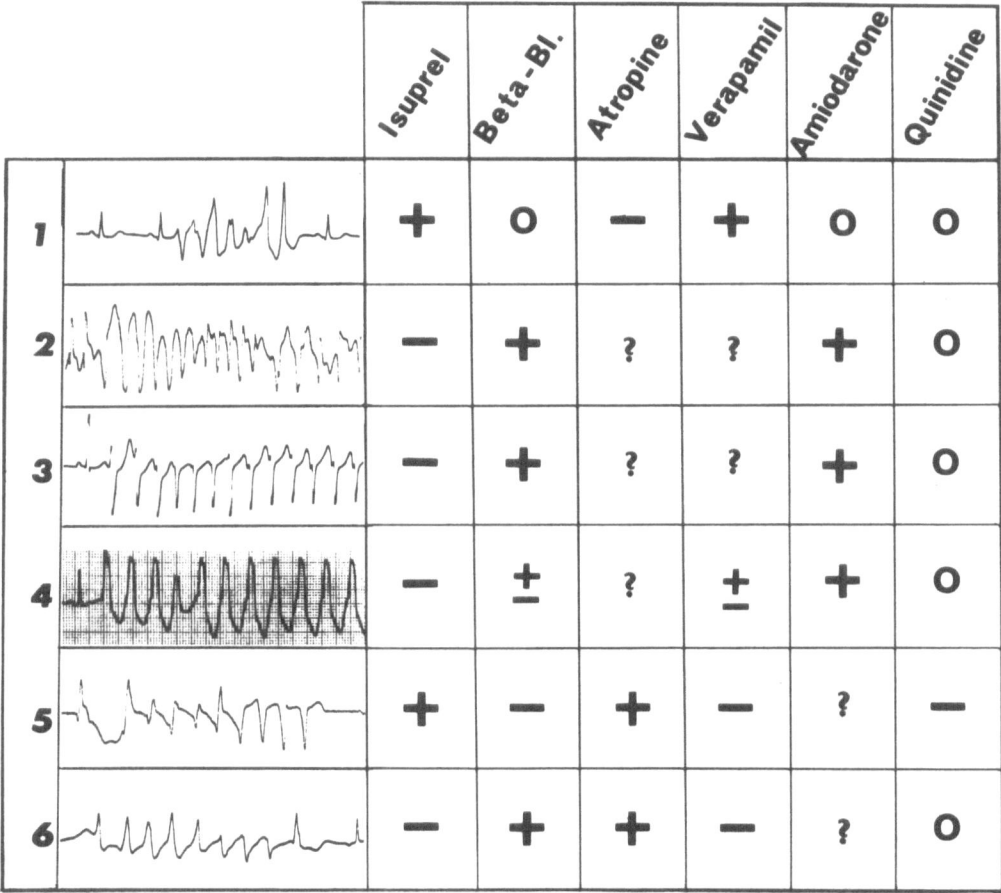

Figure 12. Effects of different drugs on these unusual ventricular tachy-arrhythmias. The effect of drugs is schematically indicated as good (+), poor (−), doubtful (±) or unexplored (?)(see text for further comments).

A-V block but surprising in the long QT syndrome. In Cases 2, 3 and 4, the role of the parasympathetic system was not explored, but the beneficial effect of beta-blockade was without question. In Case 1, the favourable effect of isoprenaline was quite surprising but unquestionable, making this patient similar to Case 5. The effect of atropine was however deleterious, which again is most surprising.

Finally, the exclusive role of the autonomic nervous system is also suggested by another of the characteristics of these cases, i.e., the complete absence of efficacy of quinidine and quinidine-like drugs. This feature is well known in patients such as Cases 5 and 6 but it was initially unexpected in patients 1 to 4. As far as other drugs are concerned, amiodarone was effective in Cases 2, 3 and 4 (possibly because of its beta-adrenergic diminishing effect) but not in Case 1; it was not tried in Cases 5 and 6. Verapamil was surprisingly effective in Case 1 and not completely ineffective in Case 4; we have already discussed the possible vagotonic action of this drug.

What are the possible electrocardiographic similarities between these patients? The similarity between Cases 5 and 6 is obvious. The problem is more difficult regarding Case 1 in which the "torsade de pointes" pattern is without question, but the extremely short coupling interval of the first ectopic beat is unusual as compared to the electrocardiographic pattern which is commonly seen in this syndrome. We ignore the exact electrophysiologic mechanism which is operative, but have to note that the opposite effect of vagal stimulation and blockade in Case 1 as compared to Cases 5 and 6 may not be coincidental.

Case 4 has in common with Cases 5 and 6 the prolongation of the QT interval, or at least the absence of QT interval shortening during the sinus acceleration preceding the onset of tachycardia: it must be underlined that this phenomenon was paroxysmal as well as the tachycardia itself. That the QT prolongation is also transient in the "torsade de pointes" associated with AV block is well-known and its spontaneous variations in the congenital long QT syndrome have been frequently observed.

Finally, the clinical features in Cases 2 and 3 are very similar, the severity of the phenomena being the only difference, so that we can consider Case 3 as a forme fruste of Case 2. We think that there may be no differences in nature between the catecholamine-induced ventricular tachycardias in children (Case 2) and the Jervell and Lange-Nielsen or Romano-Ward syndrome, but only differences in the mode of expression of the disease, the former being paroxysmal and the latter more or less chronic. Sudden stress such as arousal from sleep (15) has been reported to induce the attacks in the long QT syndrome, although not constantly. The same applies to isoprenaline infusion. In at least one report of authentic Jervell and Lange-Nielsen syndrome (16), the tachycardias were readily obtained by this method and the tracings published in that paper cannot be differentiated from our Case 2.

In conclusion, an attractive hypothesis would be to think that all these apparently so different idiopathic paroxysmal ventricular arrhythmias might represent various expressions and modalities of a same syndrome characterized by a vagosympathetic imbalance and related to focal cardioneural lesions which remain to be identified.

REFERENCES

1. Robles De Medina EO et al: WHO/ISFC Task Force, Definition of terms related to cardiac rhythm. Europ J Cardiol 8:127–144, 1978.
2. Dessertenne F, Fabiato A and Coumel Ph: Un chapitre nouveau d'électrocardiographie: les variations progressives de l'amplitude de l'électrocardiogramme. Actual Card Angeiol Intern 15:241-258, 1966.
3. Motte G, Coumel Ph, Abitbol G, Dessertenne F and Slama R: Le syndrôme QT long et syncopes par torsades de pointes. Arch Mal Coeur 63:831–853, 1970.
4. Lown B and Verrier RL: Neural factors and sudden death. In: Neural mechanisms in cardiac arrhythmias. Schwartz PJ, Brown AM, Malliani A and Zanchetti A (eds), Raven Press, New York NY 1979, p 87.
5. Rossi L: Histopathology of cardiac arrhythmias, Casa Editrice Ambrosiana, Milano 1978, p 32.
6. Coumel Ph, Leclercq JF and Attuel P: Drug-resistant paroxysmal ventricular tachycardia: approach to drug management by intracardiac electrography and ambulatory electrocardiographic monitoring. In: Management of ventricular tachycardia. Role of Mexiletine. Sandoe E, Julian DG and Bell JW (eds), Excerpta Medica, Amsterdam-Oxford 1978, p 433.
7. Coumel Ph, Leclercq JF, Attuel P, Lavallee JP and Flammang D: Autonomic influences: sympathetic drive

and the genesis of ventricular arrhythmias in "Cardiac arrhythmias. Electrophysiology, diagnosis and management." Varula OS. Ed. Baltimore. Williams and Wilkins, 1979, p. 243.

8. Coumei Ph, Fidelle J, Lucet V, Attuel P and Bouvrain Y: Catecholamine-induced severe ventricular arrhythmias with Adams-Stokes syndrome in children: report of four cases. Brit Heart J suppl XL p 28, 1978.

9. Boudoulas H, Wooley CF, Reynolds J and Mazzaferri E: Mitral valve prolapse syndrome. Evidence for a hyper-adrenergic state. Amer J Cardiol 43:368, 1979 (abstr).

10. Slama R, Motte G, Vanetti A and Temkine J: Hypokaliémie avec troubles du rythme syncopaux chez une malade entraînée par stimulateur intracorporel. Pr Medic 1978:61, 1970.

11. Schwartz PJ, Periti M and Malliani A: The long QT syndrome. Am Heart J 89:378–390, 1975.

12. Baudouy Ph, Andreassian B, Attuel P, Greze M, Soulie J and Fruchaud J: Syndrôme de Romano-Ward et stellectomie gauche. Revue de la littérature à propos d'un nouveau cas. Arch Mal Coeur 70:645–652, 1977.

13. James TN, Froggatt P, Atkinson WJ, Lurie PR, McNamara DG, Miller WW, Schloss GT, Carroll JF and North RL: De subitaneis mortibus. XXX. Observations on the pathophysiology of the long QT syndromes with special reference to the neuropathology of the heart. Circulation 57:1221–1231, 1978.

14. Steffens TG, Pierce PL and Zegerius RJ: Multiple ventricular premature beats in five adolescents. Eur. J Cardiol 8:177–184, 1978.

15. Wellens HJJ, Verneulen A and Durrer D: Ventricular fibrillation occurring on arousal from sleep by auditory stimuli. Circulation 46:661–665, 1972.

16. Pernot C, Henry M and Carre JC: Syndrôme cardio-auditif de Jervell et torsades de pointes. Arch Mal Coeur 65:261–274, 1972.

SECTION 3
THE INDICATORS OF HIGH RISK FOR SUDDEN DEATH

SECTION 3A
CLINICAL PROFILE OF HIGH RISK INDIVIDUALS

3.1. PREHOSPITAL CARDIAC ARREST: EARLY AND LONG-TERM CLINICAL AND ELECTROPHYSIOLOGIC CHARACTERISTICS

R.J. MYERBURG, C.A. CONDE, R.J. SUNG, S.M. MALLON, D.S. SHEPS, R. APPEL and A. CASTELLANOS

Unexpected cardiac arrest in an out-of-hospital environment is a worldwide problem of enormous magnitude. Estimates for the United States alone suggest that 300,000 to 600,000 sudden deaths occur each year, with the broad range of estimates reflecting various definitions of "sudden death" (1). Until recently, studies of the nature and characteristics of sudden death victims remained entirely in the realm of epidemiologists and pathologists, since prehospital cardiac arrest was virtually 100 % fatal. The clinical characteristics of patients dying suddenly and unexpectedly in the community were derived retrospectively from pathologic data, and the electrophysiologic characteristics were speculated upon from other clinical settings. The development of community-based emergency medical systems during the past decade, however, has led to the survival of a significant percentage of prehospital cardiac arrest victims; and, at the same time, has provided clinical investigators with the ability to study the clinical and electrophysiologic characteristics of individuals who have survived an unexpected, out-of-hospital cardiac arrest (2–4). Moreover, since survivors of prehospital cardiac arrest are at high risk for a recurrent cardiac arrest (approximately 30 %) in the first year after the initial event (3, 4), it is also possible to study the characteristics of patients at risk for a future event.

1. MECHANISMS OF PREHOSPITAL CARDIAC ARREST AND IMMEDIATE PROGNOSIS

While many of the studies of "prehospital cardiac arrest" were limited to patients in whom ventricular fibrillation was the initial electrophysiologic mechanism recorded by emergency medical rescue personnel, other electrophysiologic mechanisms contribute to the total population of prehospital cardiac arrest victims. Both the immediate prognosis at the scene of the cardiac arrest, and the risk of subsequent in-hospital death, are related to the initial electrical mechanism recorded. A total of 352 prehospital cardiac arrests, defined as sudden and unexpected loss of consciousness in the community, and responded to by the City of Miami and Metropolitan Dade County emergency medical systems during the 3 year period 1975–1978 (Table 1), have been analyzed. Of the 352 victims, ventricular fibrillation was the initial mechanism recorded by emergency medical system personnel in 220 persons (62 %); 24 persons (7 %) had ventricular tachycardia as the initial mechanism recorded; and 108 persons (31 %) had various forms of severe bradyarrhythmias or asystole. Of the overall group of 352 patients, 117 patients (33 %) were successfully resuscitated and admitted to the hospital alive, with the remaining 235 patients (67 %) dying

Table 1. Mechanism of cardiac arrest vs. prognosis. (Modified from (12) with permission of the American Journal of Medicine.)

	PREHOSPITAL CARDIAC ARRESTS	RESUSCITATED OUT-OF-HOSPITAL AND ADMITTED TO HOSPITAL ALIVE	DISCHARGED FROM HOSPITAL ALIVE
Ventricular Fibrillation	220 $\xrightarrow{(40\%)}$	87 $\xrightarrow{(59\%)}$	51
Ventricular Tachycardia	24 $\xrightarrow{(88\%)}$	21 $\xrightarrow{(76\%)}$	16
Asystolic Arrest or Severe Bradyarrhythmias	108 $\xrightarrow{(9\%)}$	9 $\xrightarrow{(0\%)}$	0
TOTAL	352 $\xrightarrow{(33\%)}$	117 $\xrightarrow{(57\%)}$	67

before hospitalization. As shown in Table 1, the earliest prognosis (i.e., the ability to successfully resuscitate a patient in the field and admit the patient to the hospital alive) is related closely to the initial electrophysiologic mechanism recorded. The best prognosis for prehospital resuscitation was observed in the ventricular tachycardia group, in which 21 of 24 patients (88 %) were admitted to the hospital alive, while the worst prehospital prognosis occurred in the bradyarrhythmia group – only 9 of 108 patients (9 %) were admitted to the hospital alive. In the ventricular fibrillation group, 87 patients (40 %) were admitted to the hospital alive, and 133 patients (60 %) died before hospitalization. The figures for ventricular fibrillation patients are consistent with those from other centers studying prehospital ventricular fibrillation, but excluding other mechanisms (2, 3).

The bradyarrhythmia and asystole data must be interpreted cautiously because these mechanisms may occur as an end-stage after primary ventricular fibrillation or ventricular tachycardia; or, conversely, may occur as a primary event. The City of Miami emergency medical system is deployed in a fashion such that rescue personnel can arrive at the scene of a cardiac arrest within 4 minutes in 80 % of summons (3). Moreover, a sub-group within the bradyarrhythmia and asystole group can be identified in which the time between the onset of the cardiac arrest and the arrival of emergency medical rescue personnel is known. We studied 37 bradyarrhythmia/asystole events in which 1) the loss of consciousness was witnessed, 2) summons of emergency medical personnel could be documented to have occurred without significant delay, and 3) arrival time of rescue personnel was 4 minutes or less from time of summons. Under these rigidly defined circumstances, bradyarrhythmias or asystole are more likely to be primary events. The prognosis in this subgroup is not statistically different from the total bradyarrhythmia group, in that only 5 arrests (14 %) occurring by this mechanism were admitted to the hospital alive (compared to 9 % of the total group), and there were no long-term survivors.

The in-hospital prognosis for patients who are successfully resuscitated and admitted to the hospital alive also relates quite well to the electrical mechanism initially recorded by emergency medical system personnel (Table 1). Of the overall group of 117 patients who were admitted to the hospital alive, 67 patients (57 %) survived hospitalization and were discharged, and 50 patients (43 %) died in the hospital. Of the 87 ventricular fibrillation patients who were admitted to the hospital alive, 51 were discharged alive (59 %), and 36 died. These 51 survivors represent 76 % of the overall survivors. Of 21 ventricular tachycardia patients admitted to the hospital alive, 16 were discharged alive (76 %) and there were 5 deaths in the hospital. The 16 long-term survivors in this group represent the remaining 24 % of the 67 overall survivors. None of the 9 bradyarrhythmia or asystole patients admitted to the hospital alive survived hospitalization.

The early outcome, after successful resuscitation from prehospital cardiac arrest, may be improving, although the factors responsible have not been clearly identified yet. When the experience of the Miami emergency medical systems from the 1971–1973 period (2) is compared to the 1975–1978 experience, using the same emergency medical system and the same base hospital, an interesting trend appears to be evolving (Table 2). Despite the fact that there is not a significant difference between the two time periods in terms of successful initial resuscitation and hospitalization (34 % in 1971–1973 vs. 40 % in 1975–1978, $p < 0.20$), those who have been successfully resuscitated and hospitalized had a better chance of long-term survival and discharge from the hospital in the later study period (42 % in 1971–1973 vs. 59 % in 1975–1978, $p < 0.03$). Furthermore, when the overall chances of successful resuscitation, hospitalization, and discharge alive are compared for the entire prehospital ventricular fibrillation group for the two study periods (Table 2), there was a significant improvement, from 14% in 1971–1973 (42 of 301 events) to 23% in 1975–1978 (51 of 220 events), $p < 0.01$. This analysis was restricted to only those events in which ventricular fibrillation was the initial mechanism recorded by emergency medical rescue personnel since the 1971–1973 observations did not include ventricular tachycardia or bradyarrhythmia patients (2).

Although activities in the field by emergency medical personnel do not appear to be contributing directly to the improved survival, based upon the absence of a statistically significant increase in the number of prehospital ventricular fibrillation patients reaching the hospital alive, one cannot exclude the possibility that the overall improvement may relate in part to improved activities in the field. *Improved training and technology, plus civilian bystander intervention, may be resulting in the early survivors reaching the hospital*

Table 2. Early outcome – prehospital ventricular fibrillation 1971-73 vs. 1975–78. (Modified from (12) with permission of the American Journal of Medicine.)

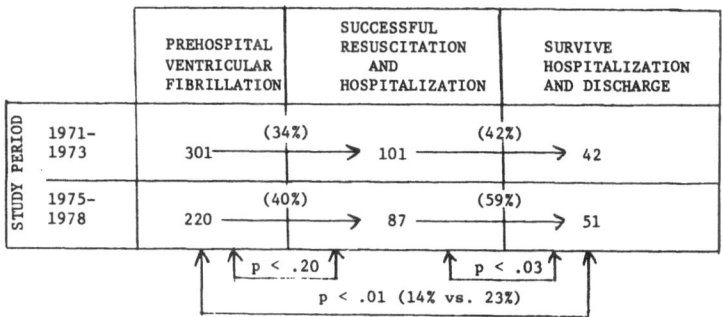

in a condition more favorable to long-term survival. The importance of the clinical state of patients reaching the hospital alive has been emphasized in the study by Copley et al. (5), in which clinical characteristics compatible with long-term survival were related to the rapidity and effectiveness of the institution of resuscitative efforts (Table 3). Those in-

Table 3.

	RESUSCITATIONS	
	EARLY	LATE
PAEDP ...... mmHg	15	29
CI ......1/min/m^2	3.1	2.2
CPK ...... IU/liter	501	5700
VENTILATOR HOURS	2	53
HOSPITAL DAYS ...	19	31
COMA ..... %	29	92
SURVIVAL	6/7	6/12

Early = Resuscitative efforts initiated within 5 minutes by bystanders or rescue personnel; Late = Resuscitative efforts initiated more than 5 minutes after arrest. PAEDP = Pulmonary artery end-diastolic pressure; CI = Cardiac Index; CPK = Creatinine Phosphokinase; (From data reported by Copley et al (5)).

dividuals in whom the response was early (< 5 min) had lower pulmonary artery end-diastolic pressures at the time of hospitalization (15 mmHg vs. 29 mmHg.), a higher cardiac index (3.1 vs. 2.2 L/mm/M^2), lower peak CPK (501 vs. 5700), much less time requiring ventilatory support (2 hours vs. 53 hours), a shorter hospital stay, better central nervous system function (29 % coma vs. 92 % coma), and a better survival rate (6/7 vs. 6/12). While these investigators were emphasizing the value of both early resuscitative efforts and bystander intervention in outcome (5), their data also points out some clinical factors which relate to early (in-hospital) deaths in resuscitated patients. Data on in-hospital deaths among survivors of initial resuscitative efforts in the Miami system are consistent with Copley's observations. Among 48 patients who died after successful resuscitation and hospitalization, but before discharge from the initial event, the importance of central nervous system damage is highlighted by the fact that 18 of the 48 deaths (38 %) were directly attributable to anoxic encephalopathy, and another 10 deaths (21 %) were directly attributed to sepsis in patients who had anoxic encephalopathy and/or were respirator-dependent. Fifteen of the 48 died of cardiogenic shock (31 %), while only 5 patients died because of recurrent or uncontrollable arrhythmias (10 %). Both Copley's observations and the Miami studies underscore the importance of rapid effective field action for salvaging central nervous system function, the importance of central nervous system damage as a cause of death in resuscitated patients, and the importance of proper management of cardiac functional abnormalities in influencing ultimate discharge from the initial event. Finally, changes in the patterns of intensive cardiac care during the past decade are very likely playing a role in the improved overall survival (Table 2), either in concert with, or independent of, the field activities.

2. CLINICAL, HEMODYNAMIC, AND ELECTROPHYSIOLOGIC CHARACTERISTICS OF SUCCESSFULLY RESUSCITATED PREHOSPITAL CARDIAC ARREST VICTIMS

Coronary heart disease is the most common etiologic entity identified in survivors of prehospital cardiac arrest. In Miami, 70 % of those patients who survive the initial event and have studies adequate to determine etiology with certainty have had coronary heart disease. Twenty-five percent of the coronary heart disease group have evidence of an acute myocardial infarction by electrocardiographic and enzymatic criteria during the early post-arrest phase of hospitalization. It is not possible to determine how many of the myocardial infarctions preceded cardiac arrest and how many were a consequence. Of the remaining prehospital cardiac arrests, 16 % have cardiomyopathies, 7 % have valvular heart disease as a primary underlying etiology, and in the remaining 7 %, either no specific abnormality had been identified or studies were not sufficient to determine a diagnosis. It must be recognized, however, that etiologic distributions may be different in this patient population than in populations derived from epidemiologic or pathologic studies, or from studies of non-survivors of the initial event.

Hemodynamic studies have revealed evidence of left ventricular dysfunction in the majority, but not all, of the patients studied. The mean left ventricular end-diastolic pressure was 14.90 mmHg. $\pm$ 7.68, with a range of 3 to 35 mmHg, and 10 of 30 patients having a value of 12 mmHg or less. The mean cardiac index was 2.64 L/min/M^2 $\pm$ 0.73, with a range of 1.6 to 4.6 L/min/M^2, and 12 of 30 patients having an index of 2.6 L/min/M^2 or more. The mean ejection fraction was 37.14 % $\pm$ 17.99 %, varying from 15 to 78 %, and 7 patients > 50 %.

Angiographic studies in 30 patients revealed left ventricular dysfunction in 23 (77 %), the dysfunction being limited to a single segment in 4, involving multiple segments in 8, and manifest as diffuse hypokinesis in 11. Discrete left ventricular aneurysms were present in 4 of the angiographic left ventricular dysfunction patients, all of whom were among the patients who presented with ventricular tachycardia. The left ventricular contraction pattern was normal in 5 patients. Five patients had valvular abnormalities. Two of the 5 had primary valvular disease as the dominant underlying etiologic factor, and the other 3 had either trivial valve disease or a valve dysfunction secondary to papillary muscle dysfunction. There were 2 patients with incomplete studies. Coronary arteriograms in the same 30 patients revealed one or more lesions > 60 % in 21, < 60 % in 2, and normal coronary arteries in the remaining 7 patients. Seventeen of the 21 patients with > 60 % coronary artery lesions had 2 or more vessels involved with lesions of this extent (81 %). The distribution of significantly diseased arteries (> 60 % lesions) was nearly equally distributed among the left anterior descending (36 % of the lesions), left circumflex (26 % of the lesions), and right coronary artery (28 % of the lesions). In addition, the left main coronary artery was involved with > 60 % occlusive lesions in 5 patients (9 % of the > 60 % lesions).

Several electrophysiologic markers of instability and risk for recurrent arrest and early mortality become evident shortly after the initial resuscitation. Liberthson et al. (2) reported a relationship between the immediate post-resuscitation heart rate and early mortality in patients resuscitated from ventricular fibrillation. Those patients who reverted to a bradycardia (< 60/min) had a 73 % chance of a recurrent arrest and death before hospitalization and an overall 95% chance of not surviving to or through hospitalization. Patients with a heart rate of 60–100/min did better, and those with an immediate post-resuscitative rate > 100/min did best (17% prehospital mortality and 57% overall mortality from arrest through hospitalization). It is conceivable, although not proven, that transient involvement of the specialized conducting system, with or without electrophysiologic disturbance of ventricular muscle, accounts for the relationship between post-ventricular bradycardia and early death.

Electrophysiologic instability, characterized by complex forms of ventricular ectopic activity which does not respond uniformly to various forms of antiarrhythmic therapy, is observed very frequently during the first 24 to 48 hours after resuscitation from prehospital cardiac arrest. Among a group of 53 resuscitated and hospitalized prehospital cardiac arrest victims, 11 were never stabilized hemodynamically and died early deaths due to low cardiac output states. Of the remaining 42 patients, 38 had complex ventricular arrhythmias and 4 had infrequent unifocal ventricular ectopic beats. Among the 38 patients having complex ventricular ectopic activity, 10 had a recurrent cardiac arrest within 72 hours of the initial event, and 28 did not (see Table 4). The characteristics of the arrhythmias,

Table 4.

		RECURRENT CARDIAC ARREST AFTER HOSPITALIZATION (< 72 HOURS)		
		NO	YES	
A-V Block, Intraventricular Conduction	NO	25	1	26
Disturbance, or Both	YES	3	9	12
		28	10	38

p < .001

the response to antiarrhythmic therapy, ventricular function, and the nature and extent of underlying heart disease did not separate those with recurrent cardiac arrests from those who did not have such events. Among the same 38 patients, however, 12 had AV block, intraventricular conduction disturbances, or both, either at the time of admission or developing during the first 24–48 hours. Nine of these 12 were among the 10 recurrent cardiac arrest victims and only 1 recurrent cardiac arrest patient did not have AV block or intraventricular conduction disturbances. Conversely, of the 28 patients admitted with complex ventricular arrhythmias who did not have recurrent cardiac arrest, 25 had no AV block or intraventricular conduction disturbances, and 3 had one or the other. The *mechanism* of cardiac arrest in the 10 patients having recurrent arrest was *ventricular fibrillation*, despite the relationship between conduction disturbances and recurrent cardiac arrest. Thus, the presence of complex ventricular arrhythmias alone did not appear to discriminate between those who did and those who did not have an *early* recurrent cardiac arrest. Rather, various specialized conducting system abnormalities appear to be the better discriminating factor. The mechanism by which conduction disturbances, interacting with an unstable myocardium, leads to a high incidence of recurrent ventricular fibrillation has not yet been determined, but may parallel the observations of Liberthson et al. (2) (see above) regarding post-resuscitation bradyarrhythmias and very early recurrent arrest and death. The occurrence of conduction disturbances in early survivors of prehospital cardiac arrest, regardless of the electrophysiologic interactions at play, appears to be of some *prognostic* value for identifying those patients who will have an early recurrent cardiac arrest in-hospital, and is independent of the severity, extent, or etiology of the underlying heart disease.

Intracardiac electrophysiologic studies, consisting of programmed extra-stimulus studies and incremental pacing of the right atrium and right ventricle (6), were carried out in a total of 17 survivors of prehospital cardiac arrest 72 hours after the event. The right atrium and/or the right ventricle were stimulated at 1 or more cycle lengths, and atrial and ventricular extra-stimuli were delivered from late diastole to early diastole, following every eighth atrial or ventricular paced beat, until the atrial or ventricular refractory period was encountered. In addition, the atrium and the ventricle were paced at rates up to 250 beats/min for a few seconds to test the effect of tachyarrhythmias. The pertinent findings in these studies were as follows: 1) no patient had prolonged sinus node recovery time; 2) minimal to moderate degrees of AV node dysfunction was present in 4 patients (AV nodal Wenckebach occurring at atrial pacing rates between 100 and 120 beats/min); 3) His-Purkinje conduction time, measured as the HV interval, was prolonged (> 55 msec) in 3 patients (60, 62, and 67 msec respectively), 2 of the 3 having associated complete left bundle branch block; 4) no patient developed sustained supraventricular tachycardia during programmed atrial premature stimulation; 5) the phenomenon of repetitive ventricular responses to a single premature stimulus delivered to the right ventricular apex was observed at short ventricular premature coupling intervals in 7 of the 17 patients (41 %); 6) sustained ventricular tachycardia could be induced during programmed ventricular extra-stimulation in 5 of the 6 patients presenting with ventricular tachycardia, 4 of the 5 having ventricular aneurysms and the other having cardiomyopathy; and 7) no patient had ventricular fibrillation triggered by ventricular premature stimulation or rapid ventricular stimulation up to 250 beats/min, and only patients who presented with ventricular tachycardia as the initial mechanism had sustained ventricular tachycardia inducible during studies. These data suggest that studies carried out 72 hours or longer after the occurrence of prehospital cardiac arrest yield useful information only in patients whose mechanism of presentation is sustained ventricular tachycardia. The ventricular fibrillation patients have limited findings during intracardiac studies at this time period, and the incidence of repetitive responses during ventricular driving and ventricular extra-stimulation may not be significantly different from normal. It is possible, nonetheless, that the electrophysiologic disturbance making the myocardium vulnerable to unexpected ventricular fibrillation may be a transient phenomenon which has reversed by 72 hours after the event, and that earlier electrophysiologic studies may yield more meaningful information. In addition, different methods of programmed stimulation particularly for eliciting repetitive responses may yield different forms of information (7).

3. POST-HOSPITAL ARRHYTHMIAS AND THEIR MANAGEMENT IN SURVIVORS OF PRE-HOSPITAL CARDIAC ARREST

Asymptomatic complex ventricular arrhythmias occur nearly universally in survivors of prehospital cardiac arrest. Among a cohort of 52 patients who have been followed with 24-hour Holter monitor recordings on a monthly basis after discharge from the hospital, 44 patients have had asymptomatic complex ventricular arrhythmias on 1 or more of the monthly recordings (85 %). In addition, 75 % of the total tapes recorded in this patient population have had frequent (> 10 ventricular ectopic beats/hour) or complex (Lown's Grades III, IV, or V) ventricular ectopic beats during the recordings. These chronic arrhythmias, while asymptomatic, tend to be resistant to therapy with standard membrane-active antiarrhythmic drugs and with some experimental drugs. Figure 1 demonstrates two types of responses which we have observed in these patients. In Panel A, an expected therapeutic response to quinidine gluconate was observed, characterized by progressive decrease in the frequency and grade of ventricular ectopic activity as therapeutic blood levels are achieved. In Panel B, there is little change and high grade activity remains despite therapeutic blood levels of procainamide. It was this latter response, shown in Panel B, that was observed in most of the patients with asymptomatic complex ventricular arrhythmias during long-term follow-up (8, 9). Since various standard and/or experimental antiarrhythmic drugs, and combinations of drugs, did not suppress the arrhythmias, and they were considered a risk factor for sudden death in these patients, a new therapeutic strategy was developed. The approach was based upon close monitoring of plasma levels of antiarrhythmic drugs, with the end-point being maintenance of stable therapeutic plasma levels of standard membrane-active antiarrhythmic drugs, rather than mandatory eradication of chronic asymptomatic arrhythmias (8, 9). Oral dosages of the antiarrhythmic drugs were adjusted in an attempt to maintain stable therapeutic levels of the drugs. The mean and median frequencies of ventricular ectopic beats, expressed as ectopic beats/hour on a 24-hour Holter monitor tape, were matched to plasma levels of antiarrhythmic drugs measured during the 1 hour period before a scheduled dose on the day the monitor tape was recorded. Table 5 demonstrates that those tapes recorded when plasma levels were in the therapeutic range had somewhat fewer ventricular ectopic beats than those recorded when plasma levels were sub-therapeutic, but that the differences were not significant. There was marked skewing in both groups, and mean ventricular ectopic beats were well within the definition of "frequent" in both groups. The lack of a predictable relationship between plasma levels of drugs and ectopic beats is further underscored in Figure 2 in which hour-to-hour variations of both plasma levels and

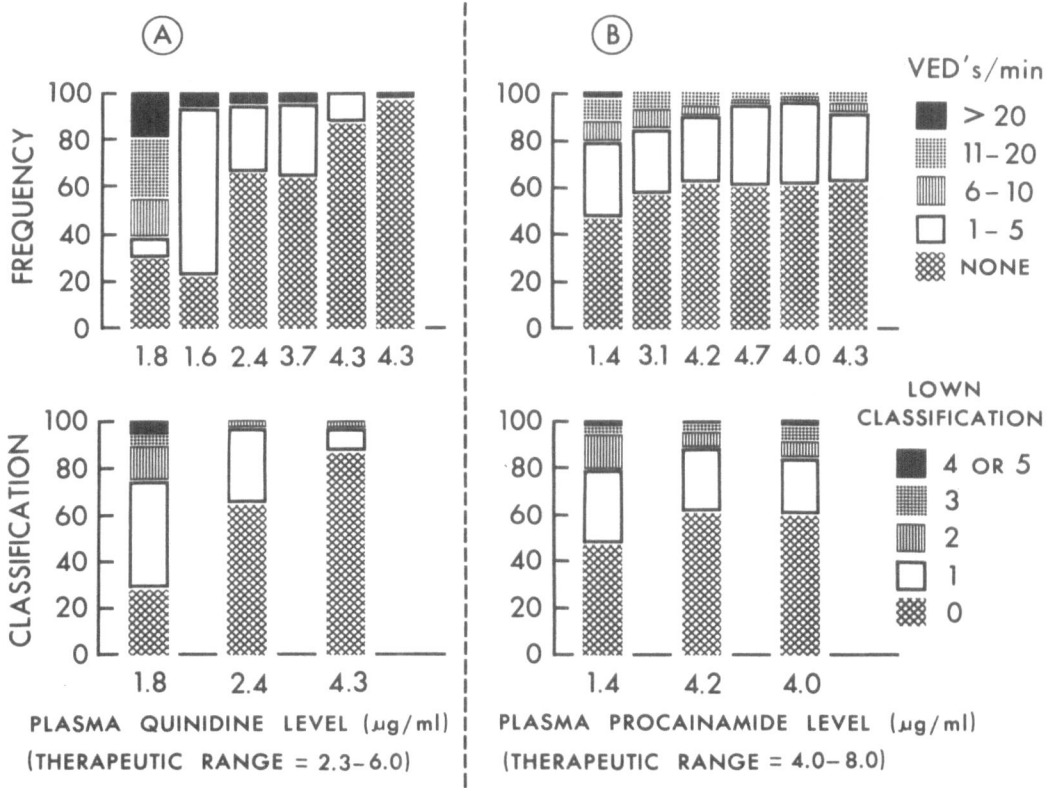

Figure 1. Frequency and grades of ventricular ectopic depolarizations (VEDs) on 24-hour Holter monitor tapes. VEDs during the first 32 seconds of each 10-minute segment of 24-hour Holter tapes are counted and extrapolated to VEDs/min. The number of segments free of VEDs, and those having 1–5, 6–10, 11–20, and > 20 are collated and plotted as percent of total segments (top graph on each panel). Similarly, grades according to the Lown classification are plotted on the lower half of each panel. Each bar demonstrates fequency distribution (top) or grade classification distribution (bottom) on one 24-hour Holter tape, at monthly intervals on the top and every other month below. In Panel A, a patient receiving quinidine demonstrated the expected dose-response relationship as the plasma level of the drug increased from subtherapeutic to therapeutic levels (see text). This type of response was observed in only 3 patients. The data in Panel B was recorded from a patient receiving procainamide. At the time of the first 2 tapes, plasma levels were subtherapeutic, and the last 4 were therapeutic (see text). The lack of a predictable relationship between blood levels and suppression of frequency of VEDs occurred in the majority of the patients. (From (9) reproduced with permission of the American Heart Association, Inc.)

Table 5.

	VED'S/hr ON 24 hr. HOLTER TAPES	
	MEAN ± SD	MEDIAN
THERAPEUTIC BLOOD LEVELS	104 (±234)	6
SUB-THERAPEUTIC BLOOD LEVELS	184 (±566)	21

(0.2 > p > 0.1)

VED'S = Ventricular Ectopic Depolarizations

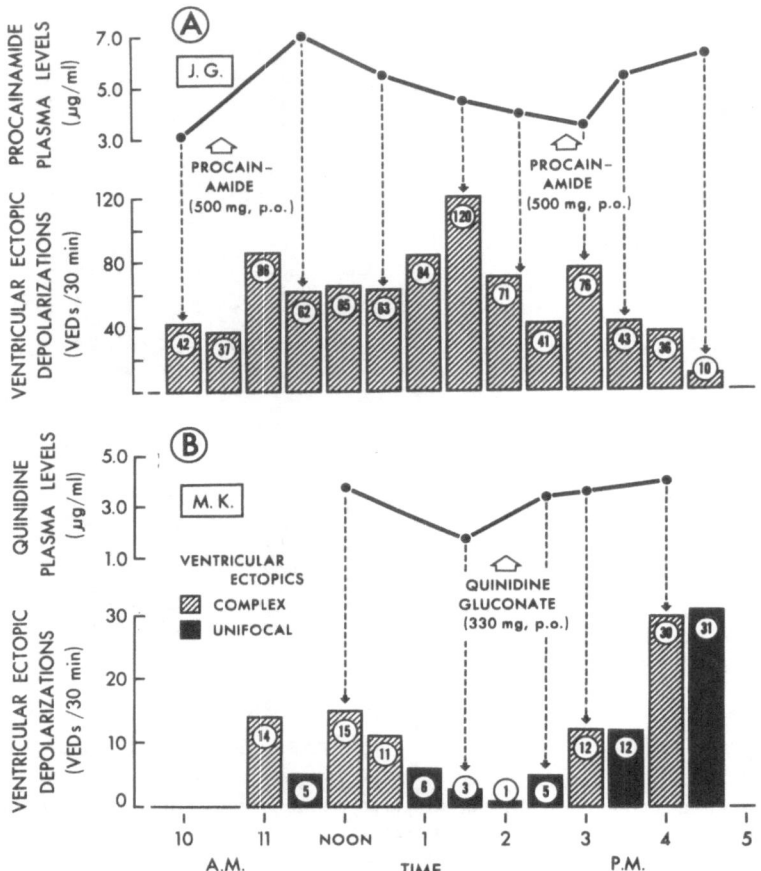

Figure 2. Plasma levels of antiarrhythmic drugs and corresponding frequencies of ventricular ectopic depolarizations between oral doses. Each bar represents a 30-minute period from a Holter tape, with the figure inserted representing the total number of VEDs. Serial plasma levels were obtained at the times indicated. The cross-hatched bars indicate complex VEDs (Lown Grade 3-5), and the solid bars indicated unifocal VED. Panel A was recorded from patient JG (procainamide), and Panel B from patient MK (quinidine gluconate) (see text for details). (From (9) reproduced with permission of the American Heart Association, Inc.)

frequency of ectopics are often out of phase. Thus, the relationship between plasma drug levels and suppression of *chronic asymptomatic ventricular arrhythmias* is not a simple one, at least in this patient population and probably in others (10) because of spontaneous variation of ventricular ectopic beats. Moreover, examples of month-to-month intra-patient variations in the relationship between plasma levels and frequency and complexity of ventricular ectopic beats is shown in Table 6. The unpredictable relationship between plasma levels of antiarrhythmic drugs and ectopic activity in individual patients is evident.

Among 16 patients who have been treated with a dose-adjusted plasma level monitored

Table 6.

RECURRENT CARDIAC ARREST					LONG–TERM SURVIVORS				
AGE	SEX	DX	PLASMA LEVEL (µg/ml)	VED's (beats/hr)	AGE	SEX	DX.	PLASMA LEVEL (µg/ml	VED's (beats/hr)
66	M	CAD	PA = 0.3	2	73	F	CAD	QU = 2.7	0
			PA = 7.0	56			ASH	QU = 3.3	9
			PA = 4.5	20				QU = 4.6	0
			PA = 3.7	94				QU = 2.8	3
21	M	CM	QU = 1.8	1	60	F	CAD	QU = 4.0	1
			QU = 1.1	2				QU = 6.0	1
			QU = 2.4	2				QU = 4.1	13
			QU = 1.4	3				QU = 4.6	91
55	M	CAD	PA = 7.1	435	74	M	CAD	PA = 9.0	88
			PA = 4.0	692				PA = 6.3	54
			PA = 3.0	19				PA = 4.7	56
			PA = 1.3	19				PA = 5.0	144
60	M	AI	PA = 2.8	3	59	F	CM	QU = 4.2	6
			PA = 1.5	26				QU = 2.6	2
			PA = 2.1	180				QU = 4.4	60
			PA = 4.8	8				QU = 3.2	3

Examples of the relationship between plasma levels of quinidine (QU) or procainamide (PA) and average hourly frequency of ventricular ectopic beats (VED's) in survivors of prehospital cardiac arrest. Patterns in 4 selected patients who had a recurrent cardiac arrest (left panel) are compared to 4 selected patients who continue as long-term survivors for > 12 months (right panel). See text.
Therapeutic levels: QU = 2.3 - 6.0 µg/ml; PA = 4.0 - 8.0 µg/ml.
Modified from Myerburg et al [9].

antiarrhythmic drug regimen, 8 have survived for 12 months or more, and 8 have had recurrent cardiac arrests as of late 1978. Plasma levels of antiarrhythmic agents were measured during the 30 to 60 minute period before a scheduled dose on the same day that monthly Holter monitor tapes were recorded. The tapes recorded during the 4 months prior to the 8 recurrent cardiac arrests were compared to tapes matched for time of entry and duration of follow-up in the 8 patients who had not had a recurrent cardiac arrest. Among these tapes, transient or persistent complex ventricular arrhythmias were recorded on 47 of the 63 monthly tapes (75 %). The difference between ventricular ectopic beats in the recurrent cardiac arrest patients, and ventricular ectopic beats in patients who have not had a recurrent cardiac arrest, was not significant ($p > 0.2$) (see Table 7). In contrast, all 8 recurrent cardiac arrest patients had unstable plasma levels of antiarrhythmic agents during the 4 months prior to their recurrent cardiac arrests (21 of 31 determinations subtherapeutic – see Table 7), while 6 of the 8 patients who have not had recurrent cardiac arrests had consistently therapeutic blood levels (27 of 32 determinations therapeutic – see Table 7), $p < 0.01$. Thus, therapeutic plasma levels of antiarrhythmic agents may be antifibrillatory, despite their failure to predictably suppress chronic asymptomatic ventricular ectopic activity. This hypothesis of a dissociation between predictable suppression of chronic ventricular ectopic activity and protection against recurrent cardiac arrest by membrane-active drugs suggests that clinical effectiveness of antiarrhythmic agents may not necessarily be measured only by their effect on chronic ventricular ectopic activity (9).

Table 7.

	PLASMA LEVELS		VED'S/HR. ON 24 HR. HOLTER TAPES
	THERAPEUTIC	SUB-THERAPEUTIC	
RECURRENT CARDIAC ARREST	10	21	Mean = 153/hr. Median = 19/hr.
LONG-TERM SURVIVORS	27	5	Mean = 122/hr. Median = 8/hr.
	p < .01		p > .20
	x^2; 2 X 2 table with Yates correction		Wilcoxan 2 sample rank test

4. CONCLUSIONS

A complete analysis of the problem of prehospital cardiac arrest requires the inclusion of all electrophysiologic mechanisms by which prehospital cardiac arrest victims may present. When this is done, 3 distinct groups evolve: 1) those who present with ventricular fibrillation, in whom the chances of successful resuscitation and hospitalization are about 40 %, with 59 % of the hospitalized patients ultimately being discharged alive; 2) those who present with ventricular tachycardia, in whom the chances of both initial resuscitation and ultimate discharge from the hospital are considerably better than the ventricular fibrillation group; and 3) those who present with various forms of bradyarrhythmias or asystole in whom the chances of initial resuscitation are dismal (9 %), and the chances of long-term survival virtually nil.

In the ventricular fibrillation group, the overall chances for successful resuscitation, hospitalization and subsequent discharge from the hospital alive, appear to be improving. Statistically, the improvement appears to be during the hospital phase, but improved field activities are very likely providing the hospital with patients in better condition, and, therefore, having a better chance for long-term survival.

There is some evidence that acute injury to the specialized conducting system influences very early prognosis. Bradyarrhythmias after resuscitation and the presence of AV block and/or intraventricular conduction disturbances are bad prognostic indicators during the prehospital phase and the first 24 to 48 hours after hospitalization. In the latter group, despite evidence of intraventricular conduction abnormalities, recurrent cardiac arrests occur by the mechanism of ventricular fibrillation.

The vast majority of in-hospital deaths (as opposed to early recurrent cardiac arrests in resuscitated patients) occur in those patients with central nervous system involvement and its consequences, and in those patients with severe cardiac functional abnormalities.

Clinical and hemodynamic data demonstrate that, while long-term survivors as a group have severe heart disease, a significant percentage of the long-term survivors have normal hemodynamics and mild to moderate abnormalities of left ventricular contraction patterns.

In patients who present with ventricular fibrillation, currently available techniques suggest that the electrophysiologic disturbance predisposing to the index event are transient, not demonstrable after 72 hours by either intracardiac or non-invasive techniques. Further studies are necessary in this area.

Data on long-term survivors of prehospital arrest who have frequent and complex asymptomatic ventricular ectopic activity suggests that there may be a dissociation between the ability or inability of membrane-active antiarrhythmic drugs to suppress chronic asymptomatic ventricular arrhythmias, and the ability or inability of the same drugs to protect against recurrent cardiac arrest. The hypothesis derived from the data presented, which requires further validation, is that stable therapeutic levels of antiarrhythmic agents may be antifibrillatory at times when they are not necessarily antiarrhythmic, "arrhythmic" referring to chronic ventricular ectopic activity.

ACKNOWLEDGEMENT

We are grateful to the personnel of the City of Miami and Metropolitan Dade County Fire Department Emergency Rescue Crews for cooperating in our efforts, and to Mrs. Thelma L. Gottlieb for secretarial and administrative support.

This work was supported by a Grant-in Aid from the National Heart, Lung and Blood Institute, NIH, NHLBI-HL-18769-04.

REFERENCES

1. Myerburg RJ: Sudden death. In: The heart, Hurst JW, Logue RB, Schlant RC, and Wenger NK, 4th edition, New York, McGraw Hill, 1978 chapter 49, p 727–733.
2. Liberthson RR, Nagel EL, Hirschman JC, Nussenfeld SR: Prehospital ventricular defibrillation. Prognosis and followup course. N Eng J Med 29:317–321, 1974.
3. Baum RS, Alvarez H, Cobb LA: Survival after resuscitation from out-of-hospital ventricular fibrillation. Circulation, 50:1231–1235, 1974.
4. Schaefer WA, Cobb LA: Recurrent ventricular fibrillation and modes of death in survivors of out-of-hospital ventricular fibrillation. N Eng J Med 293:259–262, 1975.
5. Copley DP, Mantle JA, Rogers WJ, Russell RO Jr, Rackley CE: Improved outcome for prehospital cardio-pulmonary collapse with resuscitation by bystanders. Circulation, 56:901–905, 1977.
6. Myerburg RJ, Sung RJ, Conde CA, Mallon SM, Castellanos A: Intracardiac electrophysiologic studies in patients resuscitated from unexpected cardiac arrest outside the hospital. Amer J Cardiol 39:275, 1977.
7. Greene HL, Reid PR, Schaeffer AH: Repetitive ventricular response in man – a predictor of sudden death. N Eng J Med 299:729–734, 1978.
8. Myerburg RJ, Briese FW, Conde CA, Mallon SM, Liberthson RR, Castellanos A: Long-term antiarrhythmic therapy in survivors of prehospital cardiac arrest: Initial 18 months' experience. JAMA 238:2621–2624, 1977.
9. Myerburg RJ, Conde CA, Sheps DS, Appel RA, Kiem I, Sung RJ, Castellanos A: Antiarrhythmic drug therapy in survivors of prehospital cardiac arrest: Comparison of effects on chronic ventricular arrhythmias and on recurrent cardiac arrest. Circulation, 59:855–863, 1979.
10. Winkle RA: Antiarrhythmic drug effect mimicked by spontaneous variability of ventricular ectopy. Circulation, 57:1116–1121, 1978.
11. Morganroth J, Michelson EL, Horowitz LN, Josephson ME, Pearlman AS, Dunkman WB: Limitations of routine long-term electrocardiographic monitoring to assess ventricular ectopic frequency. Circulation, 58:408–411, 1978.
12. Myerburg RJ, Conde CA, Sung RJ, Mayorga-Cortes A, Mallon OM, Sheps DS, Appel RA, Castellanos A: Clinical, electrophysiologic, and hemodynamic profile of patients resuscitated from prehospital cardiac arrest. Am J Med (in press).

3.2. CCU FINDINGS USEFUL FOR IDENTIFICATION OF SUDDEN DEATH CANDIDATES IN THE POST-HOSPITAL PHASE OF MYOCARDIAL INFARCTION

K.I. LIE, V. MANGER CATS and D. DURRER

1. INTRODUCTION

Sudden death has been reported to occur in 3.7 to 18.7 % of patients discharged from the hospital after acute myocardial infarction (1–4). It is generally believed that sudden death is by far the most common cause of death outside the hospital after myocardial infarction discharge (1–4), and is probably caused by the occurrence of ventricular fibrillation. Various studies were carried out to determine the factors predisposing to its occurrence (4–6).

It was suggested that there is a possible relationship between factors such as presence and degree of ventricular arrhythmias occurring late in the hospital course, the size of infarction and degree of left ventricular dysfunction and subsequent risk for sudden death (6–10). The present study was undertaken to investigate the prognostic significance of early characteristics of patients admitted to the coronary care unit (CCU) with a diagnosis of documented myocardial infarction. Only those parameters that can easily be obtained by non-invasive methods will be taken into consideration.

2. MATERIAL AND METHODS

This study was carried out in patients consecutively admitted to the CCU in the years 1972–1976 with a diagnosis of acute myocardial infarction. Patients over 70 years of age and those who were transferred from other hospitals to our CCU were excluded from the study. The diagnosis of infarction was based on a typical history of chest pain correlated with the appearance of diagnostic Q-waves and evolutionary ST-segment or T-wave changes and a serial rise of serum enzymes (CPK, SGOT and LDH). Infarction was localized according to criteria proposed by the New York Heart Association (11). The size of infarction was estimated by measuring SGOT every 6 hours until peak value was reached.

The stay in the CCU ranged from 3 to 7 days, and during this period continuous electro-cardiographic monitoring was performed in all patients. A 14-lead electrocardiogram was obtained twice daily. Special attention was given to early major complications, which included the occurrence of major ventricular arrhythmias, supraventricular tachycardias, atrioventricular (AV) nodal conduction disturbances, bundle branch block, a pericardial friction rub and heart failure. Patients with supraventricular tachycardias or conduction disturbances on admission were included in the study only if the rhythm or conduction disturbance was either transient or not evident in an electrocardiogram taken 6 months or less before admission. Because antiarrhythmic intervention may influence the incidence of major ventricular arrhythmias (12), these arrhythmias were studied only in patients whose antiarrhythmic therapy was withheld on purpose. During the latter study (13) continuous tape recording was performed during the first 12 hours of admission. The presence and degree of heart failure were classified according to criteria proposed by Killip and Kimball (14).

After CCU discharge the patients entered a clinical rehabilitation program with a duration varying from 2–4 weeks. After hospital discharge the patients were seen at the outpatient clinic at 3-month intervals. Beta-blocking agents were not given prophylactically in asymptomatic patients. Sudden death was defined as death (preferably witnessed) occurring within 1 hour. The significance of differences between mean ages and mean peak values of SGOT were tested with the Student's t test. A chi square test was used to test the significance of differences in incidence.

3. RESULTS

During the study period 1,200 patients under the age of 70 were consecutively admitted to the CCU with a documented acute myocardial infarction. Of these 1,200, 192 (16 %) died in hospital. Incidence and the associated mortality rate of the most common major complications are presented in Table 1. Complications such as pulmonary edema, cardiogenic shock and cardiac rupture are not listed in Table 1 in view of the nature of this study. Of the 1,008 hospital survivors of myocardial infarction, 26 died suddenly within 1 year after their infarction. The CCU complications of these 26 are contrasted with those of the remaining 982 1-year survivors in Tables 2 and 3.

CCU data shown to be significantly related to a higher incidence of sudden death were; 1) anteroseptal site of infarction; 2) mean peak SGOT level (Table 2); and 3) CCU complications such as bundle branch block and moderate heart failure (Killip class II) as is evident in Table 3. All 5 patients with sudden death having bundle branch block in the setting of anteroseptal infarction also had heart failure in the CCU. In the subgroup of

Table 1. Incidence of major complications and hospital mortality.

	No.	Incidence (%)	Hospital mortality (%)
All patients	1200	100	16
Atrial fibrillation	96	8	33
AV nodal block	134	11	24
Bundle branch block	85	7	73
Primary ventricular fibrillation	36	3	12
Congestive heart failure	229	19	25

Table 2. CCU data of 26 sudden death patients and the 982 one year survivors of AMI.

	sudden death (N = 26)	1 yr survivors (N = 982)
mean age	63.8	62.9
sex male	22	390
female	4	292
previous infarction (%)	20	22
site of infarction		
anterior	5	271
inferior	5	468
ant. + inf.	2	34
anteroseptal with BBB	5	27[a]
anteroseptal without BBB	9	182[b]
mean peak SGOT	136	104[b]

[a] p < 0.01.
[b] p < 0.05.

Table 3. CCU complications in the 26 sudden death patients and in the 982 1-year survivors.

	N = 26	N = 982	p value
Atrial fibrillation	1	62	n.s.
Primary ventricular fibrillation	3	28	n.s.
AV nodal block	2	102	n.s.
Bundle branch block	5	21	0.01
Pericarditis	5	121	n.s.
Heartfailure	14	222	0.05

hospital survivors with moderate heart failure at the CCU however, the incidence of sudden death in those showing bundle branch block was approximately 20 % compared to 6 % in patients without bundle branch block.

Table 4 shows the time interval between onset of infarction and sudden death in the 26 patients classified according to their site of infarction and presence or absence of bundle branch block. It is of interest that 4 of the 5 patients with bundle branch block and anteroseptal infarction died suddenly within 6 weeks after infarction while this preference for early death was not found in the other 21 patients.

4. DISCUSSION

In this retrospective study we have attempted to evaluate some early characteristics of hospital survivors of myocardial infarction, who have a higher risk for sudden death after hospital discharge. The results of this study suggest that factors such as site of infarction, presence of bundle branch block, heart failure and large size of infarction occur more

Table 4. Time of onset of SD after AMI in the 26 patients classified according to their site of infarction and presence or absence of BBB.

time interval after AMI	anteroseptal BBB +	anteroseptal BBB −	other sites
3–6 weeks	4	2	1
6 weeks – 3 months	1	3	4
3–6 months	–	2	4
6–12 months	–	2	3

frequently in the sudden death patients. However, among the 26 sudden death patients in our study, the subset with bundle branch block and anteroseptal infarction seems to behave differently since 4 of the 5 sudden deaths with this type of infarction (Table 4) occurred within 6 weeks after the infarction. In addition 4 of 7 patients with early (< 6 weeks after onset of infarction) sudden death had the early characteristics of bundle branch block and anteroseptal infarction.

In this respect, it is of interest to note that these patients resemble those with the so-called late in-hospital ventricular fibrillation. The latter type of ventricular fibrillation occurs preferentially 2-6 weeks after infarction (15, 16). During a 5 1/2 year retro- and prospective study we found that more than 50 % of the patients with late in-hospital ventricular fibrillation had anteroseptal infarction and bundle branch block (Table 5). A predominance of this type of infarction was not encountered among patients with either primary or secondary ventricular fibrillation.

Two other interesting observations made during our prospective study of patients with late in-hospital ventricular fibrillation should also be mentioned. One of them relates to the mode of onset of late in-hospital ventricular fibrillation. Usually these patients developed ventricular fibrillation following a phase of ventricular tachycardia with a high ventricular rate which deteriorated into ventricular fibrillation. This pattern of initiation is different from that seen in primary ventricular fibrillation, where deterioration usually occurs following a short run of ventricular premature beats. The other observation relates to our findings of ventricular aneurysms during the angiographic and/or post mortem examination in our patients with bundle branch block and anteroseptal infarction.

Table 5. Incidence of different types of in-hospital ventricular fibrillation in relation to time after onset of infarction.

time interval after AMI	Type of VF primary	Type of VF secondary	late
first 6 hours	24	4	–
6–24 hours	6	6	–
1–6 days	5	15	–
2–4 weeks	–	3	16[a]
4–6 weeks	–	–	13[a]

[a] including 15 with bundle branch block and anteroseptal infarction.

In the light of the latter findings of our in-hospital study and the present observations of the early sudden death patients we may conclude that:

1) Early (3–6 weeks after AMI) sudden death after discharge may be identical to late in-hospital ventricular fibrillation.

2) These patients are often characterized in the CCU by the presence of anteroseptal myocardial infarction and bundle branch block.

3) Early development of aneurysm seems to be the anatomical substrate.

4) The electrocardiographic event prior to sudden death is probably the deterioration of ventricular tachycardia into ventricular fibrillation.

REFERENCES

1. Coronary Drug Project Research Group: Prognostic importance of premature beats following myocardial infarction. JAMA 223:1116–1124, 1973.

2. Vismara LA, Amsterdam EA, Mason DT: Relation of ventricular arrhythmias in the late hospital phase of acute myocardial infarction to sudden death after hospital discharge. Amer J Med 59:6–12, 1975.

3. Van Durme JP, Pannier RH: Prognostic significance of ventricular dysrhythmias 1 year after myocardial infarction. Amer J Cardiol (abstr) 37:178 1976.

4. Lie KI, Roels-van IJsseldijk YC, Vermeulen A, Wellens HJJ: Een prospectieve studie van de 1-jaars overleving en van de werkhervatting na het infarct. Ned Tijdschr v Geneesk. 119:1980–1893, 1975.

5. Kannel WB, Doyle JT, McNamara PM, Quickenton P, Gordon T: Precursors of sudden coronary death. Circulation 51:606–613, 1975.

6. Kuller L: Sudden death in arteriosclerotic heart disease. Amer J Cardiol 24:617–628, 1969.

7. Kotler MN, Tabatznik B, Mower MN, Tominaga S: Prognostic significance of ventricular ectopic beats with respect to sudden death in the late postinfarction period. Circulation 47:959–966, 1973.

8. Schulze RA, Strauss HW, Pitt B: Sudden death in the year following myocardial infarction. Relation to ventricular premature contractions in the late hospital phase and L.V. ejection fraction. Amer J Med 62:192, 1977.

9. Vismara LA, Vera Z, Foerster JM: Identification of sudden death risk factors in acute and chronic coronary artery disease. Amer. J Cardiol 39:821–828, 1977.

10. Multicentre international study: Improvement in prognosis of myocardial infarction by long-term beta-adrenoreceptor blockade using practolol. British Med J 3:735–740, 1975.

11. Nomenclature and Criteria for Diagnosis: The Criteria Committee of the New York Heart Association: Diseases of heart and blood vessels. Boston, Little Brown, 1973, (seventh edition), p 98–99.

12. Lie KI, Wellens HJJ, van Capelle FJ, Durrer D: Lidocaine in the prevention of primary ventricular fibrillation. N Engl J Med 291:1324–1327, 1974.

13. Lie KI, Wellens HJJ, Downar E, Durrer D: Observations on patients with primary ventricular fibrillation complicating acute myocardial infarction. Circulation 52:755–759, 1975.

14. Killip T, Kimball JT: Treatment of myocardial infarction in a coronary care unit: a two year experience with 250 patients Amer J Cardiol 20:457–464, 1976.

15. Lie KI, Liem KL, Schuilenburg RM, David GK, Durrer D: Early identification of patients developing late in-hospital ventricular fibrillation after discharge from the CCU. Amer J Cardiol 41:674–677, 1978.

6. Lie KI, Liem KL, Durrer D: Management in hospital of ventricular fibrillation complicating acute myocardial infarction. British Heart J 40:78–82, 1978.

3.3. FACTORS ASSOCIATED WITH CARDIAC DEATH IN THE POSTHOSPITAL PHASE OF MYOCARDIAL INFARCTION

A.J. MOSS, J. DE CAMILLA and H. DAVIS

During the past ten years various cardiac and epidemiologic studies (1–3) have identified a spectrum of risk factors associated with cardiac death in the posthospital phase of myocardial infarction. A number of multivariate techniques have been utilized for identifying subsets of patients who are at high risk of death in the post-infarction period (4–6). The analytic power of these techniques is limited and these multivariate approaches have provided only minimal insight into the mechanisms responsible for cardiac death in the posthospital phase of myocardial infarction. Beginning in 1973 a prospective longitudinal posthospital follow-up program was initiated in Rochester, New York, for patients discharged alive after recovery from acute myocardial infarction (7). This population serves as the basis for the current study. In this investigation the clinical and follow-up features of 96 cardiac deaths occurring in a 52-month posthospital period are presented and compared with a group of 96 matched control patients who survived. The purpose of this retrospective analysis is to identify the factors associated with cardiac mortality in the posthospital phase of myocardial infarction in order to better understand why post-coronary patients die. Such information should provide a proper data base for the development of more rational and effective secondary prevention programs.

1. METHODS

1.1. Population

The total study population consisted of 976 Monroe County residents, 796 men and 180 women less than 66 years of age, who entered coronary care units in two of Rochester's community hospitals between January 1, 1973 and December 31, 1976 with either a definite or probable acute myocardial infarction and survived the hospitalization. Definite myocardial infarction was substantiated by a combination of any two of the following: typical coronary-type chest pain, serial acute myocardial enzyme changes, or evolving Q wave abnormality with acute ST and T wave changes on ECG. Probable myocardial infarction patients had typical coronary-type chest pain with minor enzyme changes and/or acute ST and T wave changes on ECG. Patients and their private physicians were required to give informed consent before being entered into the study.

1.2. Data acquisition

The patients were interviewed during the last week of hospitalization by a nurse investigator and the hospital chart reviewed. The patients' medical history prior to entry and their clinical course during the CCU and subsequent hospitalization were recorded on prospectively developed forms as previously described (7–8). Numerous clinical variables were considered for the purposes of this study including: 1) demographic data; 2) smoking history; 3) New York Heart Association (NYHA) functional status prior to entry; 4) cardiovascular co-morbidity with ordinal classification of severity of diabetes, hypertension and other cardiovascular conditions; 5) severity of the acute coronary event in terms of hemodynamic and arrhythmic complications; 6) 12-lead ECG prior to discharge coded according to the Minnesota classification (9); and 7) a six-hour Holter ECG tape recording. The Holter recording was applied for six hours during ordinary daytime ambulatory activity in the last few days before discharge. The ECG tape recordings were analyzed manually using Avionic rapid (60 : 1) scan technique for: 1) basic rhythm; 2) maximum, minimum and average heart rate; 3) maximum ST segment shift; 4) atrial arrhythmias; and 5) ventricular arrhythmias. All ventricular premature beats (VPBs) were identified and quantitated in terms of: 1) average frequency – the total number of VPBs in the recording divided by the duration of the recording in hours; and 2) prematurity – the earliest coupling interval $(R - R')$ divided by the QT duration, i.e., $R - R'/QT$. In addition, the following VPB patterns were categorized as present or absent: 1) multiform configuration; 2) bigeminy; 3) pairs; 4) idioventricular rhythm; and 5) ventricular tachycardia. Ventricular tachycardia was defined as a run of three or more VPBs at a peak rate greater than or equal to 100 beats/min.

1.3. Follow-up

Patients were scheduled for follow-up evaluation every four months. Data collected at follow-up visits included interval cardiac history, blood pressure, medication usage, a 12-lead resting ECG, and a six-hour daytime ambulatory Holter recording which was analyzed as indicated above. The average interval (mean $\pm$ S.E.) between the last follow-up and cardiac death was 89 ± 11 days.

1.4. Mortality evaluation

When a nonsurvivor was identified during follow-up, the immediate family members, the personal physician, and witnesses of the terminal event were contacted by phone in order to obtain an accurate description of the events surrounding the terminal event. Specific questions were asked regarding prodromal symptoms, the social setting of the event, the character and duration of symptoms, the emotional and affective state of the patient, specific medications taken during the week before death, and cigarette use in the last week of life. Hospital records and postmortem examination findings were reviewed when available. The narrative data regarding the terminal event were abstracted and entered onto prospectively designed terminal event data forms as previously described (10). The major categories of the data form included the location of death, the underlying cause of death, the time interval between onset of acute symptoms and death, the immediate cause (mechanism) of death, and the medication use and cigarette smoking status in the week before death. Written criteria were established for each of the coded items.

The criteria for the underlying cause of death included: 1) definite acute myocardial infarction – either the standard clinical criteria (any two: chest pain, new Q waves in the electrocardiogram or abnormal serum enzyme elevation) or confirmation of acute infarction on postmortem examination; 2) probable acute myocardial infarction – either chest pain typical of coronary artery disease or acute ST and T wave changes in the electrocardiogram preceding death; 3) possible acute coronary event – sudden unexpected death without preceding symptoms, or an unobserved death without prior symptoms and without other apparent explanation; 4) chronic coronary heart disease – death in a patient with a chronic low cardiac output syndrome without an immediately preceding acute cardiac event; 5) death due to other cardiac causes – death related to bacterial endocarditis, pulmonary thromboembolism, coronary bypass surgery, etc.; and 6) death unrelated to cardiac disease – death due to noncardiac causes including cancer, suicide, homicide and accident.

The coding of all data on the terminal event form was reviewed by a three member mortality committee to insure uniform judgment for all categories. Differences in coding were resolved by thorough discussion, and a consensus was obtained on all items.

All patients who died before April 1, 1977 were identified. The 976 enrolled patients were exposed to the risk of dying from a minimum of four months, i.e., those who entered in December, 1976 to a maximum of 52 months, i.e., those who entered in January, 1973. The average exposure per patient to the risk of dying was 27 months. During this time, 108 patients died, and 96 of these were of cardiac cause. Postmortem examinations were performed on 20 % of the cardiac deaths.

1.5. Control group

Ninety-six controls (survivors) were matched with the 96 cases (deaths) on the basis of the initial hospital admission date (± 4 days) and the date of a survival follow-up examination (± 7 days) closest to the date of death in the mortality group.

1.6. Statistical analysis

Case-control analyses were performed using McNemar's chi square test with a correction for continuity (11) and a paired t-test in the case of continuous variables. When information regarding a variable was unavailable for a particular patient, that patient was excluded from the analysis.

2. RESULTS

2.1. Cardiac deaths, comparison with controls, and mortality chronology

Pertinent clinical characteristics of the 96 patients who died of cardiac cause are presented in Table 1 together with comparisons between the mortality group and the matched survivor controls. Mortality was not age-related in this population with an upper age limit of 65 years. Seventy-nine percent of the mortality group was male and 80 % had a definite

Table 1. Clinical characteristics of the 96 cardiac deaths and comparisons with the matched controls.

	Cardiac Deaths	Survivor Controls	Cardiac Deaths vs. Controls[†]
DEMOGRAPHIC			
Age in yrs (mean ± S.E.)	54.7 ± 0.8	52.8 ± 0.7	t = 1.78
Sex, male (%)	79	82	0.13
Social Class IV and V[‡] (%)	73	60	2.88
PREVIOUS HISTORY			
Hypertension (%)	31	27	0.21
Diabetes mellitus (%)	21	6	6.50*
Angina pectoris (%)	45	28	4.89*
Myocardial infarction (%)	34	10	14.70***
NYHA Functional Class II-IV (%)	55	30	9.88**
ACUTE HOSPITALIZATION			
Definite myocardial infarction (%)	80	76	0.26
Peel Index[‡] (mean ± S.E.)	10.0 ± 0.4	6.5 ± 0.3	t = 7.10***
Lowest systolic pressure in CCU - mmHg (mean ± S.E.)	88 ± 2	94 ± 1	t = 2.50*
Congestive heart failure[¶]	66	36	17.42***
Pulmonary congestion on X-ray[¶] (%)	43	14	18.23***
Predischarge ECG heart rate - beats/min (mean ± S.E.)	85 ± 2	78 ± 2	t = 2.85**
ECG Q/QS Pattern[¶¶] 1.11-1.12 (%)	62	39	8.82**
Holter - any VPBs (%)	70	46	8.20**
Discharge medication			
Digitalis	45	16	17.36***
Diuretics	32	15	7.31**
WORK-UP CLOSEST TO TERMINAL EVENT			
Minnesota ECG Code[¶¶]			
Q/QS Pattern 1.11-1.12 (%)	60	38	9.19**
ST Segment 4.1-4.2 (%)	32	16	7.50**
T Wave 5.1-5.2 (%)	49	31	6.24*
Holter VPBs			
Any (%)	80	54	12.03***
Multifocal (%)	41	20	8.04**

† Cardiac Deaths vs. Controls: comparisons were performed using McNemar's chi square test (11) and paired t-test in the case of continuous variables. Values are chi square unless denoted by t. Asterix indicates significance level: * $p<0.05$; ** $p<0.01$; *** $p<0.001$.

‡ Social Class IV and V: derived from the Hollingshead (12) five level occupational and educational class rank where levels IV and V are the lowest two levels of social class.

‡ Peel Index: the score was computed according to the method of Peel (13) with possible scores ranging from 1 to 28 (most severe).

¶ Congestive heart failure: significant pulmonary rales and/or pitting edema observed in CCU; Pulmonary congestion on X-ray: roentgenographic evidence of interstitial or alveolar edema in CCU.

¶¶ Minnesota ECG Code: Minnesota classification (9) in which: Q/QS pattern 1.11-1.12 indicates an anterior infarction; ST segment 4.1-4.2 categorizes $\geq$1.0mm ST depression; and T wave 5.1-5.2 denotes significant ischemic-type T inversion.

myocardial infarction on entry into the study; similar percentages were observed in the control group. Additional comparisons between the cardiac deaths and the survivors revealed that historical comorbidity, cardiac dysfunction, anterior infarction, and electrical abnormality were significantly more frequent in those who died than in the matched controls (Table 1).

Figure 1 illustrates the cumulative mortality as a function of time after infarction during the posthospital period. This mortality graph reveals the presence of two different slopes to the curve – an initial rapid, almost linear rise in the first six-months followed by a slower, exponential increase in the subsequent 7–52 months. Approximately 50 % of the cardiac deaths occurred in the early ($\leq$ 6 months) posthospital interval with the remaining half in the late (7–52 months) posthospital period.

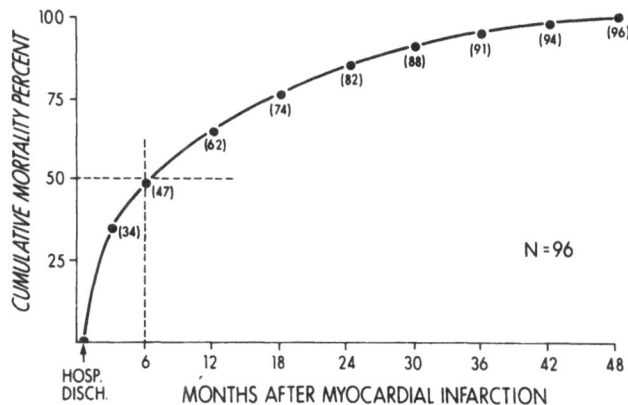

Figure 1. Cumulative mortality in 96 patients who died of cardiac cause during the posthospital phase after myocardial infarction. The parentheses at each data point contain the cumulative number of cardiac deaths which occurred in the specified posthospital interval after myocardial infarction. Fifty percent of the cardiac deaths occurred in the first six months after hospital discharge.

2.2 Comparison of early and late cardiac deaths

Those parameters which showed significant ($p < 0.05$) differences between the early ($\leq$ 6 months, n = 47) and late (> 6 months, n = 49) mortality groups are presented in Table 2. The early as contrasted with the late cardiac deaths had more anterior infarction, faster heart rates on the ECG prior to discharge, and a greater number of definite myocardial infarctions as the cause of death. The late as contrasted with the early mortality group had more patients with lower social class ranking, any VPBs on the work-up closest to the terminal event, and death occurring suddenly ($\leq$ 24 hours).

2.3. Case-control analyses of early and late cardiac deaths

Analysis of the early and late deaths with their respective controls (survivors) was carried out, and those variables which showed significant differences are presented in Tables 3

Table 2. Parameters showing significant differences between early ($\leq$ 6 mo) and late ($>$ 6 mo) cardiac deaths.

	Early (n = 47)	Late (n = 49)	Early vs. Late†
DEMOGRAPHIC			
Social Class Ranks IV and V‡ (%)	63	84	5.75*
ACUTE HOSPITALIZATION			
ECG Q/QS Pattern 1.11-1.12‡ (%)	75	47	6.49*
Predischarge ECG heart rate - beats/min (mean ± S.E.)	92 ± 3	79 ± 3	t = 2.03*
WORK-UP CLOSEST TO TERMINAL EVENT			
Holter - any VPBs (%)	71	90	3.92*
TERMINAL EVENT			
Definite myocardial infarction	34	14	4.24*
Sudden death ¶ (%)	54	73	7.34**

† Early vs. Late: values are chi square unless denoted by t. Asterix indicates significance level as in Table 1.

‡ Definitions are the same as Table 1.

¶ Sudden death: time interval $\leq$24 hours between onset of acute cardiac symptoms and demise.

Table 3. Early deaths ($\leq$ 6 mo): Case versus control comparison.

	Cardiac Deaths	Survivor Controls	Cardiac Deaths vs. Controls†
DEMOGRAPHIC			
Age in yrs (mean ± S.E.)	53.9 ± 1.2	53.6 ± 1.1	t = 0.19
Social Class Ranks IV and V‡ (%)	63	63	0.06
PREVIOUS HISTORY			
Diabetes mellitus (%)	26	4	5.79*
Angina pectoris (%)	53	32	4.35*
Previous myocardial infarction (%)	39	9	7.58**
NYHA Functional Class II-IV (%)	65	37	5.76*
ACUTE HOSPITALIZATION			
Peel Index‡ (mean ± S.E.)	10.8 ± 0.6	6.6 ± 0.5	t = 5.98***
Lowest systolic pressure in CCU - mmHg (mean ± S.E.)	85 ± 4	94 ± 2	t = 2.28*
Congestive heart failure‡ (%)	77	41	7.04**
Pulmonary congestion on X-ray‡ (%)	38	13	6.05*
Discharge medications (%)			
Digitalis	54	17	11.13***
Diuretics	28	17	1.07
WORK-UP CLOSEST TO TERMINAL EVENT			
Minnesota ECG Code‡			
Q/QS Pattern 1.11-1.12	76	44	8.52**
T wave 5.1-512	57	34	4.50*
ECG heart rate - beats/min (mean ± S.E.)	90 ± 3	77 ± 2	t = 3.57***
Holter VPBs			
Any (%)	71	46	4.50*
Multifocal (%)	39	5	10.56**

† Cardiac Deaths vs. Controls: McNemar's chi square, paired t test, and significance levels (asterix) as in Table 1.

‡ Definitions are the same as Table 1.

and 4. Both the early and late deaths had significantly more previous myocardial infarction, congestive heart failure, pulmonary congestion on x-ray, digitalis usage at discharge, high Peel index, and any VPBs (Holter) and ECG tachycardia on the work-up closest to the terminal event than their survivor controls. Early but not the late deaths had a significantly increased frequency of a history of angina pectoris, advanced NYHA classification, lower systolic blood pressure in CCU, anterior infarction, ischemic T waves, and multifocal VPBs (Holter) on the work-up closest to the terminal event than the matched controls. Late but not early deaths were significantly different from their controls with regard to an increased prevalence of lower social class, older age, and diuretic usage at discharge.

2.4. Variable combinations in early and late cardiac deaths

On the basis of the case-control analyses, historical (history of prior myocardial infarction), mechanical (congestive heart failure and/or pulmonary congestion), anatomical (anterior wall infarction), and electrical (VPBs on Holter closest to the terminal event) factors were selected to evaluate the effect of variable combinations in early and late deaths. In the early deaths (Table 5), the three most important factors were the historical, mechanical, and anatomical variables. Only 9.3 % of the cases had none of these variables, 23.3 % had one variable, and 67.4 % had two or three variables. The combination of mechanical dysfunction and anterior location of the infarction was observed in 55.8 % of the early cardiac deaths (Table 5: BC+ABC). The addition of the electrical factor (multifocal VPBs) to the other three factors did not improve the stratification process. In the late

Table 4. Late deaths (> 6 mo): Case versus control comparison.

	Cardiac Deaths	Survivor Controls	Cardiac Deaths vs. Controls†
DEMOGRAPHIC			
Age in yrs (mean ± S.E.)	55.4 ± 1.1	51.9 ± 1.1	t = 2.77**
Social Class Ranks IV and V‡ (%)	84	59	5.04*
PREVIOUS HISTORY			
Diabetes mellitus (%)	17	8	0.75
Angina pectoris (%)	38	25	1.39
Previous myocardial infarction (%)	32	11	5.82*
NYHA Functional Class II-IV (%)	45	25	3.38
ACUTE HOSPITALIZATION			
Peel Index‡ (mean ± S.E.)	9.3 ± 0.6	6.3 ± 0.5	t = 4.16***
Lowest systolic pressure in CCU - mmHg (mean ± S.E.)	91 ± 2	94 ± 2	t = 1.13
Congestive heart failure‡ (%)	61	31	9.33**
Pulmonary congestion on X-ray‡ (%)	48	15	11.25***
Discharge medication (%)			
Digitalis	38	15	5.26*
Diuretics	37	12	6.05*
WORK-UP CLOSEST TO TERMINAL EVENT			
Minnesota ECG Code‡			
Q/QS Pattern 1.11-1.12	47	33	1.44
T wave 5.1-5.2	43	29	1.57
ECG heart rate - beats/min (mean ± S.E.)	80 ± 2	71 ± 2	t = 3.01**
Holter VPBs			
Any (%)	91	63	6.75**
Multifocal (%)	43	37	0.08

† Cardiac Deats vs. Controls: McNemar's chi square, paired t test, and significance levels (asterix) as in Table 1.

‡ Definitions are the same as Table 1.

Table 5. Variable combinations in early ($\leqq$ 6 mo) cardiac death group.

Factors:

A = Historical (prior myocardial infarction)

B = Mechanical (presence of congestive heart failure and/or pulmonary congestion in the CCU)

C = Anatomical (anterior myocardial infarction by Minnesota Q/QS code 1.11-1.12)

Factor Combinations:	%
No factor	9.3
A	7.0
B	4.7
AB	9.3
C	11.6
AC	2.3
BC	37.2
ABC	18.6

Factor Grouping:	
No factor	9.3
Any one factor	23.3
Two or three factors	67.4

deaths (Table 6) the three most important factors were the historical, mechanical, and electrical variables. Less than 3 % of the late deaths had none of these variables, 27.8 % had one variable, and 69.4 % had two or three variables. The combination of mechanical and electrical dysfunction was observed in 63.9 % of the late deaths (Table 6: BC + ABC).

3. DISCUSSION

The postcoronary patients dying of cardiac cause in the posthospital period had more severe heart disease than their survivor controls. Similar observations have been noted by other investigators (1–3, 5, 6, 13, 17). Particularly striking was the predominance of prior myocardial infarction, left ventricular dysfunction (congestive heart failure and pulmonary congestion), anterior infarction, and ventricular irritability in the mortality group. Also, the distribution of the mortality over time identified the early period after hospital discharge as an interval of high risk. Fifty percent of all cardiac deaths over a four-year posthospital period (average risk exposure 27 months, range 4–52 months) occurred in the initial six months with the remaining 50 % occurring in the subsequent 7–52 months. The mortality rate (percent dying per month) is considerably higher in the early posthospital period relative to a lower rate later on. In addition, the cumulative mortality in the 7–52 month interval is almost perfectly exponential indicating a constant mortality rate in this period (14). The different mortality rates in the early and late posthospital intervals suggest that different pathophysiologic mechanisms are operative in the cause of the terminal event during these two periods. This conclusion is further supported by the fact that definite myocardial infarction and non-sudden demise were significantly more frequent in the early as opposed to the late deaths.

Table 6. Variable combinations for late (> 6 mo) cardiac death group.

```
Factors:

  A = Historical (prior myocardial infarction)

  B = Mechanical (presence of congestive heart failure and/or pulmonary
                  congestion in the CCU)

  C = Electrical (any VPB on Holter closest to terminal event)


Factor Combinations:                     %

  No factor                             2.8
  A                                     ---
  B                                     5.6
  AB                                    2.8
  C                                    22.2
  AC                                    2.8
  BC                                   33.3
  ABC                                  30.6


Factor Grouping:

  No factor                             2.8
  Any one factor                       27.8
  Two or three factors                 69.4
```

A comparison of the early and late deaths (Table 2) highlighted the relative importance of anterior infarction in the early deaths and ventricular irritability on the Holter recording closest to the terminal event in the late deaths. The case-control analyses of the early and late deaths further substantiated important differences between these two groups. Arbitrary categorization of variables into historical, mechanical, anatomical, and electrical parameters was based on clinical judgment and biostatistical significance. The combination of a history of prior infarction and left ventricular dysfunction in the CCU was common to both the early and late death groups. The combination of left ventricular dysfunction and anterior infarction was prevalent in the early deaths, and left ventricular dysfunction and ventricular irritability predominated in the late deaths. These combinations suggest important variable interactions, and more sophisticated multivariate survivorship analyses are being carried out on the total population to determine if synergistic interactions exist among these variables.

The current findings of a high frequency of certain variable combinations are of particular interest when viewed in the light of recent publications. Miller and co-workers found that anterior wall infarctions were associated with greater left ventricular dysfunction than other infarct locations (15). Furthermore, the British multicenter practolol trial observed that anterior infarcts carried a high mortality in the placebo group, and practolol produced a significant reduction in the number of deaths occurring in patients with pretrial anterior infarcts (16). Ruberman, et al. recently demonstrated that complex ventricular premature beats identified on a one hour ECG tape recording made an independent contribution to an increased risk of cardiac death after myocardial infarction (17). In their report, more than 50 % of the patients entered the study three months or longer after their last infarction – a population chronologically analagous to our late mortality group.

It should be emphasized that only 6 % (6/96) of the entire mortality group (early and late deaths) had none of the historical, mechanical, anatomical, or electrical factors. In the total population of 976 patients, there were 150 patients without these four risk factors. The mortality rate in this subset was 4 % (6/150) during an average follow-up of more than two years. Thus a low risk, low mortality group which makes up one-sixth of the total population can be identified by the absence of prior infarction, left ventricular dysfunction, anterior infarction, and ventricular premature beats.

An interesting and striking finding was the predominence of lower social classes in the late mortality group. In the early-late death comparison (Table 2) one could not differentiate between a dysfunctional role of lower social class in the late mortality group versus a beneficial effect of upper social class in the early mortality group. However, in the case-control analysis (Table 4) the association between lower social class and late cardiac death was evident. This observation raises three provocative questions: 1) Is the increased mortality of the lower social classes in the late posthospital period due to some compromise in the delivery of health services to this group? 2) Are there unmeasured environmental factors like employment activity, life stresses, financial concern, diet, habits (smoking), etc. which occur more frequently in the lower social strata of society and contribute to an increased long-term postcoronary risk of cardiac death? 3) Does a reduced educational level inhibit the application of rational secondary preventive measures in the postcoronary patient? It is interesting that a number of retrospective studies have indicated that towards the end of the coronary disease process lower socio-economic classes are at an increased risk of cardiac death (18–20). The current study provides strong documentation for this association.

This study has many implications, especially regarding the planning of intervention trials to reduce posthospital cardiac deaths after myocardial infarction. A good risk, low mortality group can be identified, and these individuals need not be included in drug trials since the potential benefit to be achieved within this group is extremely small. Reduction in mortality should be directed towards favorably influencing the remediable pathophysiological mechanisms which appear to be operative in the cause of death. Cardiac death in the first six-month posthospital interval makes up 50 % of the four year mortality. These early deaths are associated with major myocardial factors (prior myocardial infarction, congestive heart failure and/or pulmonary congestion during the acute process, anterior location to the infarction). Therapy to improve global cardiac function should be emphasized during this period, and afterload reduction drugs would seem appropriate. After the first six month, cardiac death is associated with the combination of underlying myocardial disease and VPBs recorded during follow-up, the so-called electro-mechanical subgroup (21). Therapy to reduce ischemia and improve electrical stability is indicated in this late posthospital period, and beta adrenergic blocking drugs appear to be the agent of choice. Finally, the late cardiac death group contains a significantly larger percentage of the lower social class than does the late survivor controls or the early deaths, and further investigation into this sociologic phenomenon is warranted.

ACKNOWLEDGMENT

This work was supported in part by a grant from the Gleason Memorial Fund, Inc. Rochester, New York and Research Grant HL-15790 from the USPHS.

REFERENCES

1. Norris RM, Caughey DE, Mercer CJ, Deeming LW, Scott PJ: Coronary prognostic index for predicting survival after recovery from acute myocardial infarction. Lancet 2:485–487, 1970.
2. Vedin A, Wilhelmsson C, Elmfeldt D, Save-Soderbergh J, Tibblin G, Wilhelmsen L: Deaths and non-fatal reinfarctions during two years' follow-up after myocardial infarction. Acta Med Scand 198:353–364, 1975.
3. Schulze RA, Strauss HW, Pitt B: Sudden death in the year following myocardial infarction: relation to ventricular premature contractions in the late hospital phase and left ventricular ejection fraction. Am J Med 62:192–199, 1977.
4. Moss AJ, DeCamilla J, Engstrom F, Hoffman W, Odoroff C, Davis H: The posthospital phase of myocardial infarction: Identification of patients with increased mortality risk. Circulation 49:460–466, 1974.
5. Luria MH, Knoke JD, Margolis RM, Hendricks FH, Kuplic JB: Acute myocardial infarction: prognosis after recovery. Annals of Int Med 85:561–565, 1976.
6. Coronary Drug Project Research Group: Factors influencing long-term prognosis after recovery from myocardial infarction – three-year findings of the coronary drug project. J Chron Dis 27:267–285, 1974.
7. Moss AJ, DeCamilla J, Davis H, Bayer L: The early posthospital phase of myocardial infarction: Prognostic stratification. Circulation 54:58–64, 1976.
8. Moss AJ, DeCamilla J, Mietlowski W, Greene W, Goldstein S, Locksley R: Prognostic grading and significance of ventricular premature beats after myocardial infarction. Circulation 51, 52: suppl III:III–204–III–210, 1975.
9. Blackburn H: The electrocardiographic classification for population comparison: The Minnesota code. J Electrocardiol 2:5–9, 1969.
10. Moss AJ, DeCamilla J, Davis H: Cardiac death in the first 6 months after myocardial infarction: Potential for mortality reduction in the early posthospital period. Am J Cardiol 39:816–820, 1977.
11. McNemar Q: Note on the sampling error of the difference between correlated proportions or percentages. Psychometrika 12:153–157, 1947.
12. Hollingshead AB, Redlich FC: Social class and mental illness. New York, John Wiley and Sons, 1958, pp 398–407.
13. Peel AAF, Semple T, Wang I, Lancaster WM, Dall JLG: A coronary prognostic index for grading the severity of infarction. Br Heart J 24:745–760, 1962.
14. Gehan EA: Estimating survival functions from the life table. J Chron Dis 21:629–644, 1969.
15. Miller RR, Olson HG, Vismara LA, Bogren HG, Amsterdam EA, Mason DT: Pump dysfunction after myocardial infarction: Importance of location, extent and pattern of abnormal left ventricular segmental contraction. Am J Cardiol 37:340–344, 1976.
16. Multicentre International Study: Improvement in prognosis of myocardial infarction by long-term beta-adrenoreceptor blockade using practolol. Br Med J 3:735–740, 1975.
17. Ruberman W, Weinblatt E, Goldberg JD, Frank CW, Shapiro S: Ventricular premature beats and mortality after myocardial infarction. N Engl J Med 297:750–758, 1977.
18. Croog SH, Levine S: Social status and subjective perceptions of 250 men after myocardial infarction. Public Health Rep 84:989–997, 1969.
19. Kitagawa EM, Hauser PM: Differential mortality in the United States: a study in socioeconomic epidemiology. Cambridge, Massachusetts, Harvard University Press, 1973.
20. Jenkins CD: Recent evidence supporting psychologic and social risk factors for coronary disease. N Engl J Med 294:987–994, 1976.
21. Vedin JA, Wilhelmsson C, Elmfeldt D, Tibblin G, Wilhelmsen L, Werko L: Sudden death: Identification of high risk groups. Am Heart J 86:124–132, 1973.

SECTION 3
THE INDICATORS OF HIGH RISK FOR SUDDEN DEATH

SECTION 3B
METHODS FOR DETECTION OF HIGH RISK PATIENTS

3.4. FURTHER EVALUATION OF THE REPETITIVE VENTRICULAR RESPONSE IN MAN

H.L. GREENE, PH.R. REID and A.H. SCHAEFFER

1. INTRODUCTION

Paroxysmal ventricular tachycardia and fibrillation remain a major cause of death in many countries. Despite widespread use of antiarrhythmic agents in high risk patients, the improvement in mortality has been small. This fact may be due to the trial-and-error approach to the administration of antiarrhythmic agents. Such an approach itself reflects the inability of any testing procedure to detect reliably the ventricular electrical instability which predisposes to ventricular tachycardia and fibrillation and to detect when an anti-arrhythmic agent has conferred electrical stability to a patient's heart.

Many electrophysiologic tests have been studied in animal models to evaluate ventricular electrical instability (1–13). However, most of these techniques have only limited application to man (14–15). In the past decade various tests have been used in patients to assess the electrophysiologic characteristics of the human heart and the response to various cardioactive drugs (16–29). Many of these tests have been applied to patients known to have ventricular arrhythmias, and recent reports describe serial electrophysiologic testing procedures to assess the response of a patient to pharmacologic or surgical therapy (30–32).

We have reported on the ability of an electrophysiologic test to identify those patients at risk of paroxysmal ventricular tachycardia or ventricular fibrillation (33). The repetitive ventricular response, as we have defined it, separates subjects who are normal from patients with recurrent ventricular tachycardia. The repetitive ventricular response also identifies high-risk survivors of a myocardial infarction, and it may be an indicator of response to antiarrhythmic therapy (34). This report will outline further experience with this test in these and other patient groups.

Since our initial report, there has been considerable debate surrounding the significance of the repetitive ventricular response (35–36). Much of this debate centers upon methodology and terminology as well as mechanism and significance. Many studies have shown that right ventricular premature stimulation during right ventricular pacing can produce reentry within the proximal His-Purkinje system and bundle branches, both in patients with cardiac disease and in normal subjects (18–21). Characteristics of this type of reentry have been summarized by other authors, with some of the following characteristics noted in what has been termed bundle branch reentry:

1) His bundle deflections (H_2) precede the reentry beats (V_3).

2) The time from the onset of the premature ventricular stimulus to the retrograde His bundle activation (V_2H_2 interval) is prolonged.

3) The interval from the retrograde His bundle deflection to the reentry QRS complex (H_2V_3 interval) is normal or prolonged.

4) The QRS configuration of the reentry beat (V_3) is often similar to the QRS that is induced by electrical stimulation at the apex of the right ventricle, that is, a left bundle branch block, left axis deviation morphology.

5) The premature stimulus (S_2) which induces the reentry beat (V_3) often must be closely coupled to the basic driving ventricular stimulus (S_1), presumably causing retrograde block in the right bundle branch.

6) Reentry is rarely sustained, and it most often consists of only a single reentry beat (the V_3 phenomenon).

7) Bundle branch or proximal His-Purkinje system reentry occurs commonly in any normal or abnormal subject who has normal intraventricular conduction, but this type of reentry is rare in patients who have preexisting bundle branch block.

While we have used the repetitive ventricular response to identify a predilection for spontaneous ventricular dysrhythmias, other authors have suggested that it is necessary to initiate sustained ventricular arrhythmias by other types of programmed stimulation techniques to expose ventricular electrical instability (31, 32). Initiation of sustained ventricular tachycardia by programmed stimulation most commonly occurs by a mechanism of intraventricular reentry and less commonly by sustained bundle branch reentry (28, 29). Therefore, additional questions have arisen regarding the mechanism of production of the repetitive ventricular response as we have defined it.

We report here our further experience with the use of the repetitive ventricular response to identify patients at risk of spontaneous ventricular arrhythmias. This study will also evaluate the mechanism of production of the repetitive ventricular response and the significance of the suppression of the repetitive ventricular response by an antiarrhythmic agent. In addition, we will compare the results of various programmed stimulation techniques in the same patients.

2. MATERIALS AND METHODS

2.1. Patient population

The records of all patients who underwent any type of intracardiac electrophysiologic stimulation and/or recording studies between September, 1975, and April, 1979, at the Johns Hopkins Hospital were reviewed. Two-hundred twenty two patients in this group had been tested for the repetitive ventricular response as previously described, and ninety-two of these patients had the repetitive ventricular response (Tables 1 and 2). Four different groups of patients were studied.

1) *Normal controls* (N = 22) were patients referred for evaluation of chest pain syndromes who were subsequently found to have no heart disease.

Table 1. Patient population.

| | n | Age-Yr | | M/F |
		mean ± s.d.	(range)	
Normal controls	22	50 ± 14	(25 – 71)	15/7
Recurrent VT –				
no therapy	77	53 ± 14	(21 – 77)	54/23
oral therapy	26	52 ± 10	(25 – 71)	25/1
Survivors of recent MI	61	50 ± 11	(28 – 79)	56/5
CAD without MI	36	50 ± 10	(14 – 71)	34/2

Table 2. Patient population.

| | Total | Symptomatic ventric-ular tachycardia | | Acute MI | Normal subjects | Ischemic heart disease No recent MI or arrhyth-mias |
		No drugs	Oral Drugs			
Patients tested	222	77	26	61	22	36
Repetitive ventricular response	92	66	3	22	0	1
Repetitive ventricular response with HBE or RBE recorded	30	24	0	6	0	0

MI = myocardial infarction   CAD = Coronary Artery Disease
HBE = His bundle Electrogram
RBE = Right Bundle Electrogram
VT = Ventricular tachycardia

2) *Patients with recurrent symptomatic and refractory ventricular tachycardia* (N = 77) were referred for experimental antiarrhythmic drug therapy because of refractoriness to all available conventional agents. An additional 26 patients had a recent history of ventricular tachycardia but were taking adequate doses of clinically effective antiarrhythmic agents.

A subset of the study population of the patients referred for experimental antiarrhythmic therapy for refractory ventricular tachycardia consisted of twenty-seven patients. All of these patients were refractory to treatment with conventional antiarrhythmic agents, or continued use of these agents was precluded by adverse side effects. Nine of these twenty-seven patients had been resuscitated from ventricular fibrillation. All of these patients had electrophysiologic testing for the repetitive ventricular response both before and after an intravenous antiarrhythmic agent (aprindine), and all patients had been followed for at least nine months to determine the response to the drug (or until failure of the drug or death).

Patients were initially evaluated for the presence or absence of the repetitive ventricular response. When the repetitive ventricular response was present, the right ventricular catheter was maintained in that position during the drug infusion and in subsequent· repeat attempts to induce the repetitive ventricular response. Patients were classified simply on the basis of reproducible presence or absence of the repetitive ventricular response.

Aprindine was then infused intravenously at a rate of 10–15 mg per minute with frequent monitoring of the heart rate, blood pressure, QRS duration, and symptoms. A thirty minute time period was permitted after the infusion for drug distribution, and the patient was then re-evaluated for the presence of the repetitive ventricular response. Absence of the repetitive ventricular response before and after drug administration, by definition, meant that repetitive ventricular responses could not be elicited at any stimulus interval in at least two right ventricular sites.

After the electrophysiologic evaluation, all patients were given oral aprindine as the only antiarrhythmic agent, administered in divided doses two to three times a day. After discharge from the hospital the patients were evaluated at one to four week intervals with 24 hour ambulatory electrocardiographic recordings, serum aprindine levels, and clinical assessment of response. Serum samples, run in duplicate, were obtained immediately pre-dose for measurement of aprindine concentration. The therapeutic range was considered to be 1.0 to 2.5 μg/ml. The clinical response was evaluated without knowledge of the results of the electrophysiologic testing. The criteria for a "good" clinical response were: 1) more than 75 % reduction of ventricular premature beats, or improvement in the Lown arrhythmia classification; 2) reduction of clinical episodes of symptomatic arrhythmias; and 3) maintenance of therapeutic aprindine levels without the use of additional antiarrhythmic agents.

3) *Survivors of a recent myocardial infarction* (N = 61) were evaluated as a part of a research protocol investigating risk factors and indices of long term prognosis after myocardial infarction. Patients who had survived a recent myocardial infarction were eliminated from the study if they had a history of extension of the myocardial infarction, cardiogenic shock, hypotension, thrombophlebitis, pulmonary embolism, recurrent chest pain after the infarction, or either digitalis toxicity or electrolyte imbalance. All patients who were survivors of myocardial infarction were followed clinically and with Holter monitoring at 3 months, 6 months, and 1 year. Sudden cardiac death in the follow-up period was defined as sudden cardiovascular collapse causing death or requiring cardio-pulmonary resuscitation with documented ventricular tachycardia or fibrillation within one hour of onset of symptoms in a patient who had been relatively free of symptoms to that time. Symptomatic ventricular tachycardia was defined as syncope or pre-syncope associated with electrocardiographically-documented ventricular tachycardia. Patients in whom symptoms had developed had ambulatory monitoring repeated in addition to the schedule defined above. All patients were followed for at least one year unless death occurred earlier.

4) The final group consisted of *patients with ischemic heart disease* who had neither suffered a recent myocardial infarction nor who had any history of ventricular dysrhythmias (N = 36).

2.2. Electrophysiologic techniques

All patients were post-absorptive and nonsedated at the time of the electrophysiologic study. Informed consent was obtained, and when possible, all drugs known to affect cardiac conduction or refractoriness were discontinued 48 hours prior to study. Electrode catheters were inserted via cutdown or percutaneously in the antecubital and/or femoral veins and were positioned in the right atrium and the right ventricle. In thirty of the patients, an additional catheter was positioned at the level of the His bundle or right bundle for recording electrical potentials from these structures. The ventricular catheter was positioned, usually at the apex of the right ventricle, so that there were no mechanically-induced premature beats. The pacing stimulus was 0.9 milliseconds (msec) in duration at twice diastolic threshold, never greater than 4.0 milliamperes. If the pacing threshold was greater than 2 milliamperes, the catheter was moved to another site in the right ventricle. The right atrium was either paced at a 700 msec interval, or the patient was allowed to remain in spontaneous sinus rhythm. A single ventricular extrastimulus was introduced every eighth beat, initially at the QRS complex, and it was progressively moved toward the preceding T wave by 10–20 msec intervals until the stimulus reached the end of the T wave. At that time the stimulus was further moved toward the peak of the T wave at 10 msec intervals. Electrical diastole was scanned with the ventricular stimulus in this manner until ventricular refractoriness was reached or until repetitive ventricular responses were produced. Repetitive ventricular responses were defined as two or more ventricular premature beats in response to a single ventricular stimulus, reproducible, with a stable catheter position free of mechanically-induced ventricular beats (Figures 1 and 2). At similar coupling intervals the repetitive responses were obtained at least twice, and almost always three times, in order to be considered reproducible. A second position in the right ventricle (usually the right ventricular outflow tract) was stimulated in this manner if the repetitive responses were not identified in the first position.

An additional thirty-one patients had not only the stimulation technique performed as described above, but in addition they had single ventricular premature stimulation

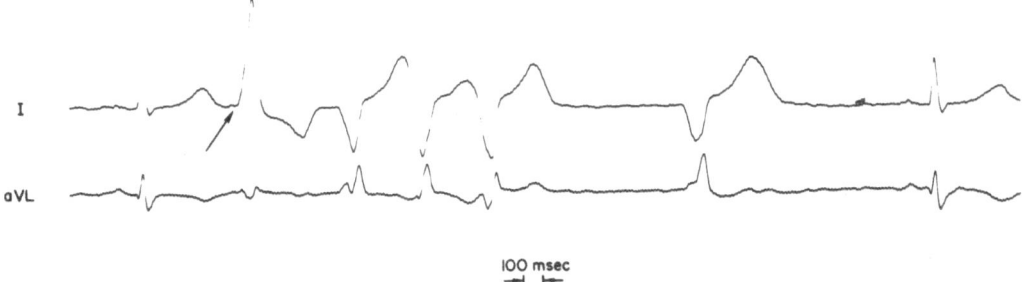

100 msec

Figure 1. Patient with the repetitive ventricular response. Surface electrocardiogram (ECG) leads I and aVL are recorded simultaneously with single ventricular extrastimulation during sinus rhythm. The ventricular extra-stimulus is denoted by the arrow. A single ventricular extrastimulus produces a QRS configuration with a left bundle branch block pattern. The subsequent four ventricular premature beats have a different configuration, and the QRS morphology changes slightly from beat to beat.

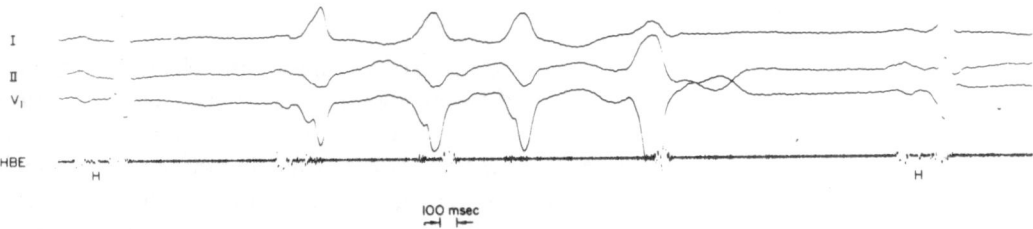

Figure 2. Patient with the repetitive ventricular response. Surface ECG leads I, II, and V₁ are recorded simultaneously with a His bundle electrogram (HBE). A single ventricular extrastimulus late in electrical diastole produces a QRS morphology with a left bundle branch block – left axis deviation pattern. The subsequent three QRS complexes are ventricular, and the QRS morphology is changing slightly, particularly on the last beat. His bundle deflections are recorded during sinus rhythm, but no His bundle deflections occur between the stimulated and repetitive beats or between subsequent repetitive beats. The last QRS is a fusion beat, but His bundle activity can be identified (H).

performed during ventricular drive (Figures 3–5). The procedure was identical to the one described above in these patients, except that testing was also performed at each right ventricular site with single ventricular extrastimulation during control of the ventricular rate with ventricular pacing at a cycle length of 600 or 700 msec. The mechanism of the reentry phenomena, whether bundle branch reentry or intraventricular reentry, was noted. Stimulation was discontinued if sustained ventricular tachycardia resulted, but otherwise the ventricular extrastimulation was continued to ventricular refractoriness at each site. Likewise, single ventricular extrastimulation during sinus rhythm or atrial drive was continued to ventricular refractoriness unless sustained ventricular tachycardia ensued, in contrast to the other 191 patients in whom extrastimulation was discontinued if simply repetitive responses occurred.

Multiple surface electrocardiograms (leads I, II, III, aVF, aVL, aVF, and V1 and/or other precordial leads) and intracardiac electrograms (right atrial, His bundle, or right bundle electrograms) were recorded simultaneously with an Electronics-for-Medicine VR-12 physiologic recorder and stored on a Hewlett Packard 3968 FM magnetic tape recorder for subsequent review. Cardiac stimulation was accomplished with a programmable digital stimulator and isolated constant current sources (Bloom Associates).

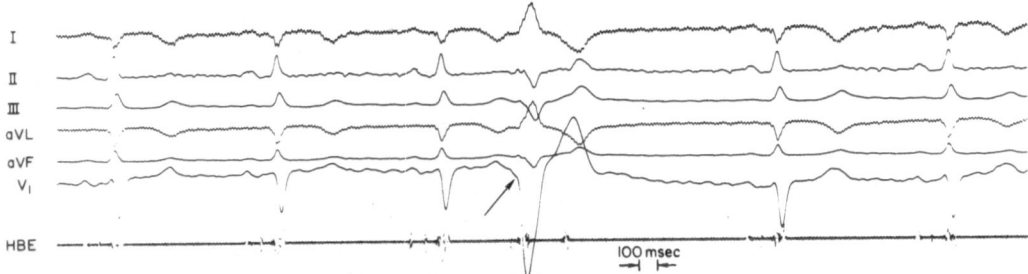

Figure 3a. Patient without the repetitive ventricular response. Surface electrocardiographic leads I, II, III, aVL, aVF, and V₁ are recorded with the His bundle electrogram (HBE). Stimulation during sinus rhythm produces only a single ventricular premature beat.

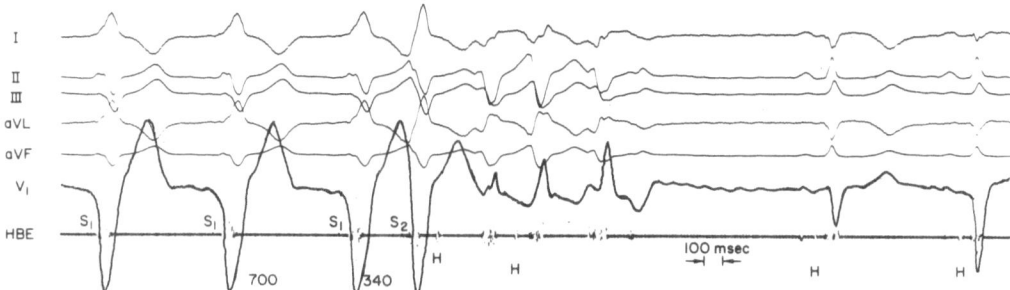

Figure 3b. Intraventricular reentry during ventricular drive and ventricular extrastimulation. During ventricular drive and ventricular extrastimulation in the same patient as Figure 3a, multiple responses occur after the single stimulated beat. A His bundle deflection occurs after the QRS induced by S_2, but it is probably only being activated coincidentally and is not responsible for the subsequent reentry beat. A His bundle deflection occurs between the first and second reentry beats, but the HV interval is short. Again this His bundle deflection is probably coincidental. A His bundle deflection is probably present *within* the QRS of the last repetitive beat just after the onset of the QRS (not marked with an H).

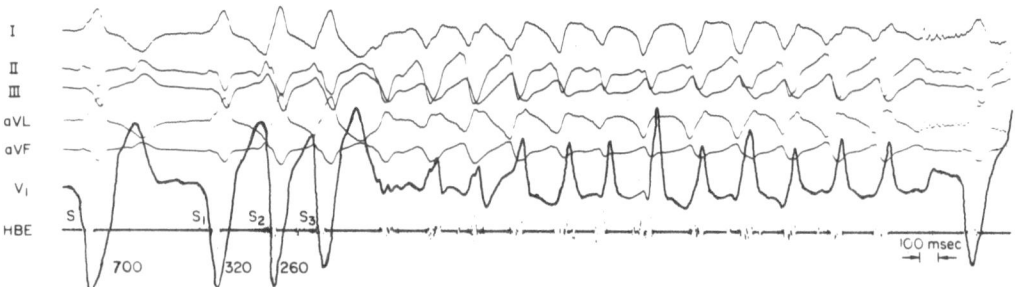

Figure 3c. Intraventricular reentry after double ventricular extrastimulation. Double ventricular extrastimulation during ventricular drive in the same patient as in Figures 3a and 3b produces multiple aRS complexes. Retrograde His bundle potentials could not be identified either between stimulated and repetitive beats or between subsequent repetitive beats. Surface QRS morphology likewise suggests intraventricular reentry as the mechanism for the repetitive beats.

2.3. Characteristics of the repetitive ventricular response

In thirty of the ninety-two patients with the repetitive ventricular response, an additional catheter had been positioned to record either His bundle and/or right bundle branch potentials during the stimulation procedures. In the other sixty-two patients who demonstrated the repetitive ventricular response, only right ventricular and right atrial stimulating catheters had been inserted. These two groups of patients were considered separately.

A. Conduction system deflections. In all thirty patients in whom either a His bundle or right bundle deflection was recorded during the stimulation technique, the presence or absence of a His bundle or right bundle deflection between the stimulated and repetitive beats was ascertained. Though absence of conduction system deflections can result from

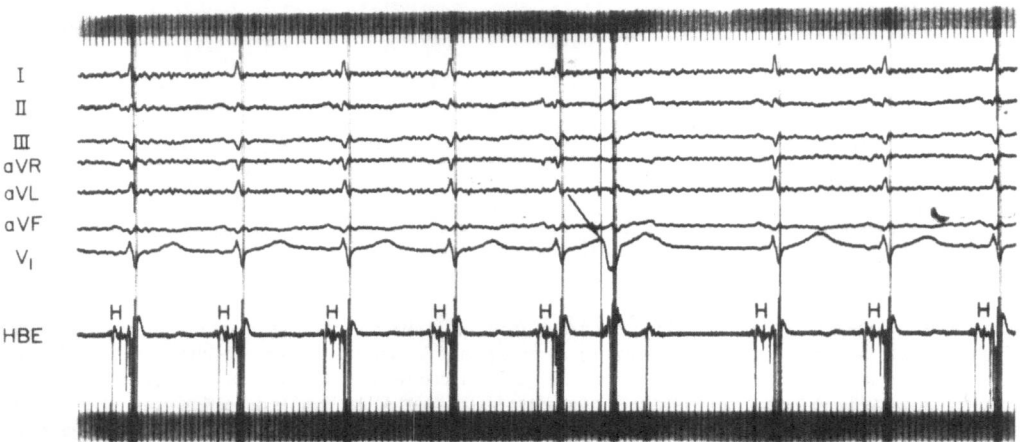

Figure 4a. Patient without the repetitive ventricular response. Surface electrocardiographic leads I, II, III, aVR, aVL, aVF, and V₁ are recorded with the His bundle electrogram. A single ventricular extrastimulus during sinus rhythm failed to elicit more than one QRS. Arrow marks the extrastimulus.

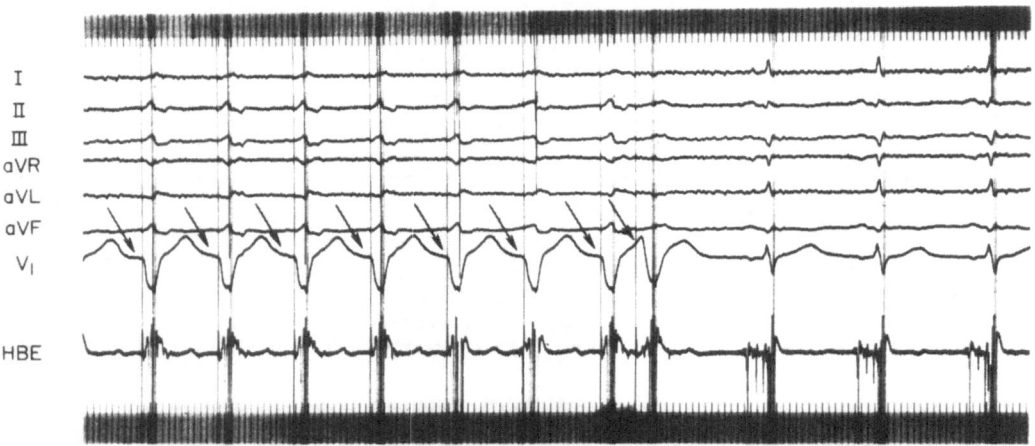

Figure 4b. No intraventricular reentry during single ventricular extrastimulation and ventricular drive. Single ventricular extrastimulation during ventricular drive in the same patient as Figure 4a produces only a single QRS complex.

catheter movement or fractionation and subsequent loss of amplitude of potentials, patients were carefully evaluated for these phenomena. All patients included in this report had reliable recordings of His bundle and/or right bundle potentials, and catheter positions were stable. Arrows mark stimuli.

B. *QRS configuration.* The frontal and/or horizontal plane QRS axis was evaluated to determine if the QRS configuration of the repetitive beat was similar to the QRS configuration of the beat induced by electrical stimulation via the right ventricular catheter.

Results were expressed as the change in degrees of frontal or horizontal plane QRS axis, whichever was greater, between stimulated and repetitive beats.

C. *Q-stimulus/QT ratio*. The prematurity of the ventricular pacemaker stimulus required to elicit the repetitive ventricular response was expressed by the ratio of the interval from the onset of the Q wave of the preceding QRS to the stimulus of the electrically induced beat (Q-stimulus) to the QT interval for that patient, measured in multiple simultaneously recorded electrocardiographic leads. Thus, if a closely coupled stimulus were required to elicit the repetitive ventricular response, the Q-stimulus/QT would be small. If a stimulus

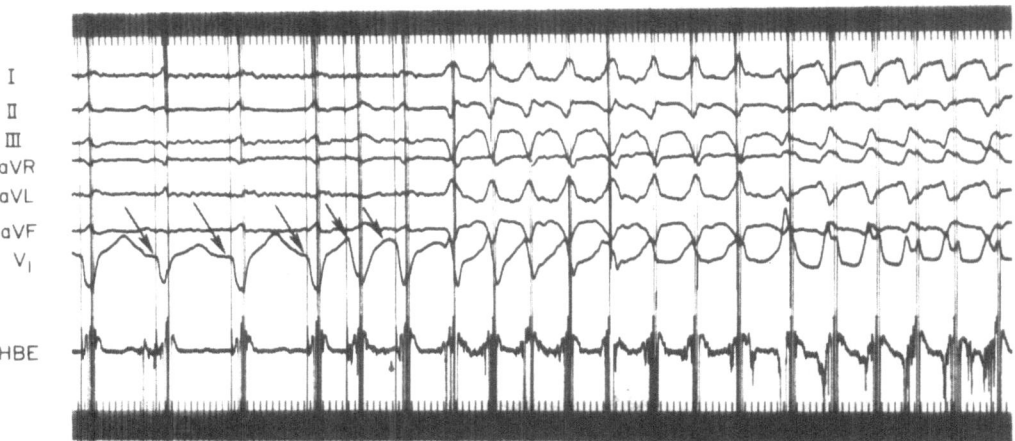

Figure 4c. Intraventricular reentry following double ventricular extrastimulation and ventricular drive. Double ventricular extrastimulation during ventricular drive in the same patient as Figure 4a and 4b produces sustained ventricular tachycardia with a change in QRS morphology. His bundle deflections cannot be identified between initiated and repetitive beats or between subsequent repetitive beats. This tachycardia most likely represents sustained intraventricular reentry.

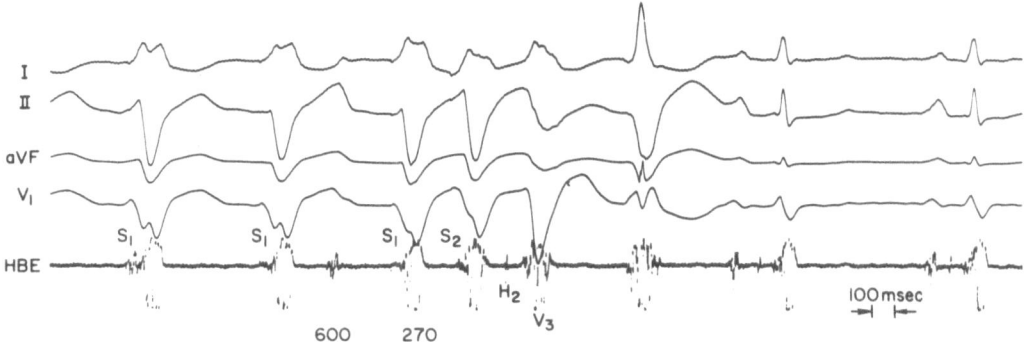

Figure 5. Bundle branch and intraventricular reentry in the same patient. Single ventricular extrastimulation during ventricular drive produces a bundle branch reentry beat. Between the stimulated beat and first reentry beat is a retrograde His bundle deflection. This first reentry beat has a left bundle branch block pattern. Another QRS follows the first reentry beat, and it has a different QRS morphology but is not preceded by a His bundle deflection. It probably represents intraventricular reentry.

late in diastole elicited the repetitive ventricular response, the Q-stimulus/QT measurement would be large.

D. *Number of sites tested*. Patients were classified according to whether the repetitive ventricular response was elicited at the first or second right ventricular pacing site. The first site was almost invariably the right ventricular apex, and in those patients in whom repetitive responses were not elicited in the first site, the second site was either the right ventricular outflow tract or the right ventricular inflow tract.

E. *Number of repetitive beats*. The maximum number of repetitive beats following the electrically induced beat were counted in each patient with attention to; 1) whether His bundle or right bundle deflections were associated with the subsequent QRS complexes; and 2) whether the QRS frontal or horizontal plane axis was changing on subsequent beats in those patients who had more than one repetitive beat.

2.4. Ventricular function

Many patients also had left ventriculography and coronary angiography performed by standard techniques. Ejection fraction was calculated from the single plane right anterior oblique ventriculogram or from a gated radioisotope blood pool scan.

3. COMPLICATIONS

Of the total 222 patients who were tested for the repetitive ventricular response or who were tested with ventricular drive and single ventricular premature stimulation who formed the basis for this report, four patients (1.8 %) developed sustained ventricular tachycardia during the testing requiring either overdrive pacing (1 patient), or external electrical cardioversion (3 patients). None of the four patients had any sequelae from these arrhythmias or cardioversion. No other complications occurred during this study.

4. STATISTICAL METHODS

Data were compared with Student's t test for paired and unpaired samples, Fisher's exact test for contingency, and the chi square test where appropriate.

5. RESULTS

5.1. Normal controls

None of these subjects had the repetitive ventricular response (Table 2). All twenty-two patients from this group were by definition normal. Seventeen of these patients had complete cardiac catheterizations, and left ventriculograms, coronary angiograms, and pressures were normal. All patients had normal 24 hour Holter monitors. All patients were alive after one year follow-up, none of them with a history of symptomatic ventricular tachycardia.

5.2. Patients with recurrent symptomatic ventricular tachycardia

Sixty-nine of these 103 patients had the repetitive ventricular response. Of the twenty-six patients taking adequate antiarrhythmic medications orally, only three had the repetitive ventricular response. Since these patients are still being evaluated in follow-up to determine if absence of the repetitive response in the face of chronic oral dosing of an antiarrhythmic agent other than aprindine predicts a good response to that agent, these patients will not be discussed further. However, the three patients who still had the repetitive ventricular response on oral antiarrhythmic therapy will be included in the evaluation of the repetitive responses themselves. Of the remaining seventy-seven patients, sixty-six had the repetitive ventricular response. Fifty of these seventy-seven patients had coronary artery disease, twenty-three patients had nonischemic cardiomyopathies of a variety of etiologies, and four patients had mitral valve prolapse. By definition, all of these patients had ventricular tachycardia on Holter monitoring at the time of entry into the study.

Twenty-seven of these patients had testing for the repetitive ventricular response both before and after intravenous aprindine therapy for their arrhythmias. Twenty-three of these patients (85 %) had the repetitive ventricular response prior to infusion of the drug. Following aprindine infusion, only six patients had the repetitive ventricular response (22 %). There was no difference in the aprindine infusion dose between those patients in whom the repetitive ventricular response was absent after aprindine (191 ± 26 mg, mean $\pm$ s.d.) compared with those in whom it remained (204 ± 9 mg). The mean dose for the entire group of twenty-seven patients was 193 mg (range 100–225 mg). The mean evaluation period after initiation of oral antiarrhythmic therapy with aprindine was 12 ± 7.3 months. A mean of twelve 24 hour Holter ambulatory electrocardiographic recordings were performed on each patient. Twenty-one of the twenty-seven patients (78 %) were judged to have a "good" clinical response. Mean daily oral dose of the drug was 119 mg (range 60–225 mg). There was no difference in daily dose between the patients with a good and a bad clinical response. Serum aprindine levels in those patients with a good response (2.1 ± 0.9 μg/ml) were not significantly different from those levels of patients who did not improve with aprindine (1.8 ± 0.4 μg/ml). Twenty of the twenty-one patients who were free of the repetitive ventricular response after the acute infusion of aprindine had a good clinical response to the oral medication, compared with only one of six patients in whom the repetitive ventricular response was present after intravenous aprindine ($p < 0.0005$). Four patients in this group of twenty-seven subjects suffered sudden cardiac death in one year follow-up. Three of these sudden deaths occurred in the group of twenty-one patients in whom the repetitive ventricular response had been abolished by intravenous aprindine. At a time when the patients were doing well without symptomatic arrhythmic episodes, their serum levels of aprindine were 1.8, 1.5, and 1.6 μg/ml. In two of these patients serum levels for aprindine were obtained after their cardiac arrest, and a serum level was obtained two weeks prior to the death of the third patient, and all were subtherapeutic (0.9, 0.8, and 0.9 μg/ml).

5.3. Survivors of myocardial infarction

All sixty-one patients in this group by definition had significant obstructive coronary artery disease, and all patients had suffered a recent myocardial infarction. The time from myocardial infarction to study ranged between 8 and 120 days, 24 ± 22 days, mean $\pm$ s.d. These patients were extensively evaluated as a part of another research protocol, and results of their nonelectrophysiologic evaluation are reported elsewhere (33). Twenty-two of these patients had the repetitive ventricular response. In one year follow-up, nineteen of these twenty-two patients had either symptomatic ventricular tachycardia or sudden death. Eight of the twenty-two patients had sudden death in the one year follow-up. Of the thirty-nine patients who did not have the repetitive ventricular response at the time of hospital discharge, only four patients had symptomatic ventricular tachycardia or sudden death in follow-up ($p < 0.001$). All four of these patients had sudden cardiac death as their manifestation of ventricular electrical instability ($p < 0.025$). There was no difference between patients with and without the repetitive ventricular response or with and without ventricular dysrhythmias in follow-up in age, male/female ratio, number of old myocardial infarctions, location of myocardial infarction, ejection fraction, number of patients with ejection fraction less than 0.30, left ventricular end diastolic pressure greater than 30 mmHg, number of vessels diseased, number of patients with left main coronary artery disease, number of patients with ventricular tachycardia recorded in the coronary care unit during the acute phase of the infarction, and number of patients with ventricular aneurysms. The patients with repetitive ventricular response had a higher incidence of Lown Class 4B and 5 arrhythmias at hospital discharge ($p < 0.02$).

5.4. Patients with ischemic heart disease without recent myocardial infarction or ventricular arrhythmias

Only one patient in this group of thirty-six patients had the repetitive ventricular response, and this patient was alive without history of symptomatic ventricular tachycardia one year after study. All other thirty-five patients were alive without symptomatic ventricular arrhythmias one year after initial evaluation.

5.4.1. Mechanism of the repetitive ventricular response

The repetitive ventricular response was present in a total of ninety-two patients. In this group, thirty patients had an additional catheter positioned to record His bundle or right bundle deflections during the stimulation studies. This group of thirty patients will be compared to the overall group of ninety-two patients with the repetitive ventricular response.

1) *Patients with the repetitive ventricular response who had His bundle or right bundle deflections evaluated.* In this group of thirty patients, twenty-four subjects had recurrent symptom-

atic ventricular tachycardia, and six patients were survivors of an acute myocardial infarction. Mean age of this group was 54 ± 16 years, ($\pm$ s.d., range 21–76 years). In the symptomatic ventricular tachycardia patients, nineteen had coronary artery disease, four had cardiomyopathies, and one patient had mitral valve prolapse. Eleven of these twenty-four patients had survived an episode of ventricular fibrillation which had not been associated with an acute myocardial infarction. An additional four patients had experienced syncope due to sustained ventricular tachycardia documented either by Holter monitoring or coronary care unit monitoring.

Table 3. Association of conduction system deflections with repetitive beats.

	Preceding QRS	Within QRS	Present in atrial rhythm, absent before repetitive beat
His	1	6	19
Right Bundle	0	3	1

In these thirty patients, twenty-nine had findings suggestive that reentry within the proximal His-Purkinje system or bundle branches was not the mechanism for the repetitive ventricular response (Table 3). In twenty-five patients the His bundle deflection was present in sinus rhythm but could not be identified between the stimulated and repetitive beats. In six of these patients the His potential could be identified within the QRS of the repetitive beat. In four additional patients in whom a right bundle branch deflection was recorded during the stimulation studies, the right bundle branch potential did not precede the repetitive beat. In three of these patients the right bundle potential could be identified *within* the QRS of the repetitive beat, and in one patient it could not be identified either before or within the repetitive beat. In one of these four patients, a His bundle deflection was also identified *within* the QRS of the repetitive beats. While recording of a right bundle potential within the repetitive beats in the three patients does not insure that bundle branch reentry is not occurring, the surface QRS pattern on the first repetitive beat had a right bundle branch block pattern, and in three of these four patients successive repetitive beats had a different QRS morphology with the right bundle deflections still located within the QRS. Though these findings remain less than absolutely confirmatory that bundle branch reentry is not occurring, their pattern does not fit the findings most commonly reported for bundle branch reentry.

In only one patient did a His bundle deflection occur between the induced and repetitive QRS complexes with retrograde $V_2 H_2$ prolongation, which would be compatible with reentry within the His-Purkinje system. However, in this patient the repetitive beat did not have a left bundle branch block configuration. Therefore, retrograde V2H2 or $V_2 RB_2$ delay was not necessary for the repetitive ventricular response in twenty-nine of thirty patients in whom it was evaluated.

The His-Purkinje system was, in fact, diseased in some of these patients. The mean HV interval ($\pm$ s.d.) for these thirty patients was 54 ± 14 msec. In only four patients, however, was the HV interval greater than 60 msec. If at any time there was ever any question regarding fractionated His bundle potentials or catheter movement, the catheter position was adjusted if necessary, and stimulation was repeated with careful attention to low voltage potentials recorded from the His bundle catheter between the stimulated and repetitive beats.

In these thirty patients who had His or right bundle potentials monitored during ventricular stimulation, four patients had preexisting right bundle branch block on the surface electrocardiogram, and three patients had preexisting left bundle branch block. The angle between the QRS axis of the electrically-induced and the repetitive beat is summarized in Table 4. In these thirty patients, the angle between induced and repetitive beats was $\geq 45°$ in twenty-four patients, and the repetitive beat had a right bundle branch block configuration in twenty-two of the thirty. The mean Q-stimulus/QT ratio was 1.19 ± 0.30 in these thirty patients.

Table 4. Angle between QRS axis[a] of electrically-stimulated and repetitive beats.

Angle	Repetitive ventricular response	
	All patients	30 patients with conduction system deflections recorded
0°−44°	19	6
45°−90°	17	4
91°−135°	18	5
136°−180°	38	15
$\geq 45°$	73	24
mean angle ±s.d.	108°±60°	122°±60°

[a] Maximum axis shift in either horizontal or frontal plane.

Eighteen of the thirty patients in this group had more than one repetitive beat, and in fourteen of these eighteen patients QRS morphology was changing from beat to beat.

In summary, all of these thirty patients with the repetitive ventricular response had one or more findings suggestive that His-Purkinje or bundle branch reentry was not the mechanism for the repetitive beats:

1) absence of His bundle or right bundle deflections preceding the repetitive beats,
2) repetitive beats $\geq 45°$ divergent from stimulated beats if stimulation was performed at the apex of the right ventricle, or not exhibiting a left bundle branch block – left axis deviation pattern if stimulation was performed elsewhere in the right ventricle,
3) right bundle branch block configuration of the repetitive beats,
4) a continually changing QRS pattern in the presence of more than one repetitive beat, and
5) lack of critical V_2H_2 prolongation necessary for His-Purkinje reentry.

The repetitive response occurred either in the presence or absence of preexisting conduction defects. It occurred both in patients who had and who had not experienced spontaneous ventricular fibrillation, but it never occurred in normal subjects. The repetitive ventricular response occurred both in the presence and absence of coronary artery disease and myocardial infarction.

2) *All patients with the repetitive ventricular response*. The total ninety-two patients with the repetitive ventricular response were found among three groups of patients: (a) asymptomatic survivors of a recent myocardial infarction (22 patients), (b) patients with recurrent symptomatic ventricular tachycardia (69 patients), and (c) patients with ischemic heart disease who had not had a recent myocardial infarction (1 patient). Mean age of all patients was 54 ± 12 years ($\pm$ s.d., range 21 to 80 years). No normal subjects had the repetitive ventricular response.

The survivors of an acute myocardial infarction with repetitive ventricular response consisted of twenty-two patients. The mean time from myocardial infarction to study was 31 ± 30 days ($\pm$ s.d., range 8 to 120 days).

In the group of sixty-nine patients with recurrent symptomatic ventricular tachycardia and the repetitive response, forty-six patients had coronary artery disease, nineteen patients had nonischemic cardiomyopathies of a variety of etiologies, and four patients had mitral valve prolapse. Prior to study, twenty-one of the sixty-nine patients with recurrent ventricular tachycardia had survived an episode of cardiac arrest with documented ventricular fibrillation or hypotensive ventricular tachycardia not associated with an acute myocardial infarction. An additional seven patients had experienced episodes of syncope due to ventricular tachycardia documented on ambulatory or continuous coronary care unit monitoring. Within the group of patients with coronary artery disease, old myocardial infarction, and recurrent symptomatic ventricular tachycardia ($N = 40$), the time from the most recent myocardial infarction to study ranged from 14 days to 24 years.

In the total group of ninety-two patients with the repetitive ventricular response, therefore, sixty-eight patients had coronary artery disease with a mean number of myocardial infarctions of 1.4 ± 1.0 (s.d., range 0 to 5). Only six patients with coronary artery disease had never had a myocardial infarction diagnosed clinically.

Mean ejection fraction ($\pm$ s.d.) in the entire study population of ninety-two patients' was 0.49 ± 0.16, $N = 55$ (range 0.20 to 0.84). In seven patients, ejection fraction could not be measured because of ventricular aneurysms. In a total of thirty patients, attempts to measure ejection fraction were not made. Only one patient had both normal overall ejection fraction and normal wall motion in all segments in those patients in whom ventricular function was analyzed. Virtually all patients, therefore, had some localized wall motion abnormalities, albeit minor. There was no difference in ventricular function between the entire group of ninety-two subjects with the repetitive response and the subset of thirty patients discussed above who had additional evaluation with catheter recording of His bundle or right bundle deflections.

In this group of ninety-two patients with the repetitive response, the mean HV interval was 52 ± 13 msec. Thirteen of these ninety-two patients had either right (8) or left (5) bundle branch block on the surface electrocardiogram during normal sinus rhythm.

Seventy-three of the ninety-two patients had $\geq 45°$ between the QRS axis of the electrically-stimulated and repetitive beats. The mean angle between the induced and repetitive beats was $108 \pm 60°$. In fifty-one of the ninety-two patients, the repetitive beats had a right bundle branch block configuration. The mean Q-stimulus/QT which produced repetitive responses was 1.14 ± 0.28. In sixty-four patients the Q-stimulus/QT ratio was ≥ 1.0; in seventy-three patients the Q-stimulus/QT ratio was ≥ 0.90. Local conduction delay (latency) was not required to produce the repetitive responses.

In thirteen of the total group of ninety-two patients (14 %) testing of a second right ventricular site was necessary to produce the repetitive response. In those thirteen patients the QRS axis between the stimulated and repetitive beats was $125 \pm 63°$. In addition, the repetitive beat had a right bundle branch block configuration in seven of these thirteen patients.

Table 5. Maximum number of repetitive beats after the induced beat.

Number of repetitive beats	Number of patients
1	48
2	11
3 – 5	17
6 – 10	2
11 – 20	1
> 20	13

Forty-eight of the ninety-two patients had only one repetitive beat after the stimulated beat. If this finding was reproducible, further stimulation was not performed. However, of the forty-four patients in whom more than one repetitive beat was present (Table 5), twenty-seven patients had QRS complexes which were changing on subsequent repetitive beats, implying that the reentry pathway or conduction was changing. More than one repetitive beat was equally common in patients who were and were not evaluated with the additional His or right bundle recordings.

5.5. *Comparison of different electrophysiologic stimulation techniques*

A total of thirty-one patients were studied both by single ventricular extrastimulation during sinus rhythm or atrial pacing and single ventricular extrastimulation during ventricular pacing. These results are summarized in Table 6. In this analysis, only intraventricular reentry was considered to be a "positive" finding. Patients who demonstrated bundle branch reentry (His-Purkinje system reentry) with the characteristics noted above were not considered to be "positive". Five patients had intraventricular reentry both during atrial drive and ventricular drive for control of the basic heart rate. Similarly, sixteen patients had no intraventricular reentry either during ventricular extrastimulation during atrial or ventricular drive. There were no patients who demonstrated intraventricular reentry during atrial drive or sinus rhythm who did not have intraventricular reentry during ventricular drive. On the contrary, ten patients had intraventricular reentry with ventricular drive but not during atrial drive or sinus rhythm ($p < 0.02$).

Table 6. Comparison of electrophysiologic techniques in eliciting intraventricular reentry.

		Ventricular drive *Single ventricular extrastimulation*	
		+	−
Atrial drive	+	5	0
Single ventricular extrastimulation	−	10	16

6. DISCUSSION

This further evaluation of the repetitive ventricular response in man supports our initial reports (33, 34). The technique is safe in patients who are clinically stable, even patients who have recently suffered a myocardial infarction. The repetitive ventricular response does not occur in normal subjects, and it is very common in patients who have already been identified as having recurrent, symptomatic, refractory ventricular tachycardia. Likewise, it can identify prospectively those patients who are at high risk of serious ventricular arrhythmias after a myocardial infarction. Suppression of the repetitive ventricular response by an antiarrhythmic agent administered acutely corresponds with the ability of that antiarrhythmic agent to suppress clinically significant ventricular arrhythmias when administered orally. Though the incidence of the repetitive ventricular response is high in certain select groups of patients, it is a relatively uncommon finding in patients who simply have ischemic heart disease with angina pectoris who have not suffered a recent myocardial infarction nor who have a history of ventricular arrhythmias. In this latter group of patients, symptomatic ventricular tachycardia or sudden death is relatively uncommon.

An electrophysiologic test which would detect the propensity of a patient to develop spontaneous symptomatic ventricular tachycardia or sudden death would be useful to apply to groups of patients already known to be at relatively high risk of these arrhythmias. Likewise, it would be useful to know when an antiarrhythmic therapy has conferred electrical stability to these patients who are at risk of potentially catastrophic ventricular arrhythmias. Until now, the selection of an antiarrhythmic agent has been based primarily upon a trial-and-error procedure. This method of drug choice primarily reflects the inability of any previously available tests to evaluate the likelihood that a patient will continue to have malignant arrhythmias after an antiarrhythmic therapy. The selection of an antiarrhythmic agent which is, in fact, ineffective in preventing ventricular arrhythmias may expose the patient to potentially life-threatening arrhythmias during the time that evaluation of the clinical responsiveness to the drug is taking place. However, repeated electrophysiologic testing may identify more rapidly those antiarrhythmic agents and dosages at which a patient is protected from his ventricular arrhythmias. In our study acute suppression of the repetitive ventricular response predicted a satisfactory response to that medication given orally. Such testing could likewise be applied to patients after chronic oral dosing when steady state has been achieved.

Many different electrophysiologic stimulation techniques have been used recently in an attempt to evaluate the likelihood that an individual patient will develop ventricular tachycardia or sudden death (22, 23, 28, 29, 31–33). Previous studies have demonstrated a high incidence of reentry phenomena after single or multiple ventricular extrastimulation during ventricular drive (18–21, 35, 36). These phenomena can occur in either normal subjects or patients with cardiac disease. Many investigators have defined the characteristics of bundle branch reentry which characterize these reentry phenomena (18–19). On the other hand, intraventricular reentry phenomena are abnormal and are associated with clinically significant ventricular arrhythmias (22, 28,37). All of these studies, using various electrophysiologic techniques, represent a form of electrophysiologic "stress testing" to expose ventricular electrical instability. Mason and Winkle (32) and Horowitz and colleagues (31) have suggested that the ability to induce sustained ventricular tachycardia by electrophysiologic techniques is necessary to classify patients with certainty as having clinically significant ventricular electrical instability. Likewise, a drug in order to be effective by their criteria must suppress the ability to induce sustained ventricular tachycardia with these electrophysiologic stimulation techniques. These techniques include ventricular pacing from both the right and the left sides of the heart in multiple sites and both single and double ventricular extrastimulation during ventricular drive. Our technique for eliciting the repetitive ventricular response to expose ventricular electrical instability perhaps represents a milder form of "stress testing" than multiple sequential ventricular extrastimuli, since sustained tachycardia is not required as an endpoint, nor is it seen commonly during our testing. With atrial pacing or sinus rhythm, simply the production of the repetitive ventricular beats following a single ventricular extrastimulus has been used as the indicator of ventricular electrical instability and has been shown to have predictive value in 1) survivors of a recent myocardial infarction and 2) patients with chronic recurrent ventricular tachycardia treated intensively with aprindine, an investigational antiarrhythmic drug. However, when applied to other groups of patients testing for the repetitive ventricular response may prove to be a less sensitive test.

Akhtar et al. (18, 19) Kastor et al. (21) and Dhatt and co-workers (20) have defined the characteristics of reentry within the His-Purkinje system which can be elicited even in normal subjects. During constant rate ventricular pacing followed by ventricular premature stimulation, reentry within the His-Purkinje system can occur when a critical delay occurs between the ventricular premature stimulus and the retrograde His-Purkinje system activation. This technique has been used to evaluate the characteristics of reentry within the His-Purkinje system and the effects of cardio-active drugs on reentry within this tissue. This type of reentry can be seen in most patients who have normal intraventricular conduction, producing a QRS configuration of left bundle branch block – left axis deviation, similar to the paced beats from the apex of the right ventricle, although other patterns of reentry have been described. Rarely does this type of reentry produce sustained ventricular tachycardia.

Josephson and colleagues (22) have demonstrated intraventricular reentry in many of their patients with chronic ventricular dysrhythmias. These investigators were reliably able to induce ventricular tachycardia in patients who had a history of recurrent sustained ventricular tachycardia. This tachycardia did not require reentry within the His-Purkinje system for its initiation or perpetuation. Retrograde conduction block in the right bundle branch was not necessary for the initiation of the ventricular tachycardia, and a retrograde V_2H_2 delay likewise was not required. The QRS configuration of the ventricular tachycardia which was induced by electrical stimulation was similar in most cases to the spontaneous ventricular tachycardia for which the patient had been referred for study. The tachycardia could be initiated and terminated reproducibly by the programmed stimulation, implying a reentry circuit. Other evidence suggested that the reentry site was a small portion of the ventricles. Sustained ventricular tachycardia could most reliably be produced with ventricular premature stimuli introduced during ventricular drive, and only rarely was sustained ventricular tachycardia induced by single or double ventricular extrastimulation during atrial drive or sinus rhythm. Likewise, ventricular fibrillation was never induced during programmed stimulation which included only ventricular drive and single ventricular extrastimulation. (38)

Our study demonstrates that the repetitive ventricular response obtained during atrial drive or sinus rhythm is not dependent upon bundle branch reentry. Retrograde V_2H_2 delay is not necessary. In only one patient out of thirty was there a retrograde His bundle deflection present prior to the repetitive beat. Even in this single patient, other characteristics of the reentry (the QRS configuration) suggested that reentry was not occurring within the bundle branches, but that the bundle branches were coincidentally being activated simultaneously while reentry was occurring elsewhere. In most patients, the surface QRS configuration of the repetitive beat suggested reentry on the left side of the heart with a right bundle branch block pattern and QRS axis dissimilar to the axis of the stimulated beat, though surface QRS patterns can be misleading when trying to ascertain the site of origin of the QRS complex. Akhtar and colleagues (19) have demonstrated differing routes of impulse propagation during reentry within the His-Purkinje system in man. However, only 15 % of their patients had reentry with a right bundle branch block pattern. In addition, thirteen of our patients had preexisting bundle branch block during sinus rhythm which would make reentry within the His-Purkinje system less likely. Furthermore, many of our patients had more than one repetitive ventricular beat, and the QRS configuration was changing from beat to beat in these patients. Likewise, a close coupling interval of the premature stimulus to the preceding QRS was not always required for the initiation of the repetitive ventricular response, a condition which is usually required for reentry within the His-Purkinje system where retrograde block in the right bundle branch is commonly necessary. Ventricular pacing with ventricular premature stimulation may establish ideal circumstances for retrograde block within the right bundle to allow His-Purkinje system reentry, whereas ventricular premature stimulation during atrial drive or sinus rhythm would tend to make His-Purkinje system reentry less likely.

We postulate that the repetitive ventricular response may represent reentry within diseased tissue, perhaps the distal Purkinje system, ventricular muscle, or in many cases a ventricular aneurysm or scar, because many of our patients have a history of recent or remote myocardial infarction. Though overall ejection fraction was normal in many patients, all but one patient had abnormal left ventricular contraction patterns with localized disease of ventricular muscle. Other patients in our study who did not have fixed myocardial disease but who had a history of ventricular dysrhythmias during certain transient phenomena which, in fact, may be responsible for most cases of sudden cardiac death, did not have the repetitive ventricular response under basal conditions. Four of our patients with coronary arterial spasm and ischemia had a history of ventricular arrhythmias during their ischemia, but repetitive responses were not present in the absence of spasm-induced ischemia. An additional four patients had ventricular tachycardia during exercise-induced ischemia, and these patients had fixed atherosclerotic narrowings of their coronary arteries. However, in the absence of pacing-induced ischemia, repetitive ventricular responses were absent. In addition, only one patient with ischemic heart disease without a recent myocardial infarction or history of ventricular dysrhythmias had intraventricular reentry as manifest by the repetitive ventricular response.

It would therefore seem that the mechanism of reentry is the important factor in the prognostic value of electrophysiologic tests. Repetitive beats characteristic of proximal His-Purkinje system reentry which are induced by any ventricular stimulation technique appear commonly in normal individuals and generally have no prognostic significance for spontaneous ventricular dysrhythmias. These repetitive beats likewise are usually not sustained to produce ventricular tachycardia. On the contrary, reentry which does not utilize the proximal His-Purkinje system and which results in sustained ventricular tachycardia during ventricular drive and ventricular premature stimulation is seen only in patients with a history of ventricular tachycardia or patients with electrically unstable ventricles. Repetitive ventricular responses during atrial drive or normal sinus rhythm occur by a mechanism of reentry most similar to intraventricular reentry. Therefore, either sustained or nonsustained intraventricular reentry elicited by various testing procedures may be of prognostic importance for 1) the prediction of symptomatic ventricular tachycardia or sudden death, and 2) the prediction of the response to antiarrhythmic medications.

The intraventricular reentry phenomenon does not occur in normal subjects, and it rarely occurs even in patients with coronary artery disease except in the survivor of a recent myocardial infarction who is at high risk of late symptomatic ventricular tachycardia or sudden death. Though it occurs in the patients with recurrent sustained ventricular tachycardia, all but one of the recent reports (37) have concentrated upon induction of sustained ventricular tachycardia as the only measure of the propensity to spontaneous ventricular arrhythmias. We therefore evaluated the similarity of the finding of intraventricular reentry phenomena in patients studied both during atrial and ventricular drive and ventricular extrastimulation. There is good agreement between the two techniques, except that it is common for patients to have intraventricular reentry during ventricular drive and ventricular premature stimulation when intraventricular reentry is absent in the same patient during atrial drive and ventricular premature stimulation. This finding would support the concept that there are various degrees of electrophysiologic "stress testing" which may expose the propensity to spontaneous ventricular arrhythmias. The "least stressful" technique is single ventricular extrastimulation during atrial drive or sinus rhythm. Single ventricular extrastimulation during ventricular drive is more likely to induce sustained ventricular arrhythmias as well as simple intraventricular reentry phenomena. Double ventricular extrastimulation during ventricular drive would be expected to produce intraventricular reentry phenomena and sustained ventricular tachycardia even more often than single ventricular extrastimulation during ventricular drive.

7. SUMMARY

The repetitive ventricular response, defined as the production of two or more ventricular premature beats in response to a single ventricular electrical stimulus during atrial pacing or sinus rhythm, was evaluated as an index of ventricular electrical instability, that is, the propensity for a patient to develop spontaneous ventricular tachycardia or ventricular fibrillation. The records of the first 222 consecutive patients tested in this manner were reviewed to determine the significance of this phenomenon. Twenty-two patients who were being evaluated for chest pain syndromes were subsequently found to be entirely normal, and they served as the control group. Seventy-seven patients had been referred for refractory symptomatic ventricular tachycardia. Twenty-six patients had recently experienced ventricular tachycardia but were taking adequate oral doses of antiarrhythmic drugs at the time of study. Sixty-one patients were survivors of an acute myocardial infarction and were followed prospectively for one year after their electrophysiologic study to determine the incidence of symptomatic ventricular tachycardia or sudden death. Thirty-six patients had coronary artery disease but had no history of recent myocardial infarction or ventricular arrhythmias.

The repetitive ventricular response was absent in all normal subjects but present in sixty-six of seventy-seven patients with recurrent refractory symptomatic ventricular tachycardia (p < 0.001). Twenty-two patients who were survivors of a recent myocardial infarction had the repetitive ventricular response, and nineteen of these patients suffered symptomatic ventricular tachycardia or sudden death in the first year after their myocardial infarction. On the contrary, thirty-nine patients who were survivors of a recent myocardial infarction did not have the repetitive ventricular response and only four patients had ventricular tachycardia or sudden death in one year follow-up (p < 0.001). Of the twenty-two patients who had survived a recent myocardial infarction who had the repetitive ventricular response, eight patients experienced sudden cardiac death, whereas only four of the thirty-nine survivors of a recent myocardial infarction who did not have the repetitive ventricular response experienced sudden death in one year follow-up (p < 0.025). Only one of the thirty-six patients with ischemic heart disease without a history of recent myocardial infarction or ventricular arrhythmias had the repetitive response, and this patient was alive at one year follow-up. No sudden deaths occurred in the other thirty-five patients in this group.

Twenty-seven patients with refractory ventricular tachycardia were evaluated to determine whether acute suppression of the repetitive ventricular response by an intravenous antiarrhythmic agent predicted a good therapeutic response to that agent. Absence of the repetitive ventricular response in twenty-one patients after intravenous aprindine correctly predicted a good therapeutic result to chronic oral aprindine in twenty of these patients.

On the contrary, only one of the six patients in whom the repetitive ventricular response was present after intravenous aprindine had a satisfactory response to oral aprindine ($p < 0.0005$).

The electrophysiologic characteristics of the repetitive ventricular response were evaluated in thirty patients in whom His bundle and/or right bundle recordings were performed at the time of ventricular stimulation. Seven of these patients had a preexisting bundle branch block. His bundle or right bundle deflections did not precede the repetitive beats in twenty-nine of the thirty patients, implying that the proximal His-Purkinje system was not involved in the reentry circuit. In twenty-four of these thirty patients the QRS axis of the repetitive beats was $\geq 45°$ divergent from the stimulated beat, and the repetitive beat had a right bundle branch block configuration in twenty-two of these thirty patients. In fourteen of eighteen patients with two or more repetitive beats, the QRS morphology was changing from beat to beat, implying that either the reentry pathway or conduction was changing. These data suggest that the repetitive response represents intraventricular, rather than bundle branch, reentry.

The technique of ventricular drive of the basic heart rate plus single ventricular premature stimulation was compared to atrial drive with single ventricular premature stimulation with respect to the presence or absence of intraventricular reentry phenomena. Thirty-one patients had testing by both of these methods. Five patients had intraventricular reentry both during atrial and ventricular drive of the basic heart rate, and sixteen patients did not have intraventricular reentry after single ventricular extrastimulation during either atrial or ventricular drive. Ten patients had intraventricular reentry phenomena with single ventricular extrastimulation during ventricular drive but not during atrial drive. No patients had intraventricular reentry from single ventricular extrastimulation during atrial drive but not with ventricular drive ($p < 0.02$).

Thus, the repetitive ventricular response identifies clinically significant ventricular electrical instability which is associated with spontaneous ventricular dysrhythmias. It has prognostic value in certain highly selected groups of patients. Suppression of the repetitive response by an antiarrhythmic agent given acutely identifies that the patient will have a good therapeutic result to the same medication given chronically orally. The repetitive ventricular response is important because it represents intraventricular reentry rather than bundle branch reentry. There is good agreement between the findings for intraventricular reentry phenomena during single ventricular premature stimulation during both atrial and ventricular drive. However, ventricular extrastimulation during ventricular drive is a more potent technique to elicit intraventricular reentry. Further evaluation will determine which technique is more reliable for detecting clinically significant ventricular electrical instability and for predicting the response to drugs.

ACKNOWLEDGMENTS

This work was supported in part by grants HL-18799 and HL-17655 from the National Heart, Lung and Blood Institute, National Institutes of Health, Bethesda, Maryland.

REFERENCES

1. Wiggers CJ, Wegria N: Ventricular fibrillation due to single localized induction and condenser shocks applied during the vulnerable phase of ventricular systole. Am J Physiol 128:500–505, 1940.
2. Gerstenblith G, Spear JF, Moore EN: Quantitative study of the effect of lidocaine on the threshold for ventricular fibrillation in the dog. Am J Cardiol 30:242–247, 1972.
3. Merx W, Han J, Yoon MS: Effects of unipolar cathodal and bipolar stimulation on vulnerability of ischemic ventricles to fibrillation. Am J Cardiol 35: 37–41, 1975.
4. Han J, de Jalon G, Moe GK: Fibrillation threshold of premature ventricular responses. Circulation Res 18:18–25, 1966.
5. Burgess MJ, Williams D, Ershler P: Influence of test site on ventricular fibrillation threshold. Am Heart J 94:55–61, 1977.
6. Merx W, Yoon MS, Han J: The role of local disparity in conduction and recovery time on ventricular vulnerability to fibrillation. Am Heart J 94:603–610, 1977.
7. Moore EM, Spear JF: Ventricular fibrillation threshold. Its physiological and pharmacological importance. Arch Int Med 135:446–453, 1975.
8. Lown B, Kleiger R, Williams J: Cardioversion and digitalis drugs: Changed threshold to electric shock in digitalized animals. Circulation Res 17:519–531, 1965.
9. Lown B: Electrical stimulation to estimate the degree of digitalization. II. Experimental studies. Am J Cardiol 22:251–259, 1968.
10. Thompson PL, Lown B: Sequential R/T pacing to expose electrical instability in the ischemic ventricle (abstr). Clin Res 20:401, 1972.
11. Axelrod PJ, Verrier RL, Lown B: Extreme vulnerability to ventricular fibrillation with acute coronary occlusion exposed by sequential R/T pulsing (abstr). Am J Cardiol 31:117, 1973.
12. Matta RJ, Verrier RL, Rabinowitz SH, et al: The repetitive extrasystole as an index of ventricular vulnerability to fibrillation (abstr). Am J Cardiol 35:156, 1975.
13. Karagueuzian HS, Ferroglio JJ, Hoffman BF, et al: Sustained ventricular tachycardia induced by electrical stimulation after myocardial infarction: relation to infarct structure (abstr). Circulation 56:III–79, 1977.
14. Engle WR, Moore EN, Spear JF et al: Limitations on the use of electrical ventricular fibrillation threshold determinations (abstr). Circulation 55:III–80, 1977.
15. Horowitz LN, Spear JF, Josephson ME, et al: Ventricular fibrillation threshold in man (abstr). Am J Cardiol 39:274, 1977.
16. Guss SB, Kastor JA, Scharf DL, et al: Effects of rate, atropine and procainamide on human ventricular refractoriness (abstract). Am J Cardiol 35: 142, 1975.
17. Engle TR, Meister SG, Frankl WS: Ventricular extrastimulation in the mitral valve prolapse syndrome. Evidence of ventricular reentry. J Electrocardiol 11:137–142, 1978.
18. Akhtar M, Damato AN, Batsford WP, et al: Demonstration of re-entry within the His-Purkinje system in man. Circulation 50:1150–1162, 1974.
19. Akhtar M, Gilbert C, Wolf FG, et al: Reentry within the His-Purkinje system. Elucidation of reentrant circuit using right bundle branch and His bundle recordings. Circulation 58:295–304, 1978.
20. Dhatt MS, Akhtar M, Reddy CP, et al: Modification and abolition of re-entry within the His-Purkinje system in man by diphenylhydantoin. Circulation 56:720–726, 1977.
21. Kastor JA, Josephson ME, Guss FB, et al: Human ventricular refractoriness. II. Effects of procainamide. Circulation 56:462–467, 1977.
22. Josephson ME, Horowitz LN, Farshidi A, et al: Recurrent sustained ventricular tachycardia. I. Mechanisms. Circulation 57:431–440, 1978.
23. Drew TM, Josephson ME, Horowitz, LN, et al: The significance of the repetitive ventricular response to programmed ventricular stimulation. (abstr). Clin Res 25:218A, 1977.
24. Wellens JH, Schuilenburg RM, Durrer D: Electrical stimulation of the heart in patients with ventricular tachycardia. Circulation 46: 216–226, 1972.
25. Wellens HJJ, Lie KI, Durrer D: Further observations on ventricular tachycardia as studied by electrical stimulation of the heart. Circulation 49:647–653, 1974.
26. Wellens HJJ, Bär FWHM, Lie KI et al: Effect of procainamide, propranolol, and verapamil on mechanism of tachycardia in patients with chronic recurrent ventricular tachycardia. Am J Cardiol 40:579–585, 1977.
27. Reddy CP, Damato AN, Akhtar M, et al: The effect of procainamide on re-entry within the His-Purkinje system in man (abstr). Am J Cardiol 37:165, 1976.

28. Josephson ME, Horowitz LN, Farshidi A: Continuous local electrical activity. A mechanism of recurrent ventricular tachycardia. Circulation 57:659–665, 1978.

29. Josephson ME, Horowitz LN, Farshidi A, et al: Recurrent sustained ventricular tachycardia. II. Endocardial mapping. Circulation 57:440–447, 1978.

30. Fisher JD, Cohen HL, Mehra R, et al: Cardiac pacing and pacemakers. II. Serial electrophysiologic-pharmacologic testing for control of recurrent tachyarrhythmias. Am Heart J 93:658–668, 1977.

31. Horowitz LN, Josephson ME, Farshidi A, et al: Recurrent sustained ventricular tachycardia. 3. Role of the electrophysiologic study in detection of antiarrhythmic regimens. Circulation 58:986–997, 1978.

32. Mason JW, Winkle RA: Electrode-catheter arrhythmia induction in the selection and assessment of antiarrhythmic drug therapy in recurrent ventricular tachycardia. Circulation 58:971–985, 1978.

33. Greene HL, Reid PR, Schaeffer AH: The repetitive ventricular response in man. A predictor of sudden death. N Engl J Med 299:729–734, 1978.

34. Schaeffer AH, Greene HL, Reid PR: Suppression of the repetitive ventricular response: An index of long term antiarrhythmic effectiveness of aprindine for ventricular tachycardia in man. Am J Cardiol 42:1007–1012, 1978.

35. Pederson DH, Troup PJ, Zipes DP: Prognostic significance of repetitive ventricular response using programmed ventricular pacing. Abstract. Clin Res 26:652A, 1978.

36. Troup PJ, Pederson DH, Zipes DP: Effects of premature ventricular stimulation in patients with ventricular tachycardia (abstr). Circulation 58 (suppl II):II-154, 1978.

37. Farshidi A, Michelson EL, Greenspan AM, et al: Repetitive responses to ventricular extrastimuli – incidence, mechanism and significance (abstr). Am J Cardiol 43:390, 1979.

38. Spielman SR, Farshidi A, Horowitz LN, et al: Ventricular fibrillation during programmed ventricular stimulation: Incidence and clinical implications. Am J Cardiol 42:913–918, 1978.

3.5. DETECTION OF PATIENTS AT HIGH RISK FOR SUDDEN DEATH: THE ROLE OF ELECTROCARDIOGRAPHIC MONITORING

R.A. WINKLE

During the past decade there has been considerable interest in ECG monitoring to identify patients at high risk of sudden cardiac death. Several studies have examined the predictive value of ventricular premature beats which occur on 12-lead electrocardiograms. There is general agreement that premature ventricular beats occurring on 12-lead electrocardiograms in the absence of clinical evidence of significant heart disease do not identify patients with an increased risk of subsequent sudden death (1–3). However, the occurrence of ventricular premature beats in patients with clinical evidence of coronary heart disease does identify a group of patients with an increased risk of subsequent sudden death (2–5).

Hinkle et al. (6, 7) have performed 6 to 24 hour ambulatory ECG recordings in a population of employed males age 35 to 65. They found that premature ventricular beats become more prevalent with increasing age and that complex ventricular beats (multiform, R on T, bigeminy, pairs, runs) all occur more frequently among men with frequent PVCs. He has noted that frequent PVCs ($> 10/1000$ complexes) occur primarily in

Table 1. Variables with prognostic importance.

	Bigger	DeBusk	DeSoyza*	Kotler*	Luria	Moss # 1	Moss # 2	Rehnqvist	Ruberman	Schulze	Vismara
	BUN	ST depression >2mm		Complex PVC's	Systolic Pressure	PVC Big/pairs	PVC's > 20 min.MF big	Enlarged heart	Complex PVC's	Complex PVC's	Complex PVC's
	Creatinine	≤ 4 METS			BUN	Age		Fct class II–IV	History of CHF	EF < 40	ST abnormally on ECG
	Uric acid				Atrial arrhythmias in CCU	PVC prematurity		Severe PVC's	ST depression on ECG		
	Enlarged heart				Angina >3 mos or prior MI	PVC frequency			Diuretic therapy		
	VT				>1 PVC/hr	Norris short					
	CPK										
	LV failure										
End Point	Cardiac death	Cardiac event	Cardiac death	Sudden death	Cardiac death	Cardiac death	Cardiac death	Reinfarction and sudden death	Sudden and cardiac death	Sudden death	Sudden death

*Study considered only arrhythmias
BUN = blood urea nitrogen
VT = ventricular tachycardia
LV = left ventricular
METS = multiples of resting energy expenditure
CCU = coronary care unit

PVC = premature ventricular complex
CHF = congestive heart failure
EF = ejection fraction
MF = multifocal
Big = bigeminy

subjects with other evidence for heart disease and that they are associated with an increased risk of coronary death and instantaneous sudden death. The occurrence of multiform PVCs and short runs of ventricular tachycardia does not add to the information gained from PVC frequency whereas premature PVCs do increase the risk. In the absence of coronary disease or risk factors, frequent PVCs did not seem to predict subsequent death.

Since there is approximately a 10 % mortality in the first year following acute myocardial infarction, numerous studies have examined the issue of whether or not cardiac arrhythmias on ambulatory ECG recordings identify coronary patients who are at increased risk of sudden cardiac death during the 1–2 years following myocardial infarction. Some studies (Table 1) have found such arrhythmias to be the most important predictor of subsequent sudden mortality (8–11). Others have found these arrhythmias to be statistically significant for identifying patients at risk for sudden death, but somewhat less valuable than other more easily and cheaply obtained clinical measurements (12, 13). Still other studies have found these arrhythmias to be either not statistically significant (14, 15) or of only borderline significance (16) for identifying patients who will die suddenly. Upon initial review one may be confused by the variety of conclusions in these studies. However, careful examination reveals that these studies vary greatly in terms of patient population (Table 2), duration of ambulatory ECG recordings (Table 3), definitions of various arrhythmia frequencies (Table 4) and complexities (Table 5), definitions of study endpoints and durations of follow-up (Table 6). Furthermore, many have been published in multiple parts and in multiple journals. In order to more fully understand the relationship between arrhythmias on ambulatory ECG recordings and sudden death during the late post infarction period, it is necessary to critically dissect each of the reported studies. The following

Table 2. Patient populations.

	Bigger	DeBusk	DeSoyza	Kotler	Luria	Moss #1	Moss # 2	Rehnqvist	Ruberman	Schulze	Vismara
No. subjects	100	90	56	160	143	100	272	160	1739	81	64
No restrictions	Yes				Yes	Yes				Yes	Yes
Age restriction		Yes**					Yes[a]	Yes[a]			
Heart failure or functional Class III or IV excluded		Yes		Yes							
Other diseases excluded		Yes		Yes							
Females excluded		Yes	Yes	Yes					Yes		
Patients entered >3 mos post MI				Yes					Yes*		

* 50% of patients
** 70 years excluded
[a] 65 years excluded

Table 3. Duration of ambulatory ECG monitoring.

	Bigger	DeBusk	DeSoyza	Kotler	Luria	Moss #1	Moss #2	Rehnqvist	Ruberman	Schulze	Vismara
1 hour									Yes		
6 hours						Yes	Yes	Yes			
8 hours				Yes							
10 hours											Yes
12 hours		Yes		Yes							
24 hours	Yes		Yes							Yes	
Sequential recordings		Yes	Yes	Yes			Yes	Yes			

Table 4. Frequency of PVCs.

	Bigger	DeBusk	DeSoyza	Kotler	Luria	Moss #1	Moss #2	Rehnqvist	Ruberman	Schulze	Vismara
Any	88%	79%	70%	80%*		72%	50%	75%	52%	65%	77%
>1/hour	55%				47%						
>10/hour	24%		26%						26%		
>20/hour							7%				
>10/1000 beats						9%					
Peak/15 minutes		Yes									
>5/min								Yes			Yes
Continuous frequency or best separation considered	Yes				Yes	Yes	Yes				
Frequency considered separately for prognosis	Yes				Yes	Yes	Yes		Yes		

*From multiple holters

summarizes the findings of major studies which have been reported to date in full manuscript form.

1. STUDY – BIGGER ET AL.

This study was published as an abstract presenting arrhythmia prevalence (17) and as a manuscript examining risk stratification for predicting death after myocardial infarction (16).

1.1. Patient population. This study involved 100 patients (71 men and 29 women) hospitalized with an acute myocardial infarction. The average age was 61 years (range 25 to 90) with 39 % being older than 65 years. Entry into the study was determined by survival beyond the ninth hospital day and willingness to participate.

1.2. Ambulatory ECG recordings. A single 24 hour ambulatory ECG monitoring was obtained on day 14.5 ± 4.0 after the onset of hospitalization. Analysis of the recordings

Table 5. Prevalence of qualitative types of PVCs.

	Bigger	DeBusk	DeSoyza	Kotler	Luria	Moss #1	Moss #2	Rehnqvist	Ruberman	Schulze	Vismara
Multiform	64%	20%	X	H	C	20%	8%	H	45%	H	C
VT	14%	1%	4%	2%*	N	4%	1%	3%	C	1%	C
Ron T	33%	X	X	H	N	9%	10%	H	12%	H	C
Bigeminy	N	17%	X	X	8%	C	4%	X	22%	H	X
Pairs	36%	12%	22%	H	C	C	3%	H	C	H	C
Complex	X	33%	43%	40%*	X	X	X	N	27%	36%	42%

X = not considered
N = considered separately but data not reported
* = from multiple recordings
H = considered but highest grade only reported
C = combined with another class

Table 6. Follow-up data.

	Bigger	DeBusk	DeSoyza	Kotler	Luria	Moss #1	Moss #2	Rehnqvist	Ruberman	Schulze	Vismara
Duration (months)	6*	24	19	30–54	24	20	12	12	24	7	26
% Dying (total cardiac)	15%	4%	14%	12%	19%	17%	9%	9%	12%	12%	25%
% Dying (sudden)	12%	3%	7%	9%	11%	4%	No Data	6%	5%	10%	19%
Correlation with all cardiac death	Yes		Yes		Yes	Yes	Yes		Yes		
Correlation with sudden death				Yes					Yes	Yes	Yes
Correlation with cardiac events		Yes									
Correlation with reinfarction and sudden death								Yes			
Definitional sudden death (hours)	24	No Data	1	1	1	No Data	12	2	Minutes	1	6

* 12 month data collected, but 6 used

was done in unusual detail with each 24 hour recording printed on a Grass polygraph and detection of complex arrhythmia forms by hand analysis.

1.3. Arrhythmia definitions. Arrhythmias were categorized according to PVC frequency per hour and the presence or absence of each of the following: bigeminy, fusion beats, multiform beats, R on T, pairs or ventricular tachycardia.

1.4. Arrhythmia prevalence. Eighty-eight percent of patients had at least one PVC. Fifty-five percent had greater than one PVC per hour, 24 % had greater than 10 per hour and 30 % had 30 or more in at least one hour. Multiform beats occurred in 64 % of patients and in 64 of 82 patients with more than one PVC per recording. Thirty-three of the 64 patients with multifocal premature beats had 3 or 4 configurations. Pairs were observed in 36 % of patients, ventricular tachycardia in either 13 or 14 % of patients and R on T premature beats in either 26 or 33 %.

1.5. Follow-up. Survival data were collected over a one year period. There were 21 deaths including 2 of non-cardiac origin. Fifteen of the 19 cardiac deaths occurred during the first six months and 12 of these 15 deaths were sudden (defined as death within 24 hours). Determination of prognostic significance of various variables was for overall cardiac death during the first six months only. The authors state that data analysis using one year period did not significantly alter their conclusions.

1.6. Conclusions.
    1.6.1. From ambulatory ECG monitoring. Using univariate analysis, ventricular tachycardia on an ambulatory ECG recording was of borderline significance ($> 0.05\,p < 0.10$) for identifying patients with subsequent cardiac death. Patients with one or more PVC/hour or with R on T beats had a higher death rate than patients without these characteristics, but the differences were not statistically significant.
    1.6.2. Other conclusions. A series of univariate predictors of cardiac death, several of which were better than ambulatory ECG findings, were found in this study. In order of decreasing importance they were: BUN greater than 20 mg/dl, creatinine greater than 1.4 mg/dl, elevated uric acid, enlarged heart on chest x-ray at 2 weeks, creatine kinase greater than 580 IU, and requirement of digoxin or left ventricular failure in the Coronary Care Unit. This study showed no relation between early CCU arrhythmias or age and cardiac death.

2. STUDY – DE BUSK ET AL. (14, 18)

Prelimininary conclusions from this study were published in abstract (18) form and the final manuscript is now in press (14).

2.1. Patient population. This study was performed on 90 males with a mean age of 52 with all patients being less than 70 years. An important difference of this study from most others published is that the patient population was selected as one with a low incidence of clinically evident left ventricular dysfunction. All patients were required to be suitable candidates for treadmill exercise testing. Patients were excluded from the study if they had any one of the following: 1) rest angina or unstable angina, 2) clinical evidence of congestive heart failure, 3) the presence of an S_3 gallop heard by a single observer or 4) associated medical conditions such as significant valvular heart disease, hypertension, or limiting pulmonary disease or musculoskeletal abnormalities. Only 21 % of patients had anterior infarctions and only 11 % had a prior history of a myocardial infarction. Cardiomegaly was present by x-ray during hospitalization in only 12% of the 90 patients.

2.2. Ambulaiory ECG recordings. Twelve hour recordings and exercise treadmill tests were done at 3, 11, 26, and 62 weeks following onset of myocardial infarction.

2.3. Arrhythmia definitions. PVC frequency was determined as the maximal number occurring during any 15 minute interval on the recording. PVCs were termed complex if they occurred as bigeminy, pairs, multiform or ventricular tachycardia. R on T was not analyzed.

2.4. Arrhythmia prevalence. The prevalence of each type of ventricular ectopic beat is given for each of the four test periods. The presence of any PVCs was constant at 80 % whereas any complex PVCs were recorded on from 33 to 56 % of the recordings. The prevalence of multifocal beats ranged from 20 to 40 %, bigeminy from 18 to 32 %, pairs from 10 to 20 % and ventricular tachycardia from 1 to 2 %.

2.5. Follow-up. Patients were followed for 24 months after initial testing at 3 weeks. Eleven patients experienced recurrent coronary events during this period. Only 3 were sudden coronary deaths, however, and 8 were recurrent infarctions, one of which was fatal.

2.6. Conclusions.

2.6.1. From ambulatory ECG. Although a previous abstract (18) reporting preliminary data from this study suggested there was an increase of arrhythmias on ambulatory ECG between 3 and 11 weeks, the final data did not confirm this widely quoted finding. The study showed no change over one year in the prevalence of peak PVCs per 15 minutes, any PVCs or the presence of complex PVCs. The study showed a strong association between bigeminy, couplets, and multiform premature beats, but these were not associated with the presence of ventricular tachycardia. However, the total number of episodes of ventricular tachycardia was relatively small. Most importantly this study shows that patients relatively free of clinically evident left ventricular dysfunction do not show a relationship between the presence of any PVCs or complex PVCs and subsequent coronary events.

2.6.2. Other findings. This study showed a relatively low rate of sudden cardiac death in a patient population free of clinically evident left ventricular dysfunction. It also showed that the ambulatory ECG was more sensitive to detect any PVCs and to detect complex PVCs than was the exercise treadmill; however, there was little overlap for the detection of ventricular tachycardia. The only findings predictive of subsequent coronary events were greater than 2 mm of ST depression on the exercise treadmill test and an inability to achieve 4 multiples of resting oxygen consumption work load during the 3 week exercise test.

3. STUDY – DE SOYZA ET AL. (15)

3.1. Patient population. This study examined 56 patients hospitalized for acute myocardial infarction. Although the exact age of the study population is not given, they were selected from patients with an average age of 54 years (range 24 to 73).

3.2. Ambulatory ECG recordings. Twenty-four hour recordings were made early in the Coronary Care Unit period and a second 24-hour recording was made 24 hours prior to discharge during the third post infarction week. An additional 38 surviving patients had 6 hour follow-up ambulatory ECG recordings performed, an average of 19 months after their entry into the study.

3.3. Arrhythmia definitions. Frequent PVCs were defined as greater than 10 per hour. Tapes were also analyzed for the presence of pairs and ventricular tachycardia. Multifocal, bigeminal and R on T beats were not considered. Complex PVCs were defined as those occurring greater than 10 per hour, in pairs or as ventricular tachycardia.

3.4. Arrhythmia prevalence. No premature beats were detected in 30 % of patients. Twenty-six percent had greater than 10 per hour, 22 % pairs, and 4.3 % had ventricular tachycardia. Complex PVCs were identified in 43 %.

3.5. Follow-up. The average follow-up was 19 months ranging from 5 to 31 months. There were 11 deaths including 8 cardiac deaths and 3 noncardiac deaths. Of the cardiac deaths, 4 were sudden and 2 died within 24 hours of the onset of symptoms of recurrent myocardial infarction. All cardiac deaths were used in data analysis.

3.6. Conclusions.
   3.6.1. From ambulatory ECG monitoring. This study showed a relationship between the presence of ventricular tachycardia in the early phases of an acute myocardial infarction and complex premature beats both at the time of hospital discharge and at the 19 month follow-up. However, neither the presence of ventricular tachycardia early after myocardial infarction nor the presence of complex premature beats on the predischarge ECG recording predicted subsequent cardiac death. Of the 6 patients who died within 24 hours of the onset of symptoms, only one had complex PVCs at the time of hospital discharge. It should be noted that this negative study was in a small number of patients and had a less comprehensive definition of complex arrhythmias than other similar studies.

4. STUDY – KOTLER ET AL. (19)

4.1. Patient population. This study was performed in 160 males under the age of 65 who were in New York Heart Association Functional Class I or II. All patients had had a previous myocardial infarction at least 3 months prior to entry into the study. They were free of recent deterioration of their cardiac disease, were free of a list of life threatening diseases and were neither on insulin nor on anticoagulant therapy.

4.2. Ambulatory ECG recordings. The patients had a total of 717 12-hour ambulatory ECG recordings. The recordings were repeated at 8 month intervals and in some instances more frequently.

4.3. Arrhythmia definitions. The following grading system was utilized: Grade 0 = no ventricular ectopic beats, Grade 1 = less than 10 uniform ventricular ectopic beats per hour, Grade 2 = greater than 10 uniform ventricular ectopic beats per hour, Grade 3 = multiform ventricular ectopic beats, Grade 4 = ventricular ectopic beats in pairs, Grade 5 = three or more successive ventricular ectopic beats. R on T premature ventricular beats were not considered. Tapes were scored as to the highest grade achieved on the tape and each patient's score was the highest grade achieved on any of the sequential recordings. Ventricular ectopic beats were considered complex when they were Grades 2 through 5.

4.4. Arrhythmia prevalence. At the time of follow-up each patient had four or five recordings and 80 % of the patients showed ventricular ectopic beats on at least one recording. Because patients were classified by the highest grade of arrhythmia achieved, it is difficult to determine the exact prevalence of each of the individual grades on these recordings. However, the number of patients achieving each maximal grade were: Grade 1 – 22.5 %, Grade 2–17.5%, Grade 3–17.5%, Grade 4–20%, Grade 5–2.5%. Forty percent were classified as having complex premature ventricular beats.

4.5. Follow-up. These patients were followed from 30 to 54 months. There were 21 deaths, 20 of which were cardiac, including 14 sudden deaths (defined as occurring instantaneously or within an hour of onset of symptoms). Relationship between ambulatory ECG characteristics was made with the occurrence of sudden death.

4.6. Conclusions.
  4.6.1. Ambulatory ECG. The sudden death rate in the patients with Grade 0 and 1 arrhythmias was 3 % compared to a sudden death rate of 13.8 % in patients with Grades 2 through 5. This difference was statistically significant. It was of interest that there were no deaths in the 30 patients with paired ventricular ectopic beats (Grade 4), a finding which the authors attributed to the high rate of parasystole in this Grade.

5. STUDY – LURIA ET AL. (12)

5.1. Patient population. This study was of 143 patients with acute myocardial infarction who were admitted to the hospital and were discharged alive. The average age was approximately 60 years.

5.2. Ambulatory ECG recordings. Single 8-hour ambulatory ECG recordings were performed on the 17th to 24th hospital day approximately one to four days prior to hospital discharge.

5.3. Arrhythmia definitions. PVC frequency is given as number per hour. Ventricular ectopy was also classified according to whether or not it occurred as bigeminy, pairs, multiform, or ventricular tachycardia and prematurity was also categorized.

5.4. Arrhythmia prevalence. The exact prevalence of arrhythmias is not given for each of the individual arrhythmia categories. However, from data provided it can be determined that 43 of 143 (30%) patients had pairs or multifocal premature ventricular beats, 67 of 143 (47%) had greater than one PVC per hour and 12 of 143 (8.4%) patients had bigeminy. Ventricular ectopic beat frequency was characterized as a continuous variable and also as a discrete variable with cut offs ranging from 0.5 to 6 per hour.

5.5. Follow-up. Patients were followed for a period of 2 years. There were 33 deaths of which 27 were of cardiac causes and 16 were sudden (defined as within one hour of the onset of symptoms). Correlation of various ambulatory ECG and clinical variables were done with regard to all cardiac deaths.

5.6. Conclusions.
  5.6.1. Ambulatory ECG recordings. PVC frequency did not relate to the occurrence of cardiac death when considered as a continuous variable. However, when considered as a discrete variable there was a relationship between ventricular ectopic beats greater than 0.5, 1.0, 1.5, and 2 per hour. The combination of paired or multiform ventricular ectopic beats was also associated with occurrence of subsequent sudden death. Ventricular bigeminy and the prematurity of the ventricular ectopic beats was not related to the occurrence of cardiac death.
  5.6.2. Other. Several other clinical variables were predictive of subsequent cardiac death including high admission systolic blood pressure, elevated BUN, elevated temperature, and a high Peel index. Several Coronary Care Unit arrhythmias were predictive of subsequent death including any atrial arrhythmia and atrial premature beats. Patients who survived had a higher rate of sinus rhythm without any significant cardiac arrhythmia and interestingly a higher rate of occurrence of accelerated idioventricular rhythm. The use of digitalis at the time of hospital discharge was associated with subsequent cardiac death. Other unfavorable factors included the occurrence of an anterior transmural

infarction or a history of previous angina pectoris or myocardial infarction. In this study a history of diabetes, hypertension or congestive heart failure were not significant indicators of subsequent cardiac death.

6. STUDY – MOSS ET AL. NUMBER 1 (8, 20)

An initial series of 100 patients was published in two articles in 1971 (20) and 1974 (8). This will be considered as Moss study number 1. A subsequent study was published in two parts in 1975 (21) and 1977 (22) and will be considered as Moss study number 2.

6.1. Patient population. The patient population consisted of 100 patients aged 33 to 78 (mean 57). There were 79 men and 21 women. Patients were hospitalized for definite acute myocardial infarction and were later discharged from the hospital.

6.2. Ambulatory ECG recordings. A 6-hour ambulatory ECG recording was performed approximately 3 days prior to hospital discharge. The time interval from hospital admission to obtaining the recording was 21 ± 7 days.

6.3. Arrhythmia definitions. Arrhythmia analysis was according to PVC frequency per 1000 beats and the presence or absence of multifocal beats, ventricular tachycardia, R on T beats and the combined category of pairs or bigeminy.

6.4. Arrhythmia prevalence. One or more premature ventricular beats were seen in 72 % of patients. Twenty percent had multifocal beats, 18 % pairs or bigeminy, 4 % ventricular tachycardia and 9 % R on T. Nine percent of the population had 10 or more premature ventricular beats per 1000 premature beats.

6.5. Follow-up. Follow-up averaged 1.8 ± 0.3 years (range 1-1/2 to 2). Twenty-one patients died during follow-up, 17 of these from cardiac causes. Only 4 of the deaths were sudden.

6.6. Conclusions.
   6.6.1. Ambulatory ECG. Among patients with premature ventricular beats the findings of prematurity, increasing frequency, and presence of bigeminy or pairs were predictive of subsequent cardiac death.
   6.6.2. Other. Among patients with PVCs on the discharge ambulatory ECG monitoring age, white count, and the Peel and Norris indices were predictive of subsequent sudden death by univariate analysis. In this group 91 % of survivors and nonsurvivors were correctly identified by a discriminant combination of arrhythmia parameters and age. For patients without ventricular arrhythmias the Norris short index, age and level of SGOT were predictive of subsequent death by univariate analysis.

7. STUDY – MOSS ET AL. NUMBER 2 (21, 22)

This study was published in two parts. The first 193 patients entered during the year 1973 up to and including September 15, 1973 were published and subsequently the entire year's group of 272 patients were published.

7.1. Patient population. The patient population was 272 patients (different from the 100 in the preceding study) admitted to the hospital with a diagnosis of definite or probable myocardial infarction and who were discharged alive. Patients were less than age 65 and had not had two or more previous myocardial infarctions. The average age of the patients was 56 years and there were 155 men and 38 women.

7.2. Ambulatory ECG recordings. Each patient underwent a 6-hour recording prior to hospital discharge and 231 patients returned at 5 months post infarction for a repeat 6-hour recording.

7.3. Arrhythmia definitions. Arrhythmia frequency was determined as number of premature ventricular beats per hour. Each tape was analyzed for the presence or absence of pairs, multifocality, bigeminy, ventricular tachycardia and R on T premature beats. Based on the results of univariate and bivariate analysis, Grade 1 premature ventricular beats were defined as those with a frequency of less than 20 per hour and without multiform or bigeminal patterns, and Grade 2 premature ventricular beats were those with a frequency of greater than or equal to 20 per hour or with multiform or bigeminal patterns, or both.

7.4. Arrhythmia prevalence. Arrhythmia prevalence on the predischarge ambulatory ECG recording showed 50 % of patients having one or more ventricular ectopic beats, 7 % greater than 20 per hour, 8 % multiform, 10 % R on T, 4 % bigeminy, 3 % pairs, 1 % ventricular tachycardia and 14 % Grade 2 ectopic beats. The 5 month recordings revealed that 63 % had one or more ventricular ectopic beat, 17 % greater than 20 per hour, 18 % multiform, 16 % R on T, 20 % bigeminy, 11 % pairs, 1 % ventricular tachycardia and 32 % Grade 2.

7.5. Follow-up. During the one year follow-up 18 patients died of cardiac causes. Eleven of these deaths occurred during the first four months after discharge. The number of deaths which were sudden is not specified.

7.6. Conclusions. Univariate analysis of predischarge ECG data revealed that only PVCs which were greater than 20 per hour or multiform or bigeminal were associated with an increased risk of death and this association was valid during the first four months only. These factors did not predict cardiac mortality from 0 to 12 months. Neither ventricular pairs nor prematurity predicted mortality at any time. No findings on the five month ambulatory ECG recording predicted mortality during the subsequent 7 months. Bivariate analysis showed that separating arrhythmias into Grade 1 and 2 allowed a much better prediction of death during the first 4 months. The recordings showed a strong association between the PVC frequency and the occurrence of pairs, multifocality and bigeminy. There was an increase in the number of patients with PVCs and an increase in prevalence of each complex type of premature ventricular beats except ventricular tachycardia when the 5 month data were compared to the discharge ambulatory ECG recordings.

8. STUDY – REHNQVIST ET AL. (13, 23, 24)

This study has been published as 3 manuscripts. Two initial manuscripts describe the arrhythmias and long-term follow-up in the first 100 patients and a subsequent paper summarizes the data for 160 patients.

8.1. Patient population. The patient population is 160 (127 men and 33 women) consecutive Coronary Care Unit treated acute myocardial infarction patients under the age of 66 years who were in sinus rhythm and without bundle branch block at the time of discharge. The average age was 59.7 years (range 44 to 65) and 77 patients were older than 59 years.

8.2. Ambulatory ECG recordings. Six hour telemetry recordings were done prior to discharge and again after one year.

8.3. Arrhythmia definitions. Arrhythmias were graded according to whether they were absent, infrequent and uniform, greater than 5 per minute, multiform, paired, R on T or occurred as ventricular tachycardia. Tapes were scored as to the highest grade achieved. It was noted that all patients with a frequency of premature beats greater than 5 per minute always had higher grades. "Severe" arrhythmias were taken as multiform, pairs, R on T or ventricular tachycardia.

8.4. Arrhythmia prevalence. Because tapes were scored as the highest grade achieved, it is difficult to determine the prevalence of each type of arrhythmia in this study. However, 75 % of the patients had one or more ventricular ectopic beats on their recordings at the time of hospital discharge. Thirty-nine percent had infrequent uniform premature beats as the highest grade achieved, 22 % had multiform, 10 % pairs, 2 % R on T, and 3 % ventricular tachycardia as their highest grade.

8.5. Follow-up. Follow-up was one year after the acute event. There were 127 men and 33 women with an age range of 44 to 65. During the follow-up year, 9 patients died suddenly (within 2 hours of onset of symptoms), 2 patients had cardiac arrest but were resuscitated, and 20 patients suffered reinfarction which was fatal in five. The endpoints for follow-up were reinfarction and sudden death.

8.6. Conclusions
   8.6.1. Ambulatory ECG. The presence of "severe" arrhythmias as compared to no

arrhythmia or infrequent uniform ventricular ectopic beats was related to cardiac events (both sudden death and reinfarction). The presence of these "severe" arrhythmias was statistically associated with increased age, a past history of congestive heart failure, a poor functional class and an increased heart size on chest x-ray. From the data provided it is unclear whether arrhythmias became worse at the one year follow-up when compared to the prehospital discharge recordings.

8.6.2. Other. The strongest prognostic factor was the presence of cardiomegaly on chest x-ray. Diabetes was also predictive of subsequent reinfarction, but not necessarily sudden death.

9. STUDY – RUBERMAN ET AL. (9, 25)

This study has been published in two parts. One manuscript (25) reports on results in 1,217 patients with regard to prognosis and provides detailed data concerning the relationship between PVC frequency and complexity and the interrelationship between each of the complex types of PVCs. The second manuscript (9) provides a detailed evaluation of premature ventricular beats and mortality in a larger group of 1,739 patients.

9.1. Patient population. The study evaluates 1,739 men with a history of previous myocardial infarction. Their ages range from 35 to 74 years. Fifty percent had a myocardial infarction less than 3 months prior to entry into the study, 30 % had a myocardial infarction 3 to 8 months before entering and 20 % had a myocardial infarction at least 9 months or more prior to entering the study.

9.2. Ambulatory ECG recordings. Each patient underwent one hour of continuous ECG recording.

9.3. Arrhythmia definitions. The total number of ventricular ectopic beats occurring in the hour was determined. PVCs were also classified as to whether or not they were R on T, multiform or bigeminal. Runs of premature beats were defined as 2 or more in a row; thus, combining pairs and ventricular tachycardia as defined in most other studies. Complex PVCs were defined as those occurring as R on T, runs, multiform or bigeminy.

9.4. Arrhythmia prevalence. There were no ventricular premature beats in 48.5 % of the patients. Of the remaining patients, 25.4 % had less than 10 premature beats per hour and 26.1 % had greater than 10 per hour. Complex premature beats were recorded in 26.6 % of patients. Of these, 6.3 % had less than 10 PVCs per hour and 20.3 % had greater than 10 per hour. Prevalence for the first 1,217 men was runs 18.5 %, multiform 44.8 %, R on T 12.0 % and bigeminy 22.2 %.

9.5. Follow-up. Follow-up ranged from 6 months to 4 years and averaged 24.4 months. There were a total of 208 deaths from all causes with 85 sudden (within minutes) deaths. All data analysis considered total mortality and sudden deaths individually.

9.6. Conclusions

9.6.1. Ambulatory ECG monitoring. This study showed an approximate threefold increase in risk of sudden death for patients with complex premature ventricular beats as
compared to those without complex beats. Of the 462 patients with complex premature
beats, the increased mortality was most striking among the 353 patients who also had
greater than 10 premature beats in the recorded hour. Simple premature beats, even when
they were greater than 10 per hour, did not identify patients at increased risk of death.
There was a marked association found for the occurrence of each of the types of complex
premature beats and it was difficult to determine the exact prognostic significance of each
qualitative type. It was possible to determine that runs or R on T beats were worse than
bigeminy or multiformal beats.

9.6.2. Other. The authors found that risk factors for sudden coronary death were similar
to those for deaths from all causes. Presence of congestive heart failure, treatment with
diuretics, ST segment depression and heart rate of more than 90 were all associated with
an approximate doubling of the risk of death when age and presence of complex ventricular
beats were controlled. This study clearly demonstrated that the presence of complex
premature beats was a risk factor even in the presence of congestive heart failure, since
among patients with congestive heart failure, mortality was approximately twice as high
if they also had associated complex premature beats. It should be noted that a large portion
of patients taking part in this study were well away from the acute phase of their myocardial
infarction and had already passed the period of highest risk for death. This study also used
a much shorter period of recording than most other published studies.

10. STUDY – SCHULZE ET AL. (10, 26)

This study was published as two manuscripts. An initial manuscript (26) was published
relating the relationship between left ventricular function as judged by gated blood pool
scans to the presence or absence of complex arrhythmias on 24-hour ambulatory ECG
recordings. A second manuscript (10) was published for a larger group of patients after a
period of follow-up.

10.1. Patient population. Eighty-one patients were studied approximately two weeks after
admission for a definite myocardial infarction. The average age of the patients is approximately 60 years and 55 were male.

10.2. Ambulatory ECG recordings. Twenty-four hour recordings were performed 2 weeks
post myocardial infarction.

10.3. Arrhythmia definitions. The authors used the Lown classification. In their preliminary
study relating arrhythmias and ventricular function, an earlier version of the Lown classification was utilized and in the final manuscript the following classification was used:
Class 0' = no premature ventricular beats, Class 1 = unifocal beats less than 30 per hour,

Class 2 = unifocal beats greater than 30 per hour in any hour, Class 3 = multifocal premature beats, Class 4 = coupled, bigeminal or runs of ventricular beats, Class 5 = R on T ventricular premature beats. Uncomplicated arrhythmias were taken as Classes 0, 1 and 2 complicated arrhythmias defined as Classes 3, 4, and 5.

10.4. Arrhythmia prevalence. Twenty-eight patients (35 %) had no premature ventricular beats identified. Because patients were classified as to the highest grade of arrhythmia achieved it is impossible to determine the exact prevalence of each type of arrhythmia except for ventricular tachycardia which was 1 %. Twenty-nine patients (36 %) were classified as complex.

10.5. Follow-up. The follow-up averaged 7 months with a range of 2 to 16 months. There were 10 cardiac deaths in the study, 8 of which were sudden (less than 1 hour). Correlations were made with sudden death.

10.6. Conclusions.

10.6.1. Ambulatory ECG recordings. The presence of complex premature ventricular beats was predictive of subsequent sudden death. There was a strong association between the occurrence of complex ventricular arrhythmias and an ejection fraction (measured by gated blood pool scan) of less than 0.40. The data suggest that sudden death is common in patients with reduced ejection fraction and complex arrhythmias since all deaths occurred in this subgroup of 26 patients. The study suggests that the low ejection fraction, while perhaps predictive of a poor prognosis, is not as important as the occurrence of complex ventricular arrhythmias.

11. STUDY – VISMARA ET AL. (11)

11.1. Patient population. The patient population is 64 patients admitted with acute myocardial infarction and discharged from the hospital with an average age of 61 years ranging from 39 and 85 years. There were 49 men and 15 women.

11.2. Ambulatory ECG recordings. Patients underwent 10-hour ambulatory ECG recordings from 5 to 14 (average 11) days after Coronary Care Unit discharge.

11.3. Arrhythmia definitions. A specific measure·of PVC frequency was not performed in this study. However, PVCs greater than 5 per minute were considered along with multiform PVCs, R on T, pairs, and presence of ventricular tachycardia as identifying a patient with complex premature beats.

11.4. Arrhythmia prevalence. Because of the method of arrhythmia definition, it is difficult to determine the exact prevalence of each type of complex premature beat. However, 27 of the 64 patients (42 %) had arrhythmias which were classified as complicated, 22 (34 %) had uncomplicated premature beats and 15 (23 %) exhibited no ventricular arrhythmias.

11.5. Follow-up. Patients were followed for an average of 25.8 months. Twelve patients died suddenly and 8 died of other causes, 4 of which were cardiac. Analysis of survival was made with regard to the occurrence of sudden death.

11.6. Conclusions.

11.6.1. Ambulatory ECG recordings. All sudden deaths occurred in patients with complex arrhythmias. This was a statistically significant observation.

11.6.2. Other findings. There was a relation between subsequent sudden death and the extent of ST segment abnormalities on an electrocardiogram obtained late in the hospitalization. Important negative findings in this study were that there was no relation between sudden death and patient age, sex, location of infarction, presence of coronary risk factors, severity of acute myocardial infarction, serum cholesterol levels, evidence of cardiomegaly on chest x-ray, presence of ventricular gallop and drug therapy received. The occurrence of sudden death was not significantly related to the occurrence of arrhythmias in the early hospital phase of myocardial infarction.

12. OTHER STUDIES

Several other studies have been published in abstract form and support the concept of frequent and complex premature ventricular beats as predictors of subsequent death (27–29).

13. DISCUSSION

13.1. Difficulties in comparing studies.

After careful analysis of the above described studies, it becomes apparent that it is difficult to compare one study to another. The studies differ markedly with regard to patient population, definitions of ventricular arrhythmias, duration of ambulatory monitoring, endpoints of data analysis and duration of follow-up.

It is difficult to compare even simple parameters such as prevalence of different types of complex premature ventricular beats recorded on the ambulatory ECGs (Table 5). Studies have used different definitions of complex premature beats and in some instances (15) bigeminy, R on T or multifocality are not even considered as complex premature beats. In others (12, 16) not all individual categories of complex beats which were considered separately in data analysis are reported in the manuscript. Other studies have combined (8, 9, 11, 12) (often arbitrarily) various grades of arrhythmias in the final data analysis. An important shortcoming of several studies (10, 13, 19) was that arbitrary classification schemes such as the Lown classification were utilized and data reported only as the highest grade recorded. This causes an important loss of information about the prevalence and significance of lesser grades of arrhythmias. Finally, some studies (19) report arrhythmia prevalence from sequential recordings and do not give isolated data for each recording period. Definitions of PVC frequency have also varied considerably and are summarized in Table 4. There has been little uniformity of duration of ECG recording with recordings ranging from as short as one hour to as long as 24 hours (Table 3).

Another factor which makes it difficult to compare studies is the differences in patient populations (Table 2). Only 5 of the 11 studies had no restrictions on entry criteria. Three studies excluded elderly patients and 2 excluded patients with heart failure, high functional class or other underlying diseases. Only 7 of the studies entered subjects of both sexes. In 2 of the 11 studies patients were entered who were greater than 3 months post myocardial infarction.

Duration of the follow-up (Table 6) ranged from 6 to 54 months. Surprisingly only 4 of the 11 studies correlated cardiac arrhythmias with *sudden* cardiac death with the remainder of studies correlating arrhythmias with all cardiac deaths (Table 1). Two of the studies did not even define sudden death and in the others definitions ranged from "within minutes" to as long as 24 hours after the onset of cardiac symptoms (Table 6).

Some studies considered only arrhythmias (19, 22) and others compared the predictive value of arrhythmias to multiple other clinical variables (Table 1). Statistical techniques also varied considerably from study to study.

13.2. Relation between arrhythmias on ambulatory ECG and subsequent sudden death

In the 11 studies summarized above 8 concluded that arrhythmias identified on ambulatory ECG monitoring were important for predicting subsequent death. Five (9, 10, 11, 13, 19) of these 8 studies considered only sudden death or considered sudden death as a separate category from cardiac death. The others (8, 12, 22) 3 correlated arrhythmias with any cardiac death. Six of these 8 studies considered multiple clinical characteristics as well as the ambulatory ECG findings in determining predictors of subsequent sudden death. Four (8, 9, 10, 11) of the 6 studies showing a relation between ambulatory ECG arrhythmias and subsequent death found that arrhythmias on the ambulatory ECG recording were the most important predictors of subsequent sudden death and the other two studies (12, 13) found one or more types of clinical information to be more important than findings on the ECG monitorings. It is of note that a large number of the other predictive clinical measures other than arrhythmias relate either directly or indirectly to left ventricular function, i.e., enlarged heart, elevated BUN, poor functional class, history of heart failure, low ejection fraction, etc. (Table 1). Two of the studies (19, 22) which showed that ambulatory ECG arrhythmias were important for identifying subsequent sudden death did not consider other clinical factors, so it is difficult to compare the relative importance of clinical factors to that of ambulatory ECG arrhythmias.

Since the majority of studies found arrhythmias on ambulatory ECG monitoring to be important predictors of subsequent sudden death it is important to critically review the 3 studies (14–16) which did not. The study of DeBusk et al. failed to show a relation between arrhythmias and subsequent cardiac events. However, the study of DeBusk et al. (14)

involved only patients free of clinical evidence of ventricular dysfunction. This occurred because patients taking part in this study were participants in a rehabilitation program and were required to be able to exercise on a treadmill at 3 weeks post myocardial infarction. This study overall had a very low occurrence rate of cardiac mortality. It is quite likely that the exclusion of patients with severe left ventricular dysfunction accounted for the inability to show a relationship between ventricular premature beats and subsequent cardiac events. Additionally, the study of DeBusk et al. only examined presence or absence of premature beats and did not use some measure of arrhythmia frequency.

The study of de Soyza (15) also found no relationship between ventricular arrhythmias on ambulatory monitoring and the occurrence of subsequent sudden death. However, this study can be criticized on several grounds. It included the smallest number of patients of any of the studies. Perhaps most importantly it had the least comprehensive definition of complex premature ventricular beats. These authors did not consider multifocal, R on T, or bigeminal premature beats to be complex. Thus, they excluded most of the categories that other authors found to be important for predicting subsequent cardiac mortality.

It is more difficult to explain why the study of Bigger et al. (16) did not find a correlation between ambulatory ECG arrhythmias and subsequent sudden death. Bigger's study was larger than several others which did find significant relationships between arrhythmias and sudden death. Although in this study arrhythmias were correlated with cardiac death rather than sudden death, it is unlikely that this is the explanation since 12 of the 15 deaths in that series were sudden. One possible explanation may relate to the duration of monitoring and the method utilized to detect ventricular arrhythmias. Rather than relying on automated techniques to detect arrhythmias, these authors printed out the entire ambulatory ECG recordings on a Grass polygraph. This technique should be more accurate for detecting rare episodes of complex arrhythmias than more automated techniques. In fact, these authors found a higher prevalence of any premature beats, and each of the complex forms of ventricular premature beats than any of the other 10 studies summarized above. Furthermore, their study was one of only 3 to use a full 24-hours of ECG recording. It is possible that this study used too sensitive an analysis technique and too long a duration of monitoring in order to optimally detect patients at risk of sudden death. It may be that these arrhythmias are only important when they are extraordinarily frequent and easily detected by less thorough methods of arrhythmia detection or with shorter periods of monitoring. While this explanation is purely speculative, if correct it would create problems as technology permits longer periods of recording and more accurate arrhythmia detection. The most likely explanation for the different findings of this study is a difference in patient populations.

Overall it seems likely that a strong relationship exists between arrhythmias on ambulatory ECG monitorings and subsequent death (including sudden death) in patients with coronary heart disease. However, due to difficulties in comparing studies it is impossible to determine a consensus opinion as to which specific type of complex premature ventricular beat is most important for identifying high risk patients. Not only is this difficulty due to different methods of data reporting, but several studies have commented on the strong association among different types of complex premature beats and among such complex beats and PVC frequency.

Anderson et al. (30) examined the prognostic value of ventricular tachycardia in 66 post infarction patients with sequential 6-hour recordings over 4-48 months. He found that compared to a control group without ventricular tachycardia they had a 2-fold increased risk of dying, however, the difference was not significant. Furthermore, the patients with VT had more severe cardiac disease and more ventricular irritability than the control group. The relative importance of PVC frequency as compared to the presence of complex forms of premature beats is also difficult to determine. Only 5 of the 11 studies (8, 9, 12, 16, 22) considered PVC frequency separately from complexity (Table 4). Conversely, of the 4 studies (9, 10, 11, 19) showing "complex" PVCs to be predictive of subsequent sudden death, only one (9) separately considered PVC frequency.

There also seems to be controversy over how long the ambulatory ECG remains of value to predict subsequent death following a myocardial infarction. Kotler et al. (19) entered patients only after 3 months had elapsed from the time of their myocardial infarction. During the follow-up period they performed sequential ambulatory ECG monitorings and found the arrhythmias on these monitorings to be predictive of subsequent death. On the other hand, Moss et al. (22) found that in contrast to the predictive value of arrhythmias on a 3 week post infarction Holter, a recording done 5 months later was of no value for predicting subsequent mortality.

13.3. Day to day variability of complex arrhythmias

We have recently examined the day to day variability of the occurrence of complex ventricular arrhythmias in the late hospital postinfarction period. Fifty-six patients underwent 3 consecutive 24-hour ambulatory ECG recordings. Each recording was examined for the presence of each type of complex ventricular arrhythmia. The results are summarized in Table 7. There was complete agreement (all days with or without a given type of arrhythmias) in about two-thirds of patients for each complex form. However, for some patients each type of complex arrhythmia was variable from one day to the next. This was most striking for ventricular tachycardia. Of 12 patients with ventricular tachycardia, 9 had it on only one day and only one patient had it on all three days of recording. It is of note that 44 of 56 (82 %) of patients had some type of complex arrhythmia recorded during the total of 72 hours of recording. With such a high prevalence it seems likely that complex arrhythmias detected during longer periods of monitoring may lose their predictive value.

Table 7. Number of patients with complex ventricular arrhythmias on three consecutive 24 hour ambulatory ECG recordings (total: 56 patients).

Days	Multiform	pars	bigeminy	R on T	ventricular tachycardia	any complex
none	20	35	38	26	44	12
one only	12	8	7	15	9	8
two only	9	9	5	7	2	13
all three	15	4	6	8	1	23

13.4. Relationship between arrhythmias detected on ambulatory ECG and angiographic findings

Although there appears to be a relationship between the presence and extent of coronary heart disease, left ventricular dysfunction and the occurrence of ventricular arrhythmias, the data in the literature are conflicting. Calvert et al. (31) examined 24-hour ambulatory ECG recordings in 124 patients. They found the prevalence and grade of ventricular premature beats were increased in patients with multi-vessel disease compared to patients with single vessel disease. The group with single vessel disease did not differ significantly from those without coronary heart disease. They also found a relationship between elevated left ventricular end-diastolic pressure and asynergy and ventricular ectopic beats. Vismara et al. (32) examined 10-hour ECG recordings in 115 patients undergoing arteriography. They found ventricular arrhythmias to be more common in patients with coronary heart disease as compared to normal subjects. They found the prevalence of serious premature ventricular contractions significantly greater in patients with multi-vessel disease than in those with one vessel obstruction. In contrast to the study of Calvert, Vismara did not find a relation between the presence of ventricular arrhythmias and segmental ventricular dyssynergy in the patients with coronary heart disease.

Two additional studies found no relation between asymptomatic PVCs on ambulatory ECG recording and degree of coronary artery obstruction. Califf et al. (33) performed 24-hour ambulatory ECG recordings in 244 patients undergoing arteriography. They found the presence of myocardial fibrosis as indicated by both abnormal left ventricular contraction patterns and abnormal initial QRS on electrocardiogram to be the only predictors of both frequent and complex ventricular ectopic beats. In fact, the prevalence of ventricular premature beats was directly related to the number of abnormally contracting segments on the left ventricular angiogram. The number of diseased vessels was dependent upon abnormal left ventricular contractility in its relation to ventricular ectopic beats. Similarly, Sharma et al. (34) reported that there was no relation between frequency and character of ventricular premature beats on an 8-hour ambulatory ECG recording and the number of coronary arteries diseased. They did note a relationship between these arrhythmias and the presence of asynergy on the left ventriculogram.

Schultz et al. (10, 26) have noted a strong association between depressed left ventricular ejection fraction as determined by gated blood pool scanning and the presence of complex ventricular arrhythmias on 24-hour ambulatory ECG recordings. However, subsequent data reported that sudden deaths occurred primarily in the group with both arrhythmias and low ejection fractions.

Thus, although the data are somewhat conflicting, it would appear that the occurrence of ventricular arrhythmias on ambulatory ECG recordings in patients with coronary heart disease is related to either the number of vessels diseased or the degree of left ventricular dysfunction or asynergy or both.

14. SUMMARY

1. In population studies frequent and/or complex PVCs on 12-lead ECG or ambulatory ECG seem to predict sudden death only in patients with "heart disease".

2. The presence of premature ventricular beats which are "complex and frequent" on an ambulatory ECG recording in patients with coronary heart disease appears to be a strong predictor of subsequent cardiac and sudden death.

3. It is difficult to determine the independent contribution of each type of complex premature beat and of PVC frequency in predicting this sudden death.

4. There appears to be a relationship between the occurrence of premature ventricular beats and the extent of coronary heart disease and left ventricular asynergy on angiography.

5. Other clinical factors are important in conjunction with the presence of PVCs especially those related directly or indirectly to left ventricular function.

6. There is a need for more complete data reporting and analysis and less lumping of arrhythmia categories prior to data analysis in order to facilitate comparison of studies.

REFERENCES

1. Blackburn H, de Backer G, Crow R, Prineas R and Jacobs D: Epidemiology and prevention of ventricular ectopic rhythms. Adv Cardiol 18:208–216, 1976.
2. Chiang BN, Perlman LV, Ostrander LD Jr, Epstein FH: Relationship of premature systoles to coronary heart disease and sudden death in the Tecumseh epidemiologic study. Ann Int Med 70(6):1159–116, 1969.
3. Rodstein M, Wolloch L, Gubner RS: Mortality study of the significance of extrasystoles in an insured population. Circulation 44:617–625, 1971.
4. Tominaga S, Blackburn H: Prognostic importance of premature beats following myocardial infarction: Experience in the coronary drug project. JAMA 223:1116–1124, 1973.
5. Desai DC, Hershberg PI, Alexander S: Clinical significance of ventricular premature beats in an outpatient population. Chest 64:564–569, 1973.
6. Hinkle LE, Carver ST, Stevens M: The frequency of asymptomatic disturbances of cardiac rhythm and conduction in middle-aged men. Am J Cardiol 24:629–650, 1969.
7. Hinkle LE, Carver ST, Argyros DC: The prognostic significance of ventricular premature contractions in healthy people and in people with coronary heart disease. Acta Cardiologica (suppl) 18:5–32, 1974.
8. Moss AJ, DeCamilla J, Engstrom F, Hoffman W, Odoroff C, Davis H: The posthospital phase of myocardial infarction: Identification of patients with increased mortality risk. Circulation 49:460–466, 1974.
9. Ruberman W, Weinblatt E, Goldberg J, Frank CW, Shapiro S: Ventricular premature beats and mortality after myocardial infarction. New Engl J Med 297:750–757, 1977.
10. Schulze RA Jr, Strauss HW, Pitt B: Sudden death in the year following myocardial infarction. Am J Med 62:192–199, 1977.
11. Vismara LA, Amsterdam EA, Mason DT: Relation of ventricular arrhythmias in the late hospital phase of acute myocardial infarction to sudden death after hospital discharge. Am J Med 59:6–12, 1975.
12. Luria MH, Knoke JD, Margolis RM, Hendricks FH, Kuplic JB: Acute myocardial infarction: Prognosis after recovery. Ann Int Med 85:561–565, 1976.
13. Rehnqvist N: Ventricular arrhythmias after an acute myocardial infarction. European J Cardiol 7/2–3:169–187, 1978.
14. DeBusk RF, Davidson DM, Houston N, Fitzgerald JW: Serial ambulatory electrocardiography and treadmill exercise testing following uncomplicated myocardial infarction. Circulation (in press).
15. de Soyza N, Bennett FA, Murphy ML, Bisset JK, Kane JJ: The relationship of paroxysmal ventricular tachycardia complicating the acute phase and ventricular arrhythmia during the late hospital phase of myocardial infarction to long-term survival. Am J Med 64:377–381, 1978.

16. Bigger JT, Heller CA, Wenger TL, Weld FM: Risk stratification after acute myocardial infarction. Am J Cardiol 42:202–210, 1978.

17. Wenger TL, Bigger JT Jr, Merrill GS: Ventricular arrhythmias in the late hospital phase of acute myocardial infarction. Abstract Circulation 51 and 52 (suppl II):II–110, 1975.

18. Fitzgerald JW, Houston N, DeBusk RF: Natural history of ventricular arrhythmias in post-infarction patients. Circulation 53 and 54 (suppl II):II–10, 1976.

19. Kotler MN, Tabatznik B, Mower MM, Tominaga S: Prognostic significance of ventricular ectopic beats with respect to sudden death in the late postinfarction period. Circulation 47:959–966, 1973.

20. Moss AJ, Schnitzler R, Green R, DeCamilla J: Ventricular arrhythmias 3 weeks after acute myocardial infarction. Ann Int Med 75:837–841, 1971.

21. Moss AJ, De Camilla J, Mietlowski W, Greene WA, Goldstein S, Locksley R: Prognostic grading and significance of ventricular premature beats after recovery from myocardial infarction. Circulation 51 and 52 (suppl III):III–204–210, 1975.

22. Moss AJ, DeCamilla JJ, Davis HP, Bayer L: Clinical significance of ventricular ectopic beats in the early posthospital phase of myocardial infarction. Am J Cardiol 39:635–640, 1977.

23. Rehnqvist N: Ventricular arrhythmias prior to discharge after acute myocardial infarction. European J Cardiol 4/1:63–70, 1976.

24. Rehnqvist N and Sjogren A: Ventricular arrhythmias prior to discharge and one year after acute myocardial infarction. European J Cardiol 5/5:425–442, 1977.

25. Ruberman W, Weinblatt E, Frank CW, Goldberg JD, Shapiro S, Feldman CL: Prognostic value of one hour of ECG monitoring of men with coronary heart disease. J Chron Dis 29:497–512, 1976.

26. Schulze RA Jr, Rouleau J, Rigo P, Bowers S, Strauss, Pitt B: Ventricular arrhythmias in the late hospital phase of acute myocardial infarction: Relation of left ventricular function detected by gated cardiac blood pool scanning. Circulation 52:1006–1011, 1975.

27. Kleiger RE, Martin TF, Miller JP, et al: Ventricular tachycardia and ventricular extrasystoles during the late recovery phase of myocardial infarction. Am J Cardiol 33:149, 1974.

28. Oliver GC, Nolle FM, Tiefenbrunn AJ, et al: Ventricular arrhythmias associated with sudden death in survivors of acute myocardial infarction. Am J Cardiol 33:160, 1974.

29. Van Durme JP, Pannier RH: Prognostic significance of ventricular dysrhythmias 1 year after myocardial infarction. Am J Cardiol 37:178, 1976.

30. Anderson KP, De Camilla J, Moss AJ: Clinical significance of ventricular tachycardia (3 beats or longer) detected during ambulatory monitoring after myocardial infarction. Circulation 57:890–897, 1978.

31. Calvert A, Lown B, Gorlin R: Ventricular premature beats and anatomically defined coronary heart disease. Am J Cardiol 39:627–634, 1977.

32. Vismara LA, Vera Z, Foerster JM, Amsterdam EA, Mason DT: Identification of sudden death risk factors in acute and chronic coronary artery disease. Am J Cardiol 39:821–828, 1977.

33. Califf RM, Burks JM, Behar VS, Margolis JR, Wagner GS: Relationships among ventricular arrhythmias, coronary artery disease, and angiographic and electrocardiographic indicators of myocardial fibrosis. Circulation 57:725–732, 1978.

34. Sharma SD, Ballantyne F, Goldstein S: The relationship of ventricular asynergy in coronary artery disease to ventricular premature beats. Chest 66:358–362, 1974.

3.6. DETECTION OF HIGH RISK PATIENTS FOR SUDDEN DEATH: THE ROLE OF MYOCARDIAL IMAGING WITH RADIOISOTOPES

B. PITT

Myocardial imaging with radioisotopes is finding increasing clinical application in the evaluation of patients with both ischemic and nonischemic heart disease (1–7). Although experience with these techniques for identification of patients at risk for sudden cardiac death is still limited, the data that is available, and accumulating in several centers, suggests that myocardial imaging has an important role in this, as yet, unsolved clinical problem. In this chapter the major clinically available techniques for myocardial imaging with radioisotopes will be briefly reviewed along with their application to the problem of sudden cardiac death.

1. CARDIAC BLOOD POOL IMAGING (15)

Cardiac blood pool imaging following intravenous injection of technetium-99m human serum albumin or red blood cells has been shown to be of value in identifying patients at risk for sudden cardiac death after an episode of acute myocardial infarction. Left ventricular ejection fraction and regional myocardial wall motion can be determined by monitoring the initial passage of tracer through the circulation ("first pass technique") or by waiting until the tracer has reached equilibrium within the vascular space and triggering the scintillation camera by a physiologic marker such as the R wave of the electrocardiogram. With current computer techniques, 14–56 frame/cardiac cycle nuclear angiograms can be easily obtained. Left ventricular ejection fraction can be calculated from the changes in radioactivity within the left ventricle during the cardiac cycle using the left anterior oblique projection which separates the right and left ventricular chambers. The activity within the left ventricle can be determined noninvasively or by applying semiautomatic edge detection programs. Recently completely automatic programs have been developed using "cyto" computer techniques. With these new techniques left ventricular borders can be accurately detected in images with approximately 20,000 counts in comparison to the 100,000–200,0000 counts required using currently available commercial computer programs. Because of these advances in computer processing it is now possible to obtain accurate calculations of left ventricular ejection fraction every twenty to thirty seconds. Left ventricular ejection fraction and regional myocardial wall motion obtained from the blood pool image has been found to correlate highly with data obtained by routine contrast left ventriculography both at rest and during exercise.

Schulze et al. studied patients prior to hospital discharge following an episode of acute myocardial infarction and performed blood pool imaging and 24 hour Holter ECG analysis (16–18). Arrhythmias detected by ambulatory ECG monitoring were classified according to the criteria proposed by Lown. Patients with complex ventricular arrhythmias (Lown Class III-V) were found to have a relatively low left ventricular ejection fraction and large percentage of the left ventricle that was asynergic in comparison to those without ventricular arrhythmias and those with unifocal beats (Lown Class 0-II). The association of poor ventricular function and complex ventricular arrhythmias has been since confirmed by several studies including contrast angiographic study prior to hospital discharge. These studies have also shown a high incidence of multiple vessel disease in those with low left ventricular ejection fractions and complex ventricular arrhythmias. Follow-up studies by Schulze et al. have shown that patients with low left ventricular ejection fractions and complex ventricular arrhythmias during the convalescent phase of acute myocardial infarction have a high incidence of subsequent sudden death within the next year. On subsequent follow-up studies of patients recovering from an episode of acute myocardial infarction, those with relatively good left ventricular ejection fractions and those without complex ventricular arrhythmias have also occasionally been found to have sudden cardiac death. However, there appears to be increasing evidence that patients dying suddenly after an episode of acute myocardial infarction are characterized by extensive myocardial damage and multivessel disease. Complex ventricular arrhythmias that persist on subsequent post hospital ambulatory ECG recordings appear to be markers of extensive myocardial damage and multivessel disease. Although extensive myocardial damage can often be predicted from initial serum enzyme release and signs of congestive heart failure this is not always the case. For example, patients with a previous myocardial infarction may suffer a subsequent non-transmural myocardial infarction. Serum enzyme release after these circumstances may be relatively little but total myocardial damage great. Cardiac blood pool imaging allows a better estimation of total myocardial damage under these circumstances by calculation of left ventricular ejection fraction and the percent of left ventricular akinesis. Similarly, extensive myocardial damage as evidenced by a low left ventricular ejection fraction can be present without clinical signs of manifest congestive heart failure. These factors may account for the fact that the association between extensive myocardial damage, complex ventricular arrhythmias and subsequent sudden cardiac death have only recently been recognized.

The extent of myocardial damage in a patient with acute myocardial infarction may also be established by acute infarct avid imaging with technetium-99m pyrophosphate.

2. INFARCT AVID IMAGING (8, 9)

Technetium-99m pyrophosphate is the current infarct avid agent of choice. This radiopharmaceutical is taken up by acutely infarcted myocardial tissue. The uptake of this tracer is in part related to deposition of calcium within the infarcted myocardial cells and in part to formation of complexes with the damaged myocardial cells. Uptake of tracer is dependent upon cell damage and residual myocardial blood flow to the infarcted area.

Tracer uptake by the infarcted myocardium can be detected within several hours of onset of symptoms, but is not maximum until 48 to 72 hours. If imaging is performed 48 to 72 hours after onset of symptoms, the sensitivity for detection of patients with transmural myocardial infarction is over 90 % and for nontransmural infarction approximately 75 %. With standard imaging techniques, a relatively good correlation of approximately 0.90 has been found between extent of pyrophosphate uptake and infarct size in patients with acute anterior transmural infarction. This relationship is of importance in view of the findings in both animal and human studies that the extent of infarction is directly related to the tendency for ventricular arrhythmias during the convalescent phase of acute myocardial infarction, ventricular fibrillation threshold, and sudden cardiac death. The correlation between infarct size and extent of tracer uptake is, however, not as good in patients with inferior or posterior transmural infarction nor in those patients with nontransmural infarction due to geometric limitations of conventional imaging techniques. These limitations have, however, recently been overcome through the use of tomographic imaging techniques. With current tomographic imaging techniques, an excellent correlation has been obtained in animal studies between extent of tracer uptake and infarct size in both inferior and posterior infarction as well as in anterior infarction, both transmural and nontransmural. Application of these new tomographic approaches to patients recovering from an episode of acute myocardial infarction should over the next several years provide a valuable adjunct to current estimation of infarct size by CK-MB release prediction of patients at risk for sudden death. Both of these techniques are, however, limited in regard to prognosis following myocardial infarct size as they reveal only the extent of the acute rather than the total damage as with blood pool imaging.

3. THALLIUM-201 (10)

Thallium-201 myocardial imaging is another technique to detect and evaluate patients with acute myocardial infarction. Myocardial infarction can be detected by a focal defect in tracer uptake which on serial imaging over several hours remains unchanged while areas of ischemic but viable myocardium can be detected by a defect in tracer uptake which on serial imaging over several hours tends to accumulate tracer. If imaging is performed within the first few hours of onset of infarction, over 90 % of patients with transmural and nontransmural infarction can be detected. After several hours the sensitivity for detecting patients with nontransmural infarction diminishes but remains greater than that for the electrocardiogram. The extent of the tracer defect on a thallium-201 image in a patient with acute infarction appears to correlate with subsequent cardiac death. Estimation of infarct size by thallium-201 imaging has been considerably improved by recent tomographic imaging techniques. Tomographic imaging can be accomplished with commercially available scintillation cameras by the addition of special collimators. One collimator developed by Kirsh and his colleagues in Denver, Colorado (15) consists of multiple pin holes, while another developed by Rogers et al. in Ann Arbor, Michigan (16) consists of specially drilled holes in a metal plate which passes over the detector face of the scintillation camera (coded aperture). The advantage of the coded aperture is its resolution and applicability to portable scintillation cameras. In both techniques multiple images are projected on the detector face of the camera and tomographic images reconstructed by computer processing. These tomographic techniques and new computer programs to calculate the percent of the left ventricle that is infarcted and the percent of viable myocardium have correlated closely with pathologic data from animals with myocardial infarction. Application of these tomographic approaches in conjunction with the tomographic approach to infarct avid imaging should provide a reliable clinical technique for estimating infarct size and remaining viable myocardium and should allow more accurate prediction and detection of those at risk for subsequent sudden death.

Although myocardial imaging with radioactive tracers promises to improve our ability to evaluate the extent of myocardial infarction and therefore detect patients at risk for both sudden and nonsudden cardiac death. It is unlikely that these efforts will in the end result in a major reduction in the problem of sudden cardiac death. Sudden cardiac death is often the first manifestation of ischemic heart disease. To make a major impact on the overall problem of sudden death in patients with ischemic heart disease will require early identification of patients with ischemic heart disease, prior to myocardial infarction and recognition of those at greatest risk of subsequent sudden death. Identification of patients with ischemic heart disease is the first step in a program to alter or prevent the progression of atherosclerotic coronary artery disease and to reduce or eliminate the precipitating trigger factors which initiate the process of ischemia and sudden cardiac death. To focus our attention on detection and therapy of ventricular arrhythmias following myocardial infarction as a means of preventing sudden death is shortsighted since it has been adequately demonstrated both in our previous study of sudden death following myocardial infarction and those of others that once infarction occurs the presence of complex ventricular arrhythmias during the convalescent phase suggests the presence of multivessel coronary artery disease and extensive myocardial damage.

The techniques of greatest promise for early detection of patients with ischemic heart disease are exercise thallium-201 myocardial imaging and exercise blood pool imaging. Exercise thallium-201 myocardial imaging has been shown to be a sensitive and relatively specific technique for detecting patients with myocardial ischemia (13). The appearance of a defect in thallium-201 uptake during exercise which is not present on serial imaging over several hours or on a subsequent rest image suggests myocardial ischemia and the presence of significant obstructive coronary artery disease. The location of the thallium-201 defect can be used to predict the coronary artery responsible for the myocardial ischemia. Proximal left anterior descending coronary artery lesions for example, can be predicted from a defect involving the anterior apical region on the anterior projection and the interventricular septal region on the left anterior oblique projection. Since in some studies lesions of the proximal left anterior descending coronary artery have been suggested to indicate a poor prognosis and a high incidence of sudden death, these findings on an exercise thallium-201 image may be of importance. Exercise thallium-201 imaging is also of value in evaluating patients with ventricular arrhythmias during exercise. The development of a ventricular arrhythmia during exercise does not necessarily indicate underlying myocardial disease nor conversely does the disappearance of a ventricular arrhythmia during exercise indicate the lack of ischemic heart disease. A defect in thallium-201 uptake detected during exercise in a patient developing ventricular premature beats suggest underlying myocardial ischemia even in the absence of "ischemic" ST-T wave changes on the exercise electrocardiogram.

One of the most promising applications of myocardial imaging during exercise with thallium-201 to the problem of sudden cardiac death is its application to the evaluation of asymptomatic individuals. Exercise electrocardiography has been the technique of choice to screen asymptomatic individuals for possible ischemic heart disease. It is, however, clear from the work of numerous investigators that there are major limitations to exercise electrocardiography in screening asymptomatic patients for ischemic heart disease. When used in a referral center to evaluate patients with typical angina pectoris being referred for possible coronary artery bypass graft surgery, exercise electrocardiography is extremely useful. Since there will be a relatively high prevalence of significant coronary artery disease in a center evaluating patients for coronary artery bypass graft surgery, most of the patients will be detected and there will be relatively few false positives. In an asymptomatic group of patients, however, in whom the prevalence of significant coronary artery disease is relatively low, in the order of 5%, the limited specificity of exercise electrocardiography, at best 90%, will result in a high proportion of the "positive" electrocardiographic response being falsely positive. Early and accurate detection of asymptomatic patients with atherosclerotic coronary artery disease is one of the most promising strategies for prevention of sudden cardiac death. In a pilot study of exercise thallium-201 imaging in asymptomatic individuals, we evaluated 15 patients referred with a "positive" exercise electrocardiogram (14). The individuals were evaluated as part of a risk factor screening program but were entirely asymptomatic. Of the 15 with a positive exercise electrocardiogram, 10 had a new defect in thallium-201 uptake during exercise suggesting myocardial ischemia while 5 had a normal response. Of the 10 in whom both the electrocardiogram and exercise thallium-201 studies agreed, 9 had significant obstructive coronary artery disease. In the 5 in whom there was disagreement, 4 had normal coronary arteriograms. Thus, the combination of a positive exercise electrocardiogram and a positive exercise thallium-201 test makes it likely that an asymptomatic patient has significant coronary artery disease while disagreement considerably reduces the likelihood. With further experience and the addition of exercise blood pool imaging (see below) it should be possible to be almost 100% certain of the presence of underlying ischemic heart disease in an asymptomatic individual.

Exercise thallium-201 is also being performed prior to hospital discharge following an episode of myocardial infarction. The detection of a new defect in thallium-201 uptake during exercise in a patient with myocardial infarction suggests additional vascular disease and an area of myocardium at risk for subsequent ischemia and infarction, possibly resulting in sudden death. In a number of institutions, the finding of a new thallium-201 defect on exercise prior to hospital discharge following an episode of myocardial infarction is an indication for early coronary angiography and coronary artery bypass graft surgery. Whether such an approach is justified is as yet uncertain and must await the results of careful long term follow-up.

Blood pool imaging is also finding wide application in the evaluation of patients with suspected ischemic heart disease. Contrast angiographic studies have shown that patients with normal coronary arteries and ventricular function tend to increase their left ventricular ejection fraction during exercise by at least 5 % above normal resting values. Patients with significant coronary artery narrowing either fail to increase their left ventricular ejection fractions or actually decrease their ejection fraction during exercise. The diminished response of left ventricular ejection fraction during exercise has been found to be due to an increase in left ventricular end systolic volume during exercise. Left ventricular end diastolic volume may also increase in patients with coronary artery disease but only in those with multivessel disease or extensive areas of ischemia during exercise. Similar results have been found with blood pool imaging at rest and during exercise. As with contrast left ventriculography, patients with normal coronary arteries tend to increase their left ventricular ejection fraction during supine bicycle ergometry while those with coronary artery disease either fail to increase their ejection fraction or show a decrease in left ventricular function during exercise. The presence of significant obstructive coronary artery disease may also be detected by the finding of a new abnormality of myocardial wall motion during exercise. The sensitivity for detecting patients with significant coronary artery disease with this technique has been found to be greater than 90% both in patients with development of angina pectoris during exercise and those with significant obstructive coronary artery disease who fail to develop symptoms. To achieve this relatively high sensitivity for detecting patients with coronary artery disease, careful attention must be paid to technical details. One often neglected aspect is the need to perform graded exercise. In normal individuals left ventricular ejection fraction increases and plateaus at a value of 75–80%. The response in patients with coronary artery disease is, however, more variable. As mentioned above, patients with coronary artery disease either fail to increase their left ventricular ejection fraction or have a decrease in ejection fraction during exercise. In some patients, however, left ventricular ejection fraction increases above resting values at moderate levels of exercise and then declines from peak values at maximum levels. If only the resting and maximum exercise values are recorded, the patient may be thought to have a normal response to exercise and a false negative diagnosis of ischemic heart disease made. By recording left ventricular ejection fraction at multiple levels this error can be avoided. Although the sensitivity of exercise blood pool imaging for detecting patients with ischemic heart disease is over 90%, the specificity is relatively low. Any condition that interferes with the functional integrity of the myocardium such as granuloma formation due to sarcoidosis, Chagas disease, rheumatic heart disease, or myocardial scarring due to previous viral myocarditis will result in an abnormal left ventricular ejection fraction response during exercise, although resting values may be normal. The implication of exercise blood pool imaging alone or in combination with exercise thallium-201 myocardial imaging for the problem of sudden cardiac death is enormous.

Radioactive tracer techniques may also be of value in patients with known ischemic heart disease to detect individuals at risk for cardiac death. For example, infarct avid imaging with technetium-99m pyrophosphate may have a role in detecting patients with unstable angina pectoris at risk for subsequent sudden death. Approximately 25 % of patients with unstable angina pectoris but without classic serial ECG and serum enzyme evidence of infarction have been found to have uptake of technetium-99m pyrophosphate within the myocardium. Although these patients were at first thought to have false positive pyrophosphate images, recent clinical and pathologic findings suggest that these patients have small areas of myocardial necrosis not detected by routine clinical studies. One recent study of pyrophosphate imaging by Olsen et al. (19) in 199 patients with unstable angina pectoris but without serial ECG or serum enzyme evidence of acute myocardial infarction found 67 with a positive and 132 with a negative pyrophosphate image. Those patients with a negative pyrophosphate image had a 3 % incidence of subsequent myocardial infarction and a 6 % incidence of death compared to a 21 % incidence of nonfatal infarction and a 22 % incidence of death in those with a positive pyrophosphate image. A positive pyrophosphate image in these patients may represent subclinical ongoing myocardial necrosis. If these studies are confirmed in subsequent clinical trials, this may be a way of identifying a group of patients with unstable angina pectoris at low risk for subsequent death in whom aggressive therapy is not indicated in contrast to those with a positive image with a high risk of death in whom aggressive therapy, possibly including coronary artery bypass graft surgery would be acceptable.

In conclusion, radioactive tracer technique studies have been shown to be of value in estimating the extent of myocardial damage following infarction and thereby identifying a group of patients at high risk for subsequent sudden cardiac death. The greatest promise of radioactive tracer techniques to the problem of sudden cardiac death, however, is in identifying patients with early obstructive coronary artery disease and in identifying high risk subsets for death in those with known angina pectoris. Once complex ventricular arrhythmias occur during the convalescent phase of acute myocardial infarction there is usually extensive myocardial damage and multivessel disease. The prospects for making a major impact on the problem of sudden cardiac death by use of antiarrhythmic agents along in the post infarct patient is poor. Increased emphasis must be placed on identifying patients with early ischemic heart disease and institution of therapy to prevent the progression of atherosclerosis as well as in finding subsets of patients with known ischemic heart disease at risk for sudden death prior to onset of myocardial infarction and institution of therapy to prevent or reduce the precipitation of ischemia and subsequent death. Myocardial imaging with radioactive tracers shows great promise for future advances in this problem.

REFERENCES

1. Pitt B, Strauss HW: Myocardial imaging in the noninvasive evaluation of patients with suspected ischemic heart disease. Am J Cardiol 37:797–806, 1976.
2. Strauss HW, Pitt B: Cardiovascular nuclear medicine: Its role in patients with coronary heart disease. Appl Radiol 4:57–62, 1975.
3. Pitt B, Strauss HW: Myocardial perfusion imaging and gated cardiac blood pool scanning: Clinical application. Am J Cardiol 38:739–746, 1976.
4. Strauss HW, Pitt B: Common procedures for the noninvasive determination of regional myocardial perfusion, evaluation of regional wall motion and detection of acute infarction. Am J Cardiol 38:731–738, 1976.
5. Pitt B: Right and left ventricular ejection fraction: Measurement of radionuclide angiocardiography in coronary artery disease. Chest 70:321–322, 1976.

6. Pitt B, Strauss HW: Cardiovascular nuclear medicine. Sem Nucl Med 73–6, 1977.
7. Pitt B, Thrall JH: Nuclear cardiology: A promise for improved cardiovascular diagnosis – Will it be fulfilled. Arch Intern Med (in press).
8. Bonte FJ, Parkey RW, Graham KD, Moore J, Stokely EM: A new method for radionuclide imaging of myocardial infarcts. Radiology 110:473–474, 1974.
9. Parkey RW, Bonte FJ, Stokely Em, Buja LM, Willerson JT: Acute myocardial infarct imaging with 99mTc stannous pyrophosphate. In: Nuclear cardiology – principles and methods, Serafini AN, Gilson AJ, Smoak WM (eds), Plenum Publishing Corp, 1977, p. 133–145.
10. Strauss HW, Pitt B: Thallium-201 as a myocardial imaging agent. Sem Nucl Med 7:49–58, 1977.
11. Vogel RA, Kirch DL, Lefree MT, Steele PP: Improved diagnostic results of myocardial perfusion tomography using a new rapid inexpensive technique. J Nucl Med 19:731, (abstr) 1978.
12. Rogers WL, Koral KF, Mayans R, Leonard PF, Keyes J: Coded aperture imaging of the heart. J Nucl Med 19:730, (abstr) 1978.
13. Bailey IK, Griffith LSC, Rouleau J, Strauss HW, Pitt B: Thallium-201 myocardial perfusion imaging at rest and during exercise: Comparative sensitivity to electrocardiography in coronary artery disease. Circulation 55:79–87, 1977
14. Caralis DG, Kennedy HL, Bailey IK, Pitt B: Thallium-201 myocardial perfusion scanning in the evaluation of asymptomatic patients with ischemic ST segment depression. Am J Cardiol 39:320, (Abstr) 1977.
15. Strauss HW, Pitt B: Evaluation of cardiac function and structure with radioactive tracer techniques. Circulation 57:645–654, 1978.
16. Schulze RA, Strauss HW, Pitt B: Sudden death in the year following myocardial infarction: Relation to late hospital phase VPC's and left ventricular ejection fraction. Am J Med 62:192–199, 1977.
17. Schulze RA, Humphries JO, Griffith LSC, Ducci H, Achuff S, Baird MG, Mellits ED, Pitt B: Left ventricular and coronary angiographic anatomy: Relationship to ventricular irritability in the late hospital phase of acute myocardial infarction. Circulation 55:839–843, 1977.
18. Schulze RA, Pitt B, Griffith LSC, Ducci HH, Achuff SC, Baird MG, Humphries JO: Coronary angiography and left ventriculography in survivors of transmural and non-transmural myocardial infarction. Am J Med 64:108–113, 1978.
19. Olsen H, Lyons K, Aronow WJ, Waters H: Identification of high risk unstable angina pectoris for mortality and myocardial infarction. Circulation 56 (Suppl III): 669, 1977.

SECTION 4
PREVENTION OF SUDDEN DEATH

4.1. CRITICAL ANALYSIS OF INTERVENTION STUDIES: METHODOLOGICAL PROBLEMS AND PITFALLS

D.G. JULIAN

1. INTRODUCTION

"Double-blind, randomized control trials have become the hallmark of therapeutic respectability" (1). From small beginnings some thirty years ago, clinical trials have come to take an increasingly large place in medical research and, indeed, the research budget. In their heyday, in the early 1970s, it was fashionable to suggest that all new methods of management should be submitted to this discipline and those who were reluctant to do so were castigated fiercely by statisticians and community physicians. Cardiologists, in particular, have been the butt of these complaints, notwithstanding the fact that many of the leaders of the subspeciality were early in the field in studies of anticoagulant therapy. Perhaps it was the disillusionment occasioned by this experience that made their colleagues too reluctant for a time to embark on further experiments of the same kind.

In recent years, the techniques of randomized clinical trials have been progressively refined and improved and there have been important articles on their design, analysis and pitfalls (1–5). With increasing experience, it becomes ever more apparent that new and unexpected problems occur in each area of study, so that the initial trial or trials in any particular field are found to be methodologically unsatisfactory and need to be repeated. Furthermore, it has become clear that some of the most important questions in contemporary medicine do not lend themselves to this form of assessment.

A full discussion of the problems involved is beyond the scope of a short paper and my competence. I shall largely ignore the purely statistical aspects of trials which are well discussed elsewhere (2–4). However, statisticians are frequently unaware of or do not appreciate the clinical pitfalls; this presentation is mainly concerned with those that relate to secondary prevention in ischaemic heart disease.

2. SOME STUDIES ON SECONDARY PREVENTION

2.1. The alprenolol study (6)

Post-infarction patients. Age 57–67.
Selection   – all post-infarct patients except those with contraindications to beta-blockade.
Entry   – one week after hospital discharge.
Follow-up – all patients for 2 years.

2.2. The practolol study (7)

3,038 post-infarction patients. Males aged less than 70.
Selection   – uncertain but excluded heart failure, bradycardia.
Entry   – 7 to 28 days after infarction.
Follow-up – variable, up to 2 years.

2.3. The sulfinpyrazone study (8)

1475 post-infarction patients. Age 45–70.
Selection   – Killip classes I and II.
Entry   – 25 to 35 days after infarction.
Follow-up – Variable, 1 to 20 months.

2.4. European Coronary Artery Surgery Trial (9)

790 patients with mild to moderate angina. Males – age less than 65.
Selection   – 2 to 3 arteries more than 50 % narrowed, ejection fraction more than 50 %.
Follow-up – All patients for 2 years.

3. ASKING THE WRONG QUESTION

A clinical trial is undertaken in the hope that the findings will act as a guide to the clinician in the management of cases similar to those under study. It should be designed to answer the very practical question as to whether a certain form of treatment is justified; this should be compared with what is considered to be optimal were it not available.

3.1. The treatment group

In a surgical trial, the surgical results should be on a par with those expected in any good surgical centre (however, it is unrealistic to demand results so good that they can be replicated in only one or two centres in the world). The Veterans Administration Trial (10) was justly criticised because the operative mortality was higher than is currently experienced in good centres, although this relatively high surgical mortality cannot have seriously affected the results.

In a trial of a drug, it should be given in the optimal dosage. This may be impossible to achieve if individualisation of dosage is important but complex. Furthermore, optimal dosage may not be known (e.g. the "sudden death" preventing dose of a beta-adrenergic blocking drug).

3.2. The placebo group

It is inappropriate and pointless to create a "placebo group" that is treated in a manner which would not be used in clinical practice. This situation is well illustrated by trials which aim to determine the effect of coronary artery bypass surgery on mortality. It is now clearly established that this form of surgery has a sound theoretical basis, has been demonstrated to relieve pain in randomized studies, and has been shown by exercise testing, nuclear imaging and other tests to improve the function of the heart on exercise. The control (''medical'') patient in a coronary artery surgery trial may develop intractable angina which could be helped by surgery. Is it either ethical or relevant to deny him this in order to keep him in the "medical" group?

In a beta-adrenoreceptor blocking trial after infarction, what should we do if a "placebo" patient develops angina for which the most appropriate treatment is a drug of this group? This problem has been discussed by Lovell (11) who was concerned that a disproportionately large number of patients in the Multicentre International Trial of Practolol (7) had to be withdrawn because of angina. He suggested that in such a trial one should either exclude patients who had had angina prior to the infarction or should delay the randomization of patients for 3 months after infarction and exclude those with angina at that time. Although these solutions might facilitate trial methodology, they would also result in the exclusion of patients who are known to be at particularly high risk.

I believe that these problems are the result of asking the wrong question – indeed in asking a question to which we do not wish to know the answer.

In regard to the prognostic benefit of coronary artery bypass graft surgery, the practical question which we want to answer is whether surgery should be undertaken for prognostic reasons in those who do not require it for symptomatic relief. Thus, it is reasonable to compare a group in whom surgery is used immediately for its prognostic benefit with another containing patients who are treated medically in the first place but who could be submitted to surgery if they developed intractable symptoms. Even though they receive surgery, they initially received medical treatment and can be retained in their original group. Rather than call them "medical" and "surgical" groups, we could categorize them as the "aggressive" and "conventional" surgical groups. Thus, the medical/surgical confrontation is both unnecessary and unrealistic.

Similar considerations apply to the study of beta-adrenergic blocking drugs. Nobody denies the indispensible beneficial effect of these drugs in patients with severe angina. Therefore, in the post-infarction group of patients the question we want to answer is whether beta-adrenergic blocking drugs improve prognosis in patients who would not otherwise be receiving them. Therefore, the question we want to ask is – should we be using beta-adrenergic blocking drugs prophylactically or reserve them for those patients who require them for angina? If we do this, Lovell's problems are seen to diminish substantially. Thus, patients can be randomized soon after infarction to the beta-adrenergic blocking drug or placebo. In most patients in either group, either angina will not occur or it will respond adequately to nitrates. If, however, angina does occur and a beta-adrenergic blocking drug appears necessary, it may be administered in an appropriate dose, without withdrawing the patient from the trial or breaking the code. We are conforming to what is regarded as normal clinical practice in giving a beta-adrenergic blocking drug if angina becomes severe and, if the initial dose is inadequate, increasing the dose.

4. CHOOSING THE WRONG PATIENTS

In any one condition, certain subsets of patients may improve on a given therapy whereas others may either not benefit or be made worse by it. This situation is well illustrated by beta-adrenergic blocking drugs. These are contraindicated in the presence of severe left ventricular malfunction. Thus, they are not suitable for some 20 per cent of patients after myocardial infarction although such patients are known to be at the highest risk of sudden death. However, their toxicity in other aspects is so low that it is not unreasonable to give them to all patients for whom they are not contraindicated. Similar considerations apply to the antiarrhythmic drugs but to a different subset. All the oral antiarrhythmic drugs in current use, such as quinidine, procainamide, disopyramide, mexiletine, aprindine and tocainide, have such a degree of toxicity that they cannot be recommended for routine use for low risk patients after myocardial infarction. On the other hand, they would seem to be indicated in those patients with a relatively high risk of sudden death – i.e. those with severe left ventricular malfunction particularly if associated with ventricular arrhythmias. It is apparent that beta-adrenergic blocking drugs might be most suitable for a low risk group for whom it would be unjustifiable to give relatively toxic drugs, whereas antiarrhythmic drugs might be most appropriate in those for whom beta-blockade is contraindicated. It is clear that trials which are being set up to compare directly patients treated with beta-blocking drugs with others treated with antiarrhythmic drugs, will not be solving a clinically relevant question.

5. THE EFFECT OF THE TRIAL ON OTHER THERAPY AND THE EFFECT OF OTHER THERAPY ON THE RESULTS OF THE TRIAL

There are two important aspects of concomitant therapy that are often neglected:

1. In the first place, one form of therapy in a trial may result in changes in other aspects of management that may influence outcome indirectly whilst the other may not. In the European Coronary Artery Bypass Graft Trial (9), patients allocated to surgery gave up smoking significantly more frequently than did medical patients, but more medical patients were retained on a beta-adrenergic blocking drug. Both these differences may have affected eventual mortality figures. Thus, the improvement as a result of surgery might be due to stopping smoking rather than the surgery; on the other hand, the fact that surgical patients had not received beta-blockade may have affected their mortality adversely.

2. The effect of the trial therapy may depend upon what other treatment is being used concomitantly. Thus in the alprenolol trial (6), 50 per cent of the patients were receiving digitalis. This contrasts with the sotalol study in which we are involved where only 2 per cent of the patients are on this drug. It is not improbable that digitalis has deleterious effects on some patients, encouraging arrhythmias and possibly precipitating death; alprenolol's effectiveness may be partly (or wholly) due to the prevention of death due to digitalis therapy. Alternatively, it could be argued that the giving of digitalis would prevent the adverse effects of beta-adrenoreceptor drugs and allow the safe administration of alprenolol to patients with incipient cardiac failure.

6. MISINTERPRETATION AND MISREPORTING

When a clinical trial is undertaken, it is intended that the findings should be applied in practice. In that the subset of the population at risk is often an atypical one, it is important that it should be characterised as precisely as possible so that the conclusions could be applied to an equivalent group.

In the sulfinpyrazone trial (8), only patients with the best prognosis (Killip Classes I and II) were included, yet no mention was made in the summary of the paper or in the associated editorial that the highest risk patients were excluded. Both implied that the alleged benefits from sulfinpyrazone would apply to all post-infarction patients. In fact, it is highly likely that the selection of patients was even more atypical than the report suggested, for example, in the ratio of inferior to anterior infarction being strikingly different from other studies – but this cannot be verified because of the lack of information about those who were not included.

Similar criticisms can be levelled at the Multicentre International Study of practolol. It is clear from the numbers recruited, that each centre included only a small proportion of post-myocardial infarction patients to the study. Undoubtedly patients with cardiac failure were excluded but many other factors may have been involved. Nonetheless, claims implied that practolol was of value in infarction in general.

Although the clinical material seen by a physician or by a hospital is always an atypical segment of the whole, a clearer picture of what subset is being studied can be obtained by logging all patients who are potentially eligible for the trial and explaining the reasons for all exclusions. This was done in an exemplary fashion in the alprenolol study, and is now being included in an increasing number of studies such as the sotalol trial that we are undertaking and the timolol trial being conducted in Norway.

There are three remaining problems that merit special mention – protocol deviants, false negative results and the failure to report true negative results.

6.1. Protocol deviants

In all trials, some patients who start the therapy assigned to them discontinue it prematurely. This may be for a variety of reasons, including non-cooperation, suspected side-effects or the occurrence of one of the endpoints of the study. It is a common fault to "withdraw" such patients from the study and to exclude them from the subsequent statistical analysis. However, as Lovell (11) has written "Since no cause for prematurely stopping randomized treatment can be regarded as independent of prognosis or treatment, or both, those remaining on treatment are no longer an unbiased sample of those originally randomized". Both the practolol (7) and sulfinpyrazone (8) trials failed to include "withdrawals" in their statistical analysis.

6.2. False negative results

It is a common error to conclude that because a trial has failed to demonstrate a statistically significant result in the numbers studied, the trial has shown that the therapy confers no significant benefit. However, if insufficient numbers of patients are studied, a spuriously negative result may be achieved (the beta or Type II error). Thus, in a review by Freiman et al. (5) of 71 "negative" trials reported in well-known medical journals, 67 had a greater than 10 per cent chance of missing a true 25 per cent benefit and 50 could have missed a 50 per cent improvement. Such an error may have been responsible for the negative results in the alprenolol study of Reynolds and Whitlock (12) and the practolol study of Barber et al. (13).

6.3. Non-reporting of truly negative studies

Is an investigator (or his sponsoring drug company) as likely to report a negative study as a positive one? If not, are the odds against reporting it 20 : 1 or 100 : 1? And is an editor 20 or 100 times as likely to publish a positive result as a negative one? Bearing in mind the odds against a negative report being published, what confidence can we have in the significance of a published positive report? The only solution to this problem that I can see is for all control studies supported by drug companies to be compulsarily registered so that one can be sure that the reported results are truly representative.

REFERENCES

1. Editorial – Controlled Trials: planned deception? Lancet 1:534–535, 1979.
2. Peto R: Clinical trial methodology. Biomedicine Special Issue 28:24–36, 1978.
3. Peto M, Pike MC, Armitage P, Breslow NE, Cox DR, Howard SW, Mantel N, McPherson K, Peto J, and Smith PG: Design and analysis of randomized clinical trials requiring prolonged observation of each patient. I. Introduction and design. British Journal of Cancer 34:585–612, 1976.
4. Peto M, Pike MC, Armitage P, Breslow NE, Cox DR, Howard SV, Mantel N, McPherson K, Peto J, and Smith PG: Design and analysis of randomized clinical trials requiring prolonged observation of each patient. II. Analysis and examples. British Journal of Cancer 35:1–39, 1977.
5. Freiman JA, Chalmers TC, Smith H, and Kuebler RR: The importance of beta, the Type II error and sample size in the design and interpretation of the randomized control trials. New England Journal of Medicine 299:690–694, 1978.
6. Wilhelmsson C, Vedin JA, Wilhelmsen L, Tibblin G, and Werko L: Reduction of sudden deaths after myocardial infarction by treatment with alprenolol. Lancet 2, 1157–1157, 1974.
7. Multicentre International Study: Improvement in prognosis of myocardial infarction by long-term beta-adrenoreceptor blockade using practolol. British Medical Journal 3:735–740, 1975.
8. The Anturane Reinfarction Trial Research Group: Sulfinpyrazone in the prevention of cardiac death after myocardial infarction. New England Journal of Medicine 298:289–295, 1978.
9. European Coronary Surgery Study Group. Coronary artery bypass surgery in stable angina pectoris. Lancet, 1:889–894, 1979.
10. Hultgren HN, Takaro T, Detre K and participants in the Veterans Administration Cooperative Study: Veterans Administration Cooperative Study of surgical treatment of stable angina and preliminary results. In Rahimtoola SH (ed), Coronary Bypass Surgery, FA Davis, Philadelphia, 1977.
11. Lovell RRH: Review of the present status of drug treatment for preventing sudden death. British Heart Journal, 40:(suppl) 94, 1978.
12. Reynolds JL, and Whitlock EML: Effects of a beta-adrenergic blocker in myocardial infarction treated for one year from onset. British Heart Journal 34:252–259, 1972.
13. Barber JM, Boyle DMcC, Chaturvedi NC, Singh N, and Walsh MJ: Practolol in acute myocardial infarction. Acta Medica Scandinavica (suppl) 587:213–216, 1976.

4.2. PREVENTION OF SUDDEN DEATH: THE ROLE OF BETA-BLOCKERS

Å. HJALMARSON

Ischemic heart disease is the main cause of death in the western world (8, 13, 22). Most of these deaths are sudden and occur before the patient reaches hospital (8, 11, 24). It is generally accepted that sudden death is due to ventricular fibrillation in most cases, but the pathogenesis and factors predisposing to ventricular fibrillation are not well defined (6, 26). In order to prevent deaths outside hospital one has to institute prophylactic medication in patients at high risk for cardiovascular death. During the last few years, long-term treatment with beta-blocking agents has been suggested as a potentially useful therapy to reduce morbidity and mortality in ischemic heart disease. The aim of this paper is to review the studies of chronic beta-blockade in the prevention of cardiovascular death.

1. RETROSPECTIVE STUDIES

It was first reported by Snow in 1965 (12) that oral administration of propranolol during the first weeks of acute myocardial infarction could reduce the total number of deaths as well as sudden deaths (see Table 1). This was, however, an open study including only 91 patients on short-term treatment. A few years later, Amsterdam and coworkers (2) reported that long-term treatment with propranolol of patients with angina pectoris and/or previous myocardial infarction reduced total mortality as compared to patients on long-acting nitroglycerin or following implantation of an internal mammary artery. Later, it was reported by Lambert (28) that propranolol in patients with angina pectoris and/or hypertension reduced total deaths as well as sudden deaths. All these studies were suggestive of a favorable effect of chronic beta-blockade resulting in reduction of morbidity and/or mortality in ischemic heart disease.

Table 1: Retrospective studies.

Drug	Diagnosis	Pat no.	(C–β)	Duration	Sudden death	Total death	Authors
Propranolol	Angina – MI	89	(46–43)	18 months	–	Reduced (14.5–5.7%)	Amsterdam et al. 1968
Propranolol	Angina – Hypertension	365		3 years	Reduced	Reduced	Lambert 1974
Propranolol	AMI	91	(46–45)	< 1 month	Reduced (6–3)	Reduced (35–16%)	Snow 1965

2. PROSPECTIVE STUDIES

In 1968 it was reported that treatment with propranolol compared with a placebo during the first three weeks of an acute myocardial infarction did not change total mortality (9; see Table 2). In the first study of long-term beta-blockade after myocardial infarction reported in 1972 (10), no significant effect was seen on the total death-rate but there were only 77 patients in the study and the mortality was low in both the alprenolol and the placebo groups. As can be seen from Table 2, in 1974 and 1975 three studies were published demonstrating a reduction in the number of sudden deaths in postinfarction patients (1, 3, 25).

Table 2: Prospective studies.

Drug	Diagnosis	Pat no.	(C–β)	Duration	Start	Age	Sudden death	Total death	Authors
Propranolol 200 mg × 4	AMI	454	(228–226)	3 weeks	Day 1	–	–	Not reduced (24–31)	Norris et al. 1968
Alprenolol 100 mg × 4	MI	77	(39–38)	1 year	Day 1	54	–	Low! (3–3)	Reynolds-Whitlock 1972
Alprenolol 200 mg × 2	MI	230	(116–114)	2 years	Week 5	62	*Reduced* (11–3)	*Not significant* (14–7)	Wilhelmsson et al. 1974
Alprenolol 100 mg × 4	MI	162	(93–69)	2 years	Week 3	57	*Reduced* (9–1)	*Reduced* (11–5)	Ahlmark et al. 1974
Practolol 200 mg × 2	MI	3038	(1514–1524)	14 months	Week 1–4	55	*Reduced* (52–30)	*Reduced* (73–47)	Multicentre Study 1975
Practolol 300 mg × 2	MI	298	(147–151)	2 years	Day 1	62	–	Not reduced (46–41)	Barber et al. 1975

In the Göteborg study (25), all women and men aged 57–67 years who had suffered an acute myocardial infarction and were discharged alive from hospital were included in a controlled study. Alprenolol in a daily dose of 400 mg was given to 114 patients and 116 patients received a placebo. All patients were followed-up at a special postinfarction clinic with an optimal treatment of symptoms and elimination of risk factors, such as smoking and hypertension. At entry in the trial, the patients were divided into four prognostically homogeneous subgroups including patients with no extensive cardiac damage (subgroup I), those with mechanical damage to the myocardium (subgroup II), those with significant arrhythmias (subgroup III) and those with a combination of mechanical damage and arrhythmias (subgroup IV). All deaths occurred in the subgroups II and IV consisting of patients with more marked mechanical damage of the heart. The difference between the alprenolol and placebo groups was statistically significant. The cumulative number of sudden deaths in the alprenolol study is shown in Figure 1. In this study there was no significant difference in the number of nonfatal reinfarctions between the treatment and placebo groups.

The findings in Göteborg were confirmed by a similar study performed by Ahlmark and coworkers (1). In this study, 69 patients were given alprenolol 400 mg a day for two years and there were 93 control patients. This was an open study and the patients were not followed up in a special postinfarction clinic with standardized treatment. The mean age of the patients in this study was slightly lower and there was a significant reduction both in sudden deaths and total deaths by alprenolol. In this study, there was also a significant reduction in cumulative numbers of nonfatal reinfarctions. There were only four reinfarctions in the alprenolol (6 %) compared to 15 in the control group (16 %), and this difference was significant. These

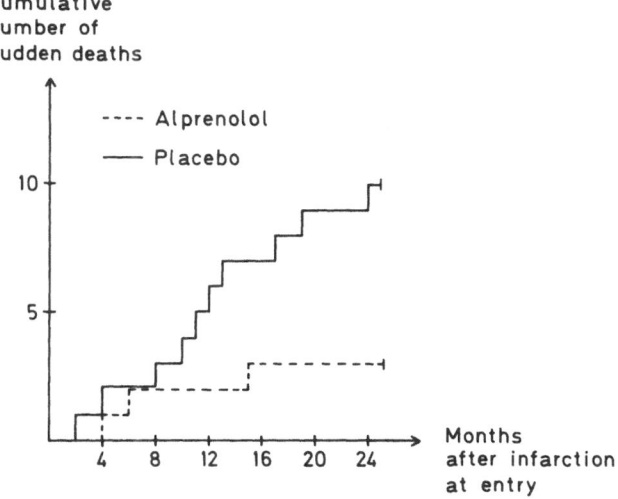

Cumulative
number of
sudden deaths

---- Alprenolol
—— Placebo

Months
after infarction
at entry

Figure 1. Cumulative numbers of sudden deaths in the group treated with alprenolol and the placebo group during two years' follow-up (Wilhelmson *et al.* 1974).

two studies demonstrated that treatment with alprenolol during two years after myocardial infarction significantly reduces the incidence of sudden death. In both studies, there was a reduction also in total mortality by approximately 50 %. The fact that there was a reduction in nonfatal reinfarctions in the study by Ahlmark and coworkers (1) and not in the Göteborg study could be due to several reasons. The Falun study was an open study with no special standardized follow-up of the patients in the postinfarction clinic with control of possible risk factors, the patients were five years younger and alprenolol was given in four daily doses compared to two in the Göteborg study. In this respect, it could be mentioned that a study in Göteborg where patients were randomly allocated to postinfarction clinic follow-up compared to nonorganized controls showed a 50 % lower incidence of nonfatal reinfarctions in the postinfarction clinic group (21). There was no significant reduction in cardiovascular deaths or all-deaths. A beneficial effect of a postinfarction clinic follow-up could be the earlier and more effective treatment of postinfarction complications, such as heart failure, chest pain and arrhythmias.

The effect of practolol was studied in a Multicentre International Study (3) including 3038 patients from 67 centers with a mean duration of follow-up of about 14 months. Patients were randomly allocated to either practolol (400 mg daily) or a placebo. There was a significantly lower incidence of sudden deaths and total deaths in the practolol group (see Table 2). In this study, there was a trend towards a lower number of nonfatal reinfarctions in the practolol group (4.5 versus 5.8 %; $p < 0.1$). There was a markedly lower incidence of number of reinfarctions also in the placebo group compared to the two studies in Sweden (9.5–13 % in 14 months). Retrospectively, it was demonstrated that patients with anterior wall infarction and low diastolic blood pressure did particularly well on practolol (Table 3). From this table it can be seen that when comparing anterior and inferior wall infarctions, a

Table 3: A Multicentre International Study (3).

Infarct site	No. of patients		Cardiac death		Sudden death		Non-sudden death	
	Practolol	Placebo	Practolol	Placebo	Practolol	Placebo	Practolol	Placebo
Anterior	764	768	22*	48*	19	33	3	15
Inferior	760	746	25	25	11	19	14	6

* p < 0.01

similar reduction in sudden deaths was found in the practolol group while contrasting results were seen in nonsudden deaths. In anterior wall infarction practolol was associated with a much lower number of nonsudden deaths while in inferior infarction, nonsudden deaths were much more frequent in the practolol group compared to the placebo group. Analyzing the time of the deaths in the study, a high incidence of fatal complications were found during the first four weeks among patients with wall infarction in the practolol group (K G Green, personal communication). When treatment was started four weeks after infarction there was no difference between patients with different sites of infarction.

In a study from Belfast (4), patients were randomly allocated to practolol (600 mg daily) or a placebo, and the treatment was started immediately on arrival in hospital. This study comprised 298 patients with myocardial infarcts with two years of follow-up (see Table 2). In this study there was no significant difference in mortality between the practolol and the placebo groups at any time (Table 4). A retrospective analysis of 53 patients with initial heart rates higher than 100 beats/minute showed significantly lower mortality in the practolol group compared to the placebo group. This was mainly due to a beneficial effect during the first three months. Despite the fact that a high daily dose of practolol was given from the first day of acute myocardial infarction and that patients with clear signs of congestive heart failure were included, the treatment was generally well tolerated with a low drop-out rate. The total three-month mortality for all patients in the study was 16 % and the three months to two years mortality was 13 % which can be compared to a 10 % three-month mortality in a similar study on metoprolol in Göteborg and a three months to two years mortality of 8.7 % in the alprenolol study in Göteborg. It could be speculated that the in-

Table 4: Practolol in AMI and post-MI (4).

Mortality at (time)	All patients (n = 298)				Patients with $HR > 100$ beats/min (n = 53)			
	Practolol	(n = 151)	Placebo	(n = 147)	Practolol	(n = 23)	Placebo	(n = 30)
24 hours	2	(1 %)	6	(4 %)	0		4	(13 %)
2 weeks	9	(6 %)	14	(10 %)	1	(4 %)	7	(23 %)
3 months	23	(15 %)	25	(17 %)	1	(4 %)	10	(33 %)
1 year	30	(20 %)	37	(25 %)	2	(9 %)	13	(43 %)
2 years	41	(27 %)	46	(31 %)	5	(22 %)	14	(47 %)

clusion of more severely ill patients in the practolol study in Belfast could have counteracted the beneficial effect of practolol in the whole series of patients.

In view of the suggestion from the Multicentre Study that patients with anterior wall infarction did particularly well on practolol (Table 3), a new Multicentre Postinfarction Trial was started comprising 783 patients with anterior wall infarction; 60 physicians are involved in this study. Propranolol is given 40 mg t.d.s. starting one week after the onset of acute myocardial infarction. Early observations from this controlled study have been reported by Baber and coworkers (27). As can be seen from Table 5 there was no significant effect of practolol on mortality at one and three months of treatment. No details are yet available from this study.

Table 5: Multicentre Propranolol Postinfarction Trial (n = 783; anterior wall infarcts; entry time 1 week; 60 physicians) (27).

Mortality at (time)	Propanolol (40 mg t.d.s.)	Placebo
1 month	18 (n = 328)	14 (n = 343)
3 months	22 (n = 301)	21 (n = 312)

2.1. Observations in hypertension and congestive cardiomyopathy

In a recent study from Göteborg (5), it was reported that antihypertensive treatment might be effective in preventing cardiovascular death and nonfatal myocardial infarction. In a population study, 1229 persons were found to be hypertensive at screening with 1026 having a systolic blood pressure higher than 175 mm Hg or a diastolic blood pressure higher than 115 mm Hg. A repeat measurement of blood pressure two weeks later showed that 391 of the untreated patients now had a systolic blood pressure lower than 175 and a diastolic blood pressure lower than 115 mm Hg. These persons were left without medical treatment while the remaining 635 patients were given medical treatment. Most of the patients were on beta-blocking agents (78 %). As can be seen from Figure 2, during a follow-up of 4.3 years in these men aged 47 to 54 years there is a significantly lower incidence of nonfatal myocardial infarctions and cardiovascular deaths in the treatment group. There is a similar difference between the control group and the treatment group for cardiovascular deaths and nonfatal myocardial infarctions, although the numbers are too small to show a significant reduction in cardiac deaths. It can be stated that in patients with hypertension medical treatment in which the majority of patients are given beta-blocking agents can prevent serious cardiovascular complications.

In a study published in 1975 (29), it was reported that long-term treatment with beta-blocking agents could improve the clinical condition and various hemodynamic parameters in patients with heart failure due to congestive cardiomyopathy. In a prospective study comprising 28 patients with moderate to severe congestive heart failure due to congestive cardiomyopathy, a beneficial effect on heart function and clinical condition was found (14). Based on standardized noninvasive investigations including phonocardiograms, pulse

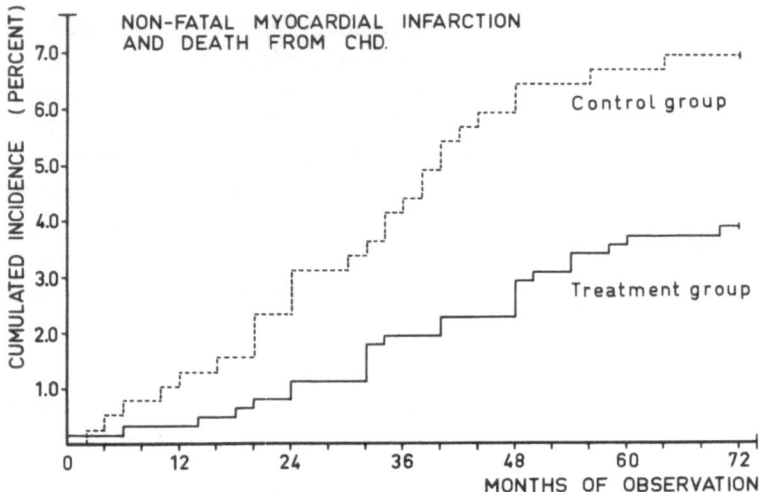

Figure 2. Cumulative incidence of nonfatal myocardial infarctions and deaths from coronary heart disease by life table analysis (Berglund *et al.* 1978).

curves and apex cardiograms, 13 patients with the same severity of congestive cardiomyopathy who were not given beta-blocking agents were compared with 28 patients treated with beta-blockade. All patients were on optimal treatment with digitalis and diuretics. Figure 3 shows that addition of beta-blocking agents to the conventional treatment resulted in a significantly better survival during a three year follow-up. After 3.2 years all patients without beta-blocking agents have died compared to 50% survival in the group of patients on chronic beta-blockade. Whether the beneficial effect of beta-blockade on survival is only secondary to the improvement in heart function or whether there is an additional prophylactic effect against fatal arrhythmias, has yet to be clarified.

2.2. Possible mechanisms of beneficial effect of beta-blocking agents in ischemic heart disease

From a large number of control studies it is known that beta-blocking agents can reduce the severity of chest pain and improve physical working capacity in patients with angina pectoris. In our own studies from Göteborg, it has been found that administration of beta-blocking agents in the early phase of acute myocardial infarction can reduce ischemic chest pain and ischemic ST-segment elevation (15–17). The possible clinical effects of beta-blockade in acute myocardial infarction are listed in Table 6. Beta-blockade reduces heart work, as indicated by a reduction in the heart rate-systolic blood pressure product. It has furthermore been suggested that early in the development of ischemia there is a marked release of noradrenaline from the sympathetic nerve endings in the ischemic area with possible deleterious effects (see 18). It has been suggested that beta-blocking agents could also reduce ventricular arrhythmias early in the infarction process, including fatal arrhythmias, and also limit infarct size. In view of these considerations, a study was started in Göteborg comparing metoprolol and a placebo to evaluate the effects on infarct size, arrhythmias and

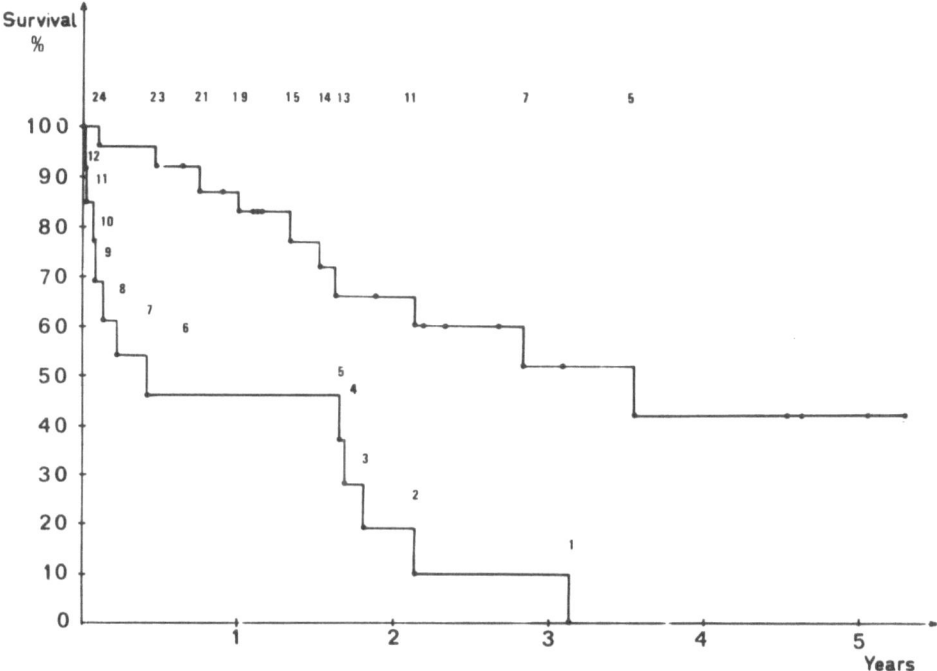

Figure 3. Numbers of cardiac deaths in patients with congestive cardiomyopathy treated with beta-blockade (upper curve) and without (lower curve) by life table analysis (Swedberg 1978).

Table 6. Possible clinical effects of β-blockade in AMI

Reduction in HR × SBP product
Reduction of ST-segment elevation
Reduction of ischemic chest pain
Reduction of ventricular arrhythmias
Reduction of infarct size
Reduction of mortality, early and late

early mortality. The patients are given, immediately after arrival in hospital, a placebo or metoprolol 15 mg i.v. and then 200 mg daily for three months. Infarct size is estimated from enzyme curves (SLDH, fractions I and II, ASAT, CPK-MB) and precordial mapping of Q and R-waves. Arrhythmias are analyzed from 24-hours of continuous electrocardiographic recording on paper. The first observations from 500 patients are summarized in Table 7. The study is still in progress and aims to include a total number of 1200 patients. Considering certain contraindications, such as a systolic blood pressure lower than 100 mm Hg, heart rate lower than 45 beats/minute, presence of basal lung rales of more than 10 cm and signs of poor peripheral circulation, there is good tolerance to metoprolol in the study. No significant effects have been seen on various ventricular arrhythmias during the

Table 7. Double-blind study of metoprolol compared to placebo in AMI or susp. AMI (15 mg i.v. +200 mg daily for 3 months).

- Good tolerance;
- No effects on ventricular arrhythmias in first 24 hours (100 pts);
- Limitation of infarct size estimated from LD I + II (360 pts);
- No effect on LD I + II in pts with high 1st LD I + II (129 pts);
- Limitation of infarct size for the whole group of pts on previous chronic beta-blockade (94 pts).

---

first 24 hours. Metoprolol was found to limit infarct size in patients in whom treatment was instituted early. These are patients whose first measurement of SLDH-I + II was normal which was the case in 75 % of the patients. In the subgroup of patients who were on chronic beta-blockade there was a significant limitation of enzyme-estimated infarct size independent from time of beginning of treatment in relation to the time of onset of infarction. From our preliminary studies, it seems that the beta-blocking agent metoprolol is well tolerated and when instituted early, seems to limit infarct size. This is in agreement with previous observations in various models (18).

Figure 4 shows the factors of importance in the development of myocardial ischemia. It seems logical that the main effect of beta-blocking agents in the prevention of myocardial ischemia is the reduction of heart work and metabolic demand. This treatment can also prevent the deleterious effects of locally released myocardial noradrenaline on metabolic demand, thrombocyte aggregation and coronary flow. A preventive effect on the development of myocardial ischemia explains the effects on pain, ST-segment changes, arrhythmias (mainly ventricular fibrillation?), depression of heart function and possibly on infarct size. It seems likely that individual properties of the myocardial cells or blood cells play an important role in the outcome of myocardial ischemia. In some patients, fatal arrhythmias and ventricular fibrillation might occur very early in the ischemic process, resulting in sudden death without myocardial damage. In others, more resistent to arrhythmias sudden severe ischemia will cause acute myocardial infarction while in still another group of patients, long-term ischemia without acute damage will cause dysfunction of cells and heart failure. It can thus be hypothesized that long-term prophylactic treatment with beta-blocking agents will reduce ischemic chest pain, sudden death, ischemic heart failure and development of acute myocardial infarction.

In the retrospective studies mentioned above, it was suggested that propranolol reduced mortality in patients with angina pectoris and hypertension as well as after myocardial infarction. However, two controlled studies (9, 27) have failed to confirm this effect. In these studies however, short term treatment was given (three weeks and three months). Norris et al. gave a low dose of propranolol (Tables 2 and 5). Although the follow-up time in the Multicentre Propranolol Postinfarction Trial is short, the three months follow-up of the anterior wall infarction in the Multicentre Study with practolol gave already a lower incidence of sudden death in the practolol group, in contrast to the findings of the propranolol group. Out of three prospective studies with alprenolol the two from Sweden (1, 15) with a larger number of patients studied during two years showed reduction in sudden death. The Multicentre International Study with practolol (3) supported the findings from the two alprenolol studies. Alprenolol is a beta$_1$- and beta$_2$-blocking agent and practolol a beta$_1$-blocking agent but both drugs have an intrinsic stimulatory activity. If it is true that a protective effect can be obtained with these two drugs and not with propranolol, one has to consider that to offer protection the beta-blocking agent should have an intrinsic stimulating activity or cardioselective beta$_1$-blocking property. Propranolol and alprenolol both have a membrane-stabilizing property, the so-called quinidine-like property, which is not the case for practolol. This would indicate that the membrane-stabilizing property is not a prerequisite for the beneficial effect of the beta-blocking agent on sudden death. Of the properties of beta-blocking agents listed in Table 8, beta$_1$-blockade and the intrinsic stimmulating activity seem to be the important ones. It is well known that the therapeutic effects of beta-blocking agents in angina pectoris, hypertension and tachyarrhythmias are due to beta$_1$-blockade. This seems also to be the case in relation to limitation of infarct size in experimental animals and man and also in experimental ventricular fibrillation.

Table 8. Properties of betablocking agents in prevention of sudden death

Beta$_1$-blockade
Beta$_2$-blockade
Intrinsic stim. activity
Membrane stabil. property

The results of a study with beta-blockade in patients with ischemic heart disease must be highly dependent upon the selection of patients (Table 9). There are definite contraindications to chronic beta-blockade, e.g. severe heart failure and hypertension. The effects of

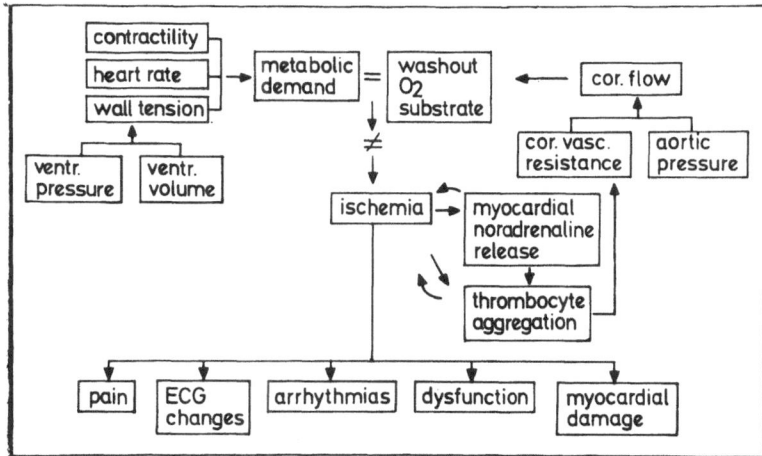

Figure 4. Factors playing a role in the development of myocardial ischemia.

Table 9. Selection of patients in sudden death prophylaxis with chron. betablockade

Tolerance
High risk
Age
Site of infarction
Other beneficial effects

beta-blockade in these patients can be harmful. It seems, however, that the majority of patients in both acute myocardial infarction and postmyocardial infarction will tolerate long-term treatment with beta-blocking agents. Even patients with mild to moderate heart failure could be given beta-blockade together with digitalis and/or diuretics. In patients at high risk for cardiac death, it seems justified to accept some mild side-effects, such as e.g. fatigue, at least for some period of time. It seems logical to institute a more aggressive prophylactic treatment in younger age groups. In our experience, beta-blockers are well tolerated also in elderly people with the recommendation of a slightly lower daily dose. There is no clear evidence that selection of patients for long-term prophylactic treatment with beta-blockade should be based on the site of infarction. Accepting the concept that long-term treatment with beta-blockade can reduce the total number of all cardiac events, cardiac deaths and nonfatal reinfarctions, all patients at some risk of cardiac events should be considered for long-term beta-blockade unless there are certain clear-cut contraindications. The presence of angina pectoris, hypertension or tachyarrhythmias would enforce the indication for beta-blockade.

3. CONCLUSION

Three different studies with the beta-blocking agents alprenolol and practolol have shown a reduced risk of sudden death after myocardial infarction. Also long-term treatment with beta-blocking agents in patients with angina pectoris, hypertension and congestive cardio-myopathy in addition seems to reduce cardiac death. Unless certain contraindications are present, it seems justified to recommend chronic beta-blockade in all cardiac patients at risk for cardiac death.

REFERENCES

1. Ahlmark G, Saetre H, Korsgren M: Reduction of sudden deaths after myocardial infarction. Lancet (abstract) 2:1563, 1974.
2. Amsterdam EA, Wolfson S, Gorlin R: Effect of therapy on survival in angina pectoris. Ann Intern Med 63:115, 1968.
3. A Multicentre International Study: Improvement in prognosis of myocardial infarction by long-term beta-adrenoreceptor blockade using practolol. Br Med J 3:735–740, 1975.
4. Barber JM, Boyle McC, Chaturvedi NC, Singh N, Walsh MJ: Practolol in acute myocardial infarction. Acta Med Scand suppl 587:213–216, 1976.
5. Berglund G, Wilhelmsen L, Sannerstedt R, Hansson L, Andersson O, Sivertson R, Wedel H, Wikstrand J:

Coronary heart disease after treatment of hypertension. Lancet 1:1–5, 1978.

6. Han J, Goel BG: Electrophysiological precursors of ventricular tachyarrhythmias. Arch Intern Med 129: 749–755, 1972.

7. Klein MS, Sobel BE: Medical management of myocardial infarction. Ann Rev Med 27:89–108, 1976.

8. Kuller L: Sudden and unexpected nontraumatic deaths in adults: a review of epidemiological and clinical studies. J Chron Dis 19:1165–000, 1962.

9. Norris RM, Caughey DE, Scott PJ: Trial of propranolol in acute myocardial infarction. Br Med J 2:398–400, 1968.

10. Reynolds JL, Whitlock RML: Effects of a beta-adrenergic receptor blocker in myocardial infarction treated for one year from onset. Br Heart J 34:252–259, 1972.

11. Romo M: Factors related to sudden death in acute ischaemic disease. Acta Med Scand suppl 547:1–92, 1973.

12. Snow PJD: Effect of propranolol in myocardial infarction. Lancet 2:551–553, 1965.

13. Stamler J: Cardiovascular diseases in the United States. Am J Cardiol 10:319–340, 1962.

14. Swedberg K, Hjalmarson AC, Waagstein F, Wallentin I: Prolongation of survival in Congestive cardiomyopathy by beta-receptor blockade. Lancet 1: 1374–1376, 1979.

15. Waagstein F, Hjalmarson ÅC: Effect of cardioselective beta-blockade on heart function and chest pain in acute myocardial infarction. Acta Med Scand suppl 587:193–200, 1976.

16. Waagstein F, Hjalmarson ÅC: Double-blind study of the effect of cardioselective beta-blockade on chest pain in acute myocardial infarction. Acta Med Scand suppl 587:201–211, 1976.

17. Waagstein F, Hjalmarson Å, Málek I: Effect of beta-blockers in reducing infarct size. In: Acute and Long-term Medical Management of Myocardial Ischaemia, Å Hjalmarson, L Wilhelmsen (eds) Astra, Sweden 1978, p 346.

18. Waldenström AP, Hjalmarson ÅC: Factors modifying ischemic injury in the isolated rat heart. Acta Med Scand 201:533–537, 1977.

19. Waldenström A, Hjalmarson Å, Thornell L: Factors of importance for infarct size in animals – Findings of the Göteborg Group. in: Acute and Long-term Medical Management of Myocardial Ischaemia, Å Hjalmarson, L Wilhelmsen, (eds) Astra, Sweden, 1978, p 221.

20. Vedin A, Wilhelmsson C, Elmfeldt D, Säve-Söderberg J, Tibblin G, Wilhelmsen L: Deaths and non-fatal reinfarctions during two years' follow-up after myocardial infarction. A follow-up study of 440 men and women discharged alive from hospital. Acta Med Scand 198:353–364, 1975.

21. Vedin A, Wilhelmsson C, Tibblin G, Wilhelmsen L: The post-infarction clinic in Göteborg, Sweden. A controlled trial of a therapeutic organization. Acta Med Scand 200:453–456, 1976.

22. Vedin JA, Wilhelmsson C, Bolander AM, Werkö L: Mortality trends in Sweden 1951–1968 with special reference to cardiovascular cause of death. Acta Med Scand suppl 515:1–76, 1971.

23. Wilhelmsen L, Wedel H, Tibblin G: Multivariate analysis of risk factors for coronary heart disease. Circulation 48:950–958, 1973.

24. Wilhelmsen L, Ljungberg S, Wedel H, Werkö L: A comparison between participants and non-participants in a primary preventive trial. J Chron Dis 29:331–339, 1976.

25. Wilhelmsson C, Vedin JA, Wilhelmsen L, Tibblin G, Werkö L: Reduction of sudden deaths after myocardial infarction by treatment with alprenolol. Lancet 2:1157–1159, 1974.

26. Vismara LA, Amsterdam EA, Mason DT: Relation of ventricular arrhythmias in the late hospital phase of acute myocardial infarction to sudden death after hospital discharge. Am J Med 59:6–12, 1975.

27. Baber NS: Multicentre propranolol post-infarction trial. Br Heart J 41:365–000, 1979.

28. Lambert DMD: Hypertension and myocardial infarction. Br Med J 3:685 (abstract), 1974.

29. Waagstein F, Hjalmarson Å, Varnauskas E, Wallentin I: Effect of chronic beta-adrenergic receptor blockade in congestive cardiomyopathy. Br Heart J 37:1022–1036, 1975.

4.3. PREVENTION OF SUDDEN DEATH: THE ROLE OF ANTIARRHYTHMIC THERAPY

J.P. VAN DURME and M.G. BOGAERT

1. INTRODUCTION

Most cases of sudden cardiac death are probably due to primary ventricular fibrillation. A prophylactic antiarrhythmic therapy thus constitutes a logical therapeutic approach in patients at high risk. There are however only few controlled data available concerning the role of antiarrhythmic treatment for the prevention of sudden death before, during and after hospitalization for acute myocardial infarction.

2. PREHOSPITAL PHASE OF ACUTE MYOCARDIAL INFARCTION

Valentine et al. (1) performed in collaboration with a large number of general practitioners a double blind randomized placebo-controlled study with lidocaine during the prehospital phase of acute myocardial infarction. Patients under the age of 70 years with suspected acute myocardial infarction were given either lidocaine (intramuscular injection of 300 mg) or saline. The end points were death or documented ventricular fibrillation occurring within two hours after the injection. Among 523 patients recruited, only 269 fulfilled the criteria for final inclusion in the study; 156 had received lidocaine and 113 a placebo. Among the 156 patients receiving lidocaine there were 2 deaths and 1 ventricular fibrillation as compared with 6 deaths and 2 ventricular fibrillations among the 113 patients receiving a placebo ($p < 0.05$). Major cardiac or neurologic side effects were not encountered in this study and the authors concluded that patients seen within one hour of the onset of symptoms should be given prophylaxis with lidocaine. However, although major risk factors were comparable in both groups the authors themselves stated that the difference between the number of patients in the lidocaine group and the placebo group could not be accounted for by random occurrence.

No other controlled studies on prophylactic antiarrhythmic treatment in the prehospital phase of acute myocardial infarction are available.

3. HOSPITAL PHASE OF ACUTE MYOCARDIAL INFARCTION

Many trials have been performed with different antiarrhythmic drugs in patients with acute myocardial infarction admitted to coronary care units. Noneman and Rogers (2) recently reviewed the data available for lidocaine. Among 13 controlled trials only 2 suggested a protective effect of lidocaine against primary ventricular fibrillation and only one study was free of major shortcomings in trial design. In the latter study (3) 212 patients under the age of 70 years were given either lidocaine (intravenous injection of 100 mg followed by an infusion of 3 mg per minute for 48 hours) or glucose 5 % in water. The study was double-blind and randomized. Both groups were comparable in age, sex, site and size of infarction and admission delay. Among 107 patients receiving lidocaine no episode of ventricular fibrillation occurred whereas among 105 patients receiving a placebo, 9 developed primary ventricular fibrillation (p < 0.002) and 2 paroxysmal ventricular fibrillation. The mortality rate was however similar in both groups (lidocaine, 8 patients; placebo, 10 patients). This is probably due to the fact that patients with primary ventricular fibrillation were successfully resuscitated in the coronary care unit and that mortality was mainly due to cardiac rupture and cardiac failure. Side effects occurred in 15 % of the patients treated with lidocaine and were more common in older patients. It should be noted however that the 212 patients included in this study were selected from a group of 716 admitted to the coronary care unit and that 13 patients were rejected for final analysis because the diagnosis of myocardial infarction could not be ascertained by subsequent serial enzyme studies. The data from this study suggest that lidocaine given during the first 48 hours after myocardial infarction can prevent primary ventricular fibrillation.

4. POSTHOSPITAL PHASE OF ACUTE MYOCARDIAL INFARCTION

As beta-blocking drugs have been extensively dealt with by Hjalmarsson et al. in this volume, their use for secondary prevention will not be discussed in this paper.

In 1971 the results of a randomized prophylactic trial with phenytoin were published (4): 568 patients under the age of 70 leaving the hospital after a proven myocardial infarction were given phenytoin, either 300 or 400 mg per day (283 patients) or for the control group phenytoin 3 to 4 mg per day (285 patients). Major characteristics of the patient population did not differ significantly in both groups. The mortality during a follow-up of 12 months was identical for both groups (8 %). During the follow-up plasma levels of phenytoin were also determined. The authors observed that in the group treated with 300 or 400 mg of phenytoin, no deaths occurred among patients with a high plasma level of phenytoin (10–20 mcg/ml); the difference with patients having low plasma levels was significant (p < 0.02). These results suggested that, provided an adequate plasma concentration was reached, phenytoin reduced sudden death during the post hospital phase of acute myocardial infarction (5). Therefore another study was designed, including a dosage adjustment procedure according to the plasma levels of phenytoin. Results of this study however, fail to show any significant mortality difference between the phenytoin treated and the control group (6).

Kosowsky et al. (7) performed a long term trial with procainamide in 78 patients recovering from acute myocardial infarction. The patients were randomly allocated to a control group or a treatment group with procaineamide 1500–2000 mg orally. After a follow-up of 18 months only 8 of the 39 patients initially receiving procainamide were still in the trial. Most of the early and late drop outs were due to toxic reactions. It was therefore concluded from this study that the high incidence of toxicity precludes the long-term prophylactic use of procainamide.

In collaboration with the Thoraxcenter (Rotterdam, The Netherlands), we have just completed a one-year double-blind randomized trial with aprindine (153 patients) versus placebo (152 patients) in patients having suffered a myocardial infarction. Selection for inclusion in the study was based on the presence of complex ventricular premature beats (VPB with peak frequency > 5/min, multifocal VPB or repetitive VPB) or ventricular tachycardia on a 24 hour Holter recording performed 10 days after admission. Details concerning the design have been published earlier (8). There was a monthly follow-up visit to the clinic for drug supply, assessment of compliance (questionnaire, pill count, urinary riboflavin, plasma level) and detection of side effects. Physical examination and 24 hour Holter tape recording were performed at months 1, 3, 6 and 12. At each follow-up visit there was a possibility of dose adjustment (up to 200 mg) without unblinding (increase dosage when ventricular arrhythmia persisted; decrease dosage if complaints suggesting side effects were present).

Data at month 12 of the follow-up indicate that the dosage in the placebo group was significantly higher than in the aprindine group. The analysis of the Holter tape recordings performed during follow-up indicates that complex ventricular arrhythmias (a requirement for inclusion in the trial) had disappeared at month 12 in 60% of the patients in the aprindine group and in 25 % of the patients in the placebo group. During the one-year follow-up 12 patients (7.8 %) died in the aprindine group (12 cardiac deaths, 10 sudden cardiac deaths) and 19 patients (12.5 %) in the placebo group (18 cardiac deaths, 13 sudden cardiac deaths). In all patients dying suddenly the last recorded Holter tape showed persistence of the complex ventricular arrhythmias. Drop-outs were more common in the aprindine group (21.6 %) than in the placebo group (13.8 %). This difference was mainly due to toxic gastro-intestinal, neurological or hematological reactions.

More recently a double-blind randomized trial with mexiletine versus placebo during three months after myocardial infarction, has been performed in the United Kingdom (9). Presence of ventricular arrhythmias was not a basis for selection in this study. So far no results from this study have been published.

5. CONCLUSION

The limited data available suggest that lidocaine may have a beneficial effect when given intramuscularly during the prehospital phase of acute myocardial infarction. Therefore its administration to patients seen within the very first hours after onset of symptoms may be advocated.

In patients hospitalized for acute myocardial infarction lidocaine was shown to prevent primary ventricular fibrillation in two studies; however the drug did not influence the early mortality. Furthermore when adequate doses for maintenance treatment were used a high incidence of side effects was encountered. Therefore systematic intravenous administration of lidocaine to all patients admitted to the coronary care unit is questionable.

As for the prevention of sudden death during the posthospital phase of myocardial infarction, some of the available data have shown the feasibility of chronic antiarrhythmic treatment. However a significant reduction of sudden death with chronic antiarrhythmic treatment has not been shown.

REFERENCES

1. Valentine PA, Frew JL, Mashford ML, Sloman JG: Lidocaine in the prevention of sudden death in the pre-hospital phase of acute infarction. N Engl J Med 291:1327–1331, 1974.
2. Noneman JW, Rogers JF: Lidocaine prophylaxis in acute myocardial infarction. Medicine 57:501–515, 1978.
3. Lie KI, Wellens HJ, Van Capelle FJ, Durrer D: Lidocaine in the prevention of primary ventricular fibrillation. N Engl J Med 291:1324–1326, 1974.
4. Collaborative Group: Phenytoin after recovery from myocardial infarction. Controlled trial in 568 patients. Lancet 2:1055–1057, 1971.
5. Vajda FJE, Prineas RJ, Lovell RRH, Sloman JG: The possible effect of long-term high plasma levels of phenytoin on mortality after acute myocardial infarction. Europ J Clin Pharmacol 5:138–144, 1973.
6. Lovell RRH: Review of the present status of drug treatment for preventing sudden death. Br Heart J 40 suppl: 94–98, 1978.
7. Kosowsky BD, Taylor J, Lown B, Ritchie RF: Long-term use of procaineamide following acute myocardial infarction. Circulation 47:1204–1210, 1973
8. Hagemeijer F, Glaser B, Van Durme J-P, Bogaert M: Design of a study to evaluate drug therapy of serious ventricular rhythm disturbances after an acute myocardial infarction. Europ J Cardiol 6/4:299–310, 1977.
9. Julian DG: Personal communication.

4.4. THE POSSIBLE ROLE OF PLATELETS IN SUDDEN CARDIAC DEATH

J.L. RITCHIE and L.A. HARKER

Endothelial injury with subsequent platelet deposition at injured sites plays a pivotal role in acute and chronic vascular diseases and their thromboembolic sequelae. The major risk factors in human coronary atherosclerosis – (i) hyperlipidemia, (ii) hypertension, and (iii) smoking – have been related experimentally to endothelial injury (1–4).

Following exposure to subendothelial collagen or other thrombogenic surfaces, platelets adhere, aggregate, and undergo the release reaction with release of platelet specific proteins from α granules (beta thromboglobulin and platelet factor 4 [PF4]), and stimulation of the arachidonate pathway to the production of thromboxane A_2 (5), a potent platelet aggregator. Thromboxane A_2 also has coronary artery vasoconstrictor properties (6). Arachidonate in the endothelial cell, by contrast, is metabolized to prostacycline (PGI_2), currently the most potent inhibitor of platelet adhesion and aggregation identified and a coronary artery vasodilator (7, 8). It has been proposed that PGI_2 plays an important role in local regulation of coronary vascular tone and may preserve the nonthrombogenicity of the normal endothelium (9). An imbalance of these competing influences of coronary vasoconstriction or dilatation, secondary to endothelial damage and/or platelet aggregation, may have a pathogenetic role in clinical syndromes, such as unstable angina, acute myocardial infarction, or sudden cardiac death.

Experimental animal studies have demonstrated that platelet mechanisms do, in fact, operate to create tissue necrosis in some models. Jorgensen (10), for example, in a basic experimental model in swine, demonstrated that intracoronary or intraventricular administration of adenosine diphosphate (ADP), one of the several agents capable of inducing platelet aggregation, produced variable hemodynamic collapse with a 20 % immediate incidence of ventricular fibrillation and myocardial infarction. Intravascular platelet aggregates were directly observed in the mesenteric circulation by cine photo microscopy and seen by histologic examination in the myocardium. Control animals, whose platelets had been rendered refractory to ADP, or who had been previously made thrombocytopenic, failed to show similar changes (10).

Similarly, patchy myocardial necrosis produced experimentally by catecholamine infusion in dogs is known to be associated with intracapillary platelet aggregates (11), and is significantly decreased by pretreatment with either of the platelet inhibitory agents – aspirin or dipyridamole (12). In the setting of experimental acute myocardial infarction in dogs, microthrombi within the subtended infarcted and ischemic zones can be demonstrated both histologically and by increased radioactivity of previously tagged ^{51}Cr platelets (13). When pretreated with either aspirin or dipyridamole, the magnitude of the zone of ischemia and microthrombi, as well as the incidence of arrhythmias (including ventricular fibrillation) was significantly reduced (13).

That platelet emboli may originate from damaged endothelium and embolize downstream has been shown by Honour and Ross (14). Following injury to the vascular endothelium with a variety of stimuli, they demonstrated repeated build-up and subsequent downstream embolization of platelet aggregates using direct microscopic examination of the live rabbit cerebral vasculature. Central nervous system ischemia has been attributed to such platelet microemboli and platelet clumps have been viewed and photographed traversing the retinal circulation during episodes of transient visual loss (15): McBrien, et al. (16) demonstrated that such antemortem retinal emboli were, on postmortem examination, primarily platelet emboli. A recently completed multicenter trial of aspirin for the prevention of transient ischemic cerebral episodes (TIAs), has been released and suggests that in the subgroup with appropriate vascular abnormalities by angiogram, the frequency of TIAs was decreased (17). The Canadian multicenter trial has also shown a reduction in stroke and mortality for male patients with TIAs following treatment with either aspirin alone or aspirin combined with sulfinpyrazone (18).

Clinical studies relating platelet inhibitory agents to coronary artery disease mortality are less well defined at present, with several multicenter trials in progress. In the syndrome of Prinzmetal angina (rest pain most commonly associated with ST segment elevation), Maseri, et al., have recently demonstrated that hemodynamic factors which might increase myocardial oxygen demands did not precede pain, and additionally, that "spontaneous" (non catheter or drug-induced) coronary artery spasm precipitated the pain syndrome (19). This group further showed that repetitive episodes of unstable pain led to myocardial infarction in some cases, and in two such autopsied cases, platelet-fibrin thrombi were found at the sites of previously identified coronary spasm (19). Oliva and Breckinridge likewise found reversible coronary artery spasm in about 40 % of all patients undergoing coronary angiography at the time of acute myocardial infarction (20). The recent description of the coronary vasoconstrictive properties of thromboxane A_2 released during platelet aggregation, raises again the possible role of abnormal platelet aggregation in contributing to the coronary artery spasm seen in pre-infarction angina or acute infarction.

In the setting of stable coronary artery disease, a variety of earlier in-vitro platelet aggregation studies gave mixed results with most recent studies reporting negative findings (21, 22, 23). Studies with in vivo ^{51}Cr labeled platelets and ^{125}I-fibrinogen have been performed in 58 men with documented coronary atherosclerosis in this laboratory (24). Compared to 26 age-matched controls, mean platelet survival time was selectively shortened (6.8 ± 1.8, s.d., days versus 9.0 ± 1.0 days; $p < 0.0001$) with no change in fibrinogen survival. Mean platelet survival time was partially normalized in nine patients following revascularization surgery (pre-op 5.1 ± 0.9 versus post-op 7.1 ± 1.5 days, $p < 0.001$) and in 13 patients after administration of dipyridamole (75 mg t.i.d.) and acetylsalicylate (ASA, 300 mg t.i.d.) (4.8 ± 0.5 versus 7.0 ± 0.8 days, $p < 0.001$). Similar results have been reported by Steele, et al. (25), and their group has shown improved platelet survival following sulfinpyrazone. Fuster has recently reported shortened platelet survival times among asymptomatic cigarette smokers with a positive family history of coronary artery disease (26). Platelet survival studies do not distinguish between coronary artery disease and atherosclerosis generally, however.

Platelet factor 4 (PF4), a platelet specific protein not normally detectable in plasma, is elevated in most patients with stable coronary artery disease (CAD) and following acute myocardial infarction (27, 28). Similar results have been obtained in this laboratory. In 30 normal subjects, plasma PF4 was 0.97 ng/ml ± 42 (serum values were 6,050 ng/ml ± 1140). In six patients with severe thrombocytopenia secondary to marrow aplasia, values were 0.62 ng/ml ± 0.34. In 20 patients with angiographically documented coronary artery disease, PF4 was 19 ± 16 (p < 0.001 compared to normals) with only a single value overlapping the normal range.

Mehta, et al., have suggested direct intracoronary consumption of platelets by establishing an aorto-coronary sinus concentration gradient in patients with coronary atherosclerosis compared to normal controls (29). Decreased coronary sinus aggregation to standard stimuli was also demonstrated in the coronary artery disease group, possibly indicative of earlier aggregation in the coronary arteries. Enhanced aggregation and shortened platelet survival following propranolol withdrawal has been reported and suggested as a contributing factor in the syndrome of enhanced angina and/or myocardial infarction in this setting (30). Clinical studies relating platelet inhibitory drugs to patients with coronary artery disease have yielded conflicting results to date. Over a quarter of a century ago, Cobb, et al. (31), suggested that patients with rheumatoid arthritis and presumed heavy aspirin intake had a disproportionately low incidence of myocardial infarction and stroke. Another retrospective study by the Boston Collaborative Drug Surveillance Group reported a negative association between regular aspirin use and myocardial infarction (32). This study has been criticized, however, in that by studying only hospitalized patients, the 60 % of patients dying of infarction before they could reach the hospital were excluded. Similarly, patients who failed to survive 72 hours upon being hospitalized were generally not included. A large, prospective study on drug use in over 1,000,000 patients failed to confirm this negative association of aspirin and coronary mortality (33). The basis for this conclusion was a single questionnaire categorizing aspirin usage as "never", "seldom", or "often", with subsequent analysis of cause of death by death certificate over the ensuing six years. The extent to which this single questionnaire reflected chronic aspirin usage over the six year follow-up is unknown, as is any indication of the amounts of aspirin ingested by those responding with "often" use. Following discharge from an initial myocardial infarction, Elwood, et al., in a randomized, prospective multicenter study, showed improved survival at one year among patients given 0.3 g aspirin daily (34). This improved survival, however, was not statistically significant. The recent report of the Anturane Reinfarction Trial Group (35), employing sulfinpyrazone, however, lends considerable support to the thesis that sudden cardiac death may be mediated in part through platelet mechanisms. In that study, the incidence of sudden death was significantly reduced by 55 % in the treated group (6.3 versus 2.7 %), although the rate of reinfarction was unaffected at a mean follow-up of eight months. The design of this study, in which a seven day wait for drug effect was required, as well as the presence of more arrhythmias in the placebo group, and the multiple temporal statistical analyses have been the subjects of some criticism.

Earlier studies with clofibrate and dipyridamole in coronary artery disease gave conflicting and negative results, respectively. Clofibrate reduced mortality in both the Scottish (36) and Newcastle Studies (37), but was ineffective in the larger Coronary Drug Research Project (38). Several additional clinical trials are in progress and results from the multi-center trial of aspirin following myocardial infarction (AMIS) are anticipated within the following year. Until this and other trials are completed, firm conclusions about clinical use of platelet active drugs in coronary atherosclerosis seem unwarranted.

Considering only sudden cardiac death, as opposed to coronary artery disease mortality generally, pathologic studies support the possible role of platelet emboli. Detailed pathologic study (sectioning of each major epicardial coronary artery every 2–3 mm with analysis of 15,000 sections) in 80 patients demonstrated an increased frequency and size of platelet aggregates in patients with coronary atherosclerosis who died suddenly when compared to patients dying of other causes (39). Pathologic study of 50 patients dying suddenly in Seattle has additionally shown evidence for patchy myocardial necrosis in 88 %. The necrosis antedated the terminal event by at least 24 hours and was present in only 6 % of hospitalized patients dying of noncardiovascular deaths (40, 41). Diffuse micro-inflammatory lesions were also described in 88 % of patients dying suddenly compared to 30 % of controls (42). The etiology of these lesions, as well as the patchy necrosis described by Reichenbach (40, 41), is uncertain, although platelet microemboli are a possible source. Only limited data concerning platelet abnormalities are available in patients who have been resuscitated from out-of-hospital ventricular fibrillation. This group represents a unique subset of patients in two senses: first, only 15–20 % have definite evidence for new transmural myocardial infarction, and second, the group without infarction at the time of ventricular fibrillation has an extraordinarily high rate of recurrent sudden death in the subsequent two years (43). That is, this subset appears to continue to be exposed to ongoing processes predisposing to sudden death – platelet microemboli are one possible factor. We have performed ^{51}Cr platelet survival measurements in 11 ambulatory patients, 5–21 months following out-of-hospital ventricular fibrillation unassociated with acute infarction (44). The mean platelet survival time of 7.7 ± 2.1 days was shortened compared to 28 normal controls of similar age (9.0 ± 1.0 days, $p < 0.03$), but not different from 56 patients with stable angina pectoris (6.85 ± 1.81 days, $p > 0.2$). One patient with a near normal survival time of 7.5 days experienced recurrent ventricular fibrillation without acute infarction one month following his platelet survival study. About half of this group had individually shortened platelet survival times. Thus, abnormal platelet survival did not distinguish ventricular fibrillation survivors from other patients with coronary artery disease. Two new approaches to the study of platelet physiology, study of the release of platelet specific proteins, such as platelet factor 4, and the organ specific localization of active platelet deposition by platelet imaging, hold the promise for more specific insights (45). Serial analysis of platelet factor 4 in primary ventricular fibrillation survivors, to the extent that the technique reflects platelet activity predominantly in the coronary vasculature, may better characterize patients at high risk. Preliminary studies from our laboratory (unpublished observations) show higher PF4 values in survivors of sudden cardiac death than in nonsudden death coronary artery disease patients, for example. Similarly, employing the ^{111}In-oxine platelet imaging technique, it is possible to detect intracavitary platelet deposition in some ventricular fibrillation survivors, although intrinsic gamma camera resolution does not allow detection of intracoronary platelet deposition. It is anticipated, however, that high resolution, quantitative platelet imaging obtainable with emission computerized positron scintigraphy, will partially resolve this problem.

In summary, considerable experimental evidence, including the documentation that platelet microemboli cause tissue damage, as well as the release of vasoactive substances capable of causing coronary artery spasm, suggests a role for platelets in sudden cardiac death. Clinico-pathologic studies, including the demonstration of platelet aggregates in the coronary arteries of some patients dying suddenly, help corroborate this thesis. Further clinical intervention trials nearing completion, as well as improved techniques for assessing abnormal platelet reactivity and deposition should more sharply define the clinical role of platelet suppressant agents in the near future.

ACKNOWLEDGEMENT

This work was supported by the Medical Research Service of the Veterans Administration by NHLBI grants HL-11775 and HL-18805; and by the Clinical Research Center of the University of Washington (Grants FR-37 and FR-133 of the National Institutes of Health).

REFERENCES

1. Ross R, Harker L: Hyperlipidemia and atherosclerosis. Science 193: 1094–1099, 1976.
2. Goldby FS, Beilin LJ: Relationship between arterial pressure and the permeability of arterioles to carbon particles in acute hypertension in the rat. Cardiovasc Res 6:384–390, 1972.
3. Goldby FS, Beilin LJ: How an acute rise in arterial pressure damages arterioles. Cardiovasc Res 6:569–584, 1972.
4. Robertson AL, Khairalloh PA: Arterial endothelial permeability and vascular disease: the trap door effect. Exp Mol Pathol 18:241–243, 1973.
5. Hamberg M, Svensson J, Samuelsson B: Thromboxanes: A new group of biologically active compounds derived from prostaglandin endoperoxides. Proc Nat Acad Sci USA 72:2994–2998, 1975.
6. Ellis EF, Oelz O, Roberts II LJ, Payne A, Sweetman BJ, Nies AS, Oates JA: Coronary arterial smooth muscle contraction by a substance released from platelets: Evidence that it is thromboxane A_2. Science 193: 1135–1137, 1976.
7. Raz A, Isakson PC, Minkes MS, Needleman P: Characterization of a novel metabolic pathway of arachidonate in coronary arteries which generates a potent endogenous coronary vasodilator. J Biol Chem 252:1123–1126, 1977.
8. Dusting GJ, Moncada S, Vane JR: Prostacycline (PGX) is the endogenous metabolite responsible for relaxation of coronary arteries induced by arachidonic acid. Prostaglandins 13:3–15, 1977.
9. Moncada S, Higgs EA, Vane JR: Human arterial and venous tissues generate prostacyclin (prostaglandin X), a potent inhibitor of platelet aggregation. Lancet 1:18–20, 1977.
10. Jorgensen L, Rowsell H, Hovig T, Glynn M, Mustard JF: Adenosine diphosphate-induced platelet aggregation and myocardial infarction in swine. Lab Invest 17:616–644, 1967.
11. Haft JI, Gershengorn K, Kranz PD, Oestreicher R: Protection against epinephrine-induced myocardial necrosis by drugs that inhibit platelet aggregation. Am J Cardiol 30:838–843, 1972.
12. Haft JI, Kranz PD, Albert F: The role of platelets in catecholamine-induced cardiac necrosis. Electron-microscopic studies. Clin Res 19:709, 1971 (abstract).
13. Moschos CB, Lahiri K, Lyons M, Weisse AB, Oldewurtel HA, Regan TJ: Relation of microcirculatory throm-

bosis to thrombus in the proximal coronary artery: Effect of aspirin, dipyridamole, and thrombolysis. Am Heart J 86:61–68, 1973.

14. Honour AJ, Russell RWR: Experimental platelet embolism. Br J Exp Pathol 43:350–362, 1962.

15. Gunning AS, Pickering GW, Robb-Smith AH, Russell RR: Mural thrombosis of the internal carotid artery and subsequent embolism. Q J Med 33:155–195, 1964.

16. McBrien DS, Bradley RD, Ashton N: The nature of retinal emboli in stenosis of the internal carotid artery. Lancet 1:697–699, 1963.

17. Fields WS, Lemak NA, Frankowski RF, Hardy RJ: Controlled trial of aspirin in cerebral ischemia. Stroke 8:301–314, 1977.

18. The Canadian Cooperative Study Group: A randomized trial of aspirin and sulfinpyrazone in threatened stroke. N Engl J Med 299:53–59, 1978.

19. Maseri A, L'Abbate A, Baroldi G, Chierchia S, Marzilli M, Ballestra AM, Severi S, Parodi O, Biagini A, Distante A, Pesola A: Coronary vasospasm as a possible cause of myocardial infarction. A conclusion derived from the study of 'preinfarction' angina. N Engl J Med 299:1271–1277, 1978.

20. Oliva PB, Breckinridge JC: Arteriographic evidence of coronary arterial spasm in acute myocardial infarction. Circulation 56:366–374, 1977.

21. McDonald L, Edgill M: Changes in coagulability of the blood during various phases of ischemic heart disease. Lancet 1:1115, 1959.

22. Nestel PS: A note on platelet adhesiveness in ischemic heart disease. J Clin Pathol 14:150–151, 1961.

23. Steele PP, Weily HS, Davies H, Genton E: Platelet function studies in coronary artery disease. Circulation 48:1194–1200, 1973.

24. Ritchie JL, Harker LA: Platelet and fibrinogen survival in coronary atherosclerosis. Response to medical and surgical therapy. Am J Cardiol 39:595–598, 1977.

25. Steele P, Rainwater J, Vogel R, Genton E: Platelet-suppressant therapy in patients with coronary artery disease. JAMA 240:228–231, 1978.

26. Fuster V, Brandenburg RO: Cigarette smoking, positive family history and shortened platelet survival as predictors of coronary artery disease under age of 50. Proc Assoc Univ Cardiologists, Phoenix, Az, 1978.

27. Marouf AA, Workman EF, White II GC: Elevation of high affinity platelet factor four (HA-PF4) in hypercoagulable states. Circulation 57, 58 (suppl II):II-116, 1978.

28. Ellis JB, Krentz LS, Levine SP: Increased plasma platelet factor 4 (PF4) in patients with coronary artery disease. Circulation 57, 58 (suppl II):II-116, 1978.

29. Mehta J, Mehta P, Pepine CJ: Platelet aggregation in aortic and coronary venous blood in patients with and without coronary disease. 3. Role of tachycardia stress and propranolol. Circulation 58:881–886, 1978.

30. Frishman WH, Christodoulou J, Weksler B, Smithen C, Killip T, Scheidt S: Abrupt propranolol withdrawal in angina pectoris: Effects on platelet aggregation and exercise tolerance. Am Heart J 95:169–179, 1978.

31. Cobb S, Anderson F, Bauer W: Length of life and cause of death in rheumatoid arthritis. N Engl J Med 249:553–556, 1953.

32. Boston Collaborative Drug Surveillance Group: Regular aspirin intake and acute myocardial infarction. Br Med J 1:440–443, 1974.

33. Hammond EC, Garfinkel L: Aspirin and coronary heart disease: findings of a prospective study. Br Med J 2:269–271, 1975.

34. Elwood PC, Cochrave AL, Burr ML, Sweetnam PM, Williams G, Welsby E: A randomized controlled trial of acetyl salicylic acid in the secondary prevention of mortality from myocardial infarction. Br Med J 1:436–441, 1974.

35. The Anturane Reinfarction Trial Research Group: Sulfinpyrazone in the prevention of cardiac death after myocardial infarction. N Engl J Med 298:289–295, 1978.

36. Research Committee of the Scottish Society of Physicians: Ischaemic heart disease: A secondary prevention trial using clofibrate. Br Med J 4:775–784, 1971.

37. Trial of Clofibrate in the treatment of ischaemic heart disease. A five-year study by a group of physicians of the Newcastle upon Tyne region. Br Med J 4:767–775, 1971.

38. Coronary Drug Project Research Group: Clofibrate and niacin in coronary heart disease. JAMA 27:360–376, 1975.

39. Haerem JW: Sudden coronary death: The occurrence of platelet aggregates in the epicardial arteries of man. Atherosclerosis 14:417–432, 1971.

40. Reichenbach DD, Moss NS: Selective myocardial necrosis in sudden death. Am J Pathol 74:75a, Feb. 1974 (abstract).

41. Reichenbach DD, Moss NS: Myocardial cell necrosis and sudden death in humans. Circulation (suppl III) 52:III-60–62, 1975.

42. Haerem JW: Myocardial lesions in sudden, unexpected coronary death. Am Heart J 90:562–568, 1975.
43. Baum RS, Alvarez H III, Cobb LA: Survival after resuscitation from out-of-hospital ventricular fibrillation. Circulation 50:1231–1235, 1974.
44. Ritchie JL, Cobb LA, Harker LA: Platelet survival in patients previously resuscitated from out-of-hospital ventricular fibrillation. J Lab Clin Med 93:310–315, 1979.
45. Thakur ML, Welch MJ, Joist JH, Coleman RE: Indium-111 labeled platelets: Studies on preparation and evaluation of in vitro and in vivo functions. Thromb Res 9:345–357, 1976.

4.5. THE AUTOMATIC IMPLANTABLE DEFIBRILLATOR: A NEW AVENUE

M. MIROWSKI, M.M. MOWER, A. LANGER and M.S. HEILMAN

The recognition by Beck et al. (1) and by Zoll and his associates (2) of the unique property of electrical countershock to terminate ventricular fibrillation in man began a new era in the treatment of cardiac arrhythmias. Within a relatively short period of time, this discovery prompted the emergence of modern coronary care and resulted in an almost complete elimination of primary ventricular fibrillation as a significant cause in hospital mortality from cardiovascular disorders.

In contrast, ventricular tachyarrhythmias occurring outside the hospital continue to present a serious threat to life. In the United States alone the number of victims is estimated at 300,000 annually (3), many under 65 years of age. The death is either instantaneous or occurs shortly after the onset of symptoms, before the patient is able to reach a medical facility. It is generally accepted that sudden cardiac death is due to electrical instability of the heart culminating in ventricular fibrillation (4, 5).

This major public health problem has hitherto been confronted almost exclusively by approaches aimed at the basic pathophysiological mechanisms underlying cardiac electrical instability. Primary prevention through identification, reduction, and eventually elimination of risk factors responsible for coronary heart disease has been seen as the preferred way to eradicate malignant arrhythmias. Secondary prevention was also advocated on the assumption that safe suppressive antiarrhythmic therapy could be developed. These strategies are difficult to implement in practice, however, and the anticipated advantages of preventive approaches to the management of malignant ventricular arrhythmias have not yet been demonstrated.

As far as therapeutic options are concerned, electrical countershock remains the only effective method available. The effectiveness of this maneuver is nevertheless limited by its complete dependence on the prompt availability of specialized personnel and equipment. The time factor is particularly critical, and, in the absence of cardiopulmonary resuscitation, only one minute or so is available (6). These inherent difficulties in dealing with ventricular fibrillation outside the hospital account for the present prohibitive toll of sudden cardiac deaths.

Since it is so often impossible to bring the fibrillating patient to a medical facility in time, efforts have been made to develop mobile coronary care units and other types of emergency services (7). While these life support systems save a larger number of patients each year, their complex logistics preclude a broad application of the approach. This limitation is compounded by the fact that the resuscitated patients, particularly those who show no evidence of acute myocardial infarction, are prone to fibrillate again, with a mortality of some 30 % in the year following the initial defibrillation (8–10).

These observations convinced us and others (11, 12) of the urgent need for an implantable defibrillator capable of accomplishing the necessary diagnostic-therapeutic tasks automatically. More specifically, such an electronic device would have to monitor the heart continuously, recognize ventricular fibrillation and deliver corrective defibrillatory shocks when indicated. When implanted in selected high-risk patients, the automatic defibrillator would provide them some protection from sudden death when and wherever they are stricken by ventricular fibrillation. Conceptually, the device can be viewed as analogous to an implantable demand pacemaker, except that ventricular fibrillation instead of asystole is sensed, and the delivered shock is of defibrillating magnitude.

Since a conventional defibrillator is an apparatus hardly lending itself to implantation in man, the idea that such a device could not only be miniaturized but also endowed with capabilities similar to those existing in a coronary care unit was recieved with skepticism. After a decade of effort, however, these objectives have been fully achieved.

The translation of the implantable automatic defibrillator concept into a small, practical, human-grade device required the development of new technology and the solution of many engineering, electrophysiological and clinical problems. The key to miniaturization was provided by the realization that the size of the defibrillator is directly related to its energy output. Our initial line of research thus centered on the design of electrode systems capable of defibrillating closed-chest subjects with only a small fraction of transthoracic energy requirements. This was achieved by developing the catheter technique of defibrillation capable of restoring normal rhythm with pulses of some 5 to 20 joules (13–16), while hundreds of joules are usually required using external paddles.

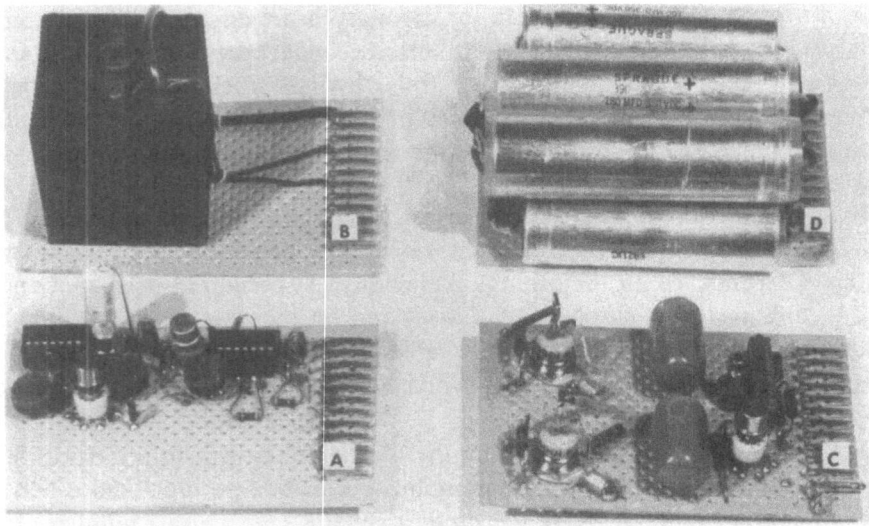

Figure 1. Original prototype of an automatic defibrillator having 50 joules capacity, displayed on 3 × 4 inch circuit boards containing the sensing circuit (**A**), high voltage converter (**B**), switching circuit (**C**), capacitor bank (**D**), and batteries (not shown). (**By permission.**)

The original laboratory prototype of the automatic defibrillator built and successfully tested by our group in 1969 is shown in Figure 1. This model (11), whose output could be set as high as 50 joules, monitored the pulsatile right ventricular pressure with a transducer attached to the tip of a transvenous right ventricular catheter. Ventricular fibrillation led to abolition of the phasic nature of the pressure which, if persisting for more than six seconds, initiated the capacitor charging cycle. When the charging process was completed, the corrective countershock was automatically delivered through a catheter-electrode wedged into the right ventricular apex and another located more proximally on the catheter, usually in the superior vena cava. The entire diagnostic-therapeutic sequence lasted some 20 seconds. The functional performance of the device is illustrated in Figure 2.

This experimental prototype was soon followed by the development of more advanced models characterized by greater miniaturization, progressive refinement of the electrode and sensing systems, increased safety and higher reliability (13–23). As a result of this innovative process, the size, structural characteristics and functional performance of the

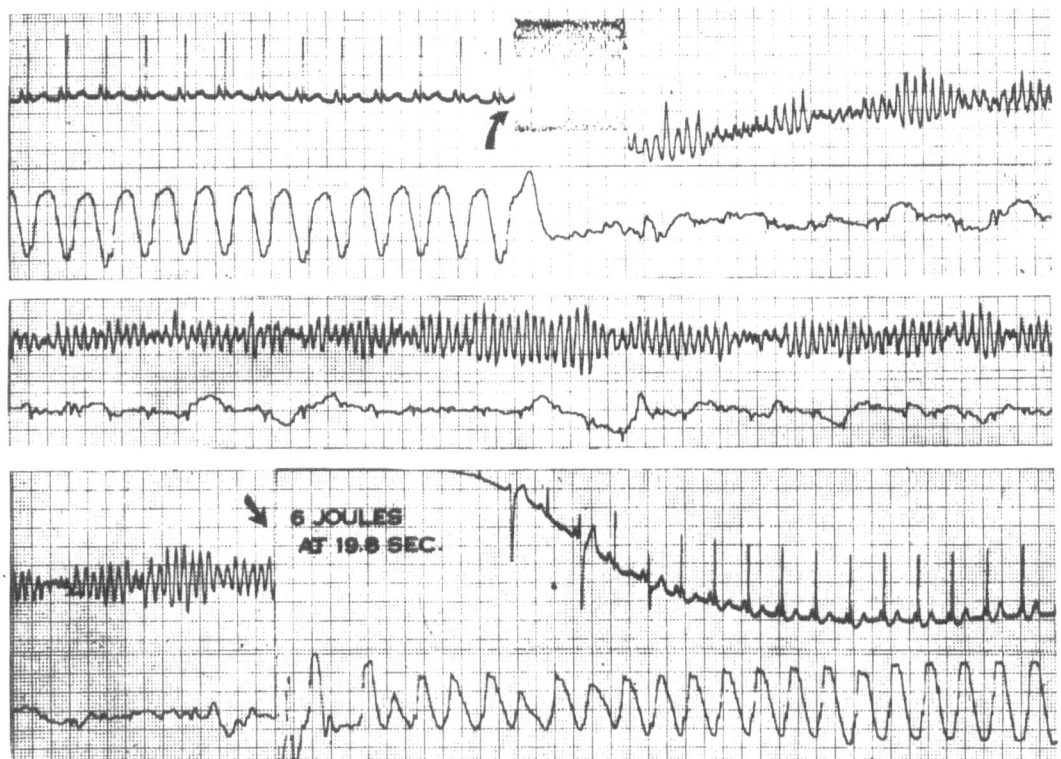

Figure 2. Functional performance of the automatic defibrillator. Simultaneous electrocardiographic and right ventricular pressure curves recorded during operating cycle of the model. Ventricular fibrillation is induced in a dog with a low-level alternating current (upper arrow); 19.8 seconds later, a shock of 6 joules is automatically delivered (lower arrow), resulting in resumption of sinus rhythm. (By permission.)

device have now reached a stage where the stringent criteria required from a clinical device have been satisfied.

The physical appearance of this recent model (19) is similar to some of the early pacemakers (Figure 3). The device[1] is encased in titanium and hermetically sealed with a laser weld; it weighs 250 grams and has a volume of 145 cc. All materials in contact with body tissue are biocompatible. The defibrillating electrodes are made from titanium and silicone rubber. One electrode is located on a catheter pervenously introduced into the distal end of the superior vena cava. For the purpose of ensuring stability, the second electrode in the form of a cup (18), is placed extrapericardially over the apex of the heart. The outside surface of the apical electrode is insulated to achieve optimum current distribution. In dogs a left thoracotomy is used for placement of this conformal apex electrode but a number of approaches aimed at obviating a thoracotomy in man are presently under study.

The ability to monitor the heart for an extensive period of time and to promptly recognize ventricular fibrillation is an essential characteristic of the automatic defibrillator. However, the development of a virtually fool-proof sensing system represented a major challenge. After experimenting with a number of approaches, singly and in combination, a system was designed which establishes the diagnosis of fibrillation by identifying a specific charac-

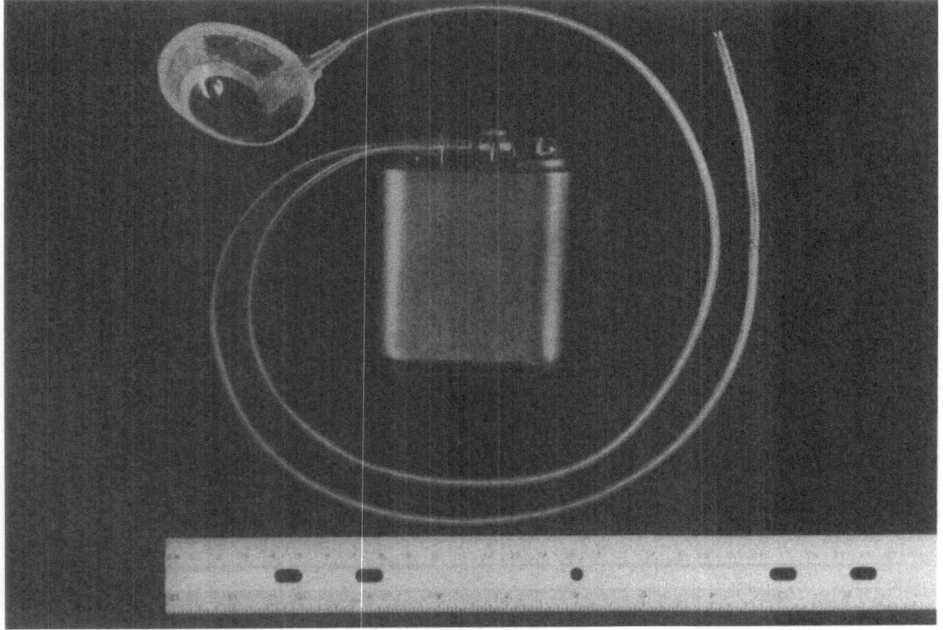

Figure 3. The clinical model of the implantable automatic defibrillator with the apical and superior vena cava electrodes.

[1] Developed in conjunction with Medrad, Inc., Pittsburgh, Pennsylvania, U.S.A.

teristic of the arrhythmia, rather than indirectly, through monitoring of such parameters as arterial pressure, R waves, electrical impedence, etc. The important advantage of this detection scheme, in addition to its reliability and low standby-power requirements, is its passive mode of failure. Passive mode of failure means that in case of sensing abnormality, theoretically possible, the device would remain passive, rather than misdiagnosing the problem as fibrillation and delivering an unwanted shock.

The principles that govern the operation of the sensor are based on continuous analysis of the probability density function of the ventricular electrical activity (20). This function

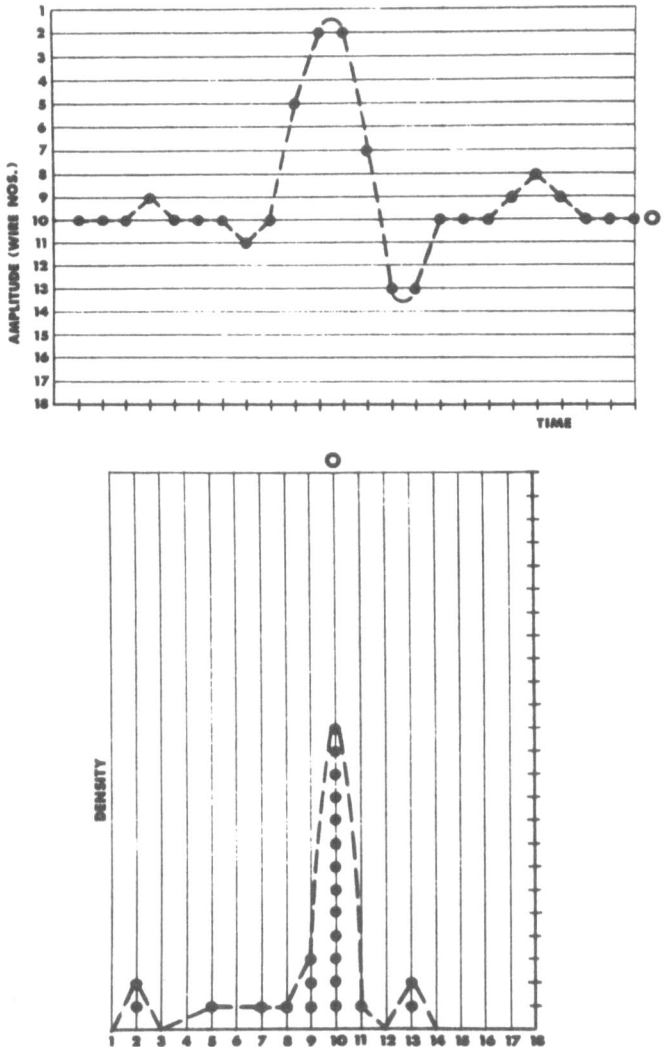

Figure 4. Diagrammatic presentation of the probability density concept. For explanation see text.

reflects the time spent by the slope of the input electrogram between two amplitude limits located, in our particular system, near zero potential. The probability density is a measure of how much time a signal spends, on average, at different amplitude levels.

This concept can be illustrated by a frame with horizontal wires and sliding beads placed upon these wires, somewhat resembling an abacus on its side (Figure 4, top). The vertical axis represents discrete amplitudes while the horizontal axis indicates time marked off in regular intervals. Let us use the beads on wires to form a crude approximation of an electrocardiogram by placing a bead on the appropriate amplitude wire at each time interval.

If this framework is now tilted sideways, the beads slide down the wires and "stack" – the height of the stack being directly proportional to the number of beads on each wire (Figure 4, bottom). For clarity, the beads are shown as not touching each other. The stack height or density value, for each amplitude, is a measure of how much time the signal spent at each of the amplitude levels. It is obvious that the density is greatest on wire number ten indicating that the signal spent most of the time at the baseline (amplitude zero).

In the automatic defibrillator, the height of the peak at amplitude zero is measured electronically from a differentiated electrogram. Initially a special filter approximates the first derivative of the input signal, recorded from the defibrillating electrodes. An additional circuit then measures the statistical distribution of the filtered signal, in effect sampling its probability density. Ventricular fibrillation is recognized by the striking absence of peak at amplitude zero, reflecting the absence of isoelectric potential segments. Panel 1 and 2 in Figure 5 show the input electrogram and its corresponding probability density curve as actually measured in a dog. The points identified by capital letters reflect the same events on both displays. Thus QRS deflections B and D, although prominent on the electrogram, represent on the average only small amounts of total time, but events such as C, close to the isoelectrical line, are reflected by a very high peak on the probability density curve. Panel 3 shows the input signal after filtering. The large ST segment has disappeared and does not appear on the corresponding probability density curve (Panel 4). The effect of the filter is thus to decrease the height of secondary peaks and to increase the height of the peak corresponding to amplitude zero. Panels 5 and 6 show filtered ventricular fibrillation and its corresponding probability density function. The absence of the peak at amplitude zero identifies ventricular fibrillation.

This sensor has been extensively tested in animals in which only paced rhythms faster than 350 beats per minute have been occasionally misinterpreted. In addition, the detector has been challenged by means of a wide range of tape-recorded human arrhythmias derived from surface body leads. Direct human testing has also been carried out during open heart surgery.

The power sources of the device are specially developed lithium batteries, characterized by high energy density to allow prolonged life in a standby mode and by high peak power density to allow charging of the capacitors in about ten or less seconds when required. Conservatively speaking, the batteries have a projected monitoring life of 3 years or a discharge capability of approximately 100 shocks.

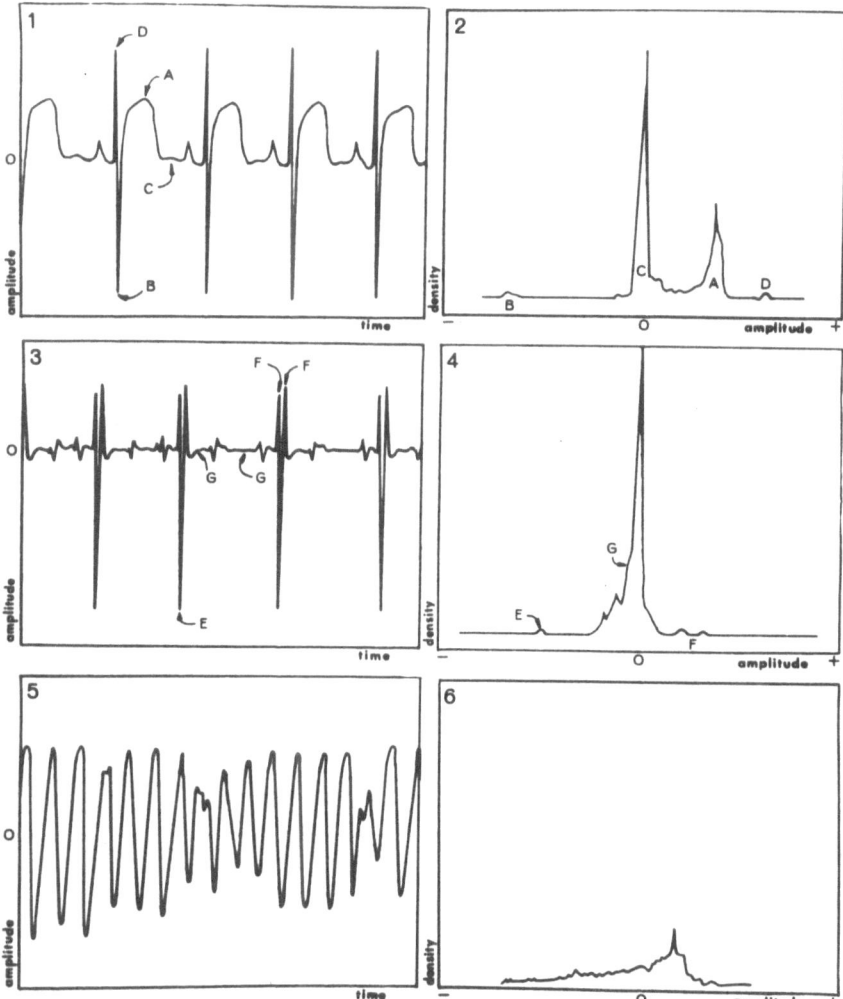

Figure 5. Selected input electrograms (Panels 1, 3, and 5) with their corresponding probability density function graphs (Panels 2, 4, and 6). Panel 1: normal input electrogram. Panel 2: the peak at zero amplitude (C), indicates that the signal spends considerable time near the baseline. Panel 3: the filtered input signal. Panel 4: filtering augments the peak at zero amplitude (G) and decreases the heights of secondary peaks. Panel 5: filtered ventricular fibrillation signal. Panel 6: the absence of peak at amplitude zero reflects the short time interval spent by the signal near the baseline and is diagnostic of ventricular fibrillation. For more detail see text.

Truncated exponential pulses described by Schuder (24) have been selected for use in the implantable defibrillator. Such pulses are simple to generate and for a given defibrillation efficacy require less peak voltage and peak current than the inductor capacitor and simple capacitor discharges. The pulse duration ranges between 3 and 8 msec as a function of the differing heart-electrode resistances.

Using these pulses, the device delivers defibrillatory shocks of up to 30 joules about

15 seconds after onset of the arrhythmia and can recycle as many as three times if the first shock is ineffective. The third and fourth shocks can be of higher delivered energy. After the fourth shock, about 35 seconds of normal rhythm are required to reset the counter and to allow a full series of pulses to be delivered again at the next episode.

Testing the functional performance of the implanted defibrillator in active, conscious dogs was made possible by designing a small, implantable, magnetically activated fibrillator (19). By placing a magnet over the skin in the area where the fibrillator is implanted, low level alternating current is generated and transmitted to the heart through a right ventricular catheter. The resulting ventricular fibrillation leads to circulatory arrest and

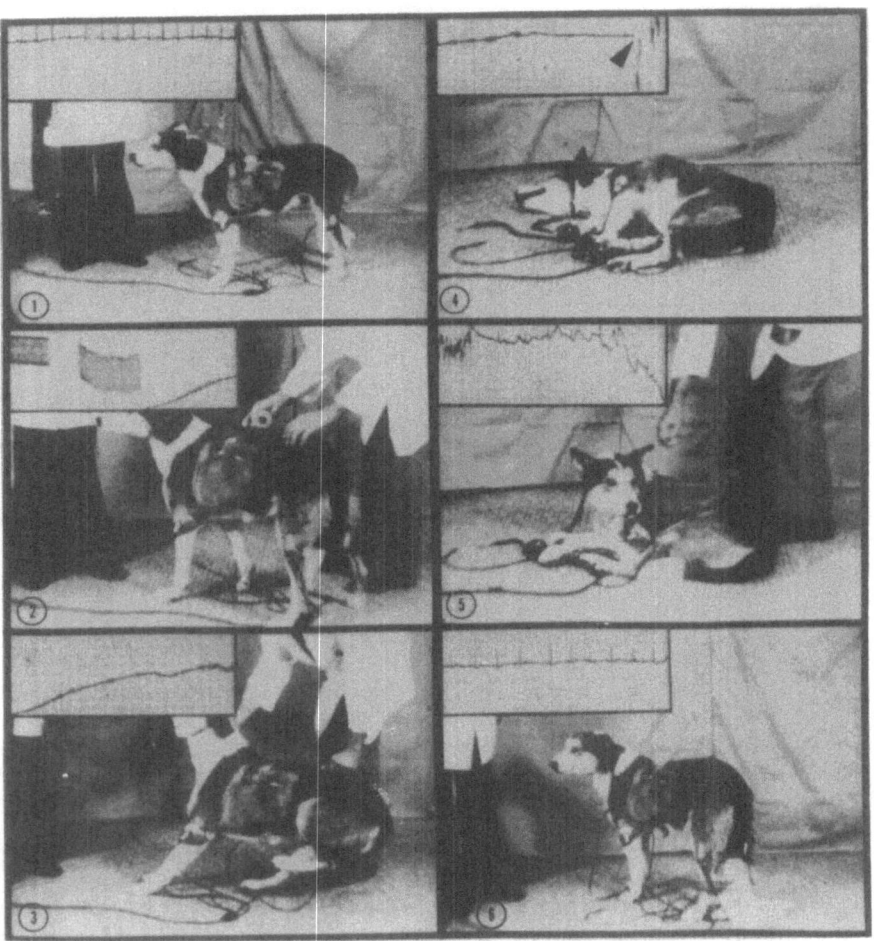

Figure 6. Selected frames from a motion picture of a typical automatic defibrillation episode. Simultaneous electrocardiographic monitoring is displayed in the left upper corner. Panel 1: the dog prior to the procedure. Panel 2: induction of ventricular fibrillation by magnetically activating the fibrillator. Panel 3: syncope secondary to the arrhythmia. Panel 4: the delivery of the defibrillatory shock 15 seconds after the onset of fibrillation (arrowhead). Panels 5 and 6: The animal at 3 and 15 seconds, respectively, following automatic defibrillation.

syncope within seconds, mimicking the clinical syndrome of sudden death. However, in striking contrast to patients stricken by ventricular fibrillation, the animals are automatically defibrillated and resuscitated by the chronically implanted defibrillator (Figure 6).

The question of how to determine the operational readiness and reliability of the device following its permanent implantation in man was solved by designing a method allowing frequent evaluation of the defibrillator function in vivo (21). The method involves triggering of the capacitor charging cycle with a magnet and then delivering the charge into a built-in test-load resistor. A specially developed analyzer measures the charging time with an electromagnetic transducer. Progressive increases of this time, normally 10 seconds or less, reflect battery depletion, while failure to initiate the cycle indicates abnormal device operation. This information is particularly important because the standby device is expected to undergo very long periods of inactivity. The simplicity and the non-invasive nature of this procedure will undoubtedly enhance the clinical applicability of the automatic defibrillator.

The anatomic effects of chronic electrode implantation and the cardiac effects of defibrillatory discharges were studied and found to be minimal. In the absence of infectious complications, only apical pericardial and epicardial fibrosis was found. Multiple shocks did not produce macro or microscopic myocardial damage (23).

This brief description of the current status of the implantable automatic defibrillator indicates that protection of patients at high risk of sudden death from ventricular fibrillation has become a practical possibility. When the intensive bench testing and animal experimentation currently underway will be completed, a pilot clinical study is scheduled to begin. Simultaneously, several important improvements to the device are being designed, including a built-in memory which would provide, in a non-invasive manner, the record of the pertinent arrhythmic events which have occurred in the patient with the implanted defibrillator and the responses of the device. In the future, pacemaking capabilities will also be incorporated into the defibrillator. These and other design changes will further increase the reliability, functional performance, and safety margin of the implanted automatic defibrillator.

REFERENCES

1. Beck CS, Pritchard WM, Feil M: Ventricular fibrillation of long duration abolished by electric shock. JAMA 125:985–986, 1947.
2. Zoll PM, Linenthal AJ, Gibson W, Paul MH, Norman LR: Termination of ventricular fibrillation in man by externally applied electric countershock. N Engl J Med 254:727–732, 1956.
3. Goldstein S: Sudden death and coronary heart disease. New York, Futura Publishing Company, Inc, 1974.
4. Lown B, Wolf M: Approaches to sudden death from coronary heart disease. Circulation 44:130–142, 1971.
5. Julian DG: Toward preventing coronary death from ventricular fibrillation. Circulation 54:360–364, 1976.
6. Stephenson Jr HE: Ventricular defibrillation: general considerations. In: Cardiac arrest & resuscitation, Stephenson Jr HE (ed), St. Louis, CV Mosby, 1974, p 337.
7. Pantridge JF, Geddes JS: A mobile intensive-care unit in the management of myocardial infarction. Lancet 2:271–273, 1967.
8. Baum RS, Alvarez II H, Cobb LA: Survival after resuscitation from out-of-hospital ventricular fibrillation. Circulation 50:1231–1235, 1974.

9. Liberthson RR, Nagel EL, Hirschman JC, Nussenfeld SR: Prehospital ventricular defibrillation. N Engl J Med 291:317–321, 1974.
10. Schaffer WA, Cobb LA: Recurrent ventricular fibrillation and modes of death in survivors of out-of-hospital ventricular fibrillation. N Engl J Med 293:259–262, 1975.
11. Mirowski M, Mower MM, Staewen WS, Tabatznik B, Mendeloff AI: Standby automatic defibrillator. An approach to prevention of sudden coronary death. Arch Intern Med 126:158–161, 1970.
12. Schuder JC, Stoeckle H, Gold JH, West JA, Keskar PY: Experimental ventricular defibrillation with an automatic and completely implanted system. Trans Am Soc Artif Int Organs 16:207–212, 1970.
13. Mirowski M, Mower MM, Staewen WS, Denniston RH, Tabatznik B, Mendeloff AI: Ventricular defibrillation through a single intravascular catheter electrode system. Clin Res 19:328, (abstract) 1971.
14. Mirowski M, Mower MM, Staewen WS, Denniston RH, Mendeloff AI: The development of the transvenous automatic defibrillator. Arch Intern Med 129:773–779, 1972.
15. Mirowski M, Mower MM, Gott VL, Brawley RK, Denniston RH: Transvenous automatic defibrillator. Preliminary clinical tests of its defibrillating subsystem. Trans Amer Soc Artif Intern Org 18:520–524, 1972.
16. Mirowski M, Mower MM, Gott VL, Brawley RK: Feasibility and effectiveness of low-energy catheter defibrillation in man. Circulation 47:79–85, 1973.
17. Mirowski M, Mower MM, Langer A, Heilman MS: Implanted defibrillators. In: Proceedings of the Cardiac Defibrillation Conference, Purdue University, West Lafayette, Indiana, 1975, p 93.
18. Heilman MS, Langer A, Mower MM, Mirowski M: Analysis of four implantable electrode systems for automatic defibrillator. Circulation 52 (suppl II): II-194, (abstract) 1975.
19. Mirowski M, Mower MM, Langer A, Heilman MS: Miniaturized implantable automatic defibrillator for prevention of sudden death from ventricular fibrillation. In: Proceedings, International Symposium on Cardiac Pacing, Tokyo, 1976, Watanabe Y (ed), Amsterdam, Excerpta Medica, 1976, p 103.
20. Langer A, Heilman MS, Mower MM, Mirowski M: Considerations in the development of the automatic implantable defibrillator. Med Instrument 10:163–167, 1976.
21. Langer A, Heilman MS, Mower MM, Mirowski M: Functional analysis of the automatic implantable defibrillator in vivo. Med Instrument 12:55, (abstract), 1978.
22. Mirowski M, Mower MM, Langer A, Heilman MS, Schreibman J: A chronically implanted system for automatic defibrillation in active conscious dogs. Experimental model for treatment of sudden death from ventricular fibrillation. Circulation 58:90–94, 1978.
23. Mirowski M, Mower MM, Bhagavan BS, Langer A, Heilman MS, Schreibman J: The automatic implantable defibrillator: toward the development of the first clinical model. In: Management of ventricular tachycardia: role of mexiletine, Proceedings of a symposium held in Copenhagen, Denmark, May 25–27, 1978. Amsterdam – Oxford, Excerpta Medica, 1978, p 655–662.
24. Schuder JC, Rahmoeller GA, Stoeckle H: Transthoracic ventricular defibrillation with triangular and trapezoidal waveforms. Circ Res 19:689–694, 1966.

SECTION 5
SUDDEN DEATH IN NONCORONARY HEART DISEASE

5.1. SUDDEN DEATH IN PATIENTS WITH HYPERTROPHIC CARDIOMYOPATHY

S.E. EPSTEIN and B.J. MARON

Natural history studies of patients with hypertrophic cardiomyopathy suggest that overall annual mortality from the disease is about 3 % per year (1, 2), with the majority of patients dying suddenly (2). However, virtually all patients included in these studies were evaluated in the 1960's, prior to the general application of echocardiography. This technique, employed in the study of hypertrophic cardiomyopathy with increasing frequency since the early 1970's, has demonstrated that the disease spectrum of hypertrophic cardiomyopathy is considerably broader than previously suspected (3). Hence, a comprehensive understanding of the natural history of this disease, and the precise incidence of sudden death in the many subgroups of patients with hypertrophic cardiomyopathy, is as yet unknown. Nonetheless, the fact remains that sudden death occurs not uncommonly. The purpose of this report is to summarize what is known about identification of the patient at risk of sudden death, and the mechanisms responsible for sudden death. The material is drawn from three studies we have previously published (4–6), with updating of the data where appropriate.

1. CLINICAL STATUS

1.1. Age at Death

Although sudden death is most frequently observed in adults with hypertrophic cardio-myopathy, it may occur during childhood as well. We followed 35 children ranging in age from 4 to 18 years at the time of initial diagnosis (4). In these patients the diagnosis of hypertrophic cardiomyopathy was established prior to the general availability of echocardiography. Over the course of one to 16 years (average 7.4 years), 11 (31 %) of the 35 patients died suddenly, yielding an annual mortality of approximately 4 % per year (Figure 1).

We also identified and studied eight families in which premature cardiac death (before 50 years of age) due to hypertrophic cardiomyopathy occurred in at least two first degree relatives (5). We have termed these "malignant" families. The age range of the 23 subjects in these families who died suddenly and unexpectedly was extremely broad; moreover, 16 of the 23 subjects were less than 20 years of age at the time of death (Figure 2).

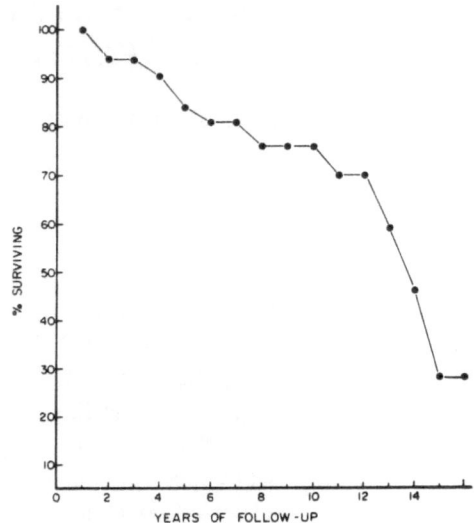

Figure 1. Percent survival with time of the 35 children with hypertrophic cardiomyopathy. The marked decrease in survival occurring after the twelfth year is due to the small numbers of patients who were followed for thirteen or more years. Reproduced with permission from the American Heart Association (4).

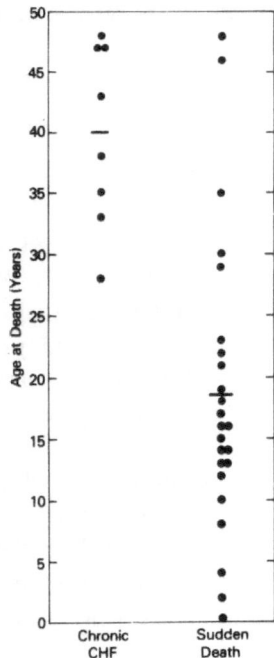

Figure 2. Age at death of patients in the 8 "malignant" families who died with chronic congestive heart failure (CHF) and of patients who died suddenly. Reproduced with permission from American Journal of Cardiology (5).

1.2. Family history

A total of 69 first degree relatives in the eight "malignant" families were identified. Of these, 41 relatives had evidence of hypertrophic cardiomyopathy and 31 (75 %) died of their heart disease. Death was sudden and unexpected in 23 of the 31 patients. Two typical family trees are depicted in Figure 3.

1.3. Symptoms

Symptomatic status was of no help in identifying patients at risk of sudden death. Thus, of the 11 deaths that occurred in children with hypertrophic cardiomyopathy, three were asymptomatic and six were in functional class II prior to sudden death (4). Likewise, of

FAMILY C.

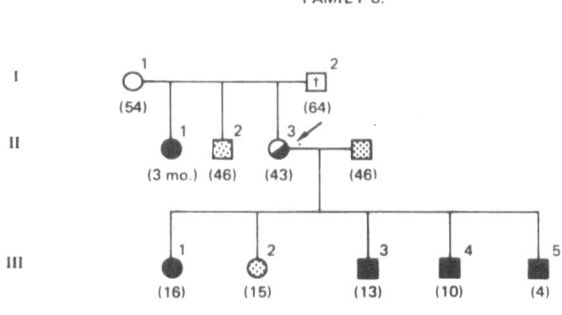

FAMILY Mo.

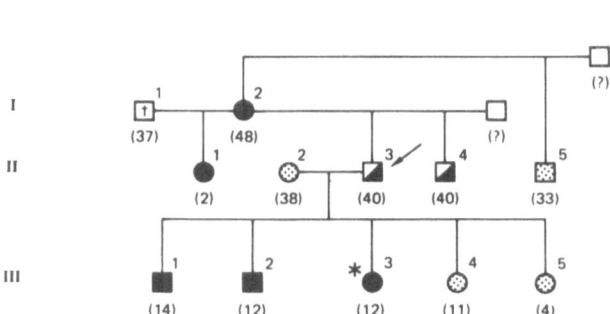

Figure 3. Pedigrees of "malignant" families C. and·Mo. Arrow = propositus; solid symbols = death probably or definitely due to hypertrophic cardiomyopathy; half-filled symbols = alive with an echocardiogram that was diagnostic of hypertrophic cardiomyopathy; clear symbols = echocardiogram not obtained. † = dead of noncardiac cause or cardiac disease other than hypertrophic cardiomyopathy; stippled symbols = alive but hypertrophic cardiomyopathy not evident in the echocardiogram; circles = female subjects; squares = male subjects. Only first degree relatives of the propositus are shown. Patients ages (yr) are shown in parenthesis below the symbols. * = episode of cardiac arrest, but has survived to date. Reproduced with permission from the American Journal of Cardiology (5).

the 23 patients from "malignant" families who died suddenly (5), 15 died without previously experiencing any symptoms whatsoever. Finally, we have recently reported 26 patients (17 of whom were not from the "malignant" families) whose *first* manifestation of hypertrophic cardiomyopathy was sudden death (6). The symptomatic status of these subjects just prior to sudden death is depicted in Table 1.

Table 1. 40 patients with sudden death.

Symptomatic status	Number of patients
No symptoms (FC.1)	30(75 %)
Mild symptoms (FC.2)	8(20 %)
Severe symptoms (FC.3)	2(5 %)
	40

From the above data the only helpful *predictor* of sudden death that can be derived from the clinical history would appear to be a *positive family history* of frequent premature deaths. However, the prevalence with which such families are found in the general population of patients with hypertrophic cardiomyopathy, or of those patients who die suddenly and unexpectedly, is quite low. Hence, the clinical history does not provide a very powerful tool for identifying the large majority of patients at risk of sudden death.

2. HEMODYNAMIC FINDINGS

Analysis of the data of the three studies cited above (4–6) yielded no hemodynamic finding that was predictive of sudden death.

2.1. Left ventricular outflow obstruction

Twelve of the 26 patients whose first manifestation of hypertrophic cardiomyopathy was sudden death had been studied hemodynamically (6). In these, half had left ventricular outflow gradients of $\geq$ 50 mm Hg under basal conditions or with provocation, and the other half had either no outflow gradient or one that was less than 20 mm Hg. Likewise, of the 19 members of "malignant" families who died without operation and in whom adequate studies were available, 7 (37 %) had evidence of marked left ventricular outflow obstruction; the remainder did not (5). In addition, elimination of outflow gradient by operation does not prevent sudden death (7). Hence, the presence or absence of a gradient does not appear to be helpful in determining which patients are at risk of sudden death. The magnitude of the left ventricular outflow tract gradient of those patients who died but were studied in all three of the previously cited investigations (4–6) is depicted in Figure 4.

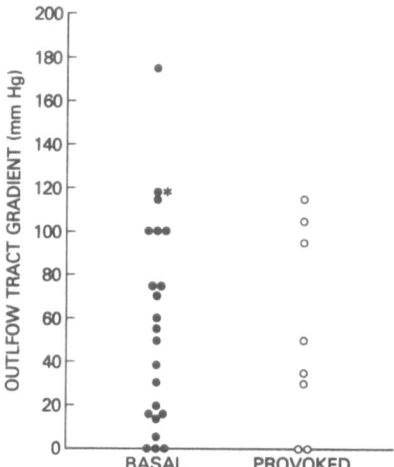

Figure 4. Composite diagram of the left ventricular outflow tract gradient of all patients who died but were studied hemodynamically in three investigations. Asterisk indicates gradient across right ventricular outflow tract (4–6).

2.2. Left ventricular end-diastolic pressure

Left ventricular end-diastolic pressure also does not appear to be a good predictor of sudden death. In the 12 patients who were studied and in whom sudden death was the first manifestation of the disease (6), left ventricular end-diastolic pressure was elevated (greater than 12 mm Hg) in 9 patients, but normal in 3 others. Moreover, while left ventricular end-diastolic pressure at initial study was elevated in 9 of the 11 (82 %) children who subsequently died (4), it was also elevated in 16 of 21 (76 %) who did not die (Figure 5).

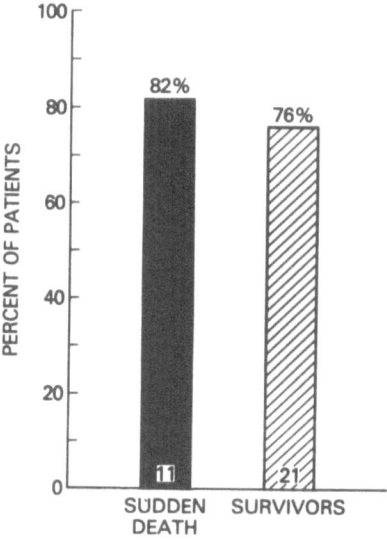

Figure 5 Percent of patients 4 to 18 years of age (4) with left ventricular end-diastolic pressure > 12 mm Hg.

3. VENTRICULAR SEPTAL THICKNESS

Echocardiographic and necropsy studies appear to provide some prognostic information in patients with hypertrophic cardiomyopathy. In the 26 patients with hypertrophic cardiomyopathy in whom death was the first manifestation of cardiac disease (6), absolute ventricular septal thicknesses ranged from 17 to 55 mm (median 25); in all but two patients septal thickness was ≥ 20 mm. The 2 patients with septal thickness < 20 mm (i.e., 17 and 18 mm) were only 11 and 12 years of age, respectively. That marked septal hypertrophy portends a greater tendency to sudden death is also reflected in our study of "malignant" families (5). The average ventricular septal thickness of those family members who died was greater than that of surviving members (25 mm vs 19 mm). In particular, 9 of 10 subjects (90 %) with a ventricular septal thickness ≥ 25 mm died while only 7 of 14 relatives (50 %) with septal thicknesses < 25 mm died (Figure 6). Thus, there appears to be a trend relating septal thickness and sudden death, although a relatively thin septum does not preclude the possibility of sudden death.

4. ELECTROCARDIOGRAPHIC FINDINGS

Of the 26 patients we studied in whom death was the initial manifestation of disease (6), 19 had had a standard 12 lead ECG obtained and in each patient the ECG was distinctly abnormal. The most common abnormalities (alone or in combination) were left ventricular hypertrophy, ST-segment and T wave abnormalities, or abnormal Q wave. Although the vast majority of patients with hypertrophic cardiomyopathy have an abnormal ECG, it is normal in about one-quarter of asymptomatic patients without obstruction (8). Such

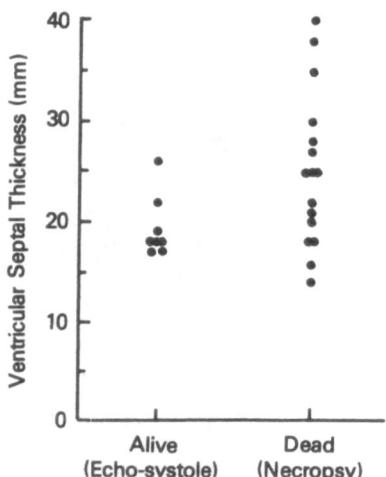

Figure 6. Ventricular septal thicknesses obtained in 8 surviving affected family members by echocardiography (echo) compared to those obtained at necropsy in 16 relatives who had died. Echocardiographic measurements shown were obtained in systole to permit comparison with necropsy measurements.

subjects may be at lower risk of sudden death. On the other hand, because the large majority of patients with hypertrophic cardiomyopathy have abnormal electrocardiograms, the mere *presence* of this sign cannot be employed as a specific predictor of sudden death.

5. IDENTIFICATION OF ARRHYTHMIAS

Ambulatory ECG monitoring has revealed that patients with hypertrophic cardiomyopathy have an alarming frequency of arrhythmias, including high grade ventricular arrhythmias (9–11). In a study from our laboratory (9), 100 patients with hypertrophic cardiomyopathy were divided into four subgroups, depending on the presence or absence of left ventricular outflow tract obstruction and the presence or absence of symptoms. Grading of VPBs (12) was performed according to the method of Lown (Table 2). Eighty-three per cent of the 100 patients had ventricular arrhythmias. Only 35 % had no or low grade ($\leq$ VPB grade 2) ventricular arrhythmia (Figure 7); 60 % had multiform VPBs, 32 % had pairs of VPBs (couplets) and 19 % had ventricular tachycardia with a rate equivalent to 100 beats per minute or more. High grade VPBs (VPB grade 3 or higher) occurred in more than 50 % of the patients in each subgroup studied – i.e., regardless of whether or not symptoms of left ventricular outflow obstruction were present (Figure 8).

Table 2. Grading of ventricular premature beats.

Grade 0 = no VPBs in 24 hours
Grade 1 = occasional VPBs, but no more than 30 in any hour of monitoring
Grade 2 = more than 30 VPBs in any hour of monitoring
Grade 3 = multiform VPBs
Grade 4a = Couplets (two consecutive VPBs)
Grade 4b = ventricular tachycardia (3 or more VPBs in succession)

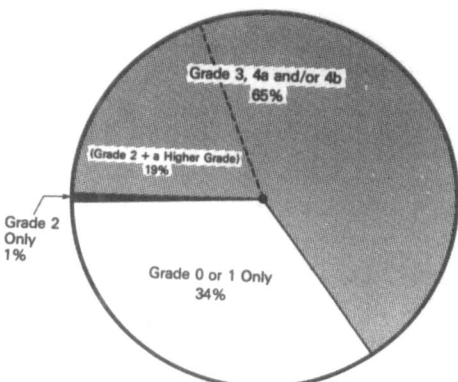

Figure 7. Prevalence of different grades of ventricular premature beats during 24-hours of ECG monitoring in 100 patients with hypertrophic cardiomyopathy. Reproduced with permission from American Heart Association (9).

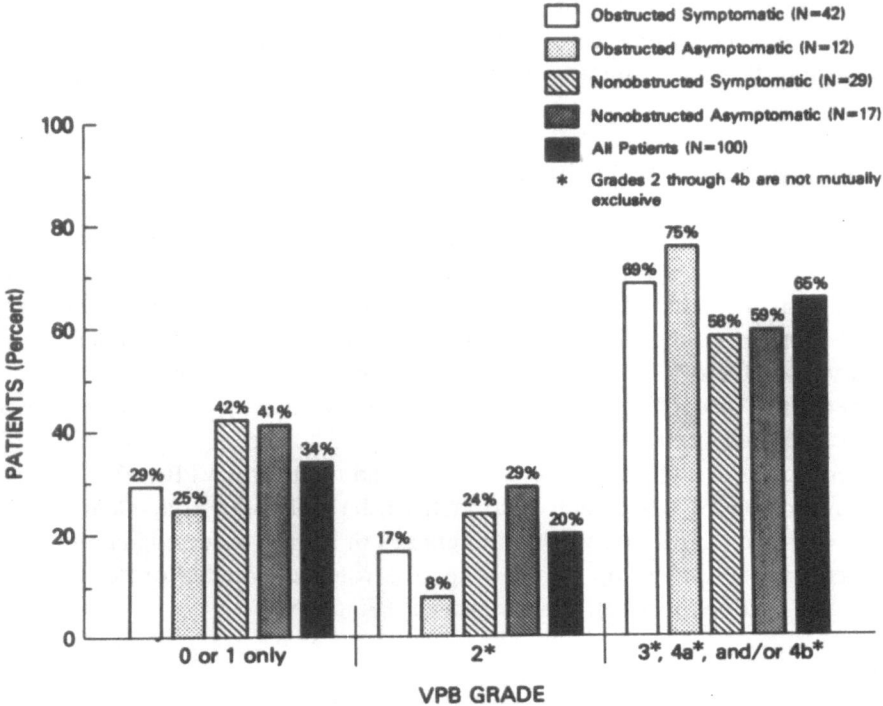

Figure 8. Prevalence of different grades of ventricular premature beats (VPB) during 24-hour monitoring in sub-groups of patients with hypertrophic cardiomyopathy. Reproduced with permission from the American Heart Association (9).

Of note, all but one patient with *frequent VPBs* (> 30 VPBs in any hour of monitoring; VPB grade 2) also had ventricular arrhythmias of grade 3 or higher (Figure 7). The converse, however, was not true. Thus, more than 30 VPBs in any hour of monitoring, or more than 100 VPBs for 24-hours were observed in only 5 of 26 patients (19 %) with multifocal VPBs (Grade III) and in only 11 of 20 patients (55 %) with couplets (Grade IVa).

No significant correlation between left ventricular outflow gradient and maximum VPB grade was found, in that high grade VPBs occurred frequently in the presence or absence of obstruction. In addition, there was no linear relation between ventricular septal thickness and frequency of VPBs. However, patients with septal thickness $\geq$ 20 mm had a greater frequency of high grade VPBs than those with septal thickness less than 20 mm. Thus, while 78 % of patients (52 of 67) with septal thickness $\geq$ 20 mm had grade III VPBs or higher, only 39 % (13 of 33) of patients with septal thickness of less than 20 mm had such arrhythmias (p < 0.005, Figure 9).

We have followed these patients over the ensuing two to three years and, although follow up is relatively brief, there have been 5 patients who experienced a cardiac arrest; two were resuscitated and three died. Of these, four had high grade (grade 3 or greater) VPBs detected during the initial period of 24-hour monitoring. In one patient, however, no VPBs whatsoever were detected on the initial study; two later periods of 24-hour

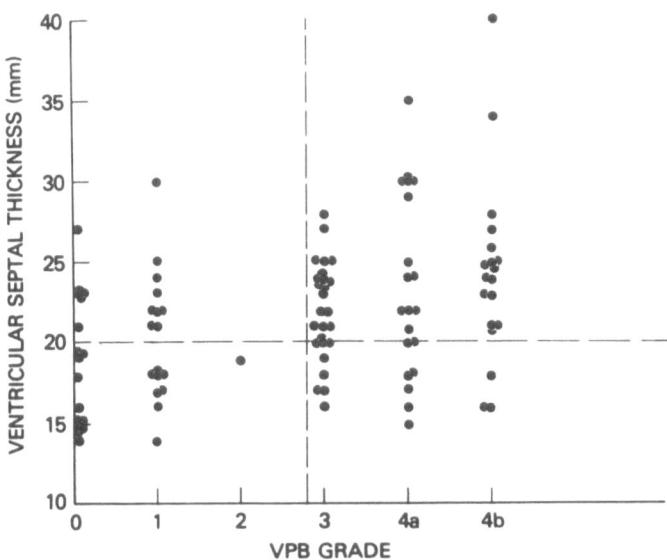

Figure 9. Ventricular premature beat (VPB) grade in relation to ventricular septal thickness. Reproduced with permission from American Heart Association (9).

monitoring disclosed only two VPBs during one period and one on a second – one of these VPBs was of the R on T type.

Exercise testing was not as sensitive as 24-hour ECG monitoring for detecting high grade ventricular arrhythmias in that we found that while 98 % of patients with high grade arrhythmias were detected by 24-hour ECG monitoring, only 73 % of the patients with VPBs were detected by exercise testing. Moreover, 57 % of patients who had high VPB grade ($\geq$ grade 3) on 24 hour monitoring had low grade or no VPBs on exercise testing. In contrast, all patients who had high VPB grade on exercise testing also had high VPB grade on 24-hour monitoring.

The above data demonstrate that ventricular arrhythmias occur frequently in all subgroups of patients with hypertrophic cardiomyopathy, and that these arrhythmias include an alarming percentage of high grade arrhythmias. Given this fact, and the association of high grade ventricular arrhythmia with sudden death in patients with coronary artery disease (13), it appears likely that 1) sudden death in many patients with hypertrophic cardiomyopathy is arrhythmic in origin and 2) patients in whom these arrhythmias are detected during life may comprise a subgroup at higher risk of sudden death than patients in whom no arrhythmia or low grade arrhythmia is detected.

While this appears to be a reasonable hypothesis, arrhythmia identification *per se* does not provide sufficient information to critically influence therapeutic decisions. The reason for this is that more than 50 % of each patient subgroup had multifocal VPBs, repetitive VPBs, or both on 24-hour ambulatory ECG monitoring (Figure 8). The identification of such a large group at risk imposes formidable practical problems for concentrating aggressive therapeutic efforts (pharmacological or surgical) on those few individuals who constitute an as yet unidentified subgroup of patients with arrhythmia at *greatest* risk of sudden death.

6. CIRCUMSTANCES OF SUDDEN DEATH

In combining the results of our three studies in which 40 patients died suddenly (4–6), approximately 35 % of such deaths occurred either during or shortly after moderate to severe exertion (Figure 10). This observation suggests that transient alterations of one or more critical factors, (including perhaps autonomic tone to the heart), in combination with a background of ventricular irritability, play an important role in evoking an environment conducive to development of a fatal ventricular arrhythmia.

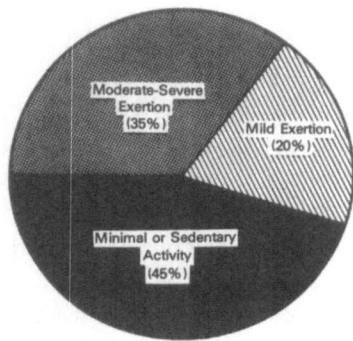

Figure 10. Activity level associated with sudden death (40 patients). Data obtained from three separate studies of patients with hypertrophic cardiomyopathy (4–6).

In summary, while sudden death in patients with hypertrophic cardiomyopathy is not common, it occurs frequently enough to be of great concern. Data are emerging that point to several areas of investigation that might help define the patient at greatest risk of sudden death. The finding that high grade ventricular arrhythmias are extremely common in patients with hypertrophic cardiomyopathy suggests that the major mechanism responsible for sudden death in such patients is ventricular fibrillation. However, since arrhythmias are so frequent, it is clear that other factors must co-exist to provide the proper electrophysiological environment for ventricular irritability to evolve into a terminal arrhythmia. On the basis of our data, some of these other factors would appear to be an excessively thick ventricular septum and a grossly abnormal baseline electrocardiogram. Genetic influences also are operative in that certain families are at particularly high risk of sudden death. However, the currently available data have not defined sensitive or specific enough predictors of sudden death to identify, with a high degree of reliability, which patients with arrhythmias, with a thick ventricular septum, and with an abnormal electrocardiogram, will die.

The observations outlined above partly define the background on which other, undoubtedly transient, factors interact to eventually precipitate a terminal arrhythmia in patients with hypertrophic cardiomyopathy. Identification of such transient aberrations leading to ventricular electrical instability may hold the key to detecting and more effectively treating those patients at high risk of sudden death.

REFERENCES

1. Hardarson T, De La Calzada CS, Curiel R, Goodwin JF: Prognosis and mortality of hypertrophic obstructive cardiomyopathy. Lancet 2:1462–1467, 1973.
2. Shah PM, Adelman AG, Wigle ED, Gobel FL, Burchell HB, Hardarson T, Curiel R, De La Calzada Cs, Oakley CM, Goodwin JF: The natural (and unnatural) course of hypertrophic obstructive cardiomyopathy. A multicenter study. Circ Res 24 and 35 (suppl II):II–179–195, 1973.
3. Epstein SE, Henry WL, Clark CE, Roberts WC, Maron BJ, Ferrans VJ, Redwood DR, Morrow AG: Asymmetric septal hypertrophy. Ann Intern Med 81:650–680, 1974.
4. Maron BJ, Henry WL, Clark CE, Redwood DR, Roberts WC, Epstein SE: Asymmetric septal hypertrophy in childhood. Circulation 53:9–19, 1976.   −
5. Maron BJ, Lipson LC, Roberts WC, Savage DS, Epstein SE: "Malignant" hypertrophic cardiomyopathy: identification of a subgroup of families with unusually frequent premature death. Amer J Cardiol 41:1133–1140, 1978.
6. Maron BJ, Roberts WC, Edwards JE, Mc Allister HA, Foley DD, Epstein SE: Sudden death in patients with hypertrophic cardiomyopathy: characterization of 26 patients without functional limitation. Amer J Cardiol 41:803–810, 1978.
7. Maron BJ, Merrill WH, Freier PA, Kent KM, Epstein SE and Morrow AG: Long-term clinical course and symptomatic status of patients after operation for hypertrophic subaortic stenosis. Circulation 57:1205–1213, 1978.
8. Savage DD, Seides SF, Clark CE, Henry WL, Maron BJ, Robinson FC, Epstein SE: Electrocardiographic findings in patients with obstructive and nonobstructive hypertrophic cardiomyopathy. Circulation 58:402–408, 1978.
9. Savage DE, Seides SF. Maron BJ, Myers DJ, Epstein SE: Prevalence of arrhythmias during 24-hour electrocardiographic monitoring and exercise testing in patients·with obstructive and nonobstructive hypertrophic cardiomyopathy (ASH). Circulation 59:866–875, 1979.
10. Ingham RE, Rossen RM, Goodman DJ, Harrison DC: Ambulatory electrocardiographic monitoring in idiopathic hypertrophic subaortic stenosis. Circulation 52 (suppl II):11–93, (abstract) 1975.
11. Lever HM, Shah PM, Reeves NC, Nanda NC: The relation of left ventricular outflow obstruction to ventricular arrhythmias in hypertrophic subaortic stenosis. Circulation 54 (suppl II):II–105, (abstract) 1976.
12. Ryan M, Lown B, Horn H: Ventricular ectopic activity in patients with coronary heart disease. N Engl J Med 292:224–229, 1975.
13. Ruberman W, Weinblatt E, Goldberg JD, Frank CW, Shapiro S: Ventricular premature beats and mortality after myocardial infarction. N Engl J Med 297:750–758, 1977.

5.2. THE LONG QT SYNDROME

P.J. SCHWARTZ

1. INTRODUCTION

The still inadequate but increasing awareness of the existence of the idiopathic long QT syndrome (LQTS) has provided ample evidence that, as suggested by many, this disease is far from being rare. This notion, coupled with the unusual pathophysiological characteristics and with the high degree of lethality in untreated patients, explains why the LQTS has a rather unique position in the more general problem of sudden death. In fact it seems to provide a mechanistic link between neural and cardiac factors in the genesis of sudden death and represents the most provocative example of neurally mediated, noncoronary sudden cardiac death.

The clinical manifestations of the LQTS have been described in detail in the many case reports published and will be simply outlined here with the addition however of some new concepts which may lead to a more comprehensive definition and to a broadening of the accepted spectrum of the disease. The main objectives of this brief review are in fact an analysis of what is currently known of the pathogenetic mechanisms and a critical evaluation of the bases for a rational management and therapy of the patients affected by the long QT syndrome.

2. HISTORICAL NOTE

The first written report on the long QT syndrome is probably dated 1856 when Meissner (1) described the case of a deaf-mute girl who collapsed and died while being publicly admonished for a misdemeanor by the director of the Leipzig Institute for the deaf. When her parents were informed they showed no surprise because two of their children had already died suddenly, one after a terrible fright and the second after a violent fit of rage.

Case-reports are often disregarded as anecdotal or repetitive of similar findings and generally thought to be of limited interest and significance. The rather satisfactory amount of knowledge recently accumulated on the LQTS would not be available, however, without the first thorough description of the disease made in 1957 by Professor Anton Jervell and his associate Dr. Fred Lange-Nielsen (2). There are not many instances in medical history of a single case report so critical for the development of the subsequent knowledge on a given disease.

In their original paper Jervell and Lange-Nielsen described four affected siblings in an otherwise healthy family. The four children were deaf-mute and had many fainting attacks induced by exercise or emotions, their only evident abnormality was a marked prolongation of the QT interval and three of them died suddenly while playing at the age of 4, 5 and 9 years. This was immediately followed in 1958 by Levine and Woodworth's description of a similar case observed in 1949 but not published until that time because "it was hoped that a similar combination of clinical findings might be met with before these extraordinary features were regarded as more than coincidental" (3). This sentence reflects well the hesitations of many physicians who eventually bury their unusual cases in a secret drawer of their desk and may explain at least in part, the "epidemic" of LQTS cases which has followed the first observations.

Another critical event was the observation by Ward in 1964 (4) of a family similar to the one described by Jervell in which, however, the hearing was normal. When an Annotation of the Lancet commented (5) on Ward's paper a hasty letter was sent by Romano (6) indicating that a similar syndrome had been observed and published the year before (7) by himself and his colleagues. Romano's paper was important also because it showed that the syncopal episodes in his 3 months old patient were due to ventricular fibrillation and because two siblings of this patient died suddenly at 44 days and at 4 months of life. The latter point is relevant to the Sudden Infant Death Syndrome that will be discussed later.

All these papers had the merit to begin the dissemination of the notion that the association between syncopal episodes and prolongation of QT interval could be causal instead of coincidental and to stimulate the description of other cases thus initiating a classic positive feed-back reaction. Data are now available on over 500 patients and it has to be noted that at this point single case reports are not written any more because most scientific journals would not publish them unless they are accompanied by some unusual feature.

3. CLINICAL ASPECTS

3.1.

There are two cardinal clinical manifestations of the syndrome: the syncopal episodes and the electrocardiographic abnormalities.

The syncopal attacks have been carefully described in the excellent paper by Fraser, Froggatt and James (8) and are usually divided into those with and those without unconsciousness. The nature of the attacks, not defined in the first reports, has been subsequently demonstrated by many authors to be ventricular fibrillation, often of the type called "torsade de pointes" (Figure 1). A few instances of asystole have also been described but, as it is the case for the sudden death of patients with ischemic heart disease (9), there is no doubt that the prevailing mechanism is ventricular fibrillation. Two points are of paramount importance in this regard: a) the syncopal attacks are almost always triggered by conditions associated with sudden increases in sympathetic activity such as violent emotions (fright or anger) or physical activity (swimming seems to be involved more often than

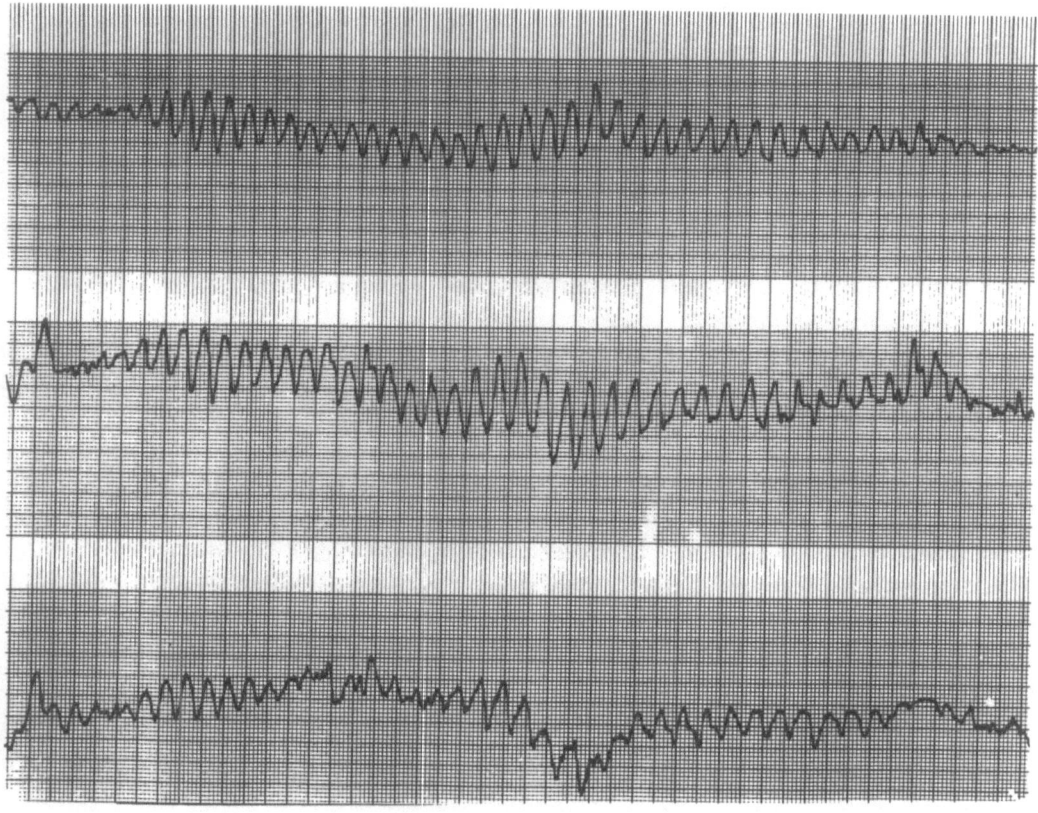

Figure 1. C.C. 6 years. Simultaneous recording in leads 1, 2 and 3 of an episode of ventricular fibrillation of the "torsades de pointe" type which occurred during an exercise stress test on a treadmill. The patient was unconscious and had convulsions. Sinus rhythm was restored by thumpversion. This patient underwent left stellectomy in 1975 and has remained free from syncopal attacks until the spring of 1979.

expected). Attacks have also been reported during sleep and in the transitional state between sleep and wakefulness. These facts are relevant to the understanding of pathophysiological mechanisms responsible for the manifestation of this disease; b) the episodes of ventricular fibrillation, if one considers the "torsades de pointe" as a type of ventricular fibrillation, are very often self-terminating (Figure 2) and it is not uncommon for a single patient, independently from his/her outcome, to have a very large number of syncopal attacks. It is indeed uncommon for these patients to die at the first attack, although this has been reported in a certain number of cases. This point is important for what concerns the management of asymptomatic patients.

There are two classic electrocardiographic abnormalities, a third is proposed here. a) A prolongation of QT interval is, appropriately, the marker of the long QT syndrome. It is idiopathic in contrast to the prolongation of QT interval which is secondary to drugs, electrolyte imbalance or other factors (10) and characterizes the acquired form of long QT syndrome which has a completely different pathogenesis and requires quite a different

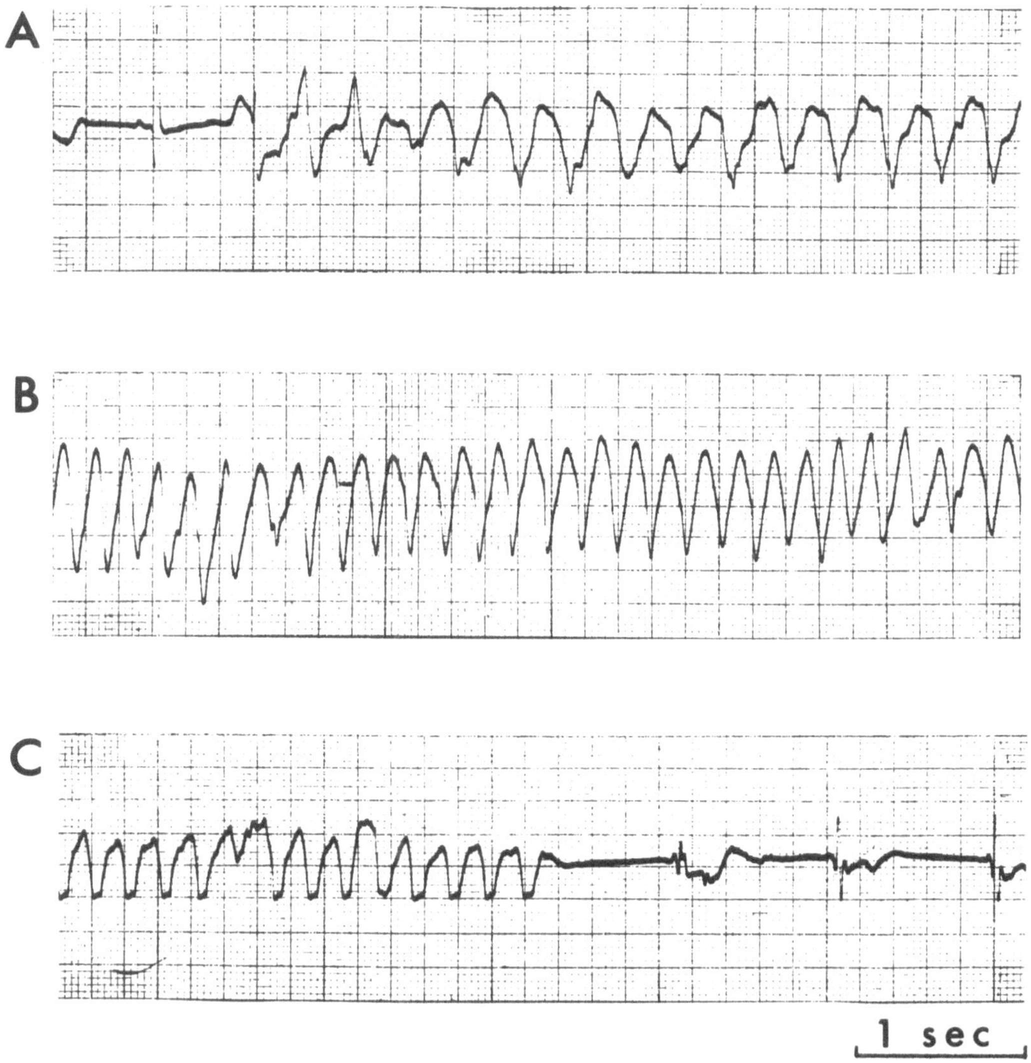

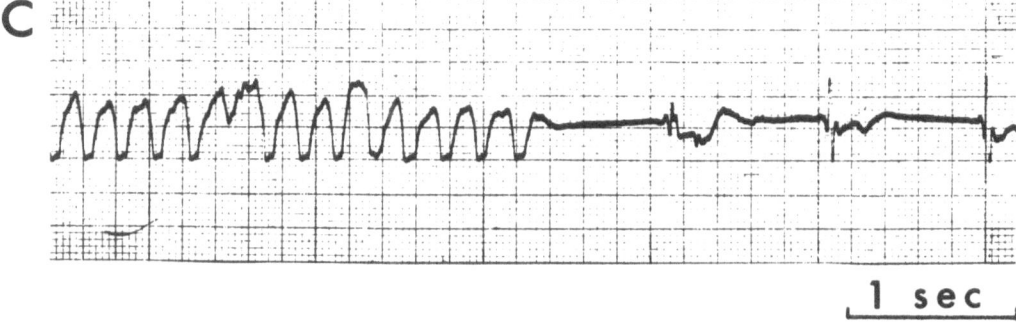

Figure 2. R.C. 5 years. The three tracings show the beginning, the intermediate phase and the spontaneous termination of an episode of "torsades de pointe" which lasted 47 seconds. This patient underwent left stellectomy in 1978 and has remained free from syncopal attacks until the spring of 1979.

treatment. The prolongation of QT interval is usually marked. Exercise often further lengthens the QT interval which also shows an unusual variability from day to day although it remains almost always in the abnormal range. The lengthening of QT interval is usually due to a large, often bizarre, T wave which is often notched, as in many cases of cerebrovascular accidents (11). The possibility of a fusion with a U wave has never been clearly discounted. b) Alternation of the T wave, in polarity or in amplitude, may be present at rest for short periods but most commonly becomes manifest during emotional or physical

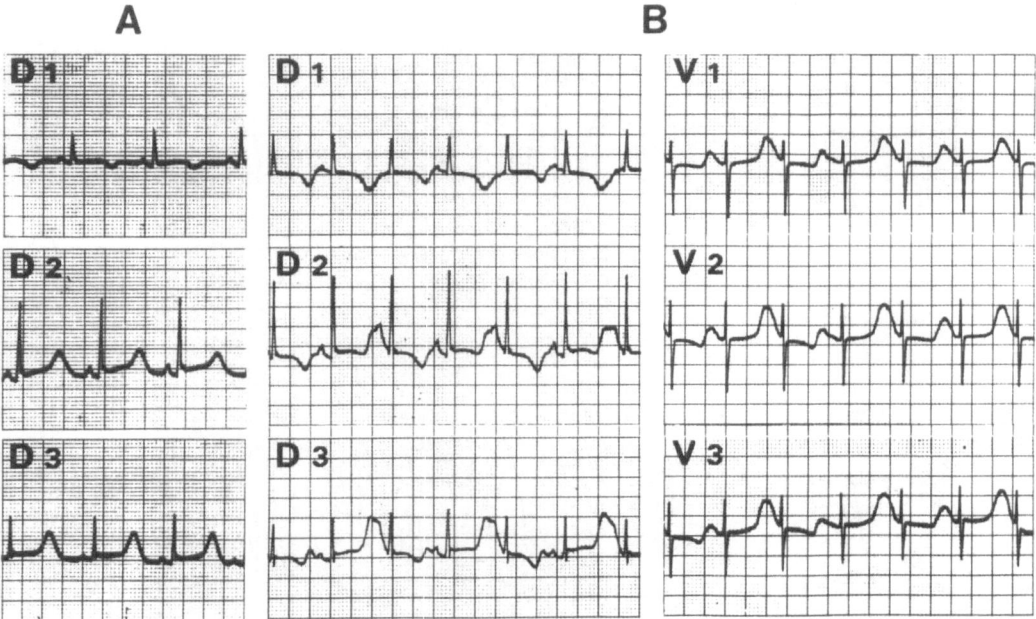

Figure 3. A.B. 9 years. In A tracing at rest showing prolongation of QT interval, QTc = 610 msec (upper limit of normal values = 440 msec). In B the two panels with simultaneous recordings after spontaneous fright show alternation of the T wave. This patient underwent left stellectomy in 1973 and has remained free from syncopal attacks until spring of 1979.

stresses (Figure 3). Schwartz and Malliani in 1975 (12) reproduced alternation of the T wave in cats by electrical stimulation of the left stellate ganglion (Figure 4) and found evidence for its occurrence in a relatively high number of LQTS patients described in the literature compared to its extreme rarity in other conditions. They suggested on the basis of clinical as well as of pathophysiological considerations, which will be discussed later, that the alternation of the T wave in LQTS patients was dependent upon the same pathogenetic mechanism responsible for the lengthening of QT interval and that its characteristic appearance under conditions of stress should be considered a specific and additional sign of the long QT syndrome. This view has been supported by the continuously growing number of LQTS patients in whom alternation of the T wave has been observed and documented (most impressive in this regard is the observation made by Froggatt and Adgey (13) of alternation of the T wave in a four-day-old baby affected by the long QT syndrome who died two years later) and has been definitively confirmed by the careful study by Crampton described in the next section. c) In some of the LQTS patients it is possible to observe during a normal sinus rhythm the sudden appearance of a long pause, greater than 1.2 seconds followed by the immediate return to the previous rhythm (Figure 5). These pauses are isolated and have no relationship with the physiological or even with an exaggerated sinus arrhythmia. It is suggested that they may represent another sign of the basic defect underlying this syndrome and that their presence may contribute to the

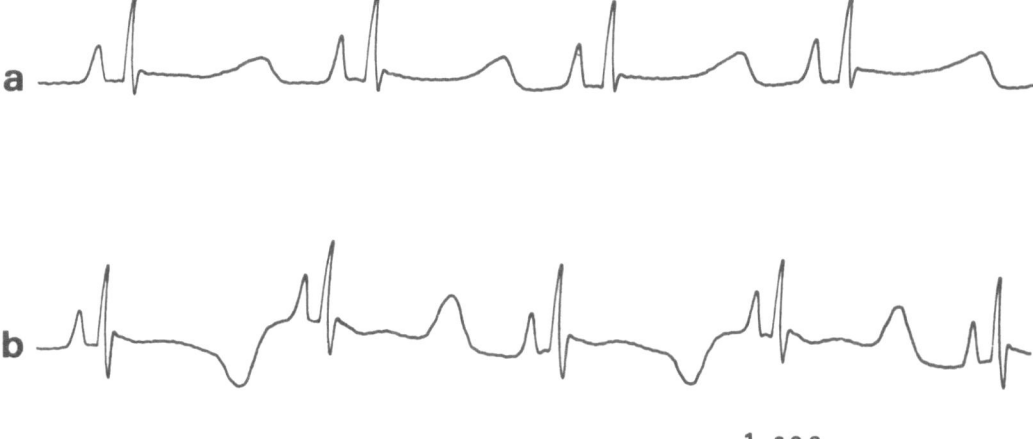

Figure 4. Anesthetized cat: ECG (D2). A, Control; B, 5 sec after the cessation of a 30 sec electrical stimulation of both stellate ganglia; (left ganglion: 20V, 2 msec, and 20 Hz; right ganglion: 10V, 2 msec, and 20 Hz). Alternation in polarity of the T-wave is evident (From (12).)

diagnosis in dubious cases. It is fair to add that for the time being this suggestion is more a personal opinion than an established fact.

3.2.

A striking aspect of the LQTS is represented by the extreme similarities of the clinical manifestations in the affected patients. The clinical history of repeated episodes of loss of consciousness under emotional or physical stress is so stereotyped and unique to be almost unmistakable. It has therefore been with increasing surprise and disbelief that in patients referred because of a history typical for the LQTS I found a normal QT interval. In some out of these cases the ECG came to my observation only after the tragic conclusion by sudden death of a long history of syncopal episodes usually triggered by psychologic stress often interpreted as of hysteric origin. I then began, in the last two months, to wonder if it could have been possible that also these patients were affected by the LQTS without, however, showing a prolongation of the QT interval in their ECG. This possibility will now be examined and discussed.

Two points, one clinical and one theoretical, which have been available for several years may support this concept. 1) The diagnosis of the LQTS has already been made in a few patients with a typical clinical history but with a normal QT at rest – in whom, however, marked prolongation of the QT interval was noted preceding the attacks (14) or during exercise (15). Notable in this regard is the patient described by Wellens whose ventricular fibrillation episodes were induced by auditory stimuli and were preceded by lengthening of the QT interval (14). Without the careful investigation which disclosed, under special circumstances, the QT prolongation these patients would not have been properly diagnosed and therefore would have not received the proper treatment. 2) As

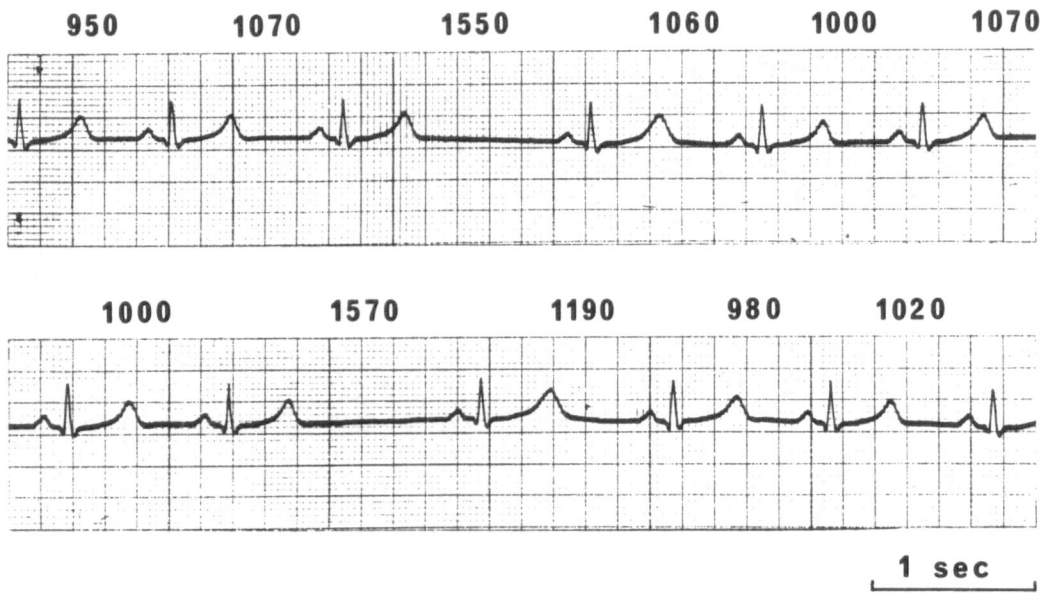

Figure 5. M.C.B. 50 years. Continuous tracing. Two sudden pauses in sinus rhythm are evident. QTc = 500 msec.

will be discussed later, the generally accepted interpretation for the prolongation of the QT interval stems from the studies by Abildskov and his associates and involves abnormalities in cardiac sympathetic innervation, the "cancellation" theory and the existence of areas of overlapping innervation (16, 17, 18). On this basis one could have already postulated the existence of cases in which the anatomical location of the hypothetical abnormality of the cardiac sympathetic nerves might have been such as to produce no changes of the QT interval in the surface electrocardiogram.

A few additional observations, probably of lesser scientific weight, will now be presented. a) Initially, as discussed above, the only patients diagnosed as affected by the LQTS were those in whom clinical history, QT prolongation, deaf-mutism and familial involvement were all present to fulfill the criteria for the diagnosis of an exceedingly rare disease. With time and more reports published it became clear that the LQTS could fully manifest itself without deaf-mutism and even without any evidence for familiar or hereditary components. The increased medical knowledge on the LQTS and the greater confidence by the physicians involved with these patients made the diagnostic criteria less stringent. b) Two families have been reported (19, 20) in which a high incidence of sudden deaths was associated with emotional stresses and in which the available ECGs apparently showed a normal QT interval. In one of these families a short PR interval and a prominent U wave were noted. The clinical history of these families does not differ from those of families with the LQTS. c) Although laboratory tests often represent useful contributions a careful analysis of the clinical history is, for the experienced physician, less misleading and generally sufficient for the proper diagnosis. When a patient with typical effort angina tells in his own precise and unforgettable words, how and when he develops that anguish called cardiac pain and how he gets relief, who would refute the diagnosis of angina pectoris because of a negative ECG? So I begin to believe that there are some patients, affected by the LQTS, who may present with an entirely normal QT interval and who should not, because of their seemingly normal ECG, be dismissed with other diagnoses and be deprived of a proper treatment which may save their lives. A possible diagnostic help may come from the important observation made by Gavrilescu and Luca (21) who found a marked prolongation of right ventricular monophasic action potentials in two patients with the LQTS. In patients suspected as affected by the LQTS and with a normal QT in the surface ECG it may be that study of the monophasic action potentials could reveal abnormalities not evident in the surface ECG because of the high degree of cancellation of repolarization (17).

Thus I am proposing, on almost purely speculative grounds and without any solid evidence, that the spectrum of the long QT syndrome may be larger than thought until now and may – or should – include those patients who have a typical clinical history of the LQTS without a long QT interval and in whom other diagnoses have been excluded. It would be extremely useful if physicians would report on such cases; we may find that they are not so uncommon.

More comprehensive clinical information on the LQTS may be found in two extensive reviews (22, 23) and in a recent editorial (10).

4. PATHOGENETIC MECHANISMS

Initially the basic defect underlying the LQTS was thought to be some unidentified abnormality in myocardial metabolism or abnormalities in the sinus node artery (8). The latter possibility was not confirmed by subsequent studies and the former does not have a single decisive point in its favour; however, as it will be seen, it is still viable.

A considerable amount of data, provided by clinical observations and by experimental studies, strongly implicates abnormalities in cardiac sympathetic innervation as responsible for the clinical picture of the LQTS. The elements in favour of this concept as well as the opposing arguments will now be examined.

The notion that the syncopal and often fatal episodes are almost always associated with sudden increases in sympathetic activity, as produced by vigorous physical activity or by emotional stresses such as fear or anger, has indicated since the beginning that a critical step is indeed represented by a sympathetic discharge.

The second essential point was to find a unitarian interpretation for the bizarre ECG changes. The single most important finding is undoubtedly provided by the experiments by Abildskov's group which showed that asymmetrical manipulation of cardiac sympathetic nerves may affect the QT interval (16). More precisely, they found that prolongation of the QT interval may be obtained by a right stellectomy or by stimulation of the left stellate ganglion; both these manoeuvres obviously result in a sympathetic imbalance with left dominance. The interpretation offered for the QT lengthening induced by left stellate stimulation was that the shortening in action potential duration in some areas of the heart was unmasking repolarization wavefronts which were previously self cancelling (17).

When Schwartz and Malliani (12) made the clinical observation that LQTS patients had frequent episodes of alternation of the T wave under the same circumstances which would provoke the syncopal episodes, it was logical to hypothesize that if the prolongation of QT interval and the T wave alternans have, in these patients, the same origin it should be possible to reproduce experimentally the alternation of the T wave by manipulating the cardiac sympathetic nerves in the same manner which was known to lenghten the QT interval. This was indeed what happened (12) by either stimulating the left stellate ganglion alone or by stimulating both stellate ganglia but with a greater intensity applied to the left (Figure 4). These experiments suggested that the LQTS patients have a congenital imbalance between right and left cardiac sympathetic innervation with a left dominance, resulting in a prolongation of QT interval at rest and in episodes of T wave alternations when sympathetic activity is increased.

An imbalance with left dominance may of course depend upon a primary increase in left activity or upon a primary reduction in right activity. The sympathetic control of heart rate is almost exclusively exerted through the right sided nerves (24); this notion coupled with the observation that most LQTS patients have an unusually low heart rate and that many of them have an impaired or even absent rate response to exercise led Schwartz et al. (23) to suggest that a lower-than-normal right cardiac sympathetic activity might be the basic defect for the LQTS. At which level – brain, sympathetic chain including the stellate ganglia or the adrenergic terminals in the myocardium – this defect would operate, could not, and cannot, be specified. Although it was immediately stated that this possibility did not need to fully apply to all LQTS cases the concept of an imbalance between right and left components of the cardiac sympathetic innervation became a useful working hypothesis which has led to a number of experimental investigations that have provided results relevant to the LQTS.

The major obstacle to the hypothesis proposed in 1975 (23) was represented by the difficulty in conceiving how a lower-than-normal right sympathetic activity could favour arrhythmias and sudden death. The available data on cardiac denervation indicated that arrhythmias were actually prevented by bilateral stellectomy (25). No one had looked at the effects of unilateral stellectomy but the only expected effect was just a somewhat less complete result than that produced by bilateral stellectomy. It was therefore a major surprise when it was found that right stellate ganglion blockade increased the incidence of ventricular arrhythmias and of ventricular fibrillation associated with short lasting coronary artery occlusion while left stellate ganglion blockade had an opposite, protective effect (26). The use of a reversible blockade by cold suggested immediately that it was not an experimental artifact but the results were odd and required confirmation. When the effects of unilateral stellectomy on the vulnerability to fibrillation were examined the same striking differences were found: while left stellectomy produced a major increase in the ventricular fibrillation threshold, right stellectomy greatly decreased it and, thus, increased the vulnerability to fibrillation (27). These findings seemed immediately relevant to the LQTS. If, as proposed, the patients with the LQTS have indeed a lower-than-normal right cardiac sympathetic activity they would probably also have a lower-than-normal threshold for ventricular fibrillation and it would become understandable why they so easily develop ventricular fibrillation. On the other hand the protective effect of left stellectomy had glaring therapeutical implications.

It remained completely obscure however by which mechanism the absence of part of the sympathetic innervation could have an arrhythmogenic effect. A collaborative effort with Verrier and Lown (28) offered a possible key for a correct interpretation. Studying the effects of unilateral stellectomy on ventricular refractoriness it was found that the paradoxical effects of right stellectomy were dependent upon an intact left stellate ganglion. It was then hypothesized that unilateral stellectomy, through a baroreceptive reflex, would increase the sympathetic activity through the contralateral ganglion. Since the left stellate ganglion is quantitatively dominant (28, 29, 30) this fact would have arrhythmogenic effects in the case of right stellectomy and antiarrhythmic effects in the case of left stellectomy. This possibility has been substantiated by data by Mc Call and associates (31) indicating that stellectomy interrupts nerve fibres which have an inhibitory effect on the contra-lateral sympathetic activity and has been further discussed recently (32).

However, the relevance of these data to the LQTS was limited by the fact that they were obtained under artificial conditions in anesthetized animals. The arrhythmogenic effect of right stellectomy was therefore evaluated under the same conditions which trigger the syncopal episodes in LQTS patients. In the first group of experiments, dogs were studied during exercise on a treadmill before and after right, left or bilateral stellectomy (32). The incidence of ventricular arrhythmias during exercise was low in the control dogs (8 %) and in the dogs with left stellectomy (11 %) but increased sharply in those with right stellectomy (86 %); dogs with bilateral stellectomy showed no arrhythmias. A similar study was performed in patients affected by Raynaud's disease who underwent stellectomy as treat-ment (33). It has to be noted that in man stellectomy produces only a partial unilateral denervation as will be discussed in the therapy section, and therefore the results would underestimate the real effects of unilateral denervation. However, these findings con-firmed those obtained in dogs: ventricular arrhythmias during exercise appeared in 3 % of healthy controls, in 5 % of patients with left stellectomy and increased to 21 % in 35 patients with right stellectomy; patients with bilateral stellectomy did not show ventric-ular arrhythmias. These two investigations, performed under natural conditions, confirm and stress the arrhythmogenic effect of the absence or incompleteness of right cardiac sympathetic innervation.

The last step in this direction is represented by the study of the effect of right stellectomy when a cat is suddenly confronted with a psychological stress (29, 34). In control conditions, cats react with a sinus tachycardia or in some instances, a sinus bradycardia; after right stellectomy, not only – as expected – the QT lengthens but also arrhythmias are induced by stress. The most frequent response is A-V nodal tachycardia but runs of ventricular tachycardia have also been observed (Figure 6). The induction of life-threatening ventric-ular arrhythmias during emotional stress in conscious cats with an intact heart whose only abnormality is the absence of the right stellate ganglion is a step towards the experimental reproduction of the LQTS. In the same study another observation was made: after right stellectomy many cats not only have a reduction in heart rate but also develop sudden long pauses during sinus rhythm (Figure 7). The similarity with the long pauses ofter.

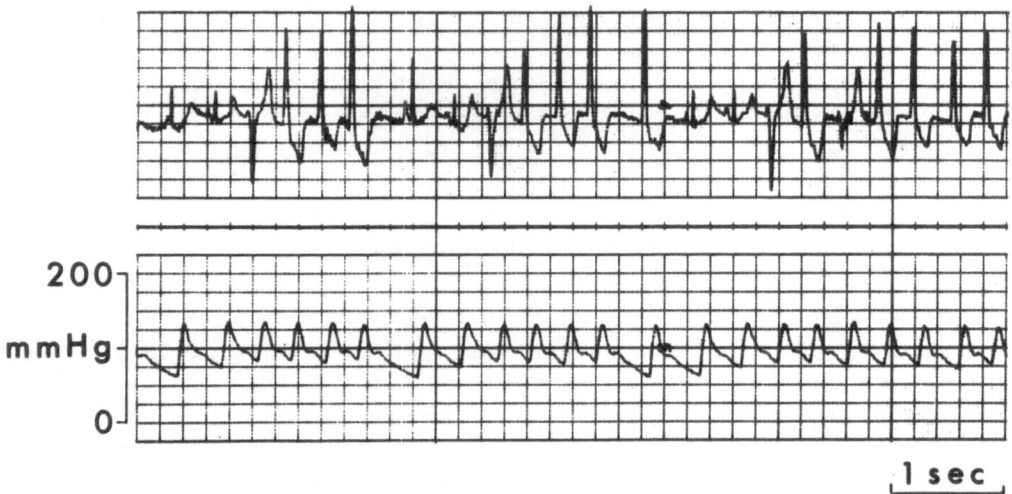

Figure 6. Conscious cat under psychological stress one week after right stellectomy. Simultaneous recording of ECG and aortic blood pressure. Several premature ventricular beats and runs of ventricular tachycardia. The noise in the ECG tracing is due to the animal movements.

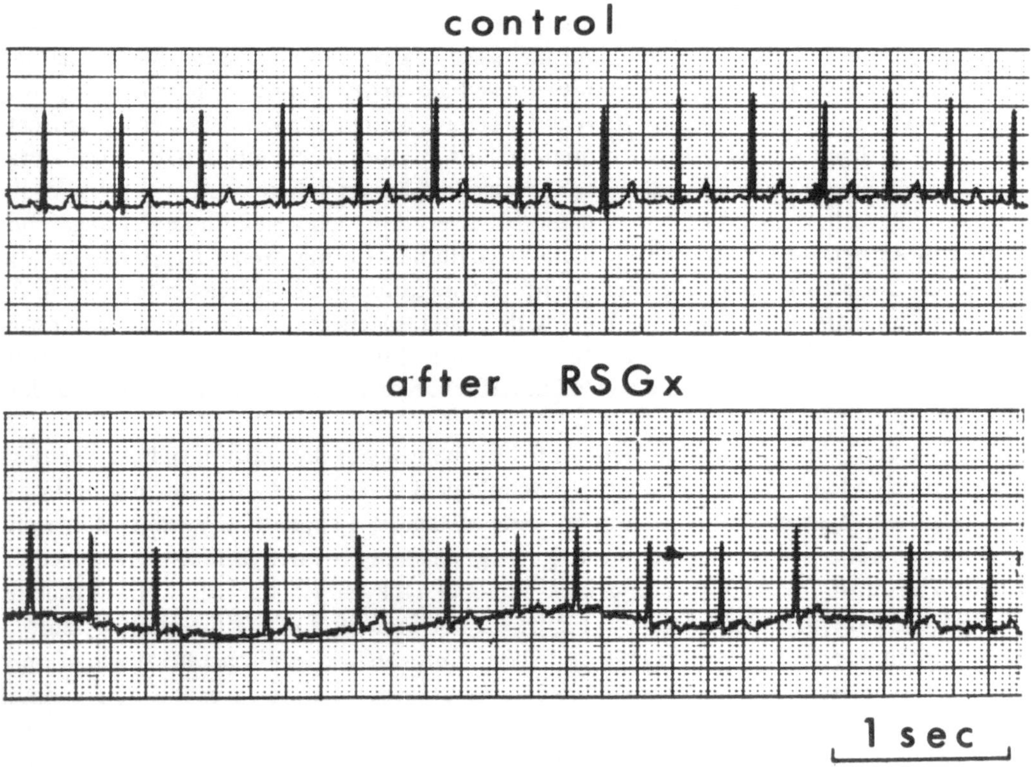

control

after RSGx

Figure 7. Conscious cat before and after right stellectomy at rest. After right stellectomy sudden long sinus pauses become evident.

observed in patients with the LQTS (Figure 5) and which have been previously called attention to, is striking and fits very well with the hypothesis that these patients have some abnormalities in the neural control of the heart which involves right sided nerves. It is therefore suggested that the long pauses in LQTS patients may be not just a chance finding but that they may actually represent another piece of the complex mosaic of this syndrome providing further information on the underlying mechanisms.

The bulk of these experimental studies has thus suggested that at the basis of the long QT syndrome there may be a congenital imbalance in the cardiac sympathetic innervation characterized by a lower-than-normal right sympathetic activity resulting in an increased activity through the left sided sympathetic nerves, which have been recently proved to be quite arrhythmogenic (26, 27, 28, 29, 30, 32, 33, 34, 35, 36, 37). We will now examine if the clinical evidence supports or discounts this possibility.

The data relative to the heart rate of LQTS patients have already been discussed. Moss and McDonald observed in a patient with the LQTS that blockade of the right stellate ganglion not only further prolonged the QT interval, but also induced alternation of the T wave (38). Almost definitive evidence comes from the very recent and thorough study by Crampton (39); he found that blockade of the right stellate ganglion and stimulation of the left in patients with the LQTS could induce T wave alternans. In the same study it was found that blockade of the left stellate ganglion was effective in interrupting T wave alternans and ventricular tachycardia and in reducing ventricular arrhythmias, thus extending a previous observation (40). This paper confirms, in a most impressive way, the data obtained in experimental animals and provides almost definitive evidence on the fact that asymmetrical sympathetic tone with left dominance exists in the LQTS.

Another impressive observation was made by Coyer et al., who induced runs of ventricular tachycardia by simply touching the left stellate ganglion in a LQTS patient, before proceeding with left stellectomy (41).

A most important finding has been reported by James et al. (42) on the neuropathology of the heart in 8 victims of the LQTS. The most important abnormality was focal neuritis and neural degeneration within the sinus node, A-V node, His bundle and ventricular myocardium. Although the etiology of these intracardiac lesions remain obscure they may – if confirmed – represent the site of the previously postulated defect in cardiac sympathetic innervation and represent a very important point in support of the hypothesis advanced in 1975 by Schwartz et al. (23). If, for instance, this degenerative process would affect more adrenergic terminals connected to right sided nerves than to left sided nerves we would have the pathologic counterpart of the functional defect hitherto postulated. It is important to note that in this study vagal as well as sympathetic nerves seemed to be involved. This finding may contribute to a better understanding of the unusual heart rate responses of these patients and also fits very nicely with the suggestion, made in this review, that abnormally long sinus pauses may in the LQTS have a specific origin related to the pathophysiology of the disease itself.

In an interesting and worth to be repeated study Curtiss et al. (43) using various autonomic manoeuvres concluded suggesting an intrinsic cardiac abnormality not better defined, but did not exclude a significant extrinsic autonomic defect. If this "intrinsic cardiac abnormality" depends on malfunction of some neural elements their conclusion would not be in contrast with the "sympathetic imbalance" hypothesis (23) nor with the finding by James et al. (41). For the time being, however, their conclusions are limited by being based on only two patients affected by the LQTS who had a quite different age, 20 and 68 years, which is a well-known factor in modifying cardiac reflexes and heart rate responses.

Thus, examining the available clinical and experimental data there seems to be overwhelming evidence in favour of a congenital imbalance in the cardiac sympathetic innervation with a left dominance likely to be secondary to a lower-than-normal right sympathetic activity. However, to a more careful analysis, the interpretation of the data may be less univocal. First of all, although the animal experiments prove that the sympathetic imbalance created by right stellectomy has a high arrhythmogenic potential – which represents a new and pathophysiologically important concept – this by no means constitutes evidence that the long QT syndrome is caused by it. As a matter of fact the recent demonstration of the arrhythmogenic role of left sided cardiac sympathetic nerves (26, 27, 28, 29, 30, 32, 33, 34, 35, 36, 37) leaves completely open the possibility that the basic defect in the LQTS is an unknown intracardiac abnormality which decreases electrical stability and sensitizes the myocardium to sympathetic discharges. Should this be the case the sympathetic nervous system, acting mostly through the dominant left stellate ganglion, would simply represent the trigger for the ventricular tachyarrhythmias which lead the LQTS patients to death. Most clinical observations, including the reports of Crampton (39) and Coyers et al. (41) might be explained on this basis. The greatest weight in supporting the "sympathetic imbalance" theory seems to still come from the fact that the characteristic ECG changes are so impressively mimicked by interrupting right cardiac sympathetic activity.

In conclusion, experimental and clinical evidence does not exclude the possibility of an unknown intracardiac abnormality which, when coupled with a sudden increase in sympathetic activity, would result in ventricular fibrillation. Nonetheless it is fair to say that for the time being the pathogenetic hypothesis which fits with all known facts and which is discounted by none remains the one proposed years ago (23): namely, a congenital imbalance between right and left cardiac sympathetic nerves – with the defect located either intra or extra cardiac – probably or often dependent upon a primary underactivity of right nerves resulting in a hyperactivity of left sympathetic nerves; this imbalance would set the stage for electrical instability of the heart which may be precipitated into ventricular fibrillation by a further and sudden increase in sympathetic activity mostly mediated through the left nerves.

5. THERAPY

Therapeutical interventions merely reflect the degree of understanding of the pathogenesis of a given disease. The initial confusion regarding the long QT syndrome has resulted in a variety of generally ineffective treatments. The previous analysis of the pathophysiological mechanisms clearly indicates that the syncopal attacks in these patients depend upon sympathetic discharges mostly mediated through the left sided cardiac nerves. It is then just an act of simple logic to expect favourable results by either annulling the effects of sympathetic discharges or preventing them from reaching the heart. Thus the two rational measures are either beta-adrenergic blocking agents or left sympathectomy. Medical history has however, plenty of rational treatments which proved to be completely unsuccessful. The evaluation of the efficacy of any therapy of an uncommon disease represents a difficult task, as already discussed (23) and certainly cannot be dealt with by using "personal experience" or published reports of single cases which almost always lack a sufficient follow-up. Only information, relative to the therapy used and to the outcome of the patients, gathered on a large number of cases and regularly updated, may provide valid and reliable information. An earlier survey of this kind, mostly based on personal contacts with physicians around the world, provided in 1975 data on 203 patients (23). The kindness and great sense of cooperation of these and other physicians have now allowed a new analysis based on 539 patients. The main data are exposed in Table 1. This table, similar to the previous one (23), still has the many limitations and shortcomings listed and discussed in the 1975 review (23). Only a major one, related to the mortality figures, will be discussed here. These figures may have only an indicative value because the necessary data on the time of exposure (time from the first syncopal attack or time from the beginning of a given therapy) is not yet known in enough cases; therefore caution is necessary in the interpretation of these data. An important point, however, which strongly suggests that the mortality figures are close to reality is represented by the fact that increasing the number of patients from 203 to 539 and increasing the follow-up has practically no effect on the percentages of mortality. Four considerations, at least, should be made in analyzing the data exposed in Table 1.

Table 1. Treatment and mortality in the long Q-T syndrome.

	Total	Outcome unknown	Deaths	Mortality
Asymptomatics	163	–	–	–
Treatment unknown	87	78	9	–
No treatment	107	13	73	78%
Miscellaneous treatment	29	8	11	52%
Beta-blockers	133	–	8	6%
Left sympathectomy	20	–	–	–
Total LQTS patients	539			

1) A large number of patients have been identified by having a prolonged QT interval and by being family members of affected individuals. The natural history of these persons is not yet clear; we certainly know that some of them will eventually begin to have syncopal episodes but we do not know in how many cases this will happen. Until harder data are available (see the Section on Perspectives) there are considerations which suggest a conservative attitude and my personal policy, at this time, is not to treat these patients but to follow them carefully for the possibility of a first syncopal episode. Treatment would in fact imply a terrible psychological burden for many persons who would otherwise lead a

completely normal life. Should a first syncopal attack occur, the patient would be under control and the proper therapy could be immediately instituted. This leaves out, however, those patients who die at the first attack; once more we need more data to know how frequently this happens; the majority of patients have in fact several episodes and sudden death at first attack seems rare. An exercise stress test may be useful in these patients. If important ventricular arrhythmias appear, this may justify a preventive treatment; if nothing happens, the patient is more likely to approach his life normally without the tremendous psychological constraints which often burden young siblings of LQTS patients.

2) The number of patients treated with drugs different from beta-blockers is small. This is largely due to the fact that these miscellaneous treatments are generally ineffective so that patients either die or continue having syncopal episodes and are eventually treated with beta-blockers. For this reason the mortality of this group is probably underestimated. A less gross data collection will certainly enable us to more precisely define the relationships between various drugs and number of syncopal attacks.

3) The mortality among the patients treated with beta-blockers has remained the same (6 %) with 4 more years of follow-up and 133 patients compared to 79; this suggests that 6 % reflects rather well the mortality of this group. Most of these patients have been treated with propranolol.

4) The number of patients treated with left stellectomy is steadily increasing. The most important point to be carefully considered is that all these patients were completely refractory to beta-blockade, which indicates that they represented the most seriously affected patients. In fact, since the surgical decision is still made only after complete failure of beta-blockers – as indicated by continuation of syncopal episodes – it is quite likely that without surgery the mortality in the group treated with beta-blockers would have been higher. At present time, to the best of my knowledge, all these 20 patients are not only alive but free from syncopal attacks. A single episode of recurrence has occurred in 4 or 5 patients. The follow-up in this group is quite variable: a group of 6–7 patients has between 4–8 years of follow-up, while the rest has of course a shorter one. Therefore it is not yet felt possible to soundly assess mortality in this group. The results are, at this time, quite favourable and rewarding especially if one keeps in mind that these patients were those with the highest frequency of attacks and those who were conducting the more miserable life, being usually restrained from most social activities. These patients are now having a completely normal life and even if their final outcome is still unknown there is no doubt that their quality of life has dramatically changed. Several of these patients are still given a moderate amount of beta-blockers, for reasons which although more visceral than rational are still very understandable. The crucial point to be made in this regard is that the same or a much larger dose of beta-blockers was ineffective in preventing the syncopal attacks before surgery.

Stellectomy in animals produces an almost complete unilateral denervation. To achieve the same in man – because of anatomical differences – it is necessary to remove the first four to five thoracic ganglia leaving intact the upper part of the stellate ganglion and thus avoiding the Horner's syndrome. This surgery, which is performed extrapleurally, is simple and almost devoid of potentially dangerous complications. It would be technically more proper to refer to it as high left thoracic sympathectomy but here it will still be referred to as left stellectomy.

The first pioneering surgical intervention in the LQTS was performed in 1970 by Moss and McDonald (38). Going only on the basis of the experiments of Yanowitz et al. (16) they performed a pharmacological blockade of right and left stellate ganglions and found that the QT interval lengthened after right blockade and shortened after left stellate ganglion blockade. On this basis they proceeded with left stellectomy which was quite successful in eliminating the syncopal episodes; the patient is still alive and in good condition. The initial objective with left stellectomy was therefore a shortening of the QT interval which was thought to correct the defect (prolongation of the QT interval) and to be the mark of a successful intervention. The basis for this intervention was, however, not considered strong enough by many and when some pharmacological blockade of the left stellate ganglion failed to shorten the QT interval the surgical procedure was abandoned. The serious limitations of stellate ganglion blockade have already been widely discussed (23). When the sympathetic imbalance theory received further support (12) another left stellectomy was performed and was successful (12); however, shortening of the QT interval was still looked upon as the necessary sign of successful therapy. A turning point was provided by the finding that stellectomy had a direct protective effect on the ventricular vulnerability to fibrillation (27). This implied that the protective effect of left stellectomy was independent of the shortening of the QT interval. As a matter of fact, in at least half of the 20 patients who underwent left stellectomy the QT interval was practically unaffected and in all of them the syncopal attacks have practically been abolished.

At present time, it seems still rational to begin the treatment of these patients with beta-adrenergic blocking agents. If propranolol is used, a dose close to 3 mg/Kg will be necessary in most cases, keeping in mind that a full protective dosage should be very rapidly achieved. Should another syncopal episode occur after institution of a full-blocking dose of beta-blockers there should be no hesitation in proceeding with left stellectomy. Attempts with other drugs not certainly effective should be avoided because of the unacceptable price of failure. "With ventricular fibrillation the physician may not have the opportunity to remedy a therapeutic error" (44).

There are some negative aspects in the use of beta-blockers which should be kept in mind and which, in some cases, may suggest left stellectomy as a first choice treatment. a) Several instances of sudden death have occurred in LQTS patients within a few weeks from the interruption of therapy; this interruption is often due to the disappearance of syncopal attacks for a while and to the consequent wrong presumption of a cure or ill advice. b) Side effects such as fatigue, nightmares and impaired sexual function may – especially in young and active patients–lead to the dangerous interruption of therapy. c) Whilst life-long treatment is psychologically detrimental, left stellectomy is done once for ever. It has no negative side effects on cardiac performance (32, 33), and still leaves completely open the possibility of adding antiarrhythmic drugs, if necessary. Stellectomy interrupts also alpha-adrenergic mediated effects with beneficial results on coronary flow (45), and does not produce post-denervation supersensitivity (46).

The apparent success of left stellectomy should not generate unwarranted expectations;

since up to now the stellectomized patients are those with the more severe manifestations of the LQTS, we cannot expect left stellectomy to represent a complete shield in all of them. Probably, sooner or later, some patients will have recurrences and some of these may ultimately prove fatal. In stellectomized patients with new syncopal episodes the addition of beta-blockers may be beneficial because of a greater protection from sympathetic discharges reaching the heart from various sources. It is possible that, in the future, these patients may become suitable candidates for the implantable automatic defibrillator proposed by Mirowski et al. in this volume, with the necessary modifications for the special requirements of the LQTS; the objective in this case would be to have a chance, after defibrillation, to modify the antiarrhythmic treatment. This "fail-safe" system may be life-saving in the most serious cases.

In conclusion, the data gathered on a very large population and updated at regular intervals, clearly indicate that anti-adrenergic measures, either pharmacological or surgical, offer the best possible protection to the LQTS patients. The analysis of these data also calls for extreme caution in accepting encouraging or discouraging conclusions based on single cases. In the last fifteen years many unwarranted claims of successful therapies have been made just to be completely disproved when the follow-ups were extended from one to 3–4 years. Typical in this regard is what has happened with digitalis. More recently some interest has been given to diphenylhydantoin and to ventricular pacing. When a more comprehensive analysis is made it appears however that in the patients treated with these two methods the mortality is still over 40 %. While diphenylhydantoin may prove valuable especially if added to beta-blockers (23), the use of a pacemaker as a maintenance therapy in a young patient has disadvantages which, coupled with the insufficient protection from ventricular fibrillation, makes the consideration of this measure justifiable only after clear-cut failure of the more rational therapies. An important exception may be represented by those patients who also have a disturbance of atrioventricular conduction. Since the LQTS patients often pay with their life the mistakes of their physicians, therapeutical decisions should be based only on the best available evidence and not on "personal experience" based on one or two cases.

6. LQTS AND THE SUDDEN INFANT DEATH SYNDROME

A pathogenetic mechanism similar to the mechanism apparently operative in the LQTS has been recently proposed (47) to be one of the possible causes of the Sudden Infant Death Syndrome (SIDS), which – excluding the first months – is the leading cause of mortality in the first year of life.

The LQTS, at least in its hereditary form, is probably not importantly implicated despite the fact that as shown by Romano (7) LQTS victims may die in the first few months of life being thus labelled as SIDS, but it is quite possible that some SIDS victims represent cases of sporadic form of the LQTS; needless to say, without a previous ECG these cases would remain undiagnosed because family examination would obviously be negative.

A developmental imbalance between right and left sides of cardiac sympathetic innervation with left dominance, or the statistical probability to be at one extreme of the normal (Gaussian) distribution for cardiac sympathetic nerves, were the main mechanisms proposed.

The attendant electrical instability could precipitate the heart into ventricular fibrillation upon a sudden sympathetic discharge produced by many of the mechanisms proposed for SIDS such as apnea, exposure to cold, changes in autonomic activity as related to sleep stages and so forth. Thus, this hypothesis is not exclusive of others, but would instead provide a final common pathway for triggering the fast and silent death of these infants. This possibility has been recently examined and discussed in detail in a comprehensive review on SIDS (48).

Initial supportive evidence comes from experimental studies which have demonstrated left sympathetic dominance in the 3-week-old puppies (49) and by the clinical observation of prolonged QT interval at birth in an infant who subsequently died of SIDS (50). Three other similar clinical observations have already been made by different investigators (48).

Since this sympathetic imbalance would probably be reflected in a prolongation of QT interval, the interesting potential of this hypothesis is that, if correct, some babies at risk may be identified by routine electrocardiography and probably protected with beta-blockers for 6–7 months. As already discussed (48, 51), studies of the so-called "near-misses" or of siblings or parents of SIDS victims cannot provide meaningful data on this possibility. The nature of this hypothesis is in fact such that it can be proved or dismissed only by a prospective study in which a large number of infants have periodic electrocardiographic examinations and are followed for possible SIDS. Such a prospective study, already with 2000 babies enrolled, is currently ongoing in Milan (52).

7. CONCLUSIONS AND PERSPECTIVES

Much progress has been made during the last decade on the understanding and on the treatment of the long QT syndrome. The most important point, on practical grounds, being represented by the knowledge that the syncopal attacks are triggered by sudden sympathetic discharges mostly mediated through the left stellate ganglion. However, a lot remains to be done if our true objective is to allow a normal life to all LQTS patients and not only to those properly diagnosed and properly treated.

Firstly, we need to know much more on the natural history of these patients, on what happens to the so-called asymptomatic patients and on what are the really long-term effects of beta-blockade and left stellectomy. With the goal to answer these and other questions a registry for the LQTS patients has been instituted by Doctors Crampton, Moss, and myself. Forms designed to gather electrocardiographic, familial and therapeutical information have been prepared for computer analysis and are available to enroll those LQTS patients who may be regularly followed for several years. With the necessary cooperation of the interested physicians we should be able, within 10–20 years to have the definitive answers to the most important clinical questions related to the LQTS.

The second point of paramount importance is represented by the right of any affected patient to be properly diagnosed and treated. This apparently simple goal, simple if one considers the unmistakable clinical picture of the LQTS, will be achieved only when the knowledge of the existence of the LQTS will be thoroughly spread through the medical world. The availability of effective therapeutic measures for a disease which, if untreated, leads to death of most of the afflicted makes unacceptable and inexcusable the existence of undiagnosed patients. Still, however, most medical students graduate without having heard a word on the LQTS; most textbooks of medicine and of pediatrics have, at best, a short paragraph or a footnote with insufficient information; neurologists and psychiatrists to whom these patients are often referred are, with few exceptions, completely unaware of the LQTS. As already written years ago (23), the diffusion of the knowledge about the long QT syndrome is an easy and imperative social measure.

ADDENDUM

Since completion of this review, a conversation with Professor Slama – witnessed by Dr. Moss – has unexpectedly provided the first documented support to the hypothesis, just advanced, of LQTS patients with an apparently normal QT interval (53). Slama and Coumel found a family with eleven children of whom five had died suddenly; examining a sixth member who had a number of syncopal attacks they found that he had a prolonged QT interval. This prompted the electrocardiographic examination of the remaining 5 siblings: 4 of them had a prolonged QT interval while one had a normal ECG. One week after this examination the sibling with a normal QT died suddenly in his bed. It seems evident that the entire family was affected by the LQTS but that in one member the surface ECG did not show any abnormality.

ACKNOWLEDGMENTS

I wish to express my deepest gratitude to the many physicians around the world who have patiently and kindly continued for several years to answer my questions on their patients thus providing invaluable data for assessing the therapeutical management of the long QT syndrome.

This work was supported in part by NIH grant HD-08976.

REFERENCES

1. Meissner FL: Taubstummenheit and Taubstummenbildung, Leipzig und Heidelberg, 1856, p 119.
2. Jervell A, Lange-Nielsen F: Congenital deaf-mutism, functional heart disease, with prolongation of the QT interval and sudden death. Am Heart J 54:59–68, 1957.
3. Levine SA, Woodworth CR: Congenital deaf-mutism, prolonged Q-T interval, syncopal attacks and sudden death. New Eng J Med 259:412–417, 1958
4. Ward OC: New familial cardiac syndrome in children. J Irish Med Ass 54:103–106, 1964.
5. Lancet, Congenital cardiac arrhythmia (annotation), 2:26, 1964.
6. Romano C: Congenital cardiac arrhythmia. Lancet 1:658–659, 1965.
7. Romano C, Gemme G, Pongiglione R: Aritmie cardiache rare dell'età pediatrica. Clinica Pediat 45:658–683, 1963.

8. Fraser GR, Froggatt P, James TN: Congenital deafness associated with electrocardiographic abnormalities, fainting and sudden deaths. Quart J Med 33:361–385, 1964.

9. Verrier RL, Lown B: Neural influences and sudden cardiac death. Adv Cardiol 25:155–168, 1978.

10. Moss AJ, Schwartz PJ: Sudden death and the idiopathic Q-T syndrome. Am J Med 66:6–7, 1979.

11. Millar K, Abildskor GA: Notched T waves in young persons with central nervous lesions. Circulation 37:597–603, 1968.

12. Schwartz PJ, Malliani A: Electrical alternation of the T wave: clinical and experimental evidence of its relationship with the sympathetic nervous system and with the long QT syndrome. Am Heart J 89:45–50, 1975.

13. Froggatt P, Adgey AA: A case of cardio-auditory syndrome (long QT interval and profound deafness) diagnosed in the perinatal period and kept under surveillance for two years. Ulster Med J 47:115–133, 1978.

14. Wellens HJJ, Vermeulen A, Durrer D: Ventricular fibrillation occurring on arousal from sleep by auditory stimuli. Circulation 46:661–665, 1972.

15. Phillips J, Ichinose H: Clinical and pathological studies in the hereditary syndrome of a long QT interval, syncopal spells and sudden death. Chest 58:236–243, 1970.

16. Yanowitz F, Preston JB, Abildskov JA: Functional distribution of right and left stellate innervation to the ventricles. Circ Res 18:416–428, 1966.

17. Burgess MJ, Millar K, Abildskov JA: Cancellation of electrocardiographic effects during ventricular recovery. J Electrocardiol 2:101–108, 1969.

18. Kralios FA, Martin L, Burgess MJ, Millar K: Local ventricular repolarization changes due to sympathetic nerve-branch stimulation. Am J Physiol 228:1621–1626, 1975.

19. Green JR, Korovetz MJ, Shanklin DR, De Vito JJ, Taylor WJ: Sudden unexpected death in three generations. Arch Intern Med 124:359–363, 1969.

20. McRae JR, Wagner GS, Rogers MC, Canent RV: Paroxysmal familial ventricular fibrillation. J Pediatr 84:515–518, 1974.

21. Gavrilescu S, Luca C: Right ventricular monophasic action potentials in patients with long QT syndrome. Brit Heart J 40:1014–1018, 1978.

22. Vincent GM, Abildskov JA, Burgess MJ: Q-T interval syndromes. Progr Cardiovasc Dis 16:523–530, 1974.

23. Schwartz PJ, Periti M, Malliani A: The long Q-T syndrome. Am Heart J 89:378–390, 1975.

24. Randall WC, Rohse WG: The augmentor action of the sympathetic cardiac nerves. Circ Res 4:470–475, 1956.

25. Harris AS, Estandia A, Tillotson RF: Ventricular ectopic rhythms and ventricular fibrillation following cardiac sympathectomy and coronary occlusion. Am J Physiol 196:505–512, 1951.

26. Schwartz PJ, Stone HL, Brown AM: Effects of unilateral stellate ganglion blockade on the arrhythmias associated with coronary occlusion. Am Heart J 92:589–599, 1976.

27. Schwartz PJ, Snebold NG, Brown AM: Effects of unilateral cardiac sympathetic denervation on the ventricular fibrillation threshold. Am J Cardiol 37:1034–1040, 1976.

28. Schwartz PJ, Verrier RL, Lown B: Effect of stellectomy and vagotomy on ventricular refractoriness in dogs. Circ Res 40:536–540, 1977.

29. Schwartz PJ, Stone HL: Unilateral stellectomy and sudden death. In: Neural mechanisms in cardiac arrhythmias, Schwartz PJ, Brown AM, Mailliani A, Zanchetti A (eds), New York, Raven Press, 1978, p 107–122.

30. Schwartz PJ: Unilateral stellectomy and dysrhythmias. Circ Res 43:939–940, 1978.

31. McCall RB, Gebber GL, Barman SM: Spinal interneurons in the baroreceptor reflex arc. Am J Physiol 232:H657–H665, 1977.

32. Schwartz PJ, Stone HL: Effects of unilateral stellectomy upon cardiac performance during exercise in dogs. Circ Res 44:637–644, 1979.

33. Austoni P, Rosati R, Gregorini L, Bianchi E, Bortolani E, Schwartz PJ: Stellectomy and exercise in man. Am J Cardiol 43:399, (abstract) 1979.

34. Schwartz PJ: Experimental reproduction of the long Q-T syndrome. Am J Cardiol 41:374, (abstract) 1978.

35. Hageman GR, Goldberg JM, Armour JA, Randall WC: Cardiac dysrhythmias induced by autonomic nerve stimulation. Am J Cardiol 32:823–830, 1973.

36. Randall WC, Thomas JX, Euler DE, Rozanski GJ: Cardiac dysrhythmias associated with autonomic nervous system imbalance in the conscious dog. In: Neural mechanisms in cardiac arrhythmias, Schwartz PJ, Brown AM, Malliani A, Zanchetti A (eds), New York, Raven Press, 1978, p 123–138.

37. Zipes D. Elharrar V, Watanabe AM, Gaum WE, Besch HR: Induction of ventricular fibrillation in probucol-treated dogs. Clin Res 25:459A, 1977.

38. Moss AJ, MacDonald J: Unilateral cervicothoracic sympathetic ganglionectomy for the treatment of long Q-T interval syndrome. N Engl J Med 285:903–904, 1970.

39. Crampton RS: Preeminence of the left stellate ganglion in the long Q-T syndrome. Circulation 59:769–778, 1979.
40. Crampton RS: Another link between the left stellate ganglion and the long Q-T syndrome. Am Heart J 96: 130–132, 1978.
41. Coyer BH, Pryor R, Kirsch WM, Blount SJ Jr: Left stellectomy in the long QT syndrome. Chest 74: 584–586, 1978.
42. James TN, Froggatt P, Atkinson WJ, Lurie PR, McNamara DG, Miller WW, Schloss GT, Carroll JF, North RL: De subitaneis mortibus. XXX. Observations on the pathophysiology of the long QT syndromes with special reference to the neuropathology of the heart. Circulation 57:1221–1231, 1978.
43. Curtiss DJ, Heibel RH, Shaver JA: Autonomic maneuvers in hereditary Q-T interval prolongation (Romano-Ward syndrome). Am Heart J 95:420–428, 1978.
44. Lown B: Sudden cardiac death: The major challenge confronting contemporary cardiology. Am J Cardiol 43:313–328, 1979.
45. Schwartz PJ, Stone HL: Tonic influence of the sympathetic nervous system on myocardial reactive hyperemia and on coronary blood flow distribution in dogs. Circ Res 41;51–58, 1977.
46. Schwartz PJ, Stone HL: Post-denervation supersensitivity and left stellectomy. Am J Cardiol 43:381, (abstract) 1979.
47. Schwartz PJ: Cardiac sympathetic innervation and the sudden infant death syndrome. A possible pathogenetic link. Am J Med 60:167–172, 1976.
48. Schwartz PJ: The sudden infant death syndrome. In: Reviews of perinatal medicine, Scarpelli EM, Cosmi EV (eds), New York, Raven Press, vol IV, (in press).
49. Kralios FA, Millar K: Functional development of cardiac sympathetic nerves in newborn dogs: Evidence for asymmetrical development. Cardiovasc Res 12:547–554, 1978.
50. Smith TA, Mason JM, Bell JS, Francisco JT: Sleep apnea and Q-T interval prolongation – a particularly lethal combination. Am Heart J 97:505–508, 1979.
51. Schwartz PJ: Near miss sudden infant death. Lancet II:853, 1976.
52. Schwartz PJ, Montemerlo M, Facchini M, Salice P, Rosti D, Poggio G, Giorgetti R. Neonatal electrocardiography and the sudden infant death syndrome. I. The QT interval through the first six months of life. (Submitted for publication.)
53. Slama R, Coumel Ph: Personal communication.

5.3. SUDDEN DEATH IN SUBJECTS WITH INTRAVENTRICULAR CONDUCTION DEFECTS

H.E. KULBERTUS, F. DE LEVAL-RUTTEN, M. DUBOIS and J.M. PETIT

The concept of bundle branch block was introduced as early as 1909 by Eppinger and Rothberger (1). Seventy years later, the prognosis of intraventricular conduction disorders still remains controversial.

Initial reports dealing primarily with hospital based populations described a very ominous outlook in patients with bundle branch block. Later studies concerned with subjects in whom bundle branch block was not associated with apparent cardiovascular disease yielded much more optimistic results.

Several investigations published in 1978 and 1979 have renewed the interest towards the prognostic significance of intraventricular conduction disturbances and indicated their association with a high risk of sudden death.

The purpose of this presentation is to review briefly this literature and to report the findings obtained in a prospective follow-up study of 696 patients in whom bundle branch block was discovered during mass screening.

1. REVIEW OF THE LITERATURE

The first report on the prognosis of bundle branch block was published in 1933 by Graybiel and Sprague (2). They followed-up 77 % of 395 cases with bundle branch block of whom most had coronary artery or hypertensive heart disease. They observed 223 fatal cases with an average survival of 14 months.

A few years later, Perera et al (3) studied 104 cases of right bundle branch block (RBBB), 95 % of whom had heart disease. Of 91 cases with adequate follow-up, one third had died over a mean follow-up period of 4 years. Their series also contained 60 instances of left bundle branch block (LBBB): 60 % were dead at one year. In the paper of Messer et al. (4), the mean survival for hospitalized patients with LBBB or RBBB was 3.3 or 3.9 years respectively. Campbell (5) obtained similar results in his follow-up study of 50 cases with bundle branch block (48 had cardiovascular disease); 39 died with a mean survival of two years.

It was realized very early that the prognosis might be influenced by the presence and severity of cardiac disease. Among their 281 cases with RBBB, Schreenivas et al. (6) found that the shortest survival was for patients with coronary or rheumatic heart disease whereas the longest was for patients without detectable cardiac abnormalities. Their impression was later confirmed by several publications (7–15) dealing with subjects who were found to have a bundle branch block with no or insignificant heart disease. These investigations indicated that acquired bundle branch block is generally associated with a good prognosis in the asymptomatic patient. For example, Rotman et al. (15) who reviewed the literature on this subject presented their own clinical and follow-up study of 394 individuals with RBBB and 125 with LBBB. Most of these subjects were asymptomatic at the time of the bundle branch block diagnosis. Complete follow-up information was available in 94 % of the RBBB group and 91 % of the LBBB group. The mean follow-up period was 10.8 ± 4.4 years in the former and 8.8 ± 4.8 years in the latter. Only 14 (4 %) RBBB and 9 (8 %) LBBB subjects died during the follow-up period.

The same contrast between studies reporting either an ominous or a favorable prognosis depending on the population from which the patients are derived still persists in the most recent literature. In 1978, Mc Anulty et al. (16) reviewed all 42,000 electrocardiograms taken at the University Medical Center of Portland from 1969 to 1971. 325 patients had LBBB or RBBB with axis deviation. In December 1974, 90 % were contacted or found to be dead. Statistical analysis revealed a high mortality rate among these subjects. Survival at 5 years of 164 LBBB patients (40.7 ± 4.1 %) was approximately equal to that of 161 patients with RBBB and axis deviation (49.5 ± 4.2 %). Patients with coronary artery disease had a particularly poor prognosis (survival at 5 years: 33.7%), especially if they had evidence of a previous myocardial infarction (survival at 5 years: 23.5 %). Primary conduction disease occurred in 20 %; with a survival of 50.6 % at 5 years, it was not without risks of its own. The same authors (17), following up prospectively 257 patients with LBBB or RBBB and axis deviation who had undergone His bundle studies, noted that during an average follow-up period of 25 months, 50 patients died, death being sudden in 27 instances. Actuarial analysis revealed an overall mortality rate of 19 ± 2.6 % at 2 years and a mortality rate from sudden death of 10.2 ± 2.6 %. In contrast with the results of Narula et al. (18), Mc Anulty et al. (17) were unable to show that the length of the HV interval could be used to determine the magnitude of risk of sudden death. Some authors have indicated that only a greatly prolonged HV time may predict a subgroup of patients at high risk of sudden death (19), especially when congestive heart failure is associated (20). This particular view is not accepted by all investigators (21). In a study also published in 1978, Dinghra et al. (22) reported on 102 patients with chronic left bundle branch followed up for 30 to 2,271 days. The cumulative mortality at 4 years approached 70 % and mortality by sudden death, 60 %. Following-up 452 patients with chronic bifascicular block for a period of $1,066 \pm 97$ days, the same group (23) noted a cumulative mortality for sudden death of $20.0 \% \pm 2.3$ at 4 years.

These recent studies which portray such an ominous outlook in bundle branch block should be contrasted with other reports dealing with patients culled from a private practice outpatient population (24) or from a screening examination done on London male civil servants (25). The former study (24) was concerned with 79 patients with RBBB and axis deviation followed-up for an average of 28 months. During the study period 10.1 % died. Only one patient died suddenly and he had had a stable electrocardiographic pattern of RBBB-LAHB for a period of almost 10 years.

The second study (25) investigated the prevalence and prognosis of electrocardiographic findings in 18,403 subjects aged 40 to 64. These subjects were followed-up for 5 years. In

LBBB, the excess coronary heart disease mortality reached the 5 % level of statistical significance but the dominant impression was the lowness of risk in the group with no symptomatic history: among 321 with ventricular conduction defect, only 2 % died of coronary heart disease.

The contrasting results obtained in hospital based series as compared to series of ambulatory patients with no or few symptoms raise a difficult practical problem. Electrocardiograms are more and more frequently recorded in ambulatory patients, for example by the general practitioner, or to assess occupational fitness, or insurability. The management of patients with bundle branch block and few or no symptoms of cardio-vascular disease remains unclear. A reassessment of these electrocardiographic findings as they arise in these conditions was felt useful.

2. PROSPECTIVE FOLLOW-UP STUDY OF BUNDLE BRANCH BLOCK DIAGNOSED AT SCREENING

2.1. Introduction

In 1972, the Medical Institute of the Province of Liège started an experimental community hypertension screening program. In order to make the best use of this experiment, it was decided to include an electrocardiogram in the screening examination and to initiate prospective follow-up studies of selected electrocardiographic abnormalities. The present report is concerned with the incidence and prognosis of bundle branch block among the first 33,001 individuals who were examined.

2.2. Material and methods

The practical details regarding this program have been described elsewhere (26). Screening was performed in mobile units. Specially equipped buses visited selected sites in urban, suburban and rural parts of the Province. The program was well advertised and all individuals aged 35 years or over were invited to submit themselves to a screening examination. Subjects under current treatment for cardiovascular disease were advised not to come. The examinations were free of charge. After proper identification, each subject was asked to fill up a questionnaire dealing with smoking habits and family or personal history of cardiovascular disease and to indicate all medications taken at the time of examination. The questionnaire proposed by Rose and Blackburn (27) for the diagnosis of effort angina was also answered with the help of a nurse. The person was then submitted to a measurement of height and weight, a chest X ray, a standard electrocardiogram and, finally, a blood pressure measurement taken after a 10 minute period of rest in supine position. Whenever the pression was found to be elevated (over 160/95 mm of Hg), the measurement was repeated after 2 minutes at both arms. The chest X ray and electrocardiogram were interpreted by trained cardiologists and radiologists. All data were transmitted to a central computer center where they were checked, edited and stored for retrieval analysis. High blood pressure was considered present when, on 2 successive readings, the systolic pressure was found to be > 160 mm of Hg and/or the diastolic pressure > 95 mm Hg.

Coronary heart disease was diagnosed when the patient gave a typical history of anginal chest pain or had electrocardiographic evidence, or a clinically well documented history of previous myocardial infarction.

Standard electrocardiographic criteria were used for diagnosing **RBBB** and **LBBB** (28).

Left anterior hemiblock was diagnosed when the following criteria were met (29):
– left deviation of the mean QRS frontal plane axis (−30° or higher);
– qR morphology in leads I and aVL;
– rS morphology in leads II, III and aVF;
– QRS duration shorter than 120 msec.

Since the diagnosis of left posterior hemiblock requires a combination of clinical and electrocardiographic criteria (30) and since the latter are still controversial, no attempt was made to identify this conduction abnormality. Follow-up data were obtained in all subjects who had been depicted to have a bundle branch block at the time of screening. In case of death, a social nurse interviewed the general practitioner and the family of the deceased. Whenever needed, the hospital files of the patient were also examined. Precise information was obtained in all but 1 case. Death was considered and called sudden when it was unattended or occurred within one hour of the onset of new symptoms.

In order to compare patients with intraventricular conduction defects to a population that had no conduction disorders, but was matched for age, sex, follow-up and presence of cardiac desease, each patient with bundle branch block was matched with two cases (or, if impossible, at least one), of same age, sex and clinical characteristics who were examined approximately at the same time, but who had normal intraventricular conduction. These people constituted the control groups.

2.3. Results

Between October 1st 1973 and June 30th, 1977, 33,001 individuals were examined (male 46.3 %; female 53.6 %). Their age and sex distribution is indicated in Table 1. In spite of the fact that subjects under treatment for cardiovascular disease had been discouraged to attend the screening program, 3.35 % of the men and 2.92 % of the women were taking drugs clas-

Table 1. Description of population under study.

Age (years)	≤ 39	40–49	50–59	60–69	≥ 70	Totals
Male	2446	3891	3857	3319	1787	15.300
Female	2101	4272	4750	4390	2188	17.701
						33.001

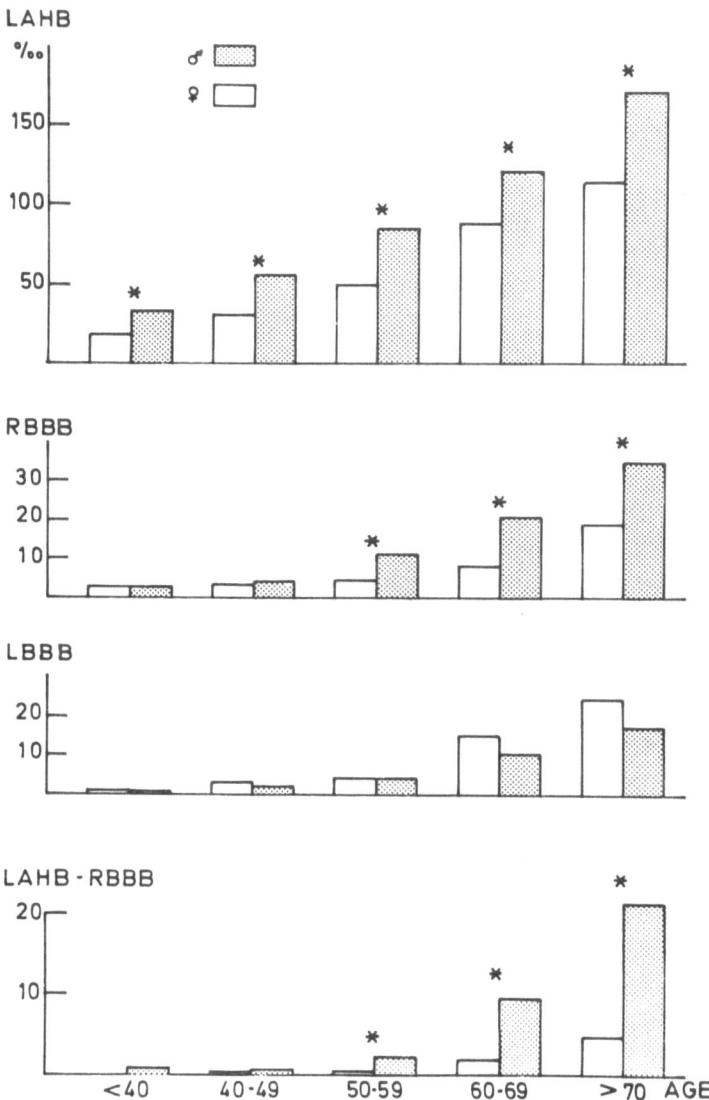

Figure 1. Age and sex distribution of left anterior hemiblock (LHAB), RBBB, LBBB and LAHB-RBBB among 33001 individuals examined during the screening program.
* indicates a significant difference between male and female.

sically administered for coronary heart disease whereas 7.10 % of the men and 15.83 % of the women were under current antihypertensive treatment. Figure 1 indicates the overall incidence and age distribution of the various types of conduction disorders. Altogether, conduction defects increased in frequency with increasing age. The age slope for LAHB was shallower than for RBBB or LBBB. Conduction disorders were more frequent in men (10.98 %) than in women (7.41 %)(p < 0.001); the male : female ratio for LAHB, RBBB and

LAHB-RBBB were 1.48 (p < 0.001), 1.95 (p < 0.001) and 4.82 (p < 0.001), respectively. On the opposite, left bundle branch block showed a slight, but statistically significant predominance in the female group (male: female ratio: 0.68, p < 0.01).

There were 319 instances of isolated right bundle branch block depicted. The 56 cases who had right bundle branch block with a QRS axis to the right of +90° were included in this subgroup. There were 197 men (age: 64.0 ± 11.3 years) and 122 women (64.6 ± 11.9 years). Coronary heart disease was present in 83 cases (26 %) and arterial hypertension in 75 (24 %). Twenty-three subjects had radiological evidence of cardiomegaly (7 %). First degree AV block was observed in 10 individuals (3 %) and ventricular ectopic beats in 26 (8 %). The mean duration of follow-up was 41.25 ± 16.6 months. During this period, 18 deaths (15 male; 3 female) were recorded. 15 occurred after the age of 70. One of them was sudden, 8 cardiac (myocardial infarction: 6; intractable heart failure: 2) and 9 noncardiac (cerebrovascular disease: 5; neoplasm: 4). An attempt was made to compare patients with right bundle branch block with a control group matched for sex, age, follow-up duration and cardiac disease (Table 2). This group contained 520 individuals (320 men; 200 women). In the male group, there was a slightly higher incidence of detectable heart disease among the RBBB patients than among controls. During follow-up 25 of the control patients died (17 men; 8 women). Fourteen of these deaths occurred after the age of 70, 7 were sudden, 5 were cardiac and 13 noncardiac. Actuarial analysis (31) (Figure 2, Table 3) disclosed no significant increase of mortality rate among patients with RBBB as compared to controls either when the total number of deaths was considered, or when only cardiac (including sudden) deaths were taken into consideration.

There were 248 cases of left bundle branch block disclosed (85 men (65.4 ± 10.2 years) and 163 women (55.9 ± 9.8 years)). Coronary artery disease was present in 139 cases (56 %) and arterial hypertension in 95 (38 %). 44 subjects had radiological evidence of cardiomegaly (18 %). First degree AV block was observed in 9 individuals (4 %) and ventricular ectopic beats in 29 (12 %). The mean duration of follow-up was 43.93 ± 15.05 months. During this period, 30 deaths (13 men; 17 women) were recorded. Nineteen occurred after the age of 70. Five were sudden, 13 were cardiac (myocardial infarction: 7; intractable heart failure: 5; pericarditis: 1) and 12 noncardiac (cerebrovascular disease: 6; neoplasm: 3; renal insufficiency: 2; road accident: 1). Patients with LBBB were compared to a control group matched for sex, age, follow-up duration and cardio-vascular disease (Table 2). This group contained

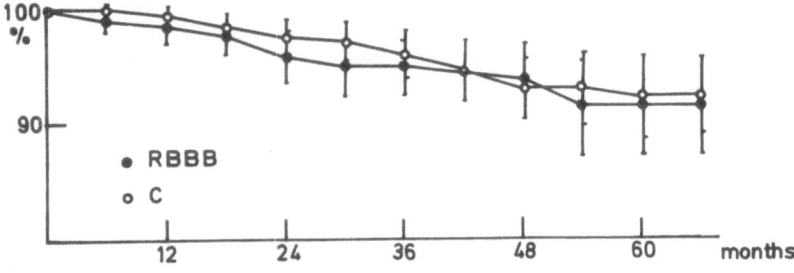

Figure 2. Actuarial survival curves (percentage, mean ± 2. SE.) of patients with RBBB and of matched controls.

Table 2. Characteristics of patients in bundle branch block and control groups.

RBBB *vs Controls*	Male			Female		
	RBBB	Controls	p	RBBB	Controls	p
Number	197	320	–	122	200	–
Age (years)	64.04 ± 11.32	62.41 ± 10.54	0.10	64.64 ± 11.9	63.43 ± 11.57	0.37
Follow-up (months)	41.08 ± 16.12	40.52 ± 16.00	0.70	41.52 ± 17.42	42.51 ± 17.87	0.62
Detectable CVD (%)	44	34 ⎱	< 0.05	56	47 ⎱	0.15
No detectable CVD (%)	56	66 ⎰		44	53 ⎰	

LBBB *vs Controls*	Male			Female		
	LBBB	Controls	p	LBBB	Controls	p
Number	85	146	–	163	292	–
Age (years)	65.4 ± 10.2	64.1 ± 9.7	0.27	65.9 ± 9.8	64.9 ± 9.1	0.33
Follow-up (months)	41.9 ± 14.6	41.7 ± 15.2	0.93	44.98 ± 15.22	45.16 ± 15.32	0.90
Detectable CVD (%)	67	59 ⎱	0.22	80	78 ⎱	0.66
No detectable CVD (%)	33	41 ⎰		20	22 ⎰	

LAHB-RBBB *vs Controls*	Male			Female		
	LAHB-RBBB	Controls	p	LAHB-RBBB	Controls	p
Number	93	165	–	36	64	–
Age (years)	68.00 ± 8.9	67.27 ± 8.93	0.53	66.59 ± 7.77	66.53 ± 6.62	0.97
Follow-up (months)	48.57 ± 14.11	48.71 ± 13.97	0.94	56.64 ± 15.45	56.61 ± 14.87	0.99
Detectable CVD (%)	59	57 ⎱	0.72	72	69 ⎱	0.72
No detectable CVD (%)	41	43 ⎰		28	31 ⎰	

438 individuals (146 men; 292 women) of whom 16 died during follow-up (7 men; 9 women). Nine of these deaths occurred after the age of 70; 3 were sudden, 4 cardiac and 9 noncardiac. Actuarial analysis (Figure 3, Table 3) of the data indicated an increased mortality rate among LBBB as compared to control patients. This held true whether all deaths, or only cardiac

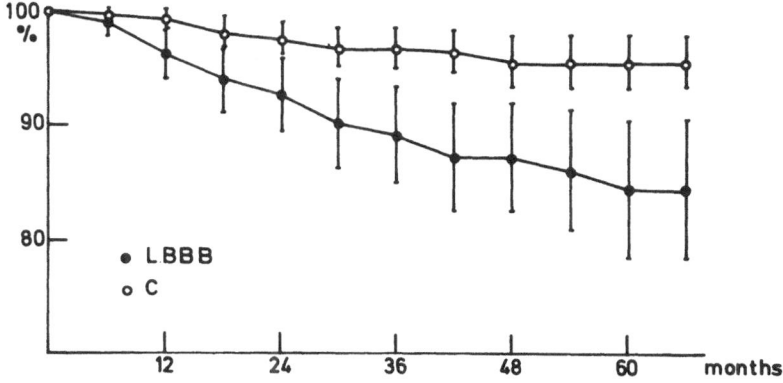

Figure 3. Actuarial survival curves (percentage, mean ± 2 S.E.) of patients with LBBB and of matched controls.

Table 3. Actuarial mortality rates (dead per thousand; mean ± SE).

Duration of follow-up	RBBB				Controls		
	Nr at risk	All deaths	Cardiac deaths		Nr at risk	All deaths	Cardiac deaths
12 months	314	15.7± 6.9	9.7± 5.6		519	5.7± 3.3	3.9± 2.8
24 months	244	41.1±11.7	17.4± 7.7		407	25.1± 7.4	10.5± 4.7
36 months	178	49.5±13.0	26.1± 9.8		292	39.6± 9.6	22.3± 7.5
48 months	105	63 ±16.0	34.0±12.5		178	67.4±14.0	34.4±10.2

Duration of follow-up	LBBB				Controls			
	Nr at risk	All deaths	Cardiac deaths	Sudden death	Nr at risk	All deaths	Cardiac deaths	Sudden deaths
12 months	238	37.4±11.9	34.0±11.8	9.0± 6.4	433	4.6± 3.2	2.3± 2.3	0
24 months	198	73.9±16.8*	47.4±14.0	9.0± 6.4	368	24.5± 7.3	12.0± 5.3	5.0±3.5
36 months	149	108.8±20.7*	63.3±15.5*	20.5±10.2	282	31.8± 8.7	12.0± 5.3	5.0±3.5
48 months	82	128.5±23.2*	84.2±20.0*	20.5±10.2	165	45.2±11.5	21.8± 8.7	10.0±6.1

Duration of follow-up	LAHB-RBBB				Controls		
	Nr at risk	All deaths	Cardiac deaths		Nr at risk	All deaths	Cardiac deaths
12 months	128	7.8± 7.7	8.6± 8.6		228	4.4± 4.4	0
24 months	119	46.7±18.6	17.4±12.2		220	9.1± 6.2	0
36 months	96	97.1±26.7	45.6±19.9		178	44.8±14.3	21.1±10.4
48 months	61	186.0±38.4	70.4±26.0		125	49.5±15.3*	21.1±10.4

The figures related to sudden death were not calculated for the **RBBB** and **LAHB-RBBB** groups in which the instances of sudden deaths were too small to permit any statistical evaluation. Cardiac deaths: sudden deaths/deaths from chronic or acute heart failure, myocardial infarction: pericarditis; endocarditis.
* Difference with controls significant at $p < 0.05$ level.

deaths, were considered. The data obtained for sudden deaths suggested the same trend but the difference did not reach statistical significance.

There were 129 instances of LAHB-RBBB diagnosed (93 men (age: 68.0±8.9 years) and 36 women (age: 67.3±8.9 years)). In this group, coronary heart disease was present in 44 cases (54%); and arterial hypertension in 39 (30%). Fifteen subjects had radiological evidence of cardiomegaly (12%). First degree AV block was observed in 4 individuals (3%) and ventricular ectopic beats in 17 (13%). The mean duration of follow-up was 50.82±14.89 months. During this period, 20 deaths (19 male, 1 female) were recorded: 14 occurred after the age of 70. One was sudden, 5 cardiac (myocardial infarction: 3; bacterial endocarditis: 1; heart failure: 1) and 14 noncardiac (neoplasm: 8; stroke: 3; chronic obstructive lung disease: 2; renal insufficiency: 1). In one, the cause of death could not be determined with certainty. The control group contained 229 individuals (165 men; 64 women) of whom 12 died during follow-up (10 men; 2 women). 10 of these deaths occurred after the age of 70; 2 were sudden; 1 cardiac and 9 noncardiac. Actuarial analysis of the data (Figure 4, Table 3)

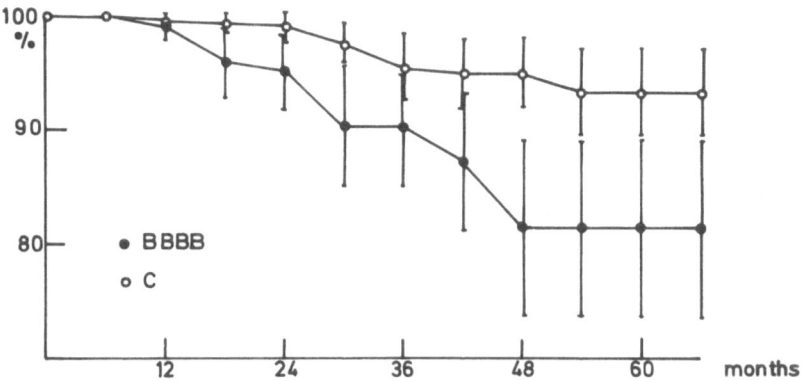

Figure 4. Actuarial survival curves (percentage, mean ±2 SE.) of patients with LABH-RBBB (i.e. partial bilateral bundle branch block, **BBBB**) and of matched controls.

indicated an increased mortality rate among patients with LAHB-RBBB as compared to controls. The same trend was observed if only cardiac (including sudden) deaths were taken into consideration, but the differences did not reach statistical significance.

An attempt was made to correlate the deaths with the presence of hypertension, cardiac enlargement and/or coronary artery disease. Considering each of these characteristics separately, no significant effect on survival could be found. On the whole, however, the number of deaths was higher among those who had one of these conditions than among those who did not. The difference reached the level of $p < 0.05$ in the **LBBB** group, of $0.1 > p > 0.05$ in the **LAHB-RBBB** group and of $0.1 < p < 0.2$ in the **RBBB** group (Table 4).

Nine patients developed complete heart block and 8 received a pacemaker during the period under survey. Three had a **LBBB** and the others **LAHB-RBBB**. The actuarial data analyzing the incidence of complete AV block in patients with **LAHB-RBBB** is indicated in Figure 5 and Table 5.

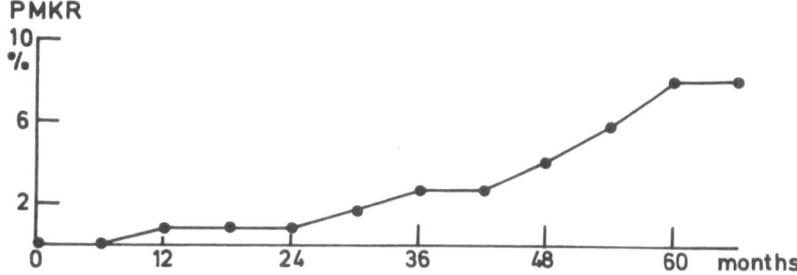

Figure 5. Cumulative annual incidence (actuarial method) of complete AV block requiring pacemaker implantation among 129 patients with LAHB-RBBB.

Table 4. Mortality in relation to presence of cardiac disease.

	(1) Number of cases with detectable cardiac disease	Number of dead in (1)	(2) Number of cases without detectable cardiac disease	Number of dead in (2)	X^2
RBBB	154	12	165	6	2.58 $0.10 < p < 0.20$
LBBB	187	27	61	3	3.92 $0.025 < p < 0.05$
LAHB-RBBB	81	16	48	4	3.64 $0.05 < p < 0.10$

2.4. Discussion

The present study is concerned with the incidence and prognosis of bundle branch block in a population including outpatient subjects from a mass screening clinic. The group under investigation cannot be directly compared with those described in previous studies, especially those dealing with hospital based series. The present group only comprizes ambulatory individuals. It clearly contains some patients with obvious cardiovascular disease. Since no physical examination was performed, an unknown number of people with valvular heart disease, cardiomyopathy and congenital heart disease might also have been included.

The study shows that conduction disorders tend, in general, to be more frequent in men than in women. LAHB, RBBB, and LAHB-RBBB were respectively and approximately 1.5, 2 and 5 times more frequent in the male than in the female group; LBBB was, on the contrary, more often found in women, at least after the age of 60. It is noteworthy that LAHB-RBBB was, in the same age group, almost exclusively observed in male individuals. The reasons for these sexual differences remain unknown.

The outlook of our patients with bundle branch block was not really ominous. Even in individuals with LBBB or LAHB-RBBB, the annual mortality rate approximated only 3.25 % and 4.5 %. These figures are considerably lower than those published recently by Mc Anulty et al. (16, 17), or by Dinghra et al. (22). They are of the same order of magnitude as the mortality rate in coronary patients with symptomatic single vessel disease (32). This data further stresses the point that the prognostic significance of an abnormal electrocardio-

Table 5. Incidence of complete AV block in LAHB-RBBB (Actuarial data).

Duration of follow-up	Number at risk	Incidence of complete AV block $(^0/_{00} + S.E.)$
12 months	127	7.8 ± 7.7
24 months	118	7.8 ± 7.7
36 months	93	27.0 ± 15.5
48 months	60	40.9 ± 20.6
60 months	37	79.6 ± 33.4

graphic finding largely depends upon the population from which the patient is derived (25). The prognostic value of most electrocardiographic abnormalities has, heretofore, been primarily studied in symptomatic patients. Reassessment of electrocardiographic findings as they arise in the setting of mass screening or population survey is needed.

If the dominant impression in this study is the relative lowness of risk, it remains that patients with LBBB and LAHB-RBBB have a decreased survival rate as compared to individuals matched for age, sex, duration of follow-up and presence of detectable heart disease. In both LBBB and LAHB-RBBB, a difference with controls could be demonstrated statistically as regards death from all causes; the difference in mortality from cardiac death-sudden death included- was significant in the LBBB group only. Sudden death was altogether uncommon in patients with bundle branch block and no statistically significant difference with controls could be demonstrated even in the left bundle branch block group where the overall figures suggested an increased mortality by sudden death.

In their series, Mc Anulty et al. (16) were unable to statistically demonstrate that cardiovascular disease significantly alters survival from sudden death or from death from all cases. In the present study, it seemed that the overall mortality was higher among bundle branch block subjects who had associated cardiovascular disease than among those who did not. The difference reached the level of statistical signivicance in left bundle branch block ($p < 0.05$). The same trend was noted among LAHB-RBBB and RBBB patients but the differences did not quite reach the level of significance. (LAHB-RBBB: $0.1 > p > 0.05$; RBBB: $0.1 < p < 0.2$). It appears therefore that hypertension, angina pectoris and cardiomegaly most probably affect the prognosis. In the absence of cardiovascular disease, no difference in mortality was noted between patients with bundle branch block and controls. The numbers are however rather small and one would wish to have larger series and longer periods of follow-up, before drawing conclusions. These remarks of caution are inspired by the observation that, among the 3 deaths which occurred in the LBBB group, one was sudden and another due to complete AV block.

In the absence of cardiovascular disease the prognosis in subjects with bundle branch block may relate to whether they develop further electrical dysfunction and AV block appears. This study confirms that progression towards complete AV block is rare among individuals with bundle branch block even in the group with LAHB-RBBB. This low percentage as well as the rarity of sudden death in the same cohort contrasts sharply with Narula and coworkers (18) who stated that elderly patients with a pattern of LAHB-RBBB should all be considered for conduction studies despite the absence of symptoms to assess the possible risk of sudden death and that they should be treated by permanent pacemaker implantation whenever the H-V time is equal or greater than 70 msec. Disagreement with this opinion has also been expressed by several investigators (17, 23).

3. CONCLUSIONS

A) There exists large differences in the prognosis of bundle branch block according to the population base from which the electrocardiograms were obtained. The diagnostic significance and prognosis of bundle branch block appear to be very different in a clinically ill population made up of hospitalized patients and in a population of asymptomatic, or at least, ambulatory individuals.

B) All studies carried out on hospital based series describe an ominous outlook in patients with LBBB and RBBB with axis deviation. The overall mortality as well as the mortality from cardio-vascular or sudden death are considerably increased in these patients. In disagreement with an opinion which was widely held until recently, it seems that the HV interval cannot be used to predict the individuals at higher risk of heart block or sudden death. However, the prognostic value of greatly prolonged HV time ($>$ 70 msec) remains controversial. At present, insertion of permanent pacemaker to prolong life does not seem warranted in individuals without documented symptomatic bradyarrhythmias.

C) In mass screening, the risk associated with bundle branch block is low and approximates the risk of symptomatic coronary heart disease involving one single artery. Yet, patients with LBBB and LAHB-RBBB have approximately a threefold increase of mortality rate as compared to controls matched for sex, age, follow-up and presence of detectable cardiovascular disease. Associated cardiovascular diseases are obviously important and mortality is the highest among patients who have hypertension, coronary heart disease and/or cardiomegaly in addition to LBBB or LAHB-RBBB.

D) Sudden death and progression towards complete AV block appears to be uncommon among subjects with bundle branch block discovered at screening. The annual risk of developing Adams-Stokes syncope is situated between 1 and 2 % in the group showing LAHB-RBBB. In view of 1) the large number of subjects with this anomaly in the elderly population, 2) the small proportion among them of high risk individuals, 3) the lack of demonstrated significance of HV interval measurements and 4) the absence of clear-cut beneficial effects of preventive pacing (33), systematic electrophysiologic investigation is not warranted in such cases.

ACKNOWLEDGMENT

The authors wish to express their gratitude to Miss M. Lejeune who, with great care and dedication, collected all the follow-up data. They are also indebted to Miss S. Smeets for her technical assistance and to Mrs Vervier who typed the manuscript.

They are thankful to the Authorities of the Government of the Province of Liège for their understanding and support.

REFERENCES

1. Eppinger H, Rothberger CJ: Zur Analyse des Elektrokardiograms. Wien Klin Wchschr 22:1091–1098, 1909.
2. Graybiel A, Sprague HB: Bundle branch block: an analysis of 395 cases. Am J Med Sci 185:395–401, 1933.
3. Perera G, Levine SA, Erlanger H: Prognosis of right bundle branch block: A study of 104 cases. Brit Heart J 4:35, 1942.
4. Messer AL, Birmingham A, Johnson RP, Schreenivas, White PD: Prognosis in bundle branch block III. A comparison of right and left bundle branch block with a note on the relative incidence of each. Amer Heart J 41:239–245, 1951.

5. Campbell M: The outlook with bundle branch block. Brit Heart J 31:575–579, 1969.
6. Schreenivas, Messer AL, Johnson RP, White PD: Prognosis in bundle branch block I. Factors influencing the survival period in right bundle branch block. Amer Heart J 40:891–902, 1950.
7. Wood FC, Jeffers WA, Wolferth CC: Follow-up study of 74 patients with a right bundle branch conduction defect. Amer Heart J 10:1056–1066, 1935.
8. Rodstein M, Gubner R Mills JP, Lovell JF, Ungerleider HE: A mortality study in bundle branch block. Arch Inter Med 87:663–668, 1951.
9. Wolfram J: Bundle branch block without significant heart disease. Amer Heart J 41:656–666, 1951.
10. Vazifdar JP, Levine SA: Benign bundle branch block. Arch Intern Med, 89:568–574, 1952.
11. Lamb LE, Johnson RC: Left bundle branch block in flying personnel. A report of 56 cases. Aerosp Med 35:97–104, 1964.
12. Massing GK, Lancaster MC: Clinical significance of acquired complete right bundle branch block in 59 patients without overt cardiac disease. Aerosp Med 40:867–971, 1969.
13. Beach TB, Gracey JG, Peter RH: Benign left bundle branch block. Ann Intern Med, 70:269–276, 1969.
14. Smith RF, Jackson DH, Harthorne JW, Sanders CA: Acquired bundle branch block in a healthy population. Amer Heart J 80:746–751, 1970.
15. Rotman M, Triebwasser JH: A clinical and follow-up study of right and left bundle branch block. Circulation 51:477–484, 1975.
16. McAnulty JH, Kauffman S, Murphy E, Kassebaum DG, Rahimtoola SH: Survival in patients with intraventricular conduction defects. Arch Intern Med 138:30–35, 1978.
17. McAnulty JH, Rahimtoola SH, MurphyES, Kauffman S, Ritzmann LW, Kanarek P, De Mots H: A prospective study of sudden death in 'high-risk' bundle branch block. New Eng J Med 299:209–215, 1978.
18. Narula OS, Gann D Samet Ph.: Prognostic value of H-V intervals in His bundle electrocardiography and clinical electrophysiology. Narula OS (ed) Philadelphia, FA Davis Company, 1975, p 437.
19. Scheinman M, Weiss A, Kunkel F: His bundle recordings in patients with bundle branch block and transient neurologic symptoms. Circulation 48:322–330, 1973.
20. Scheinman M, Peters RW, Modin G, Brennan M, Mies C, O'Young J: Prognostic value of infranodal conduction time in patients with chronic bundle branch block. Circulation 56:240–244, 1977.
21. Dinghra RC, Denes P, Wu D, Wyndham CR, Amat-y-Leon F, Twone WD, Rosen KM: Prospective observations in patients with chronic bundle branch block and marked HV prolongation. Circulation 53:600–604, 1976.
22. Dinghra RC, Amat-Y-Leon F, Wyndham C, Sridhar SS, Wu D, Denes P, Rosen KM: Significance of left axis deviation in patients with chronic left bundle branch block. Amer J Cardiol 42:551–556, 1978.
23. Dinghra RC, Wyndham C, Amat-Y-Leon F, Denes P, Wu D, Sridhar SS, Bustin AG, Rosen KM: Incidence and site of atrioventricular block in patients with chronic bifascicular block. Circulation 59:238–246, 1979.
24. Lister JW, Kline RS, Lesser ME: Chronic bilateral bundle branch block. Long term observations in ambulatory patients. Brit Heart J 39:203–207, 1977.
25. Rose G, Baxter PJ, Reid D, Mc Cartney P: Prevalence and prognosis of electrocardiographic findings in middle-aged men. Brit Heart J 40:636–643, 1978.
26. Kulbertus HE, de Leval-Rutten F, Dubois M, Petit JM: A community screening program for hypertension. Europ J Cardiol. 7:487–497, 1978.
27. Rose GA, Blackburn H: Cardiovascular population studies: Methods. WHO Press Monograph no 56, Geneva 1969.
28. Lipman BS, Massie E: Clinical scalar electrocardiography. Chicago, Year Book Medical Publishers, (5th edition) 1965, p 166.
29. Kulbertus HE, Demoulin JC: The conduction system: anatomical and pathological aspects. In: Cardiac arrhythmias: the modern electrophysiological approach. Krikler DM and Goodwin JF (eds) London, Saunders, 1975, p 16.
30. Rosenbaum MB, Elizari MV, Lazzari JO: The hemiblocks. Oldsmar, Florida, Tampa Tracings, 1970.
31. Rouquette C, Schwartz D: Méthodes en épidémiologie. Paris. Flammarion, 1970, p 252.
32. Favaloro RG: Direct myocardial revascularisation: A ten year journey. Amer J Cardiol 43:109–129, 1979.
33. Peters RW, Scheinman MM, Modin G, O'Young J, Somelofski C, Mies C.; Permanent prophylactic pacing in patients with chronic bundle branch block. Amer J Cardiol 41:385, (abstract) 1978.

5.4. SUDDEN DEATH IN THE WOLFF-PARKINSON-WHITE SYNDROME

H.J.J. WELLENS, F.W. BÄR, J. FARRE, D. ROSS and E.J. VANAGT

In the human heart the refractory period of the AV node protects the ventricle against supraventricular rhythms with a very high rate. In the presence of an accessory atrio-ventricular (AV) pathway the ventricular rate during supraventricular rhythms not only depends upon the refractory period of the AV node but also upon the refractory period of the accessory AV pathway. If the refractory period of the latter is very short atrial flutter and atrial fibrillation can become life-threatening arrhythmias. Indeed, in patients with the Wolff-Parkinson-White syndrome deterioration of atrial fibrillation into ventricular fibrillation has been reported (1–13) (see Figure 1).

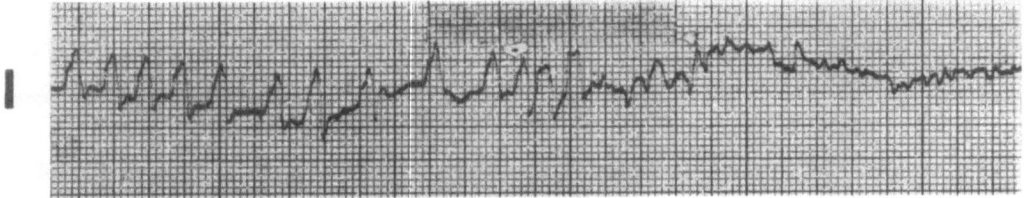

Figure 1. Deterioration of atrial fibrillation into ventricular fibrillation.

1. IDENTIFICATION OF THE WPW PATIENT AT RISK FOR SUDDEN DEATH

For the cardiologist it is important to identify the patient with WPW who is at risk for sudden death when atrial fibrillation develops. While several factors determine the ventricular rate during atrial fibrillation (Table 1), an important role is played by the duration of the refractory period of the accessory AV pathway. Three independent groups of investigators (14–16) found a correlation between the duration of the refractory period of the accessory AV pathway and the ventricular rate during atrial fibrillation. There was excellent correlation between the shortest R-R interval during atrial fibrillation and the duration of the refractory period of the accessory pathway (15, 16) (see Figure 2). Theoretically therefore the most dependable way to identify the high risk patient with the WPW syndrome would be the determination of the duration of the antegrade refractory period of the accessory pathway during programmed electrical stimulation of the heart. Because the duration of the refractory period of the accessory pathway might shorten on increasing heart rate several atrial pacing rates should be used during the study. This should preferably be followed by

Table 1. Factors determining ventricular rate during atrial fibrillation in Wolff-Parkinson-White syndrome.

Accessory pathway

1. Refractory period
2. Input, transmission and output characteristics which are influenced by the width, length and type of tissue of the accessory pathway.
3. Concealed conduction   in atrioventricular direction
                                in ventriculoatrial direction
4. Reentry

Atrioventricular nodal pathway
1. Refractory period
2. Input, transmission and output characteristics
3. Concealed conduction
4. Reentry

Ventricle
1. Refractory period

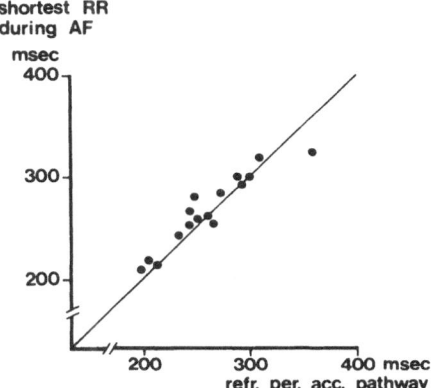

Figure 2. Relation in 16 patients between the duration of the refractory period of the accessory pathway as determined during programmed electrical stimulation of the heart (horizontal axis) and the shortest R-R interval during atrial fibrillation (vertical axis). Note the good correlation between these two values.

the induction of atrial fibrillation to ascertain the ventricular rate during this arrhythmia. From a practical point of view it is impossible to perform this type of study in all patients showing the WPW electrocardiogram. There are certain findings however that inform us about the duration of the antegrade refractory period of the accessory pathway and help us in identifying patients with a short refractory period.

1.1. The symptomatic patient

As described above in the patient with WPW suffering from tachycardia, information as to the duration of the refractory period of the accessory pathway can be obtained by determining the shortest R-R interval during atrial fibrillation. As pointed out by Klein et al. (8) all 25 patients developing ventricular fibrillation during atrial fibrillation showed their shortest R-R interval to be 250 msec or less. The same authors showed that apart from a very short R-R interval during atrial fibrillation other findings like having a history of both atrial fibrillation and reciprocal tachycardia and the presence of multiple accessory pathways were helpful in identifying the patient prone for the development of ventricular fibrillation. It is of importance that several of them were receiving digitalis at the time of occurrence of their ominous arrhythmia.

1.2. The asymptomatic patient

Because sudden death can be the first manifestation of the WPW syndrome (17, 18) information as to the duration of the antegrade refractory period of the accessory pathway is of importance in the asymptomatic patient. The following three findings point to a relatively long refractory period.

1.2.1. Intermittent pre-excitation: In our experience patients showing intermittent AV conduction over their accessory pathway never have a short refractory period of this structure in antegrade direction.

1.2.2. The ajmaline test. Recently we have demonstrated that failure to produce complete block in the accessory pathway in antegrade direction by the intravenous injection of 50 mg ajmaline given over a three minute period indicates an antegrade refractory period of the accessory pathway of 270 msec or less (19) (see Table 2). An example of complete block in the accessory pathway following ajmaline is given in Figure 3.

Table 2. Effect of 50 mg ajmaline given intravenously in relation to the length of the antegrade refractory period of the accessory pathway.

Antegrade block in AP	+	−
$ERP_{AP} > 270$ msec	25/26	1/26
$ERP_{AP} \leq 270$ msec	7/33	26/33

1.2.3. The effect of exercise. Levy et al. (20) showed that the development of complete block in the accessory pathway during exercise corresponded to a relatively long antegrade refractory period of the accessory pathway. On using this test however one should realize that exercise shortens transmission time through the AV node thereby increasing the degree of ventricular excitation over the AV node – His axis. Especially in left laterally located accessory pathways this may falsely give the impression of antegrade block in the accessory pathway.

The degree of pre-excitation during sinus rhythm has no predictive value as to the length of the refractory period of the accessory pathway. This is an important point because as shown in Figures 4 and 5 patients with little evidence of preexcitation during sinus rhythm may have life-threatening ventricular rates during atrial fibrillation.

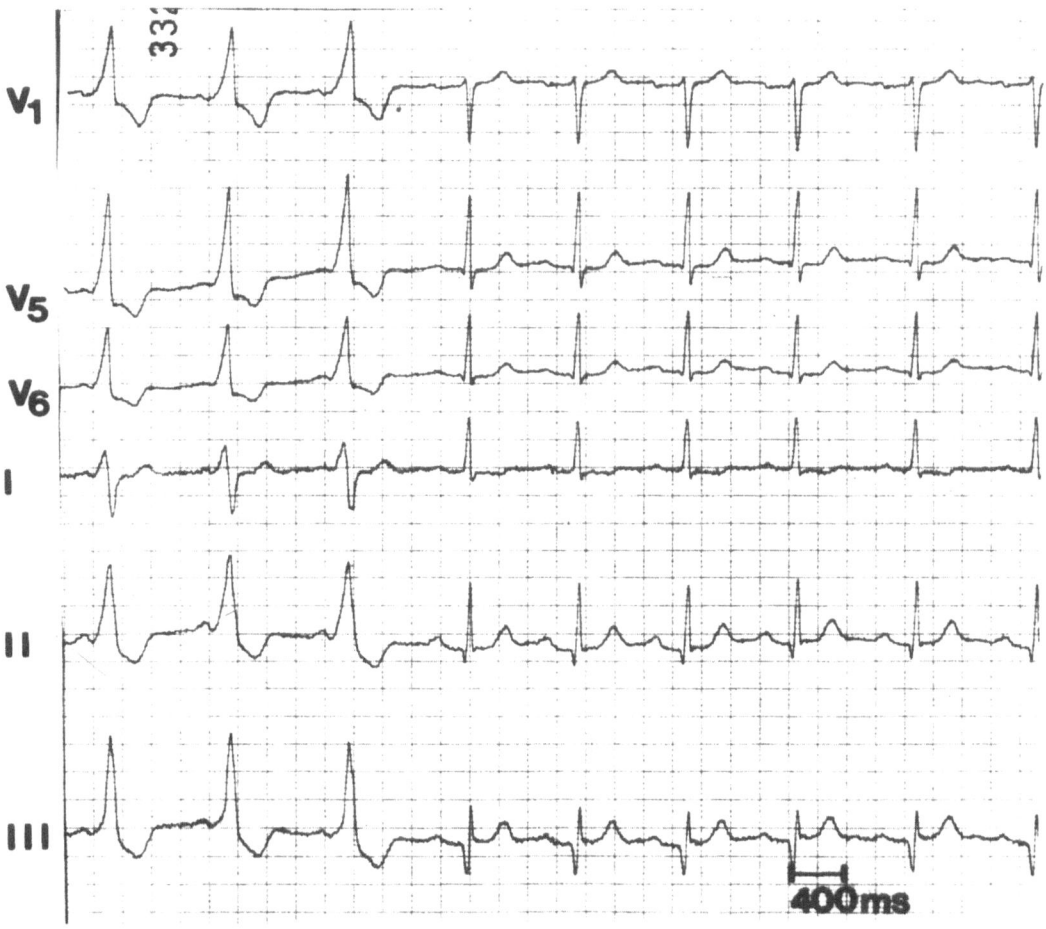

Figure 3. Development of complete antegrade block in the accessory pathway by 50 mg ajmaline given intravenously over a three minute period. Leads V_1, V_5, V_6, I, II and III were recorded simultaneously. The patient had an old inferior myocardial infarction.

2. INCIDENCE OF ACCESSORY PATHWAYS WITH A SHORT REFRACTORY PERIOD

At the present time it is not known what percentage of patients with the Wolff-Parkinson-White syndrome have such a short duration of the refractory period of their accessory pathway that they are at risk of sudden death if atrial fibrillation occurs. In our own series of 163 patients with WPW syndrome consecutively studied, 51 patients (31 %) had a refractory period of their accessory pathway of less than 250 msec with 32 patients (19 %) having a value of less than 210 msec. 155 of the 163 patients with WPW were symptomatic with tachycardia. Our group therefore represents a highly selected group of patients. No follow-up data are presently available to indicate the risk of the asymptomatic WPW patient having a short refractory period of the accessory pathway.

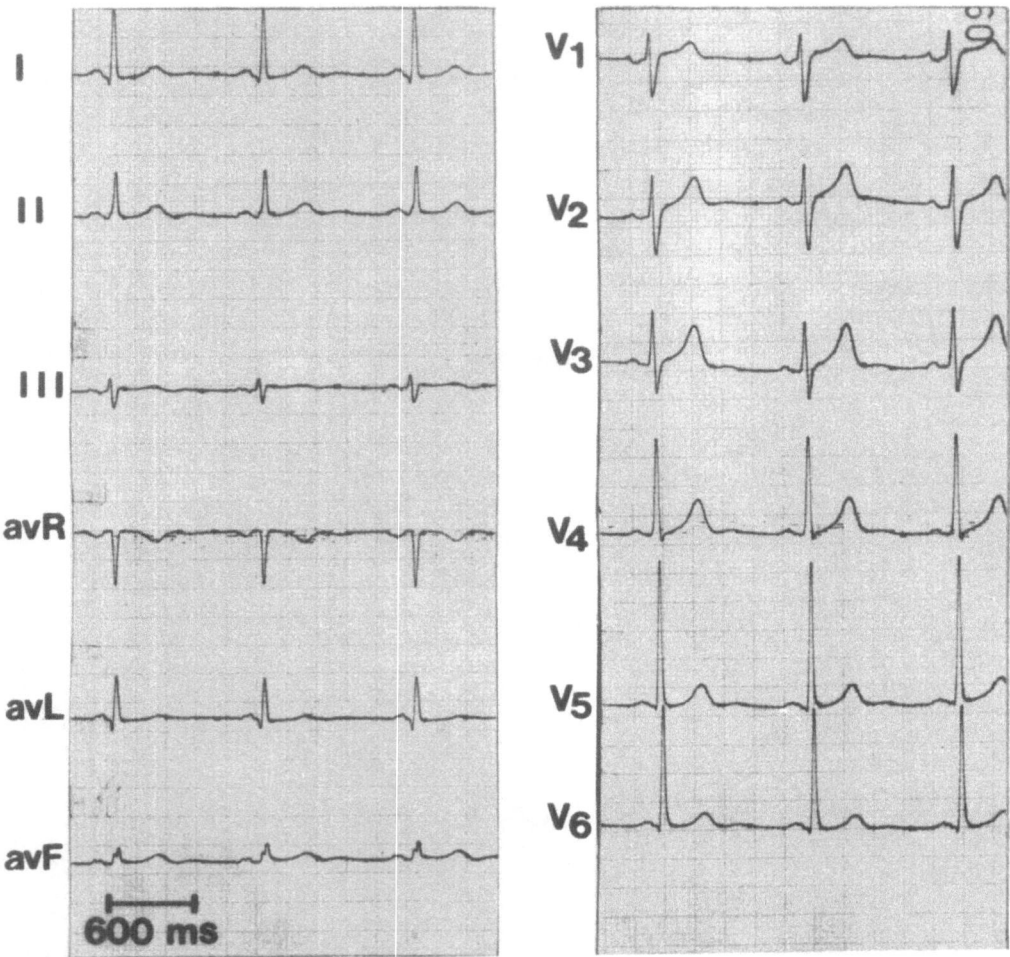

Figure 4. Twelve lead electrocardiogram showing a PQ interval of 0,14 sec, a QRS width of 0,10 sec and minimal delta waves in leads II and AVF.

3. DRUGS AND THE DURATION OF THE REFRACTORY PERIOD OF THE ACCESSORY PATHWAY

Since the mode of death unique for the WPW patient is based upon the presence of an accessory pathway with a short refractory period the most logical form of therapy would be the administration of an agent lengthening the duration of the refractory period of the accessory pathway. Recently we have reported on the relation between the initial length of the refractory period of the accessory pathway and the effect of drugs (21). As shown in Table 3 patients with a refractory period of equal to or more than 270 msec responded to administration of quinidine, procainamide, ajmaline and amiodarone by marked prolon-

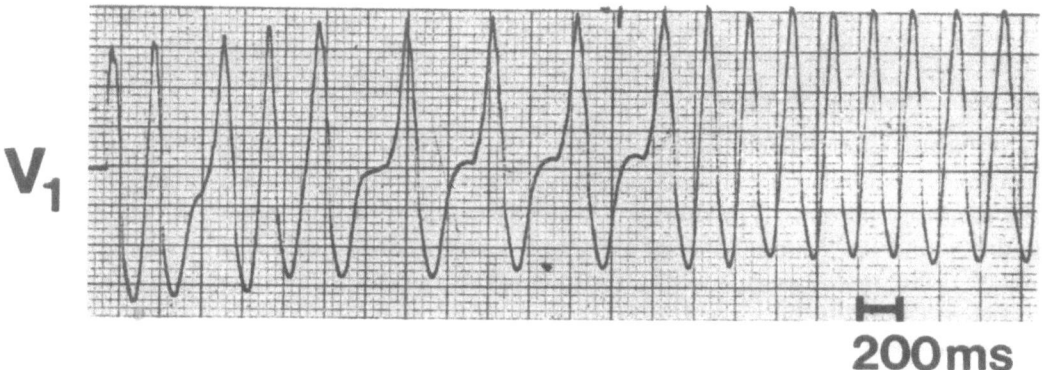

200ms

Figure 5. Same patient as Figure 4. During atrial fibrillation AV conduction over a left sided accessory pathway is seen. The shortest R-R interval during atrial fibrillation measures 200 msec.

gation of the antegrade refractory period of their accessory pathway. Of importance however in relation to the treatment of the WPW patient at risk was the observation of no or only slight lengthening of the antegrade refractory period of the accessory pathway following the administration of these drugs when the duration of the antegrade refractory period of the accessory pathway was less than 270 msec. In the latter group of patients, of the drugs investigated, amiodarone gave the greatest amount of lengthening of the duration of the antegrade refractory period of the accessory pathway. Our data indicate that the effect of drugs on the duration of the antegrade refractory period of the accessory pathway is least in patients who are most in need of prolongation of the refractory period of that structure.

Table 3. Importance of initial length of ERP_{AP} in A-V direction on effect of drugs.

| | No. Pts | $ERP_{AP} \geq 270$ msec | |
		ΔERP_{AP}	Mean
Procainamide	7	200 → 200 msec	> 268,5 msec
Quinidine Gluconate	5	20 → 300 msec	> 222,0 msec
	9	200 → 300 msec	> 262,2 msec
Amiodarone	4	50 → 300 msec	> 187,5 msec

| | No. Pts | $ERP_{AP} < 270$ msec | |
		ΔERP_{AP}	Mean
Procainamide	9	0 → 160 msec	31,1 msec
Quinidine Gluconate	5	0 → 50 msec	18,0 msec
Ajmaline	9	0 → 270 msec	51,1 msec
Amiodarone	11	20 → 200 msec	77,7 msec

Abbreviations: ERP = Effective refractory period; AP = Accessory pathway

4. PRACTICAL MANAGEMENT

4.1. The symptomatic patient

In the WPW patient with documented ventricular fibrillation or atrial fibrillation with high ventricular rates we study the effect of amiodarone on the antegrade refractory period of the accessory pathway. The duration of the antegrade refractory period of the accessory pathway and the ventricular response to electrically induced atrial fibrillation are determined before and after at least 14 days of chronic oral administration of amiodarone. As shown in Table 3 the mean increase in duration of the antegrade refractory period of the accessory pathway after amiodarone is around 70 msec. This means that a patient with a refractory period of the accessory pathway of 200 msec and a theoretical ventricular rate during atrial fibrillation of 300/min will prolong the refractory period of the accessory pathway after amiodarone administration to 270 msec and decrease the maximal ventricular rate to 230/min. This can be the difference between life and death in the patient with the WPW syndrome. Another possible advantage of giving amiodarone is suggested by our observation that the electrical induction of atrial fibrillation in the WPW patient becomes more difficult during the stimulation study following amiodarone administration. This may indicate that also the clinical incidence of this arrhythmia is less following oral amiodarone. Since the effect of amiodarone on the duration of the refractory period of the accessory pathway may be individually different, we insist upon a study with and without amiodarone in the symptomatic patient. If the results of amiodarone therapy are unsatisfactory we refer the patient for surgical interruption of the accessory pathway (17).

4.2. The asymptomatic patient

As described above, intermittent pre-excitation, the production of AV block in the accessory pathway by ajmaline and possibly the disappearance of pre-excitation on exercise identify the patient with WPW not at risk for sudden death in case of atrial fibrillation. If the WPW electrocardiogram is repeatedly present and antegrade conduction over the accessory pathway cannot be blocked by ajmaline, we determine the duration of the refractory period of the accessory pathway during a programmed stimulation study. In the asymptomatic patient with a short refractory period of the accessory pathway we do not routinely prescribe amiodarone because of the side effects of the drug. We follow these patients to get better knowledge about the natural history of the asymptomatic patient with an accessory pathway and a short antegrade refractory period. We want to make a plea to combine the results from these studies from several centres and to have this information available as soon as possible. Only then the real danger of sudden death in the patient with an accessory pathway with a short refractory period will be known and a more realistic basis for treatment will be provided.

REFERENCES

1. Dreifus LS, Haiat R, Watanabe Y: Ventricular fibrillation: A possible mechanism of sudden death in patients with Wolff-Parkinson-White syndrome. Circulation 43:520–527, 1971.
2. Laham J: Actualités electrocardiographiques 1969: Le syndrome de Wolff-Parkinson-White. Paris, Librairie Maloine SA, 1969.
3. Kaplan MA, Cohen KL: Ventricular fibrillation in the Wolff-Parkinson-White syndrome. Am J Cardiol 24:259–264, 1969.
4. Okel BB: The Wolff-Parkinson-White syndrome: Report of a case with fatal arrhythmia and autopsy findings of myocarditis, interatrial lipomatous hypertrophy and prominent right moderator band. Am Heart J 75: 673–678, 1968.
5. Castillo-Fenoy A, Goupil A, Offenstadt G, et al: Syndrome de Wolff-Parkinson-White et mort subite. Ann Med Intern 124:871–875, 1973.
6. Lem CH, Toh CCS, Chia BL: Ventricular fibrillation in type B Wolff-Parkinson-White syndrome. Aust NZ J Med 4:515, 1974.
7. Dreifus LS, Wellens HJJ, Watanabe Y, et al: Sinus bradycardia and atrial fibrillation associated with the Wolff-Parkinson-White syndrome. Am J Cardiol 38:149–156, 1976.
8. Klein GJ, Bashore TM, Sellers TD, et al: Ventricular fibrillation in the Wolff-Parkinson-White syndrome. N. Engl. J Med 301: 1080–1085, 1959.
9. Martin-Noel P, Denis B, Grundwald D, et al: Deux cas mortels de syndrome de Wolff-Parkinson-White. Arch Mal Coeur 63:1647, 1970.
10. Ahlinder S, Granath A, Holmer S, et al: The Wolff-Parkinson-White syndrome with paroxysmal atrial fibrillation changing into ventricular fibrillation, successfully treated with external heart massage. Nord Med 70:1336–1343, 1963.
11. Fox TT, Weaver J, March HW: On the mechanism of the arrhythmias in aberrant atrioventricular conduction (Wolff-Parkinson-White). Am Heart J 43:507, 1952.
12. Touche M, Touche S, Jouvet M, et al: Eléments de prognostic dans le syndrome de Wolff-Parkinson-White. Presse Méd 76:567–570, 1968.
13. Duvernoy WFC: Sudden death in Wolff-Parkinson-White syndrome. Am J Cardiol 39:472, 1977.
14. Castellanos A, Jr, Myerburg RJ, Craparo K, et al: Factors affecting ventricular rates during atrial flutter and fibrillation in preexcitation (Wolff-Parkinson-White) syndrome. Br Heart J 35:811–816, 1973.
15. Wellens HJJ, Durrer D: Wolff-Parkinson-White syndrome and atrial fibrillation: Relation between refractory period of the accessory pathway and ventricular rate during atrial fibrillation. Am J Cardiol 34:777–782, 1974.
16. Campbell RWF, Smith RA, Gallagher JJ, et al: Atrial fibrillation in the preexcitation syndrome. Am J Cardiol 40:514–520, 1977
17. Gallagher JJ, Pritchett ELC, Sealy WC, et al: The preexcitation syndromes. Progr Cardiovasc Dis 20:285–327, 1978.
18. Coumel Ph, Slama R: Syndrome de Wolff-Parkinson-White. Rev Prat 25:1821, 1975.
19. Wellens HJJ, Bär FW, Gorgels AP, et al: Use of Ajmaline in identifying patients with the Wolff-Parkinson-White syndrome and a short refractory period of their accessory pathway. Am J Cardiol 45, 63–68, 1980.
20. Levy S, Broustet JP, Clémenty J, et al: Syndrome de Wolff-Parkinson-White: Corrélations entre l'exploration électrophysiologique et l'effet de l'épreuve d'effort sur l'aspect électrocardiographique de préexcitation. Arch Mal Coeur 72:634–640, 1979.
21. Wellens HJJ, Bär FW, Gorgels AM: Effect of drugs in WPW syndrome. Importance of initial length of effective refractory period of accessory pathway. Am J Cardiol 41:372, (abstract) 1978.

INDEX